Andrology: Current and Future Developments

(Volume 1)

(Biochemistry of Andrology)

Editors

Marco G. Alves

Health Sciences Research Centre (CICS-UBI), Faculty of Health Sciences, University of Beira Interior, Covilha, Portugal

&

Pedro F. Oliveira

Department of Microscopy, Institute of Biomedical Sciences Abel Salazar UMIB - Unit for Multidisciplinary Research in Biomedicine I3S - Institute for Innovation and Health Research, University of Porto, Porto, Portugal

Andrology: Current and Future Developments

Volume # 1

Biochemistry of Andrology

Editors: Marco G. Alves & Pedro F. Oliveira

eISSN (Online): 2543-1617

ISSN (Print): 2543-1609

eISBN (Online): 978-1-68108-500-5

ISBN (Print): 978-1-68108-501-2

General:

1. Any dispute or claim arising out of or in connection with this License Agreement or the Work (including non-contractual disputes or claims) will be governed by and construed in accordance with the laws of the U.A.E. as applied in the Emirate of Dubai. Each party agrees that the courts of the Emirate of Dubai shall have exclusive jurisdiction to settle any dispute or claim arising out of or in connection with this License Agreement or the Work (including non-contractual disputes or claims).
2. Your rights under this License Agreement will automatically terminate without notice and without the need for a court order if at any point you breach any terms of this License Agreement. In no event will any delay or failure by Bentham Science Publishers in enforcing your compliance with this License Agreement constitute a waiver of any of its rights.
3. You acknowledge that you have read this License Agreement, and agree to be bound by its terms and conditions. To the extent that any other terms and conditions presented on any website of Bentham Science Publishers conflict with, or are inconsistent with, the terms and conditions set out in this License Agreement, you acknowledge that the terms and conditions set out in this License Agreement shall prevail.

Bentham Science Publishers Ltd.
Executive Suite Y - 2
PO Box 7917, Saif Zone
Sharjah, U.A.E.
Email: subscriptions@benthamscience.org

BENTHAM
SCIENCE

CONTENTS

PREFACE

Andrology is the discipline that corresponds to gynecology for men, but while the latter is a well-established discipline, the former is still an emerging field. A simple definition of andrology will include the study of all subjects that may affect the male reproductive system. In the last years, a striking large number of topics has emerged in this field and there is an increasing amount of information that may be useful for graduate, post-graduate and even well-established researchers. Herein, we summarize the available information so far in this area, presenting a review and a critical analysis of the available data on the most relevant subjects with interest to andrology, with emphasis on the biochemistry of the processes. This e-book is divided into 14 chapters, all coordinated by Dr. Marco G. Alves and Prof. Pedro F. Oliveira.

The first chapter is a brief introduction to the historical evolution of andrology and how biochemistry has emerged as a partner, contributing to the emerging relevance of this discipline. The second chapter describes general considerations on testis physiology, testicular anatomy and functional organization, as well as its embryonic development. The third chapter discusses the basic aspects of testicular cells physiology and function. The fourth chapter presents the basic aspects of spermatogenesis, a key event for species propagation, from a biochemical perspective. It is mainly focused on the mechanisms responsible for postnatal testis development but it also presents an overview on the complex events that control the spermatogenic cycle. Many of those changes are under the action and function of male-associated hormones that trigger signaling pathways thus, the fifth chapter is dedicated to those issues. The endocrine regulation of sexual maturation and sperm formation is still a matter of great debate and with an enormous interest. In the sixth chapter, the transition period between childhood and adulthood is discussed, particularly the biochemical changes that control pivotal events responsible for the sexual maturation of the individuals. There is also an overview on puberty-associated disorders, pinpointing the clinical features that should be taken into consideration and the deleterious signals that may occur until sexual maturation is achieved. In the seventh chapter, the biochemical events occurring in the epididymis that end-up in sperm maturation, are discussed. It also discussed the structural organization of epididymal epithelial cells and secretory proteins and their involvement on the spermatozoa modifications that occur during the process of maturation. The eighth chapter is dedicated to the formation and biochemical properties of seminal plasma and male accessory glands. Those changes are essential for spermatozoa to acquire fertility capacity. In the ninth chapter, the functional and physiological aspects of spermatozoa, as well as its epigenome are presented, which may have an enormous implication to the success of the pregnancy and latter to the offspring health. The male gamete is very dynamic and has to move, capacitate, migrate through the female tract, bind to the egg membrane and fuse to the oocyte, resulting in a viable embryo. The tenth chapter is dedicated to the sequential modifications and the molecular mechanisms that occur during the journey of spermatozoa through the female reproductive tract since they have a pivotal role in couple's fertility success and offspring health. Those events may be compromised by several factors that compromise male reproductive health. Congenital disorders, such as hypospadias, undescended testis, testicular atrophy and testicular cancer have increased among young males and even erectile dysfunction and sexually transmitted diseases are still problems that compromise male reproductive health. These issues are discussed in chapter eleven. The twelfth chapter discusses how the pandemic incidence of metabolic diseases is contributing for the worldwide decline in both, sperm quality and male reproductive health. The biochemical changes induced by lifestyle factors and nutrition in the testis are on spotlight to unveil the mechanisms by which metabolic diseases affect nativity rates and the offspring. There is an intense debate whether worldwide sperm quality is decreasing and the factors that may be responsible for that. Environmental contaminants have arisen as main contributors to the decline on sperm quality. Thus, the molecular mechanisms by which environmental cues alter male reproductive health remain a matter of great interest and are discussed in the thirteenth chapter. The last chapter is dedicated to the biochemical changes in the reproductive function of the aging male. Later parenting is very frequent in modern societies. Nevertheless, the quality and the altered patterns of epigenetics/gene expression in aging sperm remain to be disclosed. Thus, the biochemical changes that occur in testis and sperm and that go along with aging will be on the spotlight for the next decades.

Nowadays, there is a huge investment in reproductive healthcare that is mainly applied in assisted reproductive technologies. However, the long-term effects of these treatments and the causes for male infertility are not cautioned. Overall, this book discusses all the major topics of interest for andrology and mainly presents a focus on the biochemistry of andrology without avoiding the debate on the clinical relevance of the discussed topics. This is a fast growing discipline and thus, there is a great need to educate and prepare students, scientists and physicians for the novel challenges. As scientists working in the field, we felt that most books focused on Andrology lack a strong biochemical view on the topics. As biochemists working in the field for more than a decade, we gathered our team and prepared a book that discusses a large spectrum of topics with high relevance for andrologists all over the world. This book will be valuable for all those working on andrology that aim to understand the magnificent biochemical control of the male reproductive health. Our team had great pleasure preparing this book and we are sure that it will be very useful.

Marco G. Alves
Health Sciences Research Centre (CICS-UBI),
Faculty of Health Sciences, University of Beira Interior, Covilha,
Portugal

Pedro F. Oliveira
Department of Microscopy, Institute of Biomedical Sciences Abel Salazar,
UMIB - Unit for Multidisciplinary Research in Biomedicine,
I3S - Institute for Innovation and Health Research,
University of Porto, Porto,
Portugal

List of Contributors

Ana D. Martins Institute of Biomedical Sciences Abel Salazar and Unit for Multidisciplinary Research in Biomedicine, University of Porto, Rua de Jorge Viterbo Ferreira, 4050-313, Department of Microscopy, Laboratory of Cell Biology, Porto, Portugal

Ana M. Cardoso University of Beira Interior, Rua Marquês d'Ávila e Bolama, 6201-001, Health Sciences Research Center, Covilhã, Portugal

Bernardo C. Rodrigues University of Beira Interior, Rua Marquês d'Ávila e Bolama, 6201-001, Health Sciences Research Center, Covilhã, Portugal
Institute of Biomedical Sciences Abel Salazar and Unit for Multidisciplinary Research in Biomedicine, University of Porto, Rua de Jorge Viterbo Ferreira, 4050-313, Department of Microscopy, Laboratory of Cell Biology, Porto, Portugal

Bruno P. Moreira University of Beira Interior, Rua Marquês d'Ávila e Bolama, 6201-001, Health Sciences Research Center, Covilhã, Portugal
Institute of Biomedical Sciences Abel Salazar and Unit for Multidisciplinary Research in Biomedicine, University of Porto, Rua de Jorge Viterbo Ferreira, 4050-313, Department of Microscopy, Laboratory of Cell Biology, Porto, Portugal

João P. Monteiro Institute of Biomedical Sciences Abel Salazar and Unit for Multidisciplinary Research in Biomedicine, University of Porto, Rua de Jorge Viterbo Ferreira, 4050-313, Department of Microscopy, Laboratory of Cell Biology, Porto, Portugal

Luís Rato University of Beira Interior, Rua Marquês d'Ávila e Bolama, 6201-001, Health Sciences Research Center, Covilhã, Portugal

Marco G. Alves University of Beira Interior, Rua Marquês d'Ávila e Bolama, 6201-001, Health Sciences Research Center, Covilhã, Portugal
University of Porto, Rua de Jorge Viterbo Ferreira, 4050-313, Institute of Biomedical Sciences Abel Salazar and Unit for Multidisciplinary Research in Biomedicine, Porto, Portugal

Mário Sousa University of Porto, Rua de Jorge Viterbo Ferreira, 4050-313, Institute of Biomedical Sciences Abel Salazar and Unit for Multidisciplinary Research in Biomedicine, Porto, Portugal

Maria J. Meneses New University of Lisbon, 1150-082, ProRegeM PhD Program, CEDOC – Chronic Diseases Research Center and NOVA Medical School, Lisboa, Portugal
Institute of Biomedical Sciences Abel Salazar and Unit for Multidisciplinary Research in Biomedicine, University of Porto, Rua de Jorge Viterbo Ferreira, 4050-313, Department of Microscopy, Laboratory of Cell Biology, Porto, Portugal

Pedro F. Oliveira Institute of Biomedical Sciences Abel Salazar and Unit for Multidisciplinary Research in Biomedicine, University of Porto, Rua de Jorge Viterbo Ferreira, 4050-313, Department of Microscopy, Laboratory of Cell Biology, Porto, Portugal
University of Porto, Rua Alfredo Allen, 4200-135, i3S – Institute for Innovation and health Research, Porto, Portugal

Raquel L. Bernardino Institute of Biomedical Sciences Abel Salazar and Unit for Multidisciplinary Research in Biomedicine, University of Porto, Rua de Jorge Viterbo Ferreira, 4050-313, Department of Microscopy, Laboratory of Cell Biology, Porto, Portugal

Susana P. Almeida Institute of Biomedical Sciences Abel Salazar and Unit for Multidisciplinary Research in Biomedicine, University of Porto, Rua de Jorge Viterbo Ferreira, 4050-313, Department of Microscopy, Laboratory of Cell Biology, Porto, Portugal

Tânia R. Dias University of Beira Interior, Rua Marquês d'Ávila e Bolama, 6201-001, Health Sciences Research Center, Covilhã, Portugal
Institute of Biomedical Sciences Abel Salazar and Unit for Multidisciplinary Research in Biomedicine, University of Porto, Rua de Jorge Viterbo Ferreira, 4050-313, Department of Microscopy, Laboratory of Cell Biology, Porto, Portugal
Faculty of Pharmacy, University of Porto, Rua do Campo Alegre, 4150-755, LAQV/REQUIMTE — Laboratory of Bromatology and Hydrology, Porto, Portugal

CHAPTER 1

Introduction

Marco G. Alves[1,*] and **Pedro F. Oliveira**[2,3,*]

[1] *Institute of Biomedical Sciences Abel Salazar and Unit for Multidisciplinary Research in Biomedicine, University of Porto, Rua de Jorge Viterbo Ferreira, 4050-313, Porto, Portugal*

[2] *Department of Microscopy, Laboratory of Cell Biology, Institute of Biomedical Sciences Abel Salazar and Unit for Multidisciplinary Research in Biomedicine, University of Porto, Rua de Jorge Viterbo Ferreira, 4050-313, Porto, Portugal*

[3] *i3S – Instituto de Investigação e Inovação em Saúde, University of Porto, Rua Alfredo Allen, 4200-135, Porto, Portugal*

Abstract: Andrology has emerged since the 1950's, when gynecologists started to consistently refer to this word. However, in 1891, there was already an editorial in JAMA suggesting that andrology could evolve to become an important discipline. It was proposed that, as gynecology is a discipline that is focused on the study of genito-urinary female system, andrology could emerge as the discipline focused on the genito-urinary system of males. For many years, this issue was disregarded and there was a long period until the first societies of andrology appeared and establish it in a definitive way. This historical affirmation of andrology as a discipline will be briefly presented, together with a critical view on some aspects that are still a matter of controversy. Reproductive science is a growing discipline that needs economic support from health care systems, institutions responsible for funding research, and training centers. There was never a greater need for trained and well-prepared scientists and physicians to study human reproductive health. Most countries, developed and developing, are witnessing unprecedented rates of people seeking for assisted reproductive technologies. Decreased sperm quality and male reproductive complications are factors that unquestionably contribute to the observed decline in nativity rates. On the other hand, even though females have various contraceptive methods available, men are still limited. This could be improved if more knowledge on sperm formation, maturation and overall testicular physiology arises. In this introductory chapter, we will discuss some challenges for the upcoming years in the field of Andrology.

Keywords: Andrology, Male reproductive tract, Male fertility, Male reproductive health.

* **Corresponding authors Marco G. Alves & Pedro F. Oliveira:** Rua de Jorge Viterbo Ferreira, 4050-313, Porto, Portugal; Tel/Fax: +351967245248; E-mails: alvesmarc@gmail.com, pfobox@gmail.com

In 1891, a JAMA editorial referred to andrology as a possible specialty with difficulties in being established, since it was causing some controversy among the genito-urinary surgeons [1]. Nevertheless, it is usually considered that andrology was firstly used with authority by the gynecologist Dr. Harald Siebke from the University of Bonn in 1957 [2]. Although there was great controversy among some physicians, the first step to establish andrology as a valid specialty was taken when the Congress of American Physicians and Surgeons formed the section of Andrology. This decision was welcomed by many researchers and physicians. Andrology established itself as a growing field of research with potential to rapidly develop into a mandatory discipline to evaluate men's quality of life and health. After this, it developed within the field of dermatovenereology and gained great interest from several important researchers. Validation also came from the German Society for the Study of Fertility and Sterility that acknowledged andrology as part of its activities in 1958. Though, it was only in 1970 that an international committee of andrology was founded in Barcelona. Later, several other associations of andrology were formed, including the Nordic Association of Andrology (1973), the American Association of Andrology (1974), the German Society of Andrology (1975), and the American Society of Andrology (1976). This ended up with the formation of the International Society of Andrology in 1981. The need for a high level of formation highlighted that the training centers should be grouped and thus, in 1992, the European Academy of Andrology was formed to gather and establish the guidelines for the training in andrology at a European level. Then, all the most relevant societies involved in reproductive medicine recognized and gave attention to this specialty, including the European Society of Human Reproduction and Embryology (ESHRE). This resulted in a rapid development of the discipline in the last three decades [3]. Nevertheless, even today, there are few formal board-certified training programs in andrology. There is a parallelism between andrology and gynecology taking in consideration that the latter is dedicated to the study of the genito-urinary system of females, and the former of males. This is of particular relevance because male's fertility and the study of their reproductive system has always been overlooked when compared with females, in such a way that the term "diseases of women" is used by several physicians to summarize their specialty, while the same is rare in the case of men. Even today, the field of andrology is not widely recognized by non-experts as a clinical discipline or a research field of great interest like others such as gynecology or urology. Thus, public consciousness of the existence and relevance of this discipline is also mandatory. In summary, andrology is a young interdisciplinary specialty that deals with the male, particularly with the physiology and pathophysiology of male reproductive functions and fertility. We may go further and state that the main focus of andrology is to provide a diagnosis and treatment to males with fertility disturbances.

Andrology evolved as a branch of science that deals with male reproduction and its disorders, including erectile dysfunction, infertility and sexual development. In 1969, the first journal "Andrologie" appeared and gave visibility to this emerging field of research. A few years later, the "Andrologia" journal further contributed to the internationalization of the topic. Initially, the works published were mostly focused on the analysis of the ejaculate, particularly sperm morphology. The clinicians, veterinarians and biochemists started to publish important information on the characterization of sperm and the molecular mechanisms responsible for male fertility. Limited analytical methods, at the time, hampered the initial findings, but enormous progress was made in the first years of those journals. With the advent of molecular biology techniques, omics technologies and hormonal knowledge, andrology entered in a new era of findings. We never had so much information and ways to study testicular physiology, hormonal network, sperm physiology, testicular disorders, and the genetics of the individuals, as we have nowadays. It is also important to highlight that andrology emerged as a discipline that is forced to cooperate with others, including urology, dermatology or endocrinology and thus, it relies on a multidisciplinary work. In addition, concerning the fertility of couples and the treatment of childless couples, it is pivotal that andrologists and gynecologists cooperate and work together to solve the problems beyond the use of assisted reproductive technologies. The diagnosis and therapies of couples would greatly benefit from that. Family planning is also another important matter that benefits from the joint work of both specialties. Nowadays, there are several physicians engaged in andrology and thus, universities and research groups focused on this discipline have highly increased in the last decades. In addition, there is a high number of scientists, besides medical doctors, such as biochemists, veterinaries or biologists that focus their research interest in andrology. Training of highly qualified people is still a major need, as well as support from funding agencies to explore new methods of examination and fundamental research in this field. Basic scientists have also greatly contributed to the exponential growth of this discipline, particularly those with strong formation on biochemistry, biology, pharmacology, genetics and molecular biology. This multidisciplinary approach has allowed a rapid advancement in the understanding of the physiology and biochemical events involved in male reproduction, from the hormonal regulation to the genetic mechanisms responsible for those processes [4, 5]. Nevertheless, the translational gap between basic science and clinical practice still hampers some effective developments that could be useful to improve male reproductive health. We are witnessing an unprecedented need for scientists working on reproductive science. In fact, most developed countries present high rates of induced abortion. Notably, the oral contraceptive method was introduced in 1960, and some authors alerted to the fact that the fundamental biochemical research that served as the basis for this major step in reproductive medicine, was available since the 1920s and 1930s [6]. This clearly highlights that there is a need for a major involvement of basic researchers on translational andrology and andrologists with interest on fundamental research. To encourage both, more funds should be allocated to these areas. In addition, pharmaceutical industry should be more engaged to develop novel strategies to improve the health care of males. The general public and policymakers must be more aware of the need for andrology as an essential discipline, and special funds must be allocated to actively seek for the improvement of men's health, including the treatment of disorders (i.e. infertility, erectile dysfunction, prostate cancer) and the development of a male contraceptive. In addition, there are several societal challenges that should be considered, including the fact that men are becoming fathers later in life. As the age of father increases, there is a higher risk for miscarriage or disease in the offspring. Another important issue to be considered is the epigenetic information that can be passed along generations [7].

How genetic and environmental factors limit sperm quality and overall male reproductive health should be on spotlight for the next decades. It is of paramount importance to understand those mechanisms and to identify targets to either counteract deleterious effects or to develop a male contraceptive. The pandemic incidence of metabolic diseases and wrong dietary habits are also key factors that are now gaining momentum concerning their effect on the male reproductive health. Thus, physicians, biochemists and basic researchers should also join their efforts to study the mechanisms of action by which those factors may limit male's fertility.

There is a need for a holistic view of andrology, as an interdisciplinary medical specialty that may evolve even further with a biochemical approach. In addition, the initial problems of the discipline, such as erectile dysfunction or ejaculatory dysfunctions, developed to more dramatic issues in the worldwide trends of ageing male, including neoplastic diseases of the prostate and testis. We may postulate that andrology is still a field with a great margin of progress with the implementation of a multidisciplinary approach. This book aims to contribute to further understand this field of research from a biochemical point of view.

CONFLICT OF INTEREST

The authors confirm that they have no conflict of interest to declare for this publication.

ACKNOWLEDGEMENTS

Declared none.

REFERENCES

[1] Editorial. Andrology as a specialty. JAMA 1891; 17: 691.

[2] Schirren C. Andrology. Origin and development of a special discipline in medicine. Reflection and view in the future. Andrologia 1985; 17(2): 117-25.
[http://dx.doi.org/10.1111/j.1439-0272.1985.tb00970.x] [PMID: 3890616]

[3] Prins GS, Bremner W. Andrology in the 20th century: a commentary on our progress during the past 25 years. J Androl 2004; 25(4): 435-40.
[http://dx.doi.org/10.1002/j.1939-4640.2004.tb02812.x] [PMID: 15223830]

[4] Amory JK, Bremner WJ. Regulation of testicular function in men: implications for male hormonal contraceptive development. J Steroid Biochem Mol Biol 2003; 85(2-5): 357-61.
[http://dx.doi.org/10.1016/S0960-0760(03)00205-X] [PMID: 12943722]

[5] Matzuk MM, Lamb DJ. Genetic dissection of mammalian fertility pathways. Nat Cell Biol 2002; 4 (Suppl.): s41-9.
[http://dx.doi.org/10.1038/ncb-nm-fertilityS41] [PMID: 12479614]

[6] Aitken RJ. Age, the environment and our reproductive future: bonking baby boomers and the future of sex. Reproduction 2013; 147(2): S1-S11.
[http://dx.doi.org/10.1530/REP-13-0399] [PMID: 24194569]

[7] Schagdarsurengin U, Steger K. Epigenetics in male reproduction: effect of paternal diet on sperm quality and offspring health. Nat Rev Urol 2016; 13(10): 584-95.
[http://dx.doi.org/10.1038/nrurol.2016.157] [PMID: 27578043]

CHAPTER 2

Testis Physiology

Bruno P. Moreira[1,2], **João P. Monteiro**[2] and **Maria J. Meneses**[2,3,*]

[1] *Health Sciences Research Center, University of Beira Interior, Rua Marquês d'Ávila e Bolama, 6201-001, Covilhã, Portugal*

[2] *Department of Microscopy, Laboratory of Cell Biology, Institute of Biomedical Sciences Abel Salazar and Unit for Multidisciplinary Research in Biomedicine, University of Porto, Rua de Jorge Viterbo Ferreira, 4050-313, Porto, Portugal*

[3] *ProRegeM PhD Program, CEDOC – Chronic Diseases Research Center and NOVA Medical School, New University of Lisbon, 1150-082 Lisboa, Portugal*

Abstract: In multicellular organisms, and particularly in mammals, both gonadal and germ cell development are essential for the transmission of genetic information to the next generations. The testes are paired ovoid organs located inside the scrotum but outside the abdominal cavity. They have two major functions: spermatogenesis and steroidogenesis. The former corresponds to the production of male gametes, spermatozoa; the latter, to the production of hormones that will influence spermatogenesis and consequently male reproductive function and health. The male and female reproductive organs have the same precursor tissues. Initially, the embryo has a bipotential gonad which may have a testicular or ovarian fate. Accordingly, Müllerian ducts form the uterus and fallopian tubes in females and Wolffian ducts form the epididymis, *vas deferens*, and ejaculatory duct in males. On the other hand, male sex determination is triggered by sex-determining region Y (*SRY*), which is located on the Y chromosome and works as a master regulator, initiating *SOX9* expression. The latter causes urogenital development, a highly complex process, through a complex cascade of transcription factors and signaling events. These will promote testis differentiation and ultimately the production of hormones that will lead to male development and testicular function during adulthood. In this chapter, we will provide a brief overview of the testicular anatomy and functional organization, as well as its embryonic development.

Keywords: Genital ridge, Interstitial compartment, Leydig cells, Male reproductive tract, Peritubular myoid cells, Prenatal development, Pre-Sertoli cells, Sex-determining region Y, Sex differentiation, Testis cords, Tubular compartment.

* **Corresponding author Maria J. Meneses:** CEDOC - Chronic Diseases Research Center, Rua Câmara Pestana, nº 6, 6A, 1150-082 Lisboa, Portugal; Tel: +351 218803101; Fax:+351 218851920; E-mail: mariajoaocmo@gmail.com

Marco G. Alves and Pedro F. Oliveira (Eds.)

INTRODUCTION

Testes are the primary organs of the male reproductive system. They are central in the production of sperm and responsible for the synthesis of male sex hormones, fundamental to the normal development of male internal and external genitalia. The secondary organs of the male reproductive system support the testes in these tasks. Accessory glands produce secretions that constitute the semen. Other accessory structures support and nourish the developing germ cells. In addition, a network of ducts is responsible for storing and the transport of sperm to the female reproductive tract, where fertilization occurs.

Sexual and asexual reproduction are the two basic processes through which organisms reproduce. In the first, a male and a female are needed and each one of them equally contributes to the formation of the new individual. The egg and the spermatozoon will form a zygote, which contains genetic information from both progenitors. However, and unlike other processes of embryonic development, sex determination is a poorly conserved event among the different species, ranging from being controlled by environmental factors to being genetically determined. In mammals, sex determination is genetically determined at the time of conception, with the formation of either an XX embryo or an XY embryo. This process depends on the chromosome acquired from the father, X or Y chromosome, since the one acquired from the mother is always an X chromosome. Male and female reproductive systems are quite different and thus, evolve independently although sharing a common origin. Bipotential gonad can differentiate into testes or ovaries, depending on the stimuli received. In the male, the presence of the testis determining factor shifts the bipotential gonad into a testicular fate, leading to the development of the testes. This complex process is tightly controlled and involves the action of several different signaling molecules and transcription factors. In this chapter, we present the most relevant aspects of the male reproductive system anatomy. We also discuss the development and differentiation of the testes, from the early stages at the time of conception until they are fully developed.

ANATOMY OF THE MALE REPRODUCTIVE TRACT

The reproductive system is not essential for the survival of the individual; it is, however, required for the survival of the species. It is through the reproductive system that new individuals are born; the species are constantly repopulated and the genetic code is transmitted over generations. In humans, the sexual reproduction is the method used, which has several advantages, namely at the level of variability induced by the combination of progenitors genes. This variability ensures the evolution of the species throughout time.

The reproductive system has some unique features. Unlike any other body systems, it is not fully functional at the time of birth, and it requires the action of sex hormones around the time of puberty to be fully active and ready to perform its purpose. In addition, the gender differences between the male and female reproductive system are clearly observed, a fact that does not occur in the other body systems [1].

Structure of the Male Reproductive System

The male reproductive system has different structures that can be divided in primary and secondary sex organs. In males, the primary sex organs, also known as gonads, are the testes. They are responsible for the production of spermatozoa and the secretion of sex hormones. The secretion of sex hormones is then responsible for the development of secondary sex organs. Surrounding the testes is the scrotum, an outpouching of the abdominal wall that protects the testes. The secondary sex organs are structures responsible for the nourishment and storage or transport of the spermatozoa to the exterior or into the female reproductive tract. One of the organs responsible for this transport is the penis. The penis is the male organ used in sexual intercourse and can be divided into three structures: the root linked to the abdominal wall, the body of the penis that corresponds to the major portion of this organ and the glans, also referred as the head of the penis [2]. There are other secondary sex organs, such as the epididymis, *vas deferens*, ejaculatory ducts and urethra responsible for the storage, maturation and transport of the spermatozoa and others responsible for the secretion of fluids that are part of the ejaculate, such as seminal vesicles, prostate gland and bulbourethral glands (Fig. **2.1**). The sex hormones are also responsible for the development of the secondary sex characteristics, that appear during puberty, such as body hair, deep voice and development of the Adam's apple (see Chapter 6) [3].

Testes

The testes are the male gonads, paired ovoid organs that are responsible for the production of spermatozoa and sex hormones. They are suspended in the scrotum by the spermatic cords. Each one is about 4-5 cm long and 2.5 cm in diameter and weighs between 14-18 g in humans [4]. Both testes are covered by two tunics. The outer tunica is the tunica vaginalis and their visceral layer covers the surface of each testis, except where the testis attaches to the epididymis and spermatic cord. This tunica is a thin closed peritoneal sac that has origin on the peritoneum during the descent of the testes. The parietal layer of the tunica vaginalis covers more tissue than the previous one, extending superiorly onto the distal part of the spermatic cord. The separation between the visceral and parietal layers is filled with fluid, allowing the movement of the testis in the scrotum [1, 3, 5].

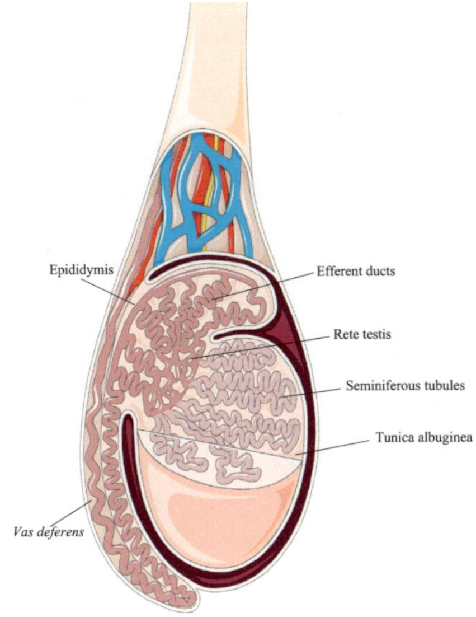

Fig. (2.1). Schematic representation of a human testis. The testis is coated by tunica albuginea, and divided in lobules. The seminiferous tubules are located inside these lobules, highly coiled and organized. The rete testis is responsible for transporting the spermatozoa from the seminiferous tubules into the efferent ducts. From this point forward, spermatozoa enter the epididymis where they go through several processes until they are ready to leave the male reproductive tract into the female reproductive tract where they are fully maturated.

The testes have also a tough fibrous outer membrane called tunica albuginea. This tunica has characteristic extensions that move to the inside of each testis dividing it into testicular lobules. Each of these lobules contains long and highly coiled seminiferous tubules that are nearly 80 cm long, if uncoiled in humans. It is inside these tubules, considered the functional unit of the testis, that spermatogenesis occurs (Fig. **2.1**). Here, spermatozoa are produced at a rate of about thousands per second. Sertoli cells, which function as a physical support to germ cells and nourish their development into sperm, form the seminiferous tubules playing a key role in this event. Between these numerous tubules is the interstitial space, home to the Leydig cells. As testes are an organ with such important and critical functions in male reproduction, it is expected that they are highly irrigated. This occurs, and the major supplier of blood are the testicular arteries, which in turn derivate from the abdominal aorta. The testicular veins are responsible for the drain of the testes. The right testicular vein enters directly into the inferior vena cava, while the left testicular vein enters into the left renal vein [6, 7]. The irrigation occurs in a similar way in the interstitial space.

Scrotum

Scrotum is the major protector of the testes, being located immediately behind the base of the penis and enclosing the testes. It regulates testes position and helps maintaining constant temperature for spermatogenesis. In this region, the skin is covered by hair and is darker when compared with other parts of the body. Depending on the activity of the scrotal muscles, in a balance between their contraction and relaxation, the external appearance of the scrotum may vary at different time periods. The scrotum is constituted by different types of muscle, specifically the dartos and the cremaster. The first is a layer of connective tissue, mostly consisting of smooth muscle. The tone of this smooth muscle is responsible for the characteristic rugose appearance of the scrotum. The cremaster is a thin layer of skeletal muscle that surrounds the testis and the spermatic cord found between the external and internal layers of spermatic fascia. These two muscles work together in response to temperature shifts moving the testes closer or farther from the abdominal cavity and adjusting the heat loss [1, 3]. This control is crucial due to the importance of temperature to spermatogenesis. The normal temperature of the testes is about 35ºC, oscillating 3-4ºC degrees below normal body temperature due to the contraction or relaxation of these two muscles.

A scrotal septum divides the scrotum into two compartments. This division is pivotal to individualize the testes so that in case of an infection the affected testis can be removed without interfering with the normal function of the other testis. Another characteristic associated with the testes is the fact that the left one is suspended lower and has a bigger size when compared with the right counterpart.

The arteries responsible for the blood supply are the anterior and posterior scrotal artery and the testicular artery. The testicular vein is responsible for the venous drainage. The scrotal nerves are principally sensory, including the pudendal nerves and the posterior cutaneous nerves of the thigh [5, 6].

FUNCTIONAL ORGANIZATION OF THE TESTES

The testes are responsible for the production of the male gametes and male sex hormones, which are processes known as spermatogenesis and steroidogenesis respectively. These two distinct processes take place in two morphologically and functionally different compartments: the seminiferous tubular compartment and the interstitial compartment. Despite being anatomically and functionally different, these two compartments function closely to one another and they are both required in order to achieve the correct parameters in sperm quality and production.

Tubular Compartment

The tubular compartment is composed by the seminiferous tubules. It is responsible for 60-80% of the testicular volume and contains the germ cells, Sertoli cells and the peritubular myoid cells (PMCs). Sertoli and germ cells are organized in a highly-polarized system in order to efficiently support the spermatogenesis. Adjacent Sertoli cells form tight junctions with each other, providing an immunoprivileged microenvironment suitable to the development of germ cells. The tight junctions formed between adjacent Sertoli cells establish the blood-testis barrier (BTB), responsible for controlling the movement of nutrients in the seminiferous tubule [8]. However, there are other types of cooperation used between adjacent Sertoli cells to strengthen the BTB, such as ectoplasmic specializations and desmosomes [9, 10]. This barrier has the function of "gate", preventing solutes and large molecules from reaching the germ cells and the function of "fence", restricting the movement of proteins and lipids generating cell polarity. BTB also divides the seminiferous tubules in basal and apical compartments where spermatogonial stem cells and spermatogonia are present in the basal compartment whereas spermatocytes reside in the apical compartment, showing distinct polarity depending on their location [11, 12]. In addition, Sertoli cell nuclei and Golgi complexes are also found in the basal compartment where early phagosomes and early processes involved in the development of the spermatids are all confined to the apical compartment. However, the most obvious form of cell polarity present in the testis is shown in the development of spermatids, where the heads of spermatids point towards the basal compartment while the tails point towards the apical compartment [13, 14].

The testis is divided by a septum of connective tissue into about 250-300 lobules, each one containing 1-3 convoluted seminiferous tubules. Generally, there are about 600 seminiferous tubules present in the human testis and each one has an average length of 30-80 centimeters which varies according to whether they are uncoiled. The total length of the seminiferous tubules is, on average, 300 meters per testis and 600 meters per man [15, 16].

Interstitial Compartment

The seminiferous tubules are surrounded by PMCs, which have several functions. In the male, three or four layers of PMCs surround the seminiferous tubules while in mice, a single layer of PMCs is present [17]. In adult testis, PMCs mediate the contraction of the seminiferous tubules and, during development of the testis and adulthood, they work together with Sertoli cells to deposit the basement membrane (composed by laminin, collagen IV and fibronectin) that surrounds the seminiferous tubules. This is a critical interaction to ensure a correct spermatogenesis and architecture of the seminiferous tubule [18 - 21]. There are other functions attributed to PMCs. In rats, these cells where shown to be an important part of the barrier function, restricting the entry of substances into the seminiferous tubules [22].

Box 2.1 | Summary

- The gender differences between the male and female reproductive system are clearly observed, unlike the other body systems.
- Testes are the primary sex organs, also known as gonads. They are responsible for the production of spermatozoa and the secretion of sex hormones.
- The secondary sex organs are structures responsible for the nourishment and storage or transport of the spermatozoa to the exterior or into the female reproductive system.
- Spermatogenesis and steroidogenesis take place in two morphologically and functionally different compartments: the tubular compartment and the interstitial compartment.
- The male reproductive system has different functions: a) production of the male gametes, spermatozoa; b) transport of these gametes into the female reproductive system through sexual intercourse; and c) production of sex hormones, essential to the proper functioning of this system.

The interstitial compartment is located between the seminiferous tubules and is filled with Leydig cells, the principal component of this compartment. In fact, there are two populations of Leydig cells, the fetal Leydig cells (FLCs) and the adult Leydig cells (ALCs) [23]. After birth, FLCs start degenerating and it is not yet clear if they give rise to ALCs. On the other hand, ALCs derive from Leydig stem cells, capable of self-renewal. These cells develop into Leydig progenitor cells, which express a number of factors such as luteinizing hormone receptors (LHR) and 3β-hydroxysteroid dehydrogenase (3βHSD) [24]. Further differentiation occurs into adult cells that no longer proliferate. In the presence of LH, these cells produce testosterone that is fundamental for the establishment and maintenance of the secondary sex characteristics and the continuation of spermatogenesis [25, 26]. There are other cell types present in the interstitium, namely the immune cells (macrophages, T-cells, dendritic cells), where they respond according to the stimuli received [27]. From this group, macrophages are the most abundant in the interstitium, corresponding to approximately 25% of the interstitial cells present in the adult rodent testis [28]. Several studies have shown that there is cross-talk between immune cells and spermatogonia, where the number of spermatogonia declines after ablation of macrophages [29]. These also establish cell junction with Leydig cells, to facilitate an eventual response. Besides this, 25-hydroxycholesterol secreted by macrophages is used by ALCs to produce testosterone. Furthermore, cytokines produced by macrophages after responding to a stimulus can be used to modulate Leydig cell production of male sex hormones [30 - 32].

PRENATAL DEVELOPMENT OF TESTES

Human reproduction requires the intervention of individuals from two genders, each of them being characterized by a distinct number of anatomic and genetic characteristics. The phenotype of the sex is dictated by the type of gonad that develops in the embryo. This event depends on the expression of the sex-determining region Y (*SRY*), located in the male-specific region of the Y chromosome that encodes the sex-determining region Y protein (SRY) [33]. The presence of SRY leads to a chain of events that culminates in the development of the testes (instead of ovaries) from the gonadal primordium [34]. The early development of the embryo is similar in both sexes. Only in later stages, the difference is manifested by the formation of testes in men or ovaries in women, according to the stimuli and genetic information received by the undifferentiated gonads [35]. Sex differentiation, characterized by the development of secondary sexual characteristics (such as external genitalia), begins when gonads start producing sex-specific hormones [36]. In early stages, the embryonic gonad has the unique ability to differentiate into one of two fully functional distinct organs, thus being called bipotential.

The pathway that leads to the formation of one or another relies on a tightly regulated network of cell signaling molecules and transcription factors [37]. Thus the phenotype of sexual differentiation is the result of several consecutive events: the appearance of the bipotential gonad, gonad development, production of sex hormones and ultimately sex differentiation [38].

Sex Determination

Sex determination refers to the key point where the bipotential gonad, particularly the somatic cells, start to differentiate either as Sertoli cells or granulosa cells during fetal life. Despite the difficulty of identifying genes involved in sex determination, some studies have made clear progresses in that field. Nowadays, several genes are already known to play a major role in that process [39, 40]. In humans, the presence of the Y chromosome, more specifically of the *SRY* gene, acts as the major male sex determinant, shifting the bipotential gonad towards a testicular fate. Several studies have shown that mice or humans carrying point mutations or deletions in this gene display an XY female sex-reversed phenotype. Moreover, XX mice where a 14-kb genomic fragment of this gene was introduced, developed sex reversal, showing that SRY is required to initiate male development [41 - 43]. One of the most important events in testis development is the differentiation of pre-Sertoli cells. This event is induced by the expression of *SRY*, which is strictly controlled by several genes. For example, embryos homozygous for the boy/girl (byg/byg) mutation show sex reversal due to a decrease in the expression of *SRY*. This mutation is an A to T transversion, which causes the appearance of a premature stop codon in the gene encoding for the mitogen-activated protein kinase kinase kinase 4 (MAP3K4), making this kinase nonfunctional [44, 45]. The decrease in *SRY* expression is partially controlled by growth arrest and DNA damage-inducible gene family 45 (GADD45γ), a protein involved in several important tasks, such as regulation of growth and apoptosis, cell cycle control and senescence [46]. Evidence towards the pattern of GADD45γ expression shows that it is quite similar to the expression pattern of *SRY* suggesting that they work together in sex determination. This pattern can explain why, in mice deficient for *GADD45γ*, sex reversal is observed due to a decrease in *SRY* expression. However, in these same mice, overexpression of MAP3K4 can prevent sex reversal, showing that MAP3K4 is also imperative for sex determination [47].

Expression of *SRY* starts in the central region of the genital ridges and occurs in a very strict time window. In mouse genital ridges, expression of *SRY* occurs around the 11th day of embryonic development, peaks on the day 11.5 of embryonic development and stops around the 12.5 day of embryonic development [48 - 51]. SRY binds to steroidogenic factor 1 (SF1), forming a complex that triggers the expression of SRY-box 9 (*SOX9*) in Sertoli cells precursors. *SOX9* expression is upregulated when expression of *SRY* is already at its highest, around the day 11.5 of embryonic development. After a short period of time, SOX9 starts downregulating *SRY* expression, leading to its interruption [52 - 54]. After being expressed, SOX9 recruits and activates several proteins that play a key role in testis development, such as prostaglandin D synthase (PGDS), an enzyme that catalyzes the isomerization of PGH_2. This event is particularly important in order to create a feedforward loop with SOX9, keeping the level of SOX9 high enough to ensure the activation of other crucial genes such as fibroblast growth factor 9 (*FGF9*) and *SF1* [55, 56].

SRY and SOX9 are members of the SOX family of developmental transcription factors that contain an amino acid motif commonly known as high mobility group (HMG-box) domain. This HMG-box is a DNA binding domain and is highly conserved among eukaryotes. SOX9 (and other transcription factors that are a part of this family) bind to the minor groove in DNA [57, 58]. The SOX transcription factors were first identified based on the molecular conservation of the 79 amino acid HMG DNA binding domain present in the *SRY* and their ability to bind to DNA in the minor groove region [59]. This highly conserved domain allows SRY and the SOX family of proteins to bind to the DNA sequence A/TA/TCAAA/TG with high affinity [60]. Several mutations found in human patients showing sex reversal (male to female) have been associated with the inability of SRY to bind to DNA [61, 62]. Additionally, *SRY* mutations in the nuclear localization signal present in the N-terminal end of the HMG-box can cause a reduction of nuclear importation, which can be the explanation for some cases of sex reversal [63, 64]. As referred before, one of these two genes individually can promote testicular differentiation. Several studies have shown that a *SOX9* transgene can promote testicular differentiation instead of *SRY* [65 - 67]. XX individuals who possess an extra copy of *SOX9* develop as male even though they have no *SRY* [68]. Those results suggest that the primordial function of *SRY* in male development is the upregulation of other transcription factors, such as *SOX9*. Other possibility is linked with the fact that the *SOX9* transgene could activate other *SRY* target genes required to induce male development making *SRY* meaningless for the testicular development. There are several genes involved in the pathway following the activation of *SRY*, however it is not yet clear if the activation of *SRY* is strictly required for the activation of these genes or if *SRY* is only required for the upregulation of *SOX9* [69].

Other genes are known to be involved in early stages of sex determination, including *NR5A1* (encoding SF1), *GATA4* (GATA-binding protein 4) and *NR0B1* (encoding DAX1, dosage-sensitive sex reversal, adrenal hypoplasia critical region, on chromosome X, gene 1) [70 - 72]. The presence or the absence of one of these genes results in significant changes in the sexual differentiation of an individual. For example, mice where SF1 is not present manifest a phenotype where one or both gonads are not formed, due to an improper gonadogenesis [73]. SF1 is linked with the transcriptional regulation of genes that encode several hormones involved in the hypothalamic-pituitary- gonadal axis [74]. SF1 is also essential to maintain the bipotential gonad and while its expression decays in the XX genital ridge of mouse embryos, in XY mouse embryos SF1 stays expressed. SF1 expression is essential in both Sertoli and Leydig cells. In Sertoli cells, SF1 works together with *SOX9* and increases the level of transcription of Anti-Müllerian hormone, essential for the degeneration of the Müllerian ducts. In Leydig cells, SF1 activates genes that will result in the production of testosterone [75, 76].

Development of the Bipotential Gonad

Formation of the Genital Ridge

In human embryos, the gonadal precursors appear on the 32nd day of embryonic development while in mice they appear earlier, on the day 10.5 of embryonic development. Unless the differentiation process starts, it is not possible to observe any morphological differences between male and female genital ridges [77]. Unlike other organs, like the lung primordium that can only differentiate into lung, the gonadal primordium can either differentiate into testes or ovaries. Before differentiation occurs, the mammalian gonad has an undifferentiated or bipotential stage and at this point it has neither male or female characteristics [78]. On the 4th week of embryonic development, the urogenital ridges appear as two raised edges, parallel to the midline of the body, in the posterior abdominal wall. This urogenital ridge arises from the intermediate mesoderm that generates the urogenital system (the kidneys, the gonads and their ducts) [79]. It develops sequentially into three sets of tubular nephric structures: the pronephros, the mesonephros and the metanephros. The pronephric tubules and part of the pronephric ducts degenerate, while the more caudal portions persist and function as an embryonic kidney, precursor of the adult kidney. The remnants of this structure form the Wolffian duct. While this occurs, the middle portion of the nephric duct induces the formation of the mesonephros that, similarly to the pronephros, has a brief existence. However, it has important functions such as being the source of hematopoietic stem cells and in male mammals, some of these tubes remain and differentiate into the adult *vas deferens* and efferent ducts. The metanephros is the result of several interactions between epithelial and mesenchymal components of the intermediate mesoderm [80 - 82]. Parallel to the development of the kidney, the gonadal primordium appears in the intermediate mesoderm around the 4th week of embryonic development and remains sexually undifferentiated until the 7th week of embryonic development. The more lateral portions of the gonadal primordium form the mesonephric ridge, while the medial portion of the gonadal primordium is constituted by coelomic epithelium and forms the genital ridge. During the indifferent stage, the coelomic epithelium in the genital ridges goes through proliferation and thickening, expanding into the coelomic cavity. This proliferation causes the invasion of the subjacent mesenchymal tissue [83]. At this point, primitive sex cords are formed and remain connected to the surface epithelium. An important player appears in this moment, laminin. The production of laminin, a glycoprotein that is the major structural component in the basal lamina of most cells, increases in the genital ridge, as the coelomic cells proliferate [84]. This glycoprotein seems to be essential for the ensuing germ cell colonization. At this point, the cell types of the genital ridge are equally capable of originating testes or ovaries. Here, *SRY* plays a key role triggering the male development leading to the development of the testis and male reproductive tract. Without interference from the *SRY* gene and the interference of other genes such as *RSPO1* and the WNT gene family, the pathway of events will lead to the formation of ovaries [85]. It is important to bear in mind that the development of a testis or an ovary involves different molecular regulation pathways that antagonize each other [86 - 88].

Testes Differentiation

The expression of a single gene, *SRY*, located on the Y chromosome, is the primary responsible for male determination [89]. It occurs in the gonadal blastema, with the coelomic-derived somatic cells, which are called supporting cells, being responsible for it [49]. Several studies have shown that a large part of this group of cells is originated from the coelomic epithelium situated above the genital ridges. However, the mechanism by which these cells enter the gonad is not clear [90]. It is known though that *SRY* is activated in the genital ridges only after these cells fully colonize the gonad, showing that their migration cannot be a consequence of the *SRY* expression [49]. The latter begins in the middle of the genital ridges with consecutive expansion to the anterior and posterior poles. After this, *SRY* expression stops in the anterior and central regions, being only expressed in the posterior region until it completely disappears from the genital ridges [91].

One of the major events in testis differentiation is the formation of the testis cords, which transforms the genital ridge into a highly-structured organ. Testis cords are specialized tubular structures and its formation is fundamental to the structure and function of the testis. They are originated from the sex cords and after sexual differentiation, particularly *SRY* expression, they differentiate into testis cords. Once this formation starts, the fate of the bipotential gonad is settled and the male sex determining pathway has overcome competitive signals trying to push the bipotential gonad into an ovarian fate [92]. This formation occurs between the day 11.5 and day 13.5 of embryonic development in mice, being that on the day 13.5 of embryonic development the number of testis cords developing into seminiferous tubules is defined. Testis cords facilitate the sheltering of germ cells from external signals. It is inside these structures that, in adult life, mature spermatogonia are nourished and given support to develop into spermatozoa, which are then guided throughout the male reproductive tract [93]. They are responsible for separating the two main functions of the testis: spermatozoa and androgen production. Moreover, they act like a shield that protects the gonocytes, also known as prospermatogonia, from retinoic acid, known to trigger meiosis. This protection is crucial to ensure that the onset of meiosis in male germ cells is delayed until after birth [94, 95]. Lastly, they are important in later stages of reproduction, as they play a role in the transport of the mature sperm from the testis. The formation of the testis cords involves the organization of pre-Sertoli cells and prospermatogonia into testis cords, which will in turn develop into the seminiferous tubules. Initially, both types of cells are evenly distributed in the genital ridge but shortly after, clusters of pre-Sertoli cells are formed and start to surround the germ cells. This aggregation occurs after *SOX9* activation. *SRY* is initially activated in the center of the testis cords which leads to *SOX9* expression and subsequent *FGF9* expression. In the center of the testis cords, a positive-feedback loop between *SOX9* and FGF9 is established, resulting in the formation of testis cords. In the pole regions, *SRY* starts to be activated after being activated in the center with a delay of approximately 4 hours. This *SRY* expression properly initiates *SOX9* expression. At the same time, *FGF9* is already expressed in the central domain, and is expected to diffuse towards the anterior and posterior poles. This diffusion of FGF9 towards the poles helps the establishment of a positive-feedback loop for *SOX9* expression in the poles that maintain *SOX9* expression, recruitment of precursor cells and proper testis cord formation in the entire gonadal area [96, 97]. From this point, the development of the clusters of pre-Sertoli cells into the future seminiferous tubules depends on the migration of endothelial precursor cells from the mesonephros [98, 99]. The endothelial precursor cells detach from the mesonephric plexus and invade the developing XY gonad, creating the characteristic coelomic vessel on the surface of the gonad. While this happens, smaller vessels originated from the coelomic vessel are formed in the interstitium of the testes. Vasculature is also a key process to a correct formation of the testis cords since its development is disrupted in cases of absence of the vasculature [100]. At this stage, testis cords start growing and are surrounded by PMCs that along with pre-Sertoli cells, deposit in the basement membrane, causing the remodeling of testis cords and his vasculature [101, 102]. PMCs contribute to the formation of the basement membrane and initiate the polarization of pre-Sertoli cells. The interaction between pre-Sertoli cells and PMCs leads to the production of various extracellular matrix proteins such as E-cadherin and P-cadherin [20, 103]. After birth, prospermatogonia develops and differentiates into spermatogonia [104, 105].

In human embryos, the precursors for male and female reproductive systems are both initially present in the mesonephros [106]. The precursors of the male duct system are the Wolffian ducts, while the precursors of the female system are the Müllerian ducts. Only one of these two ducts will advance further in development, depending if a testicular or ovarian differentiation has begun [107]. In the male gonad, the Wolffian ducts appear in small and short-term segments within the pronephros, developing to a stable and continuous tube on the urogenital ridge [108].

Pre-Sertoli Cell Differentiation

SRY expression upregulates *SOX9* expression in the supporting cells, which then start being referred as pre-Sertoli cells. *SOX9* and *SRY* share a similar expression pattern, being firstly expressed in the middle of the genital ridge and then in the anterior and posterior poles [97, 109]. The sole expression of *SRY* is not always sufficient to upregulate *SOX9* expression. In fact, a minimum level of *SRY* expression needs to be achieved, within a specific time window, to successfully upregulate *SOX9* expression [110]. In this case, both SF1 and FGF9 play a crucial role in the proliferation of pre-Sertoli cells [111, 112]. After *SRY* expression starts, FGF9 plays a major part in maintaining the required cell proliferation, namely the one that leads to the formation of pre-Sertoli cells. This proliferation is required for the formation of the sex cords [113, 114]. The expression of *SRY* upregulates the expression of *SOX9* that in turn, directly or indirectly upregulates *FGF9* expression. Consequently, FGF9 upregulates *SOX9* expression creating a positive feedback loop that maintains the high levels of*SOX9* required to induce testicular development [92]. Studies in mice lacking the FGF9 coded receptor show uncompleted sex reversal, reinforcing the importance of this gene on inducing testicular development [115]. Several other genes are activated following the activation of *SOX9*, including the hematopoietic prostaglandin D synthase (*PGDS*) that promotes the nuclear translocation of *SOX9* to induce Sertoli cell differentiation. These cells will then produce the anti-Müllerian hormone that binds to its receptor and promotes regression of Müllerian ducts through the induction of apoptosis [75, 116, 117].

Sertoli somatic cells function as a support to germ cells and nourish their development into sperm [118]. They are the first cells that differentiate from the bipotential precursors and are the first indicator that the gonad has started the development of the testis, surpassing the undifferentiated stage (Fig. **2.2**). Sertoli cells act as the organizing center of testis differentiation, influencing testis cord formation, Müllerian ducts regression and the differentiation of a large number of cell types like the germ cells, endothelial cells and fetal Leydig cells [83]. Pre-Sertoli cells can be defined as nonpolarized, scattered somatic cells that express *SRY* and *SOX9*, while Sertoli cells are polarized, have a fixed location within the testis cord and express *SOX9* [119]. The final number of Sertoli cells is an indicator of the fertility capacity of the male, the higher the number of Sertoli cells the higher the number of germ cells they will support in adulthood [120]. While the differentiation of Sertoli cells is occurring, the gonad undergoes some changes due to the expression of *SRY* [121]. These changes result from an increased proliferation and migration of cells from the adjacent mesonephros and lead to an increase in the size of the gonads [122].

Primordial Germ Cells

In contrast to the somatic cells of the fetal testes, the primordial germ cells do not arise from the genital ridges or the mesonephros. In fact, these cells originate far from their final destination, within the proximal posterior epiblast and in an initial phase of the testicular development. Indeed, they start forming cell clusters around the 6th day of embryonic development [123]. This process is mainly controlled by a growth factor secreted by the extraembryonic ectoderm, bone morphogenetic protein 4 (BMP4), which in turn activates the expression of *PRDM14* (PR domain 14) and *BLIMP1* (encoding PR domain zinc finger protein 1, PRDM1). These, along with *TFAP2c* (encoding Transcription Factor AP-2 Gamma) were shown to play a key role in primordial germ cell specification [124]. Around the 3rd week of embryonic development, they are scattered in the extraembryonic mesoderm that covers the posterior wall of the yolk sac [125]. Primordial germ cells have an ovoid shape, with a diameter between 12 and 14 µm and present a round nucleus. Due to their intense reaction to alkaline phosphatase, these cells are easily detected [126, 127]. Around the day 7.5 of embryonic development, primordial germ cells migrate from the posterior primitive streak to the developing embryonic endoderm (hindgut). Between the day 8.5 and day 10.5 of embryonic development, the hindgut invaginates into the soon-to-be abdominal cavity, towards the future genital ridges [128 - 130]. These migration events involve the interaction of several factors expressed by the genital ridges and by the primordial germ cells along with a large number of extracellular matrix proteins [131, 132]. After these successful migrations, genital ridges become colonized by the primordial germ cells, a process that involves the expression of E-cadherin and the interaction of the primordial germ cells with the rich laminin network produced by the coelomic cells [103]. The eventual failure of these germ cells to reach the genital ridge results in lack of gonad development. Once these processes of migration and colonization are complete, germ cells lose their motility and their polarized morphology and start associating with each other (Fig. **2.2**) [133].

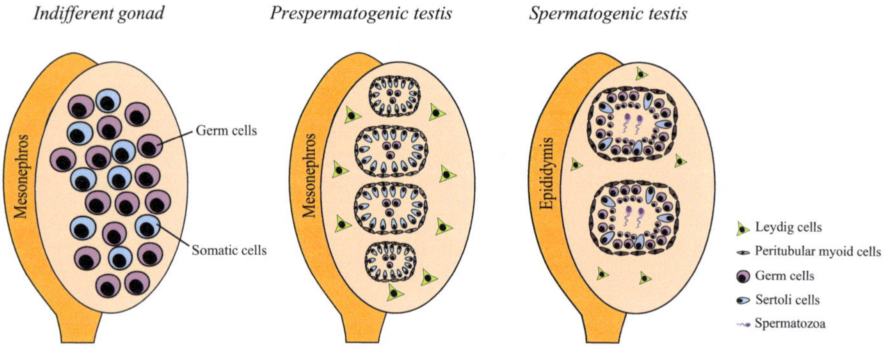

Fig. (2.2). Stages of testicular development. The undifferentiated gonad contains a pool of germ cells and somatic cells. After *SRY* expression, Sertoli cells start to proliferate and differentiate, organizing themselves into testis cords. Peritubular myoid cells also differentiate and, along with Sertoli cells, surround germ cells and deposit the basement membrane, causing the remodeling of testis cords and constituting the prespermatogenic testis. In the interstitium, Leydig cells secrete testosterone which is essential for spermatogenesis. Once every cell lineage is differentiated spermatogenesis occurs leading to the formation of the spermatozoa and testes are considered spermatogenic since they are fully functional. Abbreviations: *SRY* (sex-determining region Y).

Leydig Cell Development

Leydig cells were first discovered in 1850 by Franz Leydig. Nevertheless, the origin of Leydig cells has not yet been fully understood. Although there are several hypotheses, none fully explains and supports the origin of these cells. They differentiate in the second compartment of the testis, the interstitium and are often located near the blood vessels due to their role, the production of androgens for the fetal masculinization. These cells are considered the FLCs and it is thought that they degenerate postnatally. FLCs are responsible for the production of the androgens involved in the promotion of several mechanisms of the secondary sexual development in the fetus, in a process that started being deciphered long ago [134, 135]. These mechanisms comprise the development of the Wolffian ducts and external genitalia, testicular descent, and sex-specific brain patterning [136 - 140].

Fetal Leydig Cell Origin

Human Leydig cells are thought to differentiate from multiple progenitor cells. Early adreno-gonadal precursor cells seem to be in the origin of FLCs [141 - 143], and these may share these precursors with both, Sertoli and PMCs [36, 144]. Due to their common origin, it is suggested that adreno-gonadal precursor cells contribute to the FLCs progenitor population when genital ridge is formed [143]. However, the accurate origin of FLCs is still unknown [144]. After the occurrence of sex determination, the male genital ridge starts differentiating into the testis cords and the interstitium. In the latter, the pool of progenitor FLCs population is stored and other interstitial somatic cells such as fibroblasts. Several types of cells are found in the testicular interstitial compartment, the local of origin of FLCs, such as transcription factor MafB (MAFB) positive cells that migrate from the coelomic epithelium and MAFB and/or vascular cell adhesion protein 1 (VCAM1) positive cells that originate in the gonad-mesonephros border [145 - 147]. Additionally, the vasculature invasion in the interstitial space has a key role regulating the migration and expansion of interstitial progenitor cells in the developing testis indicating that these cells are prone to contribute to the interstitial progenitor pool where FLCs progenitors are included [100]. In summary, FLCs are derived from multiple and different cell types from the coelomic epithelium progenitor cells and are influenced by vasculature invasion.

FLC population is established relatively late during the formation of the testes: on the 14th day of embryonic development in rats, 12th day of embryonic development in mice, and on the middle of the 7th week of embryonic development in humans [148]. The increase in the FLC number was linked to the increase in plasma testosterone during the embryonic and early fetal period [149] illustrating a possible relation between these two events. Differentiation from progenitors into FLCs is thought to occur during the 8th week of embryonic development until the 14th week of embryonic development in the fetal human testes [150]. Leydig cells proliferate and gradually differentiate, attaining a development peak on the 19th week of embryonic development [24, 150]. Upon differentiation, the main function of FLCs is the production of androgens that mediate the masculinization of XY embryos [24, 36, 151]. FLCs are capable of producing androstenedione, but not testosterone, because they lack 17β-hydroxysteroid dehydrogenase. However, androstenedione can be converted to testosterone by fetal Sertoli cells, since they express that enzyme [152, 153]. This interplay between FLCs and Sertoli cells results in testosterone production, which is of extreme importance in fetal testes [154]. However, the cooperation between these types of cells in fetal testes does not end here. FLCs are able to produce Activin A, a member of transforming growth factor-β (TGF-β) protein superfamily, which regulates Sertoli cell proliferation and, in turn, modulate testes cord expansion [155].

Fetal Leydig Cell Differentiation

The differentiation and function of FLCs is subjected to a tight regulation by specific genes and signaling proteins. Sertoli cells are responsible for coordinating the testis cord formation after sex determination, an event that coincides with FLCs differentiation. In fact, differentiation of FLCs occurs under the intervention of Sertoli cells, which provide cell-derived factors [148, 156 - 158] and were reported to release pivotal factors in the differentiation of these cells. Some of them are promoting factors, such as KITL (KIT ligand, essential to ALCs survival and growth) and DHH (Desert Hedgehog, a member of the DHH/PTCH1 signal pathway that triggers FLC differentiation) while others are inhibiting factors, such as Anti-Müllerian hormone, functioning as a negative modulator of FLC function and Wilms' tumor 1 (WT1), leading to the failure of the differentiation of FLCs into ALCs [159, 160]. The platelet-derived growth factor (PDGF) is also a fetal Sertoli cell secretion that was shown to be vital for FLCs ontogeny [36, 144, 157, 161]. In addition, two other Sertoli cell-secreted peptides that have long been suggested to be involved in the regulation of Leydig cell function are TGF-β and insulin-like growth factor I (IGF1) [162]. Interestingly, upon differentiation, function of FLCs seems largely independent of Sertoli cells, but also of germ and PMCs [163].

Besides Sertoli-cell released factors, there are several FLC progenitor factors that are known to modulate FLC progenitor formation and consequently FLC differentiation. Again, some of them are promoting factors such as SF1, DAX1 and GATA4 while others are inhibiting factors such as NOTCH [164 - 167]. Nonetheless, FLC derived factors also play an important role in the regulation of

FLCs differentiation. Several of them are known, like SF1, IGF1 and myocyte enhancer factor 2 (MEF2) [168 - 170]. The development of FLCs is not a separated process from the rest of the testis development, it occurs in sync with testis cord formation, Sertoli cells differentiation and proliferation and male vasculature development, with each one of them influencing and modulating FLCs differentiation process.

Fate of Fetal Leydig Cells

The fate of FLCs was subject of some controversy. Some stated that they would disappear after birth [141], while it was later suggested that they would persist into early postnatal life as a subpopulation of Leydig cells within the testes. It is now accepted that FLCs persist in adult testes, accounting for about 20% of total Leydig cells present [171], although they undergo a gradual process of atrophy [172 - 174]. These FLCs that remain in the adult testes are hydroxysteroid 17-beta dehydrogenase 3 and hydroxy-delta-5-steroid dehydrogenase, 3 beta- and steroid delta-isomerase 6 negative, showing that they cannot produce testosterone, which further indicates that ALCs are in fact the only steroidogenic cells able to produce testosterone in adult testes [171, 175]. TGF-β, anti-Müllerian hormone (AMH), and gonadotropin-releasing hormone (GnRH) are signaling molecules that have been proposed to be involved in the degeneration of FLCs in rodents [159, 176]. It is a fact that androstenedione-producing Leydig cells are gradually replaced by testosterone-producing ones during postnatal development [158, 174], but the mechanisms involved and actual fate of FLCs remain far from being fully understood [144].

After birth, a second population of Leydig cells arises, peaking around the second to fourth month [177, 178], coinciding timewise with transient activity of the hypothalamic-pituitary-gonadal axis [179, 180]. The function of these neonatal Leydig cells is, however, largely undiscovered, although it was suggested that their short promotion of testosterone synthesis would be linked to brain development and central nervous system activity [148].

Postnatally, ALCs gradually replace FLCs, although the first do not originate from the second [171, 181]. The lineage of the ALCs includes Leydig cell progenitors, immature Leydig cells and ALCs [182 - 184]. In the postnatal testes, interaction with other cells present in the interstitium, namely macrophages and PMCs, concurs to the development and differentiation of arising ALCs [148].

Firstly, Leydig cell progenitors are formed postnatally from active proliferation of fibroblastic mesenchymal-like stem cells, in the testicular interstitium [183, 185]. Then, progenitor Leydig cells differentiate into immature Leydig cells, and, during puberty, ALCs differentiate from immature Leydig cells present in the peritubular interstitium. A peak of ALCs population is achieved by the end of puberty [186].

Box 2.2 | Summary

- The presence of the Y chromosome, more specifically the *SRY* gene, acts as the major male sex determinant, shifting the bipotential gonad towards a testicular fate.
- SRY, SOX9 and FGF9 establish a positive feedback loop that maintains the high levels of SOX9 required to induce testicular development.
- Before differentiation occurs, the mammalian gonad has an undifferentiated or bipotential stage and at this point it has neither male nor female characteristics.
- The formation of the testis cords, which transforms the genital ridge into a highly-structured organ is a major event in testis differentiation.
- Testis cords have several functions, such as, in adulthood, nourish mature spermatogonia and give them support to develop into spermatozoa, which are then guided through the male reproductive tract.
- Fetal Leydig Cells are responsible for the production of the androgens involved in the promotion of several mechanisms of the secondary sexual development in the fetus.

CONCLUDING REMARKS

Testicular development is a complex process that depends on the expression of *SRY* gene, located in the Y chromosome, and on the expression of other genes located on the autosomal genes. Around the 4th week of embryonic development, the urogenital ridge arises, further transforming into the bipotential gonad. At this stage the gonad can either differentiate into testes or ovaries, depending on the stimuli received. If *SRY* expression occurs, the gonads start differentiating towards the testes. This process is marked by the differentiation of coelomic-derived cells into pre-Sertoli cells, forming the sex cords, the precursor of testis cords. These cords are surrounded by PMCs. Hormones also play an important role, with testosterone causing testicular maturation, inducing the differentiation of pre-Sertoli cells and primordial germ cells and the development of other organs present in the male reproductive tract.

Despite the enormous advances on the understanding of testes development and function there are several questions that remain unanswered. The origin of some cells types such as FLCs is still under debate and some components, such as the PMC lineage and the tunica albuginea, remain poorly described. Also, the factors that determine the gonadal size and shape remain fairly unknown. In addition, the majority of these studies have been made in mice and the translation to human models has not yet been made due to ethical issues. In the future, understanding the detailed process and pathways involved in testis development will help to better understand some problems that remain a hot topic of research in several fields, including studying the disorders of sex development and infertility.

CONFLICT OF INTEREST

The authors confirm that they have no conflict of interest to declare for this publication.

ACKNOWLEDGEMENTS

This work was supported by the "Fundação para a Ciência e a Tecnologia"–FCT (PTDC/BIM-MET/4712/2014), UMIB (PEst-OE/SAU/UI0215/2014), CICS (UID /Multi/00709/2013); and of FEDER through the POPH and POCI - COMPETE 2020 (POCI-01-0145-FEDER-007491) funds. J. P. Monteiro (within the project PTDC/BBB-BQB/1368/2014) and M. J. Meneses (PD/BD/114256/2016) were also funded by FCT.

REFERENCES

[1] Van De Graaff KM. Human Anatomy: McGraw-Hill Higher Education. 2001.

[2] Clark RK. Anatomy and Physiology: Understanding the Human Body. Jones and Bartlett Publishers 2005.

[3] VanPutte C, Russo A, Regan J. Seeley's Anatomy & Physiology. McGraw-Hill Education 2010.

[4] Johnson L, Petty CS, Neaves WB. Influence of age on sperm production and testicular weights in men. J Reprod Fertil 1984; 70(1): 211-8.
[http://dx.doi.org/10.1530/jrf.0.0700211] [PMID: 6694139]

[5] Rizzo DC. Fundamentals of Anatomy and Physiology. Cengage Learning 2009.

[6] Gilbert SF. Developmental Biology. Sinauer 2014.

[7] Regan J, Russo A, VanPutte C. Seeley's Essentials of Anatomy and Physiology. McGraw-Hill Education 2015.

[8] Wong CH, Cheng CY. The blood-testis barrier: its biology, regulation, and physiological role in spermatogenesis. Curr Top Dev Biol 2005; 71: 263-96.
[http://dx.doi.org/10.1016/S0070-2153(05)71008-5] [PMID: 16344108]

[9] Lie PP, Cheng CY, Mruk DD. The biology of the desmosome-like junction a versatile anchoring junction and signal transducer in the seminiferous epithelium. Int Rev Cell Mol Biol 2011; 286: 223-69.
[http://dx.doi.org/10.1016/B978-0-12-385859-7.00005-7] [PMID: 21199783]

[10] Mruk DD, Cheng CY. Sertoli-Sertoli and Sertoli-germ cell interactions and their significance in germ cell movement in the seminiferous epithelium during spermatogenesis. Endocr Rev 2004; 25(5): 747-806.
[http://dx.doi.org/10.1210/er.2003-0022] [PMID: 15466940]

[11] Mruk DD, Cheng CY. The mammalian blood-testis barrier: its biology and regulation. Endocr Rev 2015; 36(5): 564-91.
[http://dx.doi.org/10.1210/er.2014-1101] [PMID: 26357922]

[12] Pelletier RM. The blood-testis barrier: the junctional permeability, the proteins and the lipids. Prog Histochem Cytochem 2011; 46(2): 49-127.
[http://dx.doi.org/10.1016/j.proghi.2011.05.001] [PMID: 21705043]

[13] Gao Y, Cheng CY. Does cell polarity matter during spermatogenesis? Spermatogenesis 2016; 6(2): e1218408.
[http://dx.doi.org/10.1080/21565562.2016.1218408] [PMID: 27635303]

[14] Gao Y, Xiao X, Lui WY, Lee WM, Mruk D, Cheng CY. Cell polarity proteins and spermatogenesis. Semin Cell Dev Biol 2016; 59: 62-70.
[http://dx.doi.org/10.1016/j.semcdb.2016.06.008] [PMID: 27292315]

[15] Griswold MD. Spermatogenesis: the commitment to meiosis. Physiol Rev 2016; 96(1): 1-17.
[http://dx.doi.org/10.1152/physrev.00013.2015] [PMID: 26537427]

[16] Xiao X, Mruk DD, Wong CK, Cheng CY. Germ cell transport across the seminiferous epithelium during spermatogenesis. Physiology (Bethesda) 2014; 29(4): 286-98.
[http://dx.doi.org/10.1152/physiol.00001.2014] [PMID: 24985332]

[17] Gardner PJ, Holyoke EA. Fine structure of the seminiferous tubule of the swiss mouse. Anat Rec 1964; 150: 391-404.
[http://dx.doi.org/10.1002/ar.1091500407] [PMID: 14248309]

[18] Bichoualne L, Thiébot B, Langris M, Barbey P, Oulhaj H, Bocquet J. Membrane associated proteoglycans in rat testicular peritubular cells. Mol Cell Biochem 1994; 140(1): 37-48.
[http://dx.doi.org/10.1007/BF00928364] [PMID: 7877596]

[19] Maekawa M, Kamimura K, Nagano T. Peritubular myoid cells in the testis: their structure and function. Arch Histol Cytol 1996; 59(1): 1-13.
[http://dx.doi.org/10.1679/aohc.59.1] [PMID: 8727359]

[20] Skinner MK, Tung PS, Fritz IB. Cooperativity between Sertoli cells and testicular peritubular cells in the production and deposition of extracellular matrix components. J Cell Biol 1985; 100(6): 1941-7.
[http://dx.doi.org/10.1083/jcb.100.6.1941] [PMID: 3889013]

[21] Verhoeven G, Hoeben E, De Gendt K. Peritubular cell-Sertoli cell interactions: factors involved in PmodS activity. Andrologia 2000; 32(1): 42-5.
[PMID: 10702865]

[22] Dym M, Fawcett DW. The blood-testis barrier in the rat and the physiological compartmentation of the seminiferous epithelium. Biol Reprod 1970; 3(3): 308-26.
[http://dx.doi.org/10.1093/biolreprod/3.3.308] [PMID: 4108372]

[23] OShaughnessy PJ, Baker PJ, Johnston H. The foetal Leydig cell differentiation, function and regulation. Int J Androl 2006; 29(1): 90-5.
[http://dx.doi.org/10.1111/j.1365-2605.2005.00555.x] [PMID: 16466528]

[24] Haider SG. Cell biology of Leydig cells in the testis. Int Rev Cytol 2004; 233: 181-241.
[http://dx.doi.org/10.1016/S0074-7696(04)33005-6] [PMID: 15037365]

[25] Smith LB, Walker WH. The regulation of spermatogenesis by androgens. Semin Cell Dev Biol 2014; 30: 2-13.
[http://dx.doi.org/10.1016/j.semcdb.2014.02.012] [PMID: 24598768]

[26] Walker WH. Testosterone signaling and the regulation of spermatogenesis. Spermatogenesis 2011; 1(2): 116-20.
[http://dx.doi.org/10.4161/spmg.1.2.16956] [PMID: 22319659]

[27] Pérez CV, Theas MS, Jacobo PV, Jarazo-Dietrich S, Guazzone VA, Lustig L. Dual role of immune cells in the testis: Protective or pathogenic for germ cells? Spermatogenesis 2013; 3(1): e23870.
[http://dx.doi.org/10.4161/spmg.23870] [PMID: 23687616]

[28] Niemi M, Sharpe RM, Brown WR. Macrophages in the interstitial tissue of the rat testis. Cell Tissue Res 1986; 243(2): 337-44.
[http://dx.doi.org/10.1007/BF00251049] [PMID: 2418975]

[29] DeFalco T, Potter SJ, Williams AV, Waller B, Kan MJ, Capel B. Macrophages contribute to the spermatogonial niche in the adult testis. Cell Reports 2015; 12(7): 1107-19.
[http://dx.doi.org/10.1016/j.celrep.2015.07.015] [PMID: 26257171]

[30] Hales DB. Testicular macrophage modulation of Leydig cell steroidogenesis. J Reprod Immunol 2002; 57(1-2): 3-18.
[http://dx.doi.org/10.1016/S0165-0378(02)00020-7] [PMID: 12385830]

[31] Lukyanenko YO, Chen JJ, Hutson JC. Production of 25-hydroxycholesterol by testicular macrophages and its effects on Leydig cells. Biol Reprod 2001; 64(3): 790-6.
[http://dx.doi.org/10.1095/biolreprod64.3.790] [PMID: 11207193]

[32] Meinhardt A, Hedger MP. Immunological, paracrine and endocrine aspects of testicular immune privilege. Mol Cell Endocrinol 2011; 335(1): 60-8.
[http://dx.doi.org/10.1016/j.mce.2010.03.022] [PMID: 20363290]

[33] Koopman P, Bullejos M, Bowles J. Regulation of male sexual development by *SRY* and *SOX9* . J Exp Zool 2001; 290(5): 463-74.
[http://dx.doi.org/10.1002/jez.1089] [PMID: 11555853]

[34] Schagdarsurengin U, Western P, Steger K, Meinhardt A. Developmental origins of male subfertility: role of infection, inflammation, and environmental factors. Semin Immunopathol 2016; 38(6): 765-81.
[http://dx.doi.org/10.1007/s00281-016-0576-y] [PMID: 27315198]

[35] Biason-Lauber A. The battle of the sexes: human sex development and its disorders. Results Probl Cell Differ 2016; 58: 337-82.
[http://dx.doi.org/10.1007/978-3-319-31973-5_13] [PMID: 27300185]

[36] Svingen T, Koopman P. Building the mammalian testis: origins, differentiation, and assembly of the component cell populations. Genes Dev 2013; 27(22): 2409-26.
[http://dx.doi.org/10.1101/gad.228080.113] [PMID: 24240231]

[37] Biason-Lauber A. Control of sex development. Best Pract Res Clin Endocrinol Metab 2010; 24(2): 163-86.
[http://dx.doi.org/10.1016/j.beem.2009.12.002] [PMID: 20541146]

[38] Flück CE, Meyer-Böni M, Pandey AV, *et al.* Why boys will be boys: two pathways of fetal testicular androgen biosynthesis are needed for male sexual differentiation. Am J Hum Genet 2011; 89(2): 201-18.
[http://dx.doi.org/10.1016/j.ajhg.2011.06.009] [PMID: 21802064]

[39] Fleming A, Vilain E. The endless quest for sex determination genes. Clin Genet 2005; 67(1): 15-25.
[http://dx.doi.org/10.1111/j.1399-0004.2004.00376.x] [PMID: 15617542]

[40] She ZY, Yang WX. *SRY* and SoxE genes: How they participate in mammalian sex determination and gonadal development? Semin Cell Dev Biol 2016.
[http://dx.doi.org/10.1016/j.semcdb.2016.07.032] [PMID: 27481580]

[41] Gubbay J, Collignon J, Koopman P, *et al.* A gene mapping to the sex-determining region of the mouse Y chromosome is a member of a novel family of embryonically expressed genes. Nature 1990; 346(6281): 245-50.
[http://dx.doi.org/10.1038/346245a0] [PMID: 2374589]

[42] Koopman P, Gubbay J, Vivian N, Goodfellow P, Lovell-Badge R. Male development of chromosomally female mice transgenic for *SRY*. Nature 1991; 351(6322): 117-21.
[http://dx.doi.org/10.1038/351117a0] [PMID: 2030730]

[43] Sinclair AH, Berta P, Palmer MS, *et al.* A gene from the human sex-determining region encodes a protein with homology to a conserved DNA-binding motif. Nature 1990; 346(6281): 240-4.
[http://dx.doi.org/10.1038/346240a0] [PMID: 1695712]

[44] Bogani D, Siggers P, Brixey R, *et al.* Loss of mitogen-activated protein kinase kinase kinase 4 (MAP3K4) reveals a requirement for MAPK signalling in mouse sex determination. PLoS Biol 2009; 7(9): e1000196.
[http://dx.doi.org/10.1371/journal.pbio.1000196] [PMID: 19753101]

[45] Gierl MS, Gruhn WH, von Seggern A, Maltry N, Niehrs C. GADD45G functions in male sex determination by promoting p38 signaling and*SRY* expression. Dev Cell 2012; 23(5): 1032-42.
[http://dx.doi.org/10.1016/j.devcel.2012.09.014] [PMID: 23102581]

[46] Yang Z, Song L, Huang C. Gadd45 proteins as critical signal transducers linking NF-kappaB to MAPK cascades. Curr Cancer Drug Targets 2009; 9(8): 915-30.
[http://dx.doi.org/10.2174/156800909790192383] [PMID: 20025601]

[47] Warr N, Carre GA, Siggers P, *et al.* Gadd45γ and Map3k4 interactions regulate mouse testis determination via p38 MAPK-mediated control of*SRY* expression. Dev Cell 2012; 23(5): 1020-31.
[http://dx.doi.org/10.1016/j.devcel.2012.09.016] [PMID: 23102580]

[48] Albrecht KH, Eicher EM. Evidence that*SRY* is expressed in pre-Sertoli cells and Sertoli and granulosa cells have a common precursor. Dev Biol 2001; 240(1): 92-107.
[http://dx.doi.org/10.1006/dbio.2001.0438] [PMID: 11784049]

[49] Bullejos M, Koopman P. Spatially dynamic expression of*SRY* in mouse genital ridges. Dev Dyn 2001; 221(2): 201-5.
[http://dx.doi.org/10.1002/dvdy.1134] [PMID: 11376487]

[50] Hacker A, Capel B, Goodfellow P, Lovell-Badge R. Expression of *SRY*, the mouse sex determining gene. Development 1995; 121(6): 1603-14.
[PMID: 7600978]

[51] Jeske YW, Bowles J, Greenfield A, Koopman P. Expression of a linear*SRY* transcript in the mouse genital ridge. Nat Genet 1995; 10(4): 480-2.
[http://dx.doi.org/10.1038/ng0895-480] [PMID: 7670499]

[52] Jakob S, Lovell-Badge R. Sex determination and the control of *SOX9* expression in mammals. FEBS J 2011; 278(7): 1002-9.
[http://dx.doi.org/10.1111/j.1742-4658.2011.08029.x] [PMID: 21281448]

[53] Jo A, Denduluri S, Zhang B, *et al.* The versatile functions of *SOX9* in development, stem cells, and human diseases. Genes Dis 2014; 1(2): 149-61.
[http://dx.doi.org/10.1016/j.gendis.2014.09.004] [PMID: 25685828]

[54] Koopman P. *SRY* and *SOX9* : mammalian testis-determining genes. Cell Mol Life Sci 1999; 55(6-7): 839-56.
[http://dx.doi.org/10.1007/PL00013200] [PMID: 10412367]

[55] Malki S, Nef S, Notarnicola C, *et al.* Prostaglandin D2 induces nuclear import of the sex-determining factor *SOX9via* its cAMP-PKA phosphorylation. EMBO J 2005; 24(10): 1798-809.
[http://dx.doi.org/10.1038/sj.emboj.7600660] [PMID: 15889150]

[56] Moniot B, Declosmenil F, Barrionuevo F, *et al.* The PGD2 pathway, independently of *FGF9* , amplifies *SOX9* activity in Sertoli cells during male sexual differentiation. Development 2009; 136(11): 1813-21.
[http://dx.doi.org/10.1242/dev.032631] [PMID: 19429785]

[57] Soullier S, Jay P, Poulat F, Vanacker JM, Berta P, Laudet V. Diversification pattern of the HMG and SOX family members during evolution. J Mol Evol 1999; 48(5): 517-27.
[http://dx.doi.org/10.1007/PL00006495] [PMID: 10198118]

[58] Schepers GE, Teasdale RD, Koopman P. Twenty pairs of sox: extent, homology, and nomenclature of the mouse and human sox transcription factor gene families. Dev Cell 2002; 3(2): 167-70.
[http://dx.doi.org/10.1016/S1534-5807(02)00223-X] [PMID: 12194848]

[59] Chew LJ, Gallo V. The Yin and Yang of Sox proteins: Activation and repression in development and disease. J Neurosci Res 2009; 87(15): 3277-87.
[http://dx.doi.org/10.1002/jnr.22128] [PMID: 19437544]

[60] Harley VR, Goodfellow PN. The biochemical role of*SRY* in sex determination. Mol Reprod Dev 1994; 39(2): 184-93.
[http://dx.doi.org/10.1002/mrd.1080390211] [PMID: 7826621]

[61] Harley VR, Jackson DI, Hextall PJ, *et al.* DNA binding activity of recombinant*SRY* from normal males and XY females. Science 1992; 255(5043): 453-6.
[http://dx.doi.org/10.1126/science.1734522] [PMID: 1734522]

[62] Mitchell CL, Harley VR. Biochemical defects in eight*SRY* missense mutations causing XY gonadal dysgenesis. Mol Genet Metab 2002; 77(3): 217-25.
[http://dx.doi.org/10.1016/S1096-7192(02)00165-8] [PMID: 12409269]

[63] Harley VR, Layfield S, Mitchell CL, *et al.* Defective importin beta recognition and nuclear import of the sex-determining factor*SRY* are associated with XY sex-reversing mutations. Proc Natl Acad Sci USA 2003; 100(12): 7045-50.
[http://dx.doi.org/10.1073/pnas.1137864100] [PMID: 12764225]

[64] Li B, Zhang W, Chan G, Jancso-Radek A, Liu S, Weiss MA. Human sex reversal due to impaired nuclear localization of *SRY*. A clinical correlation. J Biol Chem 2001; 276(49): 46480-4.
[http://dx.doi.org/10.1074/jbc.C100388200] [PMID: 11641389]

[65] Bishop CE, Whitworth DJ, Qin Y, *et al.* A transgenic insertion upstream of *SOX9* is associated with dominant XX sex reversal in the mouse. Nat Genet 2000; 26(4): 490-4.
[http://dx.doi.org/10.1038/82652] [PMID: 11101852]

[66] Qin Y, Bishop CE. *SOX9* is sufficient for functional testis development producing fertile male mice in the absence of *SRY*. Hum Mol Genet 2005; 14(9): 1221-9.
[http://dx.doi.org/10.1093/hmg/ddi133] [PMID: 15790596]

[67] Vidal VP, Chaboissier MC, de Rooij DG, Schedl A. *SOX9* induces testis development in XX transgenic mice. Nat Genet 2001; 28(3): 216-7.
[http://dx.doi.org/10.1038/90046] [PMID: 11431689]

[68] Huang B, Wang S, Ning Y, Lamb AN, Bartley J. Autosomal XX sex reversal caused by duplication of *SOX9* . Am J Med Genet 1999; 87(4): 349-53.
[http://dx.doi.org/10.1002/(SICI)1096-8628(19991203)87:4<349::AID-AJMG13>3.0.CO;2-N] [PMID: 10588843]

[69] Sekido R, Lovell-Badge R. Genetic control of testis development. Sex Dev 2013; 7(1-3): 21-32.
[http://dx.doi.org/10.1159/000342221] [PMID: 22964823]

[70] Larney C, Bailey TL, Koopman P. Switching on sex: transcriptional regulation of the testis-determining gene *SRY*. Development 2014; 141(11): 2195-205.
[http://dx.doi.org/10.1242/dev.107052] [PMID: 24866114]

[71] Ludbrook LM, Harley VR. Sex determination: a window of DAX1 activity. Trends Endocrinol Metab 2004; 15(3): 116-21.
[http://dx.doi.org/10.1016/j.tem.2004.02.002] [PMID: 15046740]

[72] Parker KL, Schimmer BP, Schedl A. Genes essential for early events in gonadal development. Cell Mol Life Sci 1999; 55(6-7): 831-8.
[http://dx.doi.org/10.1007/s000180050337] [PMID: 10412366]

[73] Luo X, Ikeda Y, Parker KL. A cell-specific nuclear receptor is essential for adrenal and gonadal development and sexual differentiation. Cell 1994; 77(4): 481-90.
[http://dx.doi.org/10.1016/0092-8674(94)90211-9] [PMID: 8187173]

[74] Köhler B, Achermann JC. Updatesteroidogenic factor 1 (SF-1, *NR5A1*). Minerva Endocrinol 2010; 35(2): 73-86.
[PMID: 20595937]

[75] Arango NA, Lovell-Badge R, Behringer RR. Targeted mutagenesis of the endogenous mouse Mis gene promoter: *in vivo* definition of genetic pathways of vertebrate sexual development. Cell 1999; 99(4): 409-19.
[http://dx.doi.org/10.1016/S0092-8674(00)81527-5] [PMID: 10571183]

[76] Ramkissoon Y, Goodfellow P. Early steps in mammalian sex determination. Curr Opin Genet Dev 1996; 6(3): 316-21.
[http://dx.doi.org/10.1016/S0959-437X(96)80008-6] [PMID: 8791510]

[77] Lucas-Herald AK, Bashamboo A. Gonadal development. Endocr Dev 2014; 27: 1-16.
[http://dx.doi.org/10.1159/000363608] [PMID: 25247640]

[78] Tanaka SS, Nishinakamura R. Regulation of male sex determination: genital ridge formation and*SRY* activation in mice. Cell Mol Life Sci 2014; 71(24): 4781-802.
[http://dx.doi.org/10.1007/s00018-014-1703-3] [PMID: 25139092]

[79] Nistal M, Paniagua R, González-Peramato P, Reyes-Múgica M. Perspectives in pediatric pathology, chapter 1. Normal development of testicular structures: from the bipotential gonad to the fetal testis. Pediatr Dev Pathol 2015; 18(2): 88-102.
[http://dx.doi.org/10.2350/12-04-1184-PB.1] [PMID: 25119266]

[80] Pietilä I, Vainio SJ. Kidney development: an overview. Nephron, Exp Nephrol 2014; 126(2): 40.
[http://dx.doi.org/10.1159/000360659] [PMID: 24854638]

[81] Joseph A, Yao H, Hinton BT. Development and morphogenesis of the Wolffian/epididymal duct, more twists and turns. Dev Biol 2009; 325(1): 6-14.
[http://dx.doi.org/10.1016/j.ydbio.2008.10.012] [PMID: 18992735]

[82] Saxén L, Sariola H. Early organogenesis of the kidney. Pediatr Nephrol 1987; 1(3): 385-92.
[http://dx.doi.org/10.1007/BF00849241] [PMID: 3153305]

[83] Wilhelm D, Palmer S, Koopman P. Sex determination and gonadal development in mammals. Physiol Rev 2007; 87(1): 1-28.
[http://dx.doi.org/10.1152/physrev.00009.2006] [PMID: 17237341]

[84] Timpl R, Rohde H, Robey PG, Rennard SI, Foidart JM, Martin GR. Laminina glycoprotein from basement membranes. J Biol Chem 1979; 254(19): 9933-7.
[PMID: 114518]

[85] Zhou L, Charkraborty T, Yu X, *et al.* R-spondins are involved in the ovarian differentiation in a teleost, medaka (Oryzias latipes). BMC Dev Biol 2012; 12: 36.
[http://dx.doi.org/10.1186/1471-213X-12-36] [PMID: 23217106]

[86] Barrionuevo F, Bagheri-Fam S, Klattig J, *et al.* Homozygous inactivation of *SOX9* causes complete XY sex reversal in mice. Biol Reprod 2006; 74(1): 195-201.
[http://dx.doi.org/10.1095/biolreprod.105.045930] [PMID: 16207837]

[87] Barrionuevo F, Georg I, Scherthan H, *et al.* Testis cord differentiation after the sex determination stage is independent of *SOX9* but fails in the combined absence of *SOX9* and Sox8. Dev Biol 2009; 327(2): 301-12.
[http://dx.doi.org/10.1016/j.ydbio.2008.12.011] [PMID: 19124014]

[88] Jameson SA, Lin YT, Capel B. Testis development requires the repression of Wnt4 by Fgf signaling. Dev Biol 2012; 370(1): 24-32.
[http://dx.doi.org/10.1016/j.ydbio.2012.06.009] [PMID: 22705479]

[89] She ZY, Yang WX. Molecular mechanisms involved in mammalian primary sex determination. J Mol Endocrinol 2014; 53(1): R21-37.
[http://dx.doi.org/10.1530/JME-14-0018] [PMID: 24928207]

[90] Karl J, Capel B. Sertoli cells of the mouse testis originate from the coelomic epithelium. Dev Biol 1998; 203(2): 323-33.
[http://dx.doi.org/10.1006/dbio.1998.9068] [PMID: 9808783]

[91] Wilhelm D, Martinson F, Bradford S, *et al.* Sertoli cell differentiation is induced both cell-autonomously and through prostaglandin signaling during mammalian sex determination. Dev Biol 2005; 287(1): 111-24.
[http://dx.doi.org/10.1016/j.ydbio.2005.08.039] [PMID: 16185683]

[92] Kim Y, Kobayashi A, Sekido R, *et al.* *FGF9* and Wnt4 act as antagonistic signals to regulate mammalian sex determination. PLoS Biol 2006; 4(6): e187.
[http://dx.doi.org/10.1371/journal.pbio.0040187] [PMID: 16700629]

[93] Cool J, DeFalco T, Capel B. Testis formation in the fetal mouse: dynamic and complex de novo tubulogenesis. Wiley Interdiscip Rev Dev Biol 2012; 1(6): 847-59.
[http://dx.doi.org/10.1002/wdev.62] [PMID: 23799626]

[94] Griswold MD, Hogarth CA, Bowles J, Koopman P. Initiating meiosis: the case for retinoic acid. Biol Reprod 2012; 86(2): 35.
[http://dx.doi.org/10.1095/biolreprod.111.096610] [PMID: 22075477]

[95] Busada JT, Kaye EP, Renegar RH, Geyer CB. Retinoic acid induces multiple hallmarks of the prospermatogonia-to-spermatogonia transition in the neonatal mouse. Biol Reprod 2014; 90(3): 64.
[http://dx.doi.org/10.1095/biolreprod.113.114645] [PMID: 24478393]

[96] Harikae K, Miura K, Kanai Y. Early gonadogenesis in mammals: significance of long and narrow gonadal structure. Dev Dyn 2013; 242(4): 330-8.
[http://dx.doi.org/10.1002/dvdy.23872] [PMID: 22987627]

[97] Hiramatsu R, Harikae K, Tsunekawa N, Kurohmaru M, Matsuo I, Kanai Y. FGF signaling directs a center-to-pole expansion of tubulogenesis in mouse testis differentiation. Development 2010; 137(2): 303-12.
[http://dx.doi.org/10.1242/dev.040519] [PMID: 20040496]

[98] Buehr M, Gu S, McLaren A. Mesonephric contribution to testis differentiation in the fetal mouse. Development 1993; 117(1): 273-81.
[PMID: 8223251]

[99] Combes AN, Wilhelm D, Davidson T, *et al.* Endothelial cell migration directs testis cord formation. Dev Biol 2009; 326(1): 112-20.
[http://dx.doi.org/10.1016/j.ydbio.2008.10.040] [PMID: 19041858]

[100] Cool J, DeFalco TJ, Capel B. Vascular-mesenchymal cross-talk through Vegf and Pdgf drives organ patterning. Proc Natl Acad Sci USA 2011; 108(1): 167-72.
[http://dx.doi.org/10.1073/pnas.1010299108] [PMID: 21173261]

[101] Buehr M, McLaren A, Bartley A, Darling S. Proliferation and migration of primordial germ cells in We/We mouse embryos. Dev Dyn 1993; 198(3): 182-9.
[http://dx.doi.org/10.1002/aja.1001980304] [PMID: 8136523]

[102] Martineau J, Nordqvist K, Tilmann C, Lovell-Badge R, Capel B. Male-specific cell migration into the developing gonad. Curr Biol 1997; 7(12): 958-68. [http://dx.doi.org/10.1016/S0960-9822(06)00415-5] [PMID: 9382843]

[103] Bendel-Stenzel MR, Gomperts M, Anderson R, Heasman J, Wylie C. The role of cadherins during primordial germ cell migration and early gonad formation in the mouse. Mech Dev 2000; 91(1-2): 143-52. [http://dx.doi.org/10.1016/S0925-4773(99)00287-7] [PMID: 10704839]

[104] Oatley JM, Brinster RL. The germline stem cell niche unit in mammalian testes. Physiol Rev 2012; 92(2): 577-95. [http://dx.doi.org/10.1152/physrev.00025.2011] [PMID: 22535892]

[105] Yoshida S. Elucidating the identity and behavior of spermatogenic stem cells in the mouse testis. Reproduction 2012; 144(3): 293-302. [http://dx.doi.org/10.1530/REP-11-0320] [PMID: 22733803]

[106] Shaw G, Renfree MB. Wolffian duct development. Sex Dev 2014; 8(5): 273-80. [http://dx.doi.org/10.1159/000363432] [PMID: 24942390]

[107] Murashima A, Xu B, Hinton BT. Understanding normal and abnormal development of the Wolffian/epididymal duct by using transgenic mice. Asian J Androl 2015; 17(5): 749-55. [http://dx.doi.org/10.4103/1008-682X.155540] [PMID: 26112482]

[108] Capel B. The battle of the sexes. Mech Dev 2000; 92(1): 89-103. [http://dx.doi.org/10.1016/S0925-4773(99)00327-5] [PMID: 10704890]

[109] Bullejos M, Koopman P. Delayed*SRY* and *SOX9* expression in developing mouse gonads underlies B6-Y(DOM) sex reversal. Dev Biol 2005; 278(2): 473-81. [http://dx.doi.org/10.1016/j.ydbio.2004.11.030] [PMID: 15680364]

[110] Hiramatsu R, Matoba S, Kanai-Azuma M, *et al.* A critical time window of*SRY* action in gonadal sex determination in mice. Development 2009; 136(1): 129-38. [http://dx.doi.org/10.1242/dev.029587] [PMID: 19036799]

[111] Ostrer H, Huang HY, Masch RJ, Shapiro E. A cellular study of human testis development. Sex Dev 2007; 1(5): 286-92. [http://dx.doi.org/10.1159/000108930] [PMID: 18391539]

[112] Willerton L, Smith RA, Russell D, Mackay S. Effects of *FGF9* on embryonic Sertoli cell proliferation and testicular cord formation in the mouse. Int J Dev Biol 2004; 48(7): 637-43. [http://dx.doi.org/10.1387/ijdb.031778lw] [PMID: 15470636]

[113] Schmahl J, Capel B. Cell proliferation is necessary for the determination of male fate in the gonad. Dev Biol 2003; 258(2): 264-76. [http://dx.doi.org/10.1016/S0012-1606(03)00122-2] [PMID: 12798287]

[114] Schmahl J, Kim Y, Colvin JS, Ornitz DM, Capel B. *FGF9* induces proliferation and nuclear localization of FGFR2 in Sertoli precursors during male sex determination. Development 2004; 131(15): 3627-36. [http://dx.doi.org/10.1242/dev.01239] [PMID: 15229180]

[115] Bagheri-Fam S, Sim H, Bernard P, *et al.* Loss of Fgfr2 leads to partial XY sex reversal. Dev Biol 2008; 314(1): 71-83. [http://dx.doi.org/10.1016/j.ydbio.2007.11.010] [PMID: 18155190]

[116] Nachtigal MW, Hirokawa Y, Enyeart-VanHouten DL, Flanagan JN, Hammer GD, Ingraham HA. Wilms tumor 1 and Dax-1 modulate the orphan nuclear receptor SF-1 in sex-specific gene expression. Cell 1998; 93(3): 445-54. [http://dx.doi.org/10.1016/S0092-8674(00)81172-1] [PMID: 9590178]

[117] Wilhelm D, Hiramatsu R, Mizusaki H, *et al.* *SOX9* regulates prostaglandin D synthase gene transcription *in vivo* to ensure testis development. J Biol Chem 2007; 282(14): 10553-60. [http://dx.doi.org/10.1074/jbc.M609578200] [PMID: 17277314]

[118] Rato L, Meneses MJ, Silva BM, Sousa M, Alves MG, Oliveira PF. New insights on hormones and factors that modulate Sertoli cell metabolism. Histol Histopathol 2016; 31(5): 499-513. [http://dx.doi.org/10.14670/HH-11-717] [PMID: 26711246]

[119] Voutilainen R. Differentiation of the fetal gonad. Horm Res 1992; 38 (Suppl. 2): 66-71. [http://dx.doi.org/10.1159/000182601] [PMID: 1292985]

[120] Orth JM, Gunsalus GL, Lamperti AA. Evidence from Sertoli cell-depleted rats indicates that spermatid number in adults depends on numbers of Sertoli cells produced during perinatal development. Endocrinology 1988; 122(3): 787-94. [http://dx.doi.org/10.1210/endo-122-3-787] [PMID: 3125042]

[121] Capel B, Albrecht KH, Washburn LL, Eicher EM. Migration of mesonephric cells into the mammalian gonad depends on *SRY*. Mech Dev 1999; 84(1-2): 127-31. [http://dx.doi.org/10.1016/S0925-4773(99)00047-7] [PMID: 10473126]

[122] Schmahl J, Eicher EM, Washburn LL, Capel B. *SRY* induces cell proliferation in the mouse gonad. Development 2000; 127(1): 65-73. [PMID: 10654601]

[123] Ying Y, Zhao GQ. Cooperation of endoderm-derived BMP2 and extraembryonic ectoderm-derived BMP4 in primordial germ cell generation in the mouse. Dev Biol 2001; 232(2): 484-92. [http://dx.doi.org/10.1006/dbio.2001.0173] [PMID: 11401407]

[124] Magnúsdóttir E, Dietmann S, Murakami K, *et al.* A tripartite transcription factor network regulates primordial germ cell specification in mice. Nat Cell Biol 2013; 15(8): 905-15. [http://dx.doi.org/10.1038/ncb2798] [PMID: 23851488]

[125] Dolci S, Campolo F, De Felici M. Gonadal development and germ cell tumors in mouse and humans. Semin Cell Dev Biol 2015; 45: 114-23. [http://dx.doi.org/10.1016/j.semcdb.2015.10.002] [PMID: 26456276]

[126] Fujimoto T, Miyayama Y, Fuyuta M. The origin, migration and fine morphology of human primordial germ cells. Anat Rec 1977; 188(3): 315-30. [http://dx.doi.org/10.1002/ar.1091880305] [PMID: 900520]

[127] Witschi E. Migration of the germ cells of human embryos from the yolk sac to the primitive gonadal folds. Contrib Embryol 1948; 67-80.

[128] Anderson R, Copeland TK, Schöler H, Heasman J, Wylie C. The onset of germ cell migration in the mouse embryo. Mech Dev 2000; 91(1-2): 61-8. [http://dx.doi.org/10.1016/S0925-4773(99)00271-3] [PMID: 10704831]

[129] Hara K, Kanai-Azuma M, Uemura M, *et al.* Evidence for crucial role of hindgut expansion in directing proper migration of primordial germ cells in mouse early embryogenesis. Dev Biol 2009; 330(2): 427-39. [http://dx.doi.org/10.1016/j.ydbio.2009.04.012] [PMID: 19371732]

[130] Molyneaux KA, Stallock J, Schaible K, Wylie C. Time-lapse analysis of living mouse germ cell migration. Dev Biol 2001; 240(2): 488-98. [http://dx.doi.org/10.1006/dbio.2001.0436] [PMID: 11784078]

[131] García-Castro MI, Anderson R, Heasman J, Wylie C. Interactions between germ cells and extracellular matrix glycoproteins during migration and gonad assembly in the mouse embryo. J Cell Biol 1997; 138(2): 471-80. [http://dx.doi.org/10.1083/jcb.138.2.471] [PMID: 9230086]

[132] Richardson BE, Lehmann R. Mechanisms guiding primordial germ cell migration: strategies from different organisms. Nat Rev Mol Cell Biol 2010; 11(1): 37-49. [http://dx.doi.org/10.1038/nrm2815] [PMID: 20027186]

[133] Donovan PJ, Stott D, Cairns LA, Heasman J, Wylie CC. Migratory and postmigratory mouse primordial germ cells behave differently in culture. Cell 1986; 44(6): 831-8. [http://dx.doi.org/10.1016/0092-8674(86)90005-X] [PMID: 3955652]

[134] Jost A. Recherches sur la differenciation sexuelle de l'embrion de lapin. Arch Anat Microsc Morphol Exp 1947; 36: 151-200.

[135] Jost A. Problems of fetal endocrinology-the gonadal and hypophyseal hormones. Recent Prog Horm Res 1953; 8: 379-418.

[136] Vilain E, McCabe ER. Mammalian sex determination: from gonads to brain. Mol Genet Metab 1998; 65(2): 74-84. [http://dx.doi.org/10.1006/mgme.1998.2749] [PMID: 9787099]

[137] Scott HM, Mason JI, Sharpe RM. Steroidogenesis in the fetal testis and its susceptibility to disruption by exogenous compounds. Endocr Rev 2009; 30(7): 883-925. [http://dx.doi.org/10.1210/er.2009-0016] [PMID: 19887492]

[138] Griswold SL, Behringer RR. Fetal Leydig cell origin and development. Sex Dev 2009; 3(1): 1-15. [http://dx.doi.org/10.1159/000200077] [PMID: 19339813]

[139] Klonisch T, Fowler PA, Hombach-Klonisch S. Molecular and genetic regulation of testis descent and external genitalia development. Dev Biol 2004; 270(1): 1-18. [http://dx.doi.org/10.1016/j.ydbio.2004.02.018] [PMID: 15136137]

[140] Nef S, Shipman T, Parada LF. A molecular basis for estrogen-induced cryptorchidism. Dev Biol 2000; 224(2): 354-61. [http://dx.doi.org/10.1006/dbio.2000.9785] [PMID: 10926772]

[141] Huhtaniemi I, Pelliniemi LJ. Fetal Leydig cells: cellular origin, morphology, life span, and special functional features. Proc Soc Exp Biol Med 1992; 201(2): 125-40. [http://dx.doi.org/10.3181/00379727-201-43493] [PMID: 1409728]

[142] Hatano O, Takakusu A, Nomura M, Morohashi K. Identical origin of adrenal cortex and gonad revealed by expression profiles of Ad4BP/SF-1. Genes Cells 1996; 1(7): 663-71. [http://dx.doi.org/10.1046/j.1365-2443.1996.00254.x] [PMID: 9078392]

[143] Val P, Lefrançois-Martinez A-M, Veyssière G, Martinez A. SF-1 a key player in the development and differentiation of steroidogenic tissues. Nucl Recept 2003; 1(1): 8. [http://dx.doi.org/10.1186/1478-1336-1-8] [PMID: 14594453]

[144] Wen Q, Cheng CY, Liu Y-X. Development, function and fate of fetal Leydig cells. Semin Cell Dev Biol 2016; 59: 89-98. [http://dx.doi.org/10.1016/j.semcdb.2016.03.003] [PMID: 26968934]

[145] DeFalco T, Takahashi S, Capel B. Two distinct origins for Leydig cell progenitors in the fetal testis. Dev Biol 2011; 352(1): 14-26. [http://dx.doi.org/10.1016/j.ydbio.2011.01.011] [PMID: 21255566]

[146] Merchant-Larios H, Moreno-Mendoza N. Mesonephric stromal cells differentiate into Leydig cells in the mouse fetal testis. Exp Cell Res 1998; 244(1): 230-8. [http://dx.doi.org/10.1006/excr.1998.4215] [PMID: 9770365]

[147] Val P, Jeays-Ward K, Swain A. Identification of a novel population of adrenal-like cells in the mammalian testis. Dev Biol 2006; 299(1): 250-6. [http://dx.doi.org/10.1016/j.ydbio.2006.07.030] [PMID: 16949566]

[148] Martin LJ. Cell interactions and genetic regulation that contribute to testicular Leydig cell development and differentiation. Mol Reprod Dev 2016; 83(6): 470-87. [http://dx.doi.org/10.1002/mrd.22648] [PMID: 27079813]

[149] Svechnikov K, Landreh L, Weisser J, *et al.* Origin, development and regulation of human Leydig cells. Horm Res Paediatr 2010; 73(2): 93-101. [http://dx.doi.org/10.1159/000277141] [PMID: 20190545]

[150] Pelliniemi LJ, Niemi M. Fine structure of the human foetal testis. I. The interstitial tissue. Z Zellforsch Mikrosk Anat 1969; 99(4): 507-22. [http://dx.doi.org/10.1007/BF00340942] [PMID: 5355846]

[151] Wainwright EN, Wilhelm D. Chapter Six - The game plan: Cellular and molecular mechanisms of mammalian testis development. In: Peter K, Ed. Curr Top Dev Biol. Academic Press 2010; pp. 231-62.

[152] OShaughnessy PJ, Baker PJ, Heikkila M, Vainio S, McMahon AP. Localization of 17β-hydroxysteroid dehydrogenase/17-ketosteroid reductase isoform expression in the developing mouse testis—Androstenedione is the major androgen secreted by fetal/neonatal Leydig cells. Endocrinology 2000; 141(7): 2631-7. [http://dx.doi.org/10.1210/endo.141.7.7545] [PMID: 28201136]

[153] Shima Y, Miyabayashi K, Haraguchi S, *et al.* Contribution of Leydig and Sertoli cells to testosterone production in mouse fetal testes. Mol Endocrinol 2013; 27(1): 63-73. [http://dx.doi.org/10.1210/me.2012-1256] [PMID: 23125070]

[154] Rabinovici J, Jaffe RB. Development and regulation of growth and differentiated function in human and subhuman primate fetal gonads. Endocr Rev 1990; 11(4): 532-57. [http://dx.doi.org/10.1210/edrv-11-4-532] [PMID: 2292242]

[155] Archambeault DR, Yao HH. Activin A, a product of fetal Leydig cells, is a unique paracrine regulator of Sertoli cell proliferation and fetal testis cord expansion. Proc Natl Acad Sci USA 2010; 107(23): 10526-31. [http://dx.doi.org/10.1073/pnas.1000318107] [PMID: 20498064]

[156] Brennan J, Tilmann C, Capel B. Pdgfr-α mediates testis cord organization and fetal Leydig cell development in the XY gonad. Genes Dev 2003; 17(6): 800-10. [http://dx.doi.org/10.1101/gad.1052503] [PMID: 12651897]

[157] Yao HH, Whoriskey W, Capel B. Desert Hedgehog/Patched 1 signaling specifies fetal Leydig cell fate in testis organogenesis. Genes Dev 2002; 16(11): 1433-40. [http://dx.doi.org/10.1101/gad.981202] [PMID: 12050120]

[158] Wen Q, Liu Y, Gao F. Fate determination of fetal Leydig cells. Front Biol 2011; 6: 12-8. [http://dx.doi.org/10.1007/s11515-011-1100-3]

[159] Rouiller-Fabre V, Carmona S, Merhi RA, Cate R, Habert R, Vigier B. Effect of anti-Mullerian hormone on Sertoli and Leydig cell functions in fetal and immature rats. Endocrinology 1998; 139(3): 1213-20. [http://dx.doi.org/10.1210/endo.139.3.5785] [PMID: 9492056]

[160] Yan W, Kero J, Huhtaniemi I, Toppari J. Stem cell factor functions as a survival factor for mature Leydig cells and a growth factor for precursor Leydig cells after ethylene dimethane sulfonate treatment: implication of a role of the stem cell factor/c-Kit system in Leydig cell development. Dev Biol 2000; 227(1): 169-82. [http://dx.doi.org/10.1006/dbio.2000.9885] [PMID: 11076685]

[161] Bergeron F, Bagu ET, Tremblay JJ. Transcription of platelet-derived growth factor receptor α in Leydig cells involves specificity protein 1 and 3. J Mol Endocrinol 2011; 46(2): 125-38. [http://dx.doi.org/10.1530/JME-10-0145] [PMID: 21289081]

[162] Lejeune H, Skalli M, Chatelain PG, Avallet O, Saez JM. The paracrine role of Sertoli cells on Leydig cell function. Cell Biol Toxicol 1992; 8(3): 73-83.
[http://dx.doi.org/10.1007/BF00130513] [PMID: 1446260]

[163] Rebourcet D, OShaughnessy PJ, Pitetti J-L, *et al.* Sertoli cells control peritubular myoid cell fate and support adult Leydig cell development in the prepubertal testis. Development 2014; 141(10): 2139-49.
[http://dx.doi.org/10.1242/dev.107029] [PMID: 24803659]

[164] Bielinska M, Seehra A, Toppari J, Heikinheimo M, Wilson DB. GATA-4 is required for sex steroidogenic cell development in the fetal mouse. Dev Dyn 2007; 236(1): 203-13.
[http://dx.doi.org/10.1002/dvdy.21004] [PMID: 17096405]

[165] Karpova T, Ravichandiran K, Insisienmay L, Rice D, Agbor V, Heckert LL. Steroidogenic factor 1 differentially regulates fetal and adult leydig cell development in male mice. Biol Reprod 2015; 93(4): 83.
[http://dx.doi.org/10.1095/biolreprod.115.131193] [PMID: 26269506]

[166] Meeks JJ, Crawford SE, Russell TA, Morohashi K, Weiss J, Jameson JL. Dax1 regulates testis cord organization during gonadal differentiation. Development 2003; 130(5): 1029-36.
[http://dx.doi.org/10.1242/dev.00316] [PMID: 12538527]

[167] Tang H, Brennan J, Karl J, Hamada Y, Raetzman L, Capel B. Notch signaling maintains Leydig progenitor cells in the mouse testis. Development 2008; 135(22): 3745-53.
[http://dx.doi.org/10.1242/dev.024786] [PMID: 18927153]

[168] Daems C, Di-Luoffo M, Paradis É, Tremblay JJ. MEF2 cooperates with forskolin/cAMP and *GATA4* to regulate star gene expression in mouse MA-10 leydig cells. Endocrinology 2015; 156(7): 2693-703.
[http://dx.doi.org/10.1210/en.2014-1964] [PMID: 25860031]

[169] Frigeri C, Tsao J, Czerwinski W, Schimmer BP. Impaired steroidogenic factor 1 (*NR5A1*) activity in mutant Y1 mouse adrenocortical tumor cells. Mol Endocrinol 2000; 14(4): 535-44.
[http://dx.doi.org/10.1210/mend.14.4.0440] [PMID: 10770490]

[170] Rouiller-Fabre V, Lecref L, Gautier C, Saez JM, Habert R. Expression and effect of insulin-like growth factor I on rat fetal Leydig cell function and differentiation. Endocrinology 1998; 139: 2926-34.
[http://dx.doi.org/10.1210/endo.139.6.6035] [PMID: 9607803]

[171] Shima Y, Matsuzaki S, Miyabayashi K, *et al.* Fetal Leydig cells persist as an androgen-independent subpopulation in the postnatal testis. Mol Endocrinol 2015; 29(11): 1581-93.
[http://dx.doi.org/10.1210/me.2015-1200] [PMID: 26402718]

[172] Prince FP. Ultrastructural evidence of mature Leydig cells and Leydig cell regression in the neonatal human testis. Anat Rec 1990; 228(4): 405-17.
[http://dx.doi.org/10.1002/ar.1092280406] [PMID: 2178325]

[173] Mendis-Handagama SM, Ariyaratne HB, Teunissen van Manen KR, Haupt RL. Differentiation of adult Leydig cells in the neonatal rat testis is arrested by hypothyroidism. Biol Reprod 1998; 59(2): 351-7.
[http://dx.doi.org/10.1095/biolreprod59.2.351] [PMID: 9687307]

[174] Wen Q, Zheng Q-S, Li X-X, *et al.* Wt1 dictates the fate of fetal and adult Leydig cells during development in the mouse testis. Am J Physiol Endocrinol Metab 2014; 307(12): E1131-43.
[http://dx.doi.org/10.1152/ajpendo.00425.2014] [PMID: 25336526]

[175] Kaftanovskaya EM, Lopez C, Ferguson L, Myhr C, Agoulnik AI. Genetic ablation of androgen receptor signaling in fetal Leydig cell lineage affects Leydig cell functions in adult testis. FASEB J 2015; 29(6): 2327-37.
[http://dx.doi.org/10.1096/fj.14-263632] [PMID: 25713029]

[176] Gautier C, Levacher C, Saez J-M, Habert R. Expression and regulation of transforming growth factor β1 mRNA and protein in rat fetal testis *in vitro*. Biochem Biophys Res Commun 1997; 236(1): 135-9. [http://dx.doi.org/10.1006/bbrc.1997.6914] [PMID: 9223440]

[177] Codesal J, Regadera J, Nistal M, Regadera-Sejas J, Paniagua R. Involution of human fetal Leydig cells. An immunohistochemical, ultrastructural and quantitative study. J Anat 1990; 172: 103-14. [PMID: 2272896]

[178] Prince FP. The triphasic nature of Leydig cell development in humans, and comments on nomenclature. J Endocrinol 2001; 168(2): 213-6. [http://dx.doi.org/10.1677/joe.0.1680213] [PMID: 11182757]

[179] Winter JS, Faiman C, Hobson WC, Prasad AV, Reyes FI. Pituitary-gonadal relations in infancy. I. Patterns of serum gonadotropin concentrations from birth to four years of age in man and chimpanzee. J Clin Endocrinol Metab 1975; 40(4): 545-51. [http://dx.doi.org/10.1210/jcem-40-4-545] [PMID: 1127071]

[180] Andersson A-M, Toppari J, Haavisto A-M, *et al.* Longitudinal reproductive hormone profiles in infants: peak of inhibin B levels in infant boys exceeds levels in adult men. J Clin Endocrinol Metab 1998; 83(2): 675-81. [http://dx.doi.org/10.1210/jcem.83.2.4603] [PMID: 9467591]

[181] Zirkin BR. Where do adult Leydig cells come from? Biol Reprod 2010; 82(6): 1019-20. [http://dx.doi.org/10.1095/biolreprod.110.084111] [PMID: 20237331]

[182] Mendis-Handagama SM, Ariyaratne HB. Differentiation of the adult Leydig cell population in the postnatal testis. Biol Reprod 2001; 65(3): 660-71. [http://dx.doi.org/10.1095/biolreprod65.3.660] [PMID: 11514326]

[183] Benton L, Shan L-X, Hardy MP. Differentiation of adult Leydig cells. J Steroid Biochem Mol Biol 1995; 53(1-6): 61-8. [http://dx.doi.org/10.1016/0960-0760(95)00022-R] [PMID: 7626518]

[184] Chen H, Stanley E, Jin S, Zirkin BR. Stem Leydig cells: from fetal to aged animals. Birth Defects Res C Embryo Today 2010; 90(4): 272-83. [http://dx.doi.org/10.1002/bdrc.20192] [PMID: 21181888]

[185] Chemes H, Cigorraga S, Bergadá C, Schteingart H, Rey R, Pellizzari E. Isolation of human Leydig cell mesenchymal precursors from patients with the androgen insensitivity syndrome: testosterone production and response to human chorionic gonadotropin stimulation in culture. Biol Reprod 1992; 46(5): 793-801. [http://dx.doi.org/10.1095/biolreprod46.5.793] [PMID: 1591335]

[186] Teerds KJ, Rijntjes E, Veldhuizen-Tsoerkan MB, Rommerts FF, de Boer-Brouwer M. The development of rat Leydig cell progenitors *in vitro*: how essential is luteinising hormone? J Endocrinol 2007; 194(3): 579-93. [http://dx.doi.org/10.1677/JOE-06-0084] [PMID: 17761897]

CHAPTER 3

Basic Aspects of Testicular Cells: Physiology and Function

João P. Monteiro*

Department of Microscopy, Laboratory of Cell Biology, Institute of Biomedical Sciences Abel Salazar and Unit for Multidisciplinary Research in Biomedicine, University of Porto, Rua de Jorge Viterbo Ferreira, 4050-313, Porto, Portugal

Abstract: Within the testes there is a considerable histological diversity, reflected in a significant variety of different circumscribed environments and cells. As is always the case regarding structures slowly forged by evolution, this translates into meaningful differences in the physiology and function for each cell type. Leydig cells are essentially known for their steroidogenic potential; Sertoli cells are known for their local support to germ cells, and peritubular myoid cells are rapidly transcending a simple structural role. They are all known to actively determine and contribute to spermatogenesis in some way. Moreover, the physiological interplay between these types of cells is known to functionally impact male fertility. However, the specific physiological mechanisms by which each cell type governs spermatozoa production are not fully accounted for, and pathways underlying the cooperative action of these cells in the process are far from being clarified. Increased knowledge regarding the function and interaction of these cells could potentially lead to important breakthroughs within the contexts of testes disease, infertility and contraception.

Keywords: Blood-testis barrier, Cell differentiation, Energetic metabolism, Hormonal regulation, Leydig cells, Paracrine regulation, Peritubular myoid cells, Sertoli cells, Spermatogenesis, Steroidogenesis.

INTRODUCTION

The continuous production of competent spermatozoa by sexually mature males is a complex, highly regulated multistep process implying an intricate interaction between different cooperating cell types present in the testes. Spermatogenesis is regulated by a large number of endocrine and testicular paracrine/autocrine factors. Classically, the process is perceived as being dependent on interactions between somatic and germ cells, involving the coordinated action of three main

* **Corresponding author João P. Monteiro:** Rua de Jorge Viterbo Ferreira, 4050-313, Porto, Portugal; Tel: +351 220 428 000; E-mail: jpspmonteiro@yahoo.com

Marco G. Alves and Pedro F. Oliveira (Eds.)

cell lineages: supporting cells, steroidogenic cells, and germ cells. Therefore, in the testes, there is a need for a provision of differentiated cells types, and the high rate of cell turnover and differentiation displayed these organs surely is associated with that.

Sertoli cells are viewed as supporting cells in the process of spermatogenesis (they are even called "nurse cells" by some researchers). They are morphological and physiologically very distinct from all other cells present in the testes, and their importance for spermatogenesis ranges from mere physical support, to immunoprotection and nutritional support of developing germ cells. Leydig cells are mostly recognized as being steroidogenic cells. Therefore, they are known to play an important role in the hormonal regulation of the spermatogenic process and, furthermore, in ensuring an adequate definition and sustenance of male secondary sexual characteristics. Peritubular myoid cells have been relatively overlooked regarding their role in spermatogenesis. Other than just a structural role in the establishment of the basement membrane, a more active role in the process has been lately disclosed, involving relevant paracrine function. These three cell types, and their respective importance and involvement in the spermatogenic process, will be the subject of this chapter, and the relative location and organization of each cell type within the testes can be perceived in Fig. (**3.1**). Aspects related to their functional relationships and interactions that are meaningful for competent spermatozoa production will be discussed. Peritubular myoid cells, through the establishment of the basement membrane, preclude direct physical proximity between Leydig and Sertoli cells. However, despite actual mechanical constrictions, these cells were all shown to interact with each other locally, through paracrine mechanisms, and these interaction mechanisms have substantiated many justified studies.

LEYDIG CELLS: STRUCTURE AND FUNCTION

Leydig cells were first characterized in the 1850's by Franz Leydig, from whom they got their name [1]. Leydig cells, located within the interstitial compartment of the testes, are arguably the most relevant cell type involved in endocrine function of the testes, being the main cells responsible for the synthesis and secretion of hormones, namely testosterone in male adults [2]. This important role of Leydig cells implies that the normal function of these cells is crucial for the reproductive activity of males. Leydig cells produce testosterone under the control of luteinizing hormone, which is produced by gonadotropic cells in the anterior pituitary gland [3] and binds to G protein-coupled receptors, activating adenylyl cyclase and therefore increasing cAMP formation [4]. Testosterone was reported to regulate a multiplicity of genes (mostly repressed) in the testes [5].

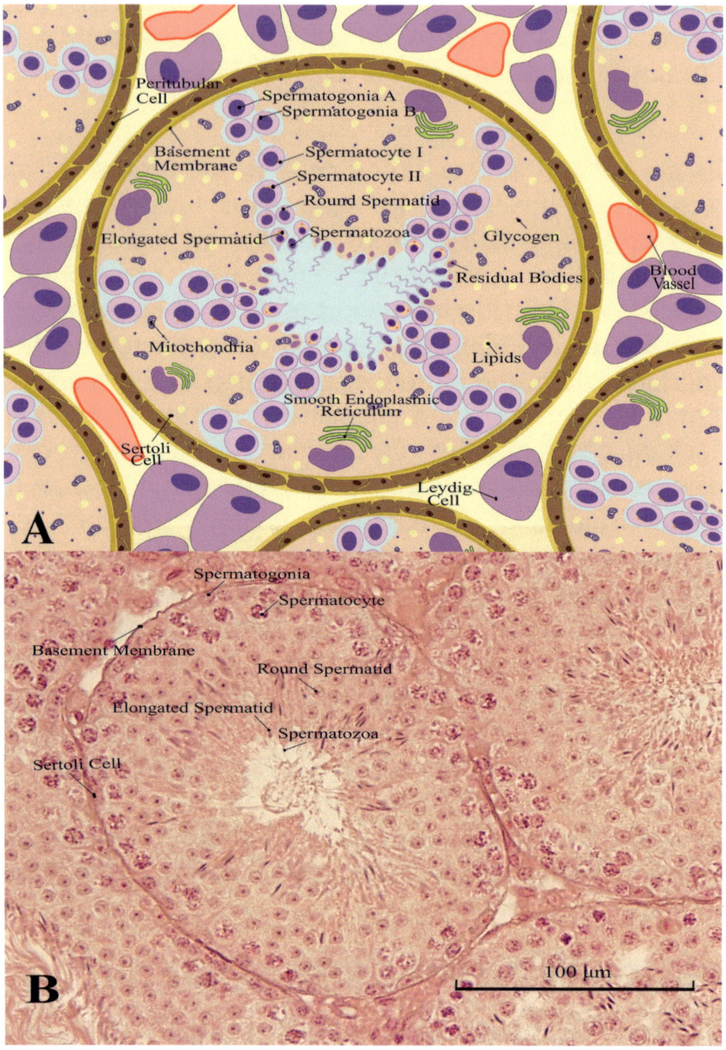

Fig. (3.1). (A) Schematic representation of a transversal cut of mouse (*Mus musculus*) seminiferous tubules, exposing the location of Leydig cells (outside the tubules), peritubular myoid cells (disposed around the tubules, in the basement membrane), and Sertoli cells (inside the basement membrane, in close contact with germ cells, at different maturation stages). **(B)** Actual microscopy image of the transversal cut shown in A), where the same cells type elements are also visible.

Leydig cells have, therefore, an important role in the definition and maintenance of the secondary sexual features defining male characteristics, intermediating testes development, maintenance of spermatogenesis and general male fertility [6, 7]. Some of the processes by which testosterone impacts spermatogenesis include the sustenance of spermatogonia population, preservation of a functional blood-testis barrier (BTB), completion of meiosis by spermatocytes, establishment of adherences between elongated spermatids and Sertoli cells, release of mature spermatozoa, and the establishment of the seminiferous tubule lumen [8].

Two different populations of Leydig cells are present in mammals. Fetal Leydig cells (FLCs) and adult Leydig cells (ALCs) are present respectively in fetal and adult testes [9], but they each have particular functions and are modulated by different regulatory mechanisms [10]. FLCs and ALCs differ in terms of morphology, capability of synthesizing androgen, and response to gonadotropins and growth factors [11 - 13]. In morphological terms, FLCs display round to oval shapes, presenting abundant lipid droplets. They preferentially aggregate in clusters, and are encircled by a basement membrane that is rich in collagen and laminin [14]. In turn, ALCs have larger size, and display a round, dense core. They also aggregate; however, they are not surrounded by a basement membrane. ALCs display higher testosterone synthesis capacity with relation to FLCs [13]. FLCs and ALCs differ in their origin, although the nature of this difference has not been elucidated yet [6, 7, 15]. Leydig cell differentiation and function has been shown to involve several hormones and signaling molecules. In humans, FLC population reaches its maximum by the 14th to 18th week of embryonic development, while ALC number expands during puberty, remaining roughly the same throughout adult life. Besides fetal and adult populations, there is also a neonatal population of Leydig cells, that peaks around 3 months after birth, making Leydig cell proliferation a "triphasic" process [16].

Differentiation of ALCs depends on a diversity of cellular cascades, resulting in the modulation of the expression of steroidogenic enzymes and androgen receptors, and guaranteeing all the specific steroidogenic machinery involved in testosterone biosynthesis [17]. For instance, 5α-androstane3α,17β-diol is the main androgen produced by rat immature Leydig cells [18] while ALCs, which unlike FLCs express 17β-hydroxysteroid dehydrogenase, predominantly produce testosterone [7]. ALCs produce testosterone at about 150 times the production of progenitor Leydig cells, and five times the production of immature Leydig cells [19]. Androgen generation by ALCs is vital for the maintenance of adequate sexual function [20] and spermatogenesis [21]. Besides testosterone, Leydig cells are able to secrete other nonsteroidal factors which can potentially influence Sertoli cell function, namely β-endorphin and α-melanocyte-stimulating hormone [22, 23]. Secretion of insulin-like 3 (INSL3) hormone is another important process mediated by ALCs that critically impacts spermatogenesis [24].

During adulthood, although maintaining high steroidogenic potential, ALCs compose a latent population almost entirely devoid of mitotic and apoptotic activities [25]. Later in life, in the aging male, Leydig cell testosterone production is progressively reduced [26, 27]. This decrease is suggested to be a result of reduced cell function or of alterations in the pulsatility of luteinizing hormone [28]. Some of the mechanisms that may be involved in this reduction of steroidogenic activity by ALCs include the decrease in luteinizing hormone-stimulated cAMP production, and possible defects in the expression and/or activity of cholesterol transport proteins, steroidogenic acute regulatory (STAR) and outer mitochondrial membrane cholesterol-binding translocator protein (TSPO), and of steroidogenic enzymes present in mitochondria or the smooth endoplasmic reticulum [29 - 33]. Moreover, intracellular redox unbalance should also be involved in age-related reduction of testosterone production in Leydig cells [29].

PERITUBULAR CELLS: LOCALIZATION AND RELEVANCE

Peritubular myoid cells are contractile smooth muscle cells that are located externally to the basement membrane, forming a layered compartment between the germinal epithelium and the interstitial compartment [34 - 36], maintaining direct contact with the basal surface of Sertoli cells [37]. From all the cell types present in human testes, these cells are probably the least studied ones, therefore holding a more obscure role in male fertility [34, 35]. The strategic position of peritubular cells within the male reproductive system, guaranteeing relative closeness with other distinctive testicular cell types (Leydig, Sertoli and even germ cells) should be a sign of meaningful interaction involving these cells, concurring for a successful spermatogenesis. In rodents, peritubular myoid cells surrounding the seminiferous tubules form a semi-permeable barrier restricting the entrance of small molecules into the tubular environment [38, 39]. In these animals, the peritubular myoid cell layer consists of a single cell structure composed of cells joined by junctional complexes, while in larger mammals it is composed by multiple layers of thin, long, spindle-shaped cells, gathered by extracellular connective tissue [34, 40, 41]. Cellular phenotypic differences between inner and outer layer cell types have been hinted [40]. The structure surrounding the seminiferous epithelium is denominated basal membrane and is composed by the peritubular cells and an extracellular matrix mainly dependent on their secretions [35, 37, 42, 43]. In humans, fibroblast cells (myofibroblasts) may also be components of the outer layers of this structure [40, 41]. Peritubular myoid cells present morphological features and express both smooth muscle and fibroblast cell-specific markers, namely abundant actin levels (that may be used to identify them), but also structural proteins as desmin/vimentin, calponin, and myosin-heavy-chain [44 - 46]. Other structural proteins produced by peritubular cells and secreted to the extracellular matrix include several collagens (I, III, IV, V, VI, XI, XII, XIV, XV, XVI, XVII), fibronectin, laminin, secreted protein acidic and rich in cysteine (SPARC), proteoglycan decorin and fibrillin-1 [44, 47 - 49].

The view of peritubular cells in the context of male fertility has evolved greatly, and they are not still seen as mere structural components, but also as active paracrine mediators. Peritubular cells are androgen-receptor positive [34], and that may represent a means of feedback communication between these cells and both Sertoli and Leydig cells. In fact, the presence of androgen receptors in peritubular cells was proven to be essential for normal differentiation and function of adult Leydig cells [50], and their importance in a putative regulation of Sertoli cells should be implicit, since in specific androgen receptor-knockout (PTM-ARKO) mice, Sertoli cell function was found to be impaired, and a 86% reduction in germ cells was found [51]. In fact, peritubular cells intimately co-operate with Sertoli cells in the development and function of seminiferous tubule, including the formation of the lamina propria [42, 52 - 54]. Moreover, peritubular cells were suggested to actively participate in the regulation Sertoli cell function, since they release PModS (peritubular factor that Modulates Sertoli cell function) [34, 55 - 59], as well as insulin-like growth factor 1 (IGF1), basic fibroblast growth factor (bFGF), heregulins and transforming growth factor β2 (TGF-β2) [60 - 63]. Also, peritubular cells produce several paracrine factors that impact Leydig cell steroidogenesis [64], as the aforementioned IGF1 [65], and transforming growth factors [53, 66]. In fact, peritubular cell–derived factors were shown to regulate testosterone production by Leydig cells in gonadotropin-deficient conditions [67]. Examples of other signaling factors produced by peritubular cells include interleukin 6 (IL-6), monocyte chemotactic protein 1 (MCP1), glial cell line-derived neurotropic factor (GDNF) and nerve growth factor (NGF) and its precursor pro-NGF [35, 68 - 70].

Moreover, peritubular cells were reported to display pluripotent and steroidogenic capacities and could, therefore, represent a reservoir for Leydig cell regeneration in men [71]. Also, peritubular cells are anatomically close to spermatogonial stem cells and this proximity is thought to have a physiological relevance, since the factors secreted by the first were suggested to contribute to the establishment of a favorable niche for the second [35, 72]. In fact, peritubular cells were reported to secrete chemokines and growth factors essential for spermatogonial stem cells maintenance, along with proteins related to cell adhesion and migration, and also vasculature development [49]. Peritubular cells also secrete pigment epithelium-derived factor (PEDF), which could be important in the establishment and maintenance of the avascular nature of seminiferous tubules [73]. This would be another way for peritubular cells to regulate spermatogonial stem cell niche, which is dependent on testicular microvessels and blood flow [74]. Peritubular myoid cells are also important for the transport of immotile sperm [75]. These cells are accountable for the creation of irregular peristaltic waves, which propel and push forward spermatozoa and testicular fluid towards the excurrent ducts and epididymis [34, 76]. The contractile ability of peritubular cells is regulated by angiotensin through specific receptors present in the membranes of these cells [77]. Endothelin 1 [78, 79], platelet-derived growth factor (PDGF) [80], prostaglandins and neurotransmitters [81, 82], hormones (including sex steroids) [83] and vasopressin [84] are factors that were reported to have the potential to modulate the contraction of peritubular cells. Peritubular myoid cells were thought to originate from the adjacent mesonephros, although their actual progeny remains unknown [85]. However, it was more recently suggested that peritubular cells may originate from intragonadal cells or from the coelomic epithelium by epithelial-to-mesenchymal transformation [86]. These cells initially develop during early fetal testes differentiation, shortly after the formation of primitive testes cords (13th day of embryonic development in mice [87] or 12th week of embryonic development in humans [88]). Peritubular myoid cells proliferate extensively after birth [89]. Expression of the characteristic smooth muscle protein actin, takes place around puberty in peritubular cells [90]. Peritubular cell differentiation is thought to exponentially increase following androgen production taking place at the beginning of puberty, and androgens should definitely play a critical role in the process [91, 92]. Besides the crucial role in spermatogenesis classically linked to an action on Sertoli cells, androgen stimulation of the peritubular myoid cells also proved to be essential for normal germ cells development [51]. The events elicited by androgens on peritubular cells remain, however, obscure [93]. Also follicle stimulating hormone (FSH) is thought to play a relevant role in peritubular cell differentiation [90]. Estrogens also seem to regulate peritubular myoid cells. This regulation is thought to be mediated by G protein-coupled estrogen receptor (GPER), and the importance of these receptors is highlighted by the fact that their expression is lost in cases of idiopathic infertility [94]. Tumor necrosis factor-α (TNF-α) is also an important regulator of peritubular cell function [68]. Peritubular myoid cells possess high cellular plasticity that may be reflected in changes in contractile and secretory properties [35]. In infertile men, typical phenotypic changes in peritubular cells, namely hypertrophy, decreased markers for contractility and accumulation of components of the extracellular matrix, were reported to occur [95 - 98]. This contractility restrictions may be a disregarded aspect concurring to male infertility [35], although it remains to be clarified whether these changes in peritubular cells are a cause or just a result of primary events related to the onset of subfertility or infertility [48]. Although the basement membrane was suggested to represent a physical barrier preventing carcinoma cells to breach the interior of the seminiferous tubules [99], peritubular cells were reported to be sources of several pro-invasive factors mediating testicular germ cell tumor progression (namely MCP-1, PDGF, IL-6, NGF and IGF) [100]. Therefore, peritubular cells were suggested to represent potential targets within testicular germ cell tumor therapies [100].

SERTOLI CELLS AND THE NUTRITIONAL/PHYSICAL SUPPORT OF SPERMATOGENESIS

Sertoli cells are unique polarized epithelial cells that are the main structural element of the seminiferous epithelium. Pivotal structural and physiological roles have been disclosed for these cells in the male reproductive function. These cells, originally described by Enrico Sertoli in the 19th century [101], only represent 3% of the population of cells within the adult testes [102] and evidence of their critical involvement in competent male fertility is piling up to this day. The use of human Sertoli cell in vitro cultures in reproductive-oriented studies has proven to be convenient since they may be long-term maintained and display satisfactory proliferation rates [103]. Moreover, they have been suggested to represent a reliable model to address BTB function [104, 105]. In addition, Sertoli cells have also been suggested as an innovative cell source for regenerative medicine. In fact, Sertoli cells derived from mesoderm may be converted into multipotent neural stem cells [106, 107], opening the way for possible applications in cell-based therapies and tissue engineering.

Sertoli cells assure a number of important functions with pivotal importance to male fertility. Those include the nourishment of developing germ cells, the establishment of the blood-testis barrier, the integration of hormonal signals, the secretion of factors and hormones essential for spermatogenesis, the modulation of the apoptosis in germ cells, the phagocytosis of apoptotic spermatogenic cells and the production and the control of the composition of the seminiferous tubular fluid [108, 109].

Sertoli cells are responsible for the compartmentalization of the seminiferous epithelium, since they are the responsible for the definition of the BTB, also known as Sertoli cell barrier, which physically separates the seminiferous epithelium into basal and apical compartments. This structure is decisive for the physical and physiological support of the proliferation and differentiation of germ cells into mature spermatids, by providing a suitable environment for spermatogenesis and for propitiating the establishment of a localized immune-privileged environment [110]. The BTB is responsible for excluding many molecules present in the interstitial fluids from permeating into the tubular lumen [111]. It allows the setting of a protected environment for the majority of the auto-antigenic germ cells, since it restricts the access by the immune system to these cells, which express singular cell surface and intracellular proteins liable of being targeted as foreign antigens [112]. Furthermore, Sertoli cells express several immunoregulatory factors able to modulate the activity of testes immune cells, guaranteeing a local tolerant environment for those germ cells not sequestered inside the BTB [112].

Adjacent Sertoli cells are interjoined by tight junctions, basal ectoplasmic specializations, basal tubulobulbar complexes, desmosome-like junctions and gap junctions, established alongside in the seminiferous epithelium [113]. These tight associations result in the establishment of a barrier that successfully prevents molecular movement (especially by large molecules) from the interstitial space to the lumen of the seminiferous tubules [38]. Occludin and claudins have been suggested to play a pivotal role in the function and dynamics of established Sertoli cells tight junctions [114 - 116]. The composition of the BTB is dynamic and subject of restructuration at specific stages of the spermatogenic cycle [117].

Morphologically, Sertoli cells are polygonal, with irregularly shaped nuclei and present filamentous processes of variable length [107]. In their basal side, Sertoli cells are in contact with the basement membrane, which plays an important role in the maintenance of the seminiferous tubules structural integrity [118]. Longitudinally, Sertoli cells acquire a columnar shape that extends towards the lumen of the tubules, and are in close contact with the surface of germ cells [119] in a very meaningful physiological functional proximity, as will be discussed later. Sertoli cells are able to protrude their cytoplasm, encasing germ cells in a plastic, dynamic 3-dimensional amoeboid structure, which ensures the support to each germ cell [120, 121]. The structural interplay between Sertoli and germ cells takes place through several types of ectoplasmic specializations [122 - 126], contributing to their structural and physiological entanglement. The physical support of germ cells by Sertoli cells is achieved through deposits of extracellular matrix components (like collagen and laminin), contributing to these specialized junctions. These structures exhibit very well organized cytoskeleton interconnections, established between both cells [127]. Desmosome-gap junctions are also present in the interface between Sertoli and germ cells, particularly in the case of spermatocytes [128].

Besides their function as structural elements in the seminiferous epithelium, providing the physical support needed for the normal development of spermatogenesis, fully differentiated Sertoli cells hold more subtle yet important roles in the process. In fact, there is significant evidence compiled over time highlighting the pivotal role of Sertoli cells in the production of competent spermatozoa. Notably, the presence of germ cells in testes demands the presence of Sertoli cells [129]. Moreover, efficient Sertoli cell function is vital for the proliferation/maturation of germ cells, and important reproductive hormones essential for spermatogenesis in higher vertebrates (FSH and testosterone) were found to exert their action on Sertoli cells rather than directly on germ cells [129]. The production of competent spermatozoa is a complex multistep process and Sertoli cells are essential in the regulation/completion of nearly every step of the way. In fact, Sertoli cells provide the nutritional support male germ cells need, through the production and release of regulatory factors and by regulating the flow of nutrients, therefore positively defining their development. In this case, each Sertoli cell is supposed to support up to 30 to 50 germ cells at different stages of development [130]. Taking into account this nourishing action towards germ cells, any problem in the maturation or function of Sertoli cells will surely constrain the capacity to support germ cell development, and therefore the spermatogenic process as a whole. Other than the support of germ cells, Sertoli cells are also responsible for the phagocytosis of residual bodies and degenerating germ cells [109].

The conventional view regarding Sertoli cells was that they were terminally differentiated and confined to a defined number by the end of puberty. However, this notion has already been questioned [131], as it was demonstrated in hamster that the adult population Sertoli cell may be in fact regulated by hormones (namely gonadotropins and FSH) [132]. Moreover, there are studies demonstrating the ability of Sertoli cells from adult animals, namely mice and humans [133, 134], to divide in culture under specific experimental conditions. Nevertheless, the dogma stating that Sertoli cell number is defined in the prepubertal period persists, given the specificities and scarcity of the defying studies. Sertoli cells are the first to differentiate in the undifferentiated fetal gonad [135]. They differentiate under the regulation of transcription factors SRY and SOX9, but recent research has put the spotlight on the *Sox9* gene as the main determinant of the differentiation of these cells [6]. Sertoli cells act as organizing centers to form the testes cords (future seminiferous tubules), which is a crucial event in testes differentiation, ensuring the sequestration of germ cells [136]. Inhibitors of neurotrophic tyrosine kinase receptors (NTRKs), expressed by pre-Sertoli cells, may be involved in testes cord formation [137 - 140], and fibroblast growth factor 9 (FGF9), also secreted by these cells, should also play a role [141]. Sertoli cell differentiation will then also have an impact the differentiation and function of other somatic cells of the testes [142].

Sertoli cells display a significant proliferative ability during both fetal and neonatal life. These stages and the peripubertal period are the only phases where Sertoli cells are known to proliferate in all species [143]. There are some elicitors presumably involved in the proliferation of Sertoli cells, namely intratesticular factors and pituitary hormones, such as FSH (a mitogenic factor for neonatal Sertoli cells) [144]. The proliferative activity of Sertoli cells may also be mediated or influenced by estrogens, since their levels are particularly significant in these stages [145]. During puberty, Sertoli cells undergo radical changes [142] and mature and immature Sertoli cells greatly differ in terms of both morphology and biochemistry [146] (this topic will be discussed in chapter 6). Only when in their mature form will Sertoli cells start to define the BTB [147]. Proliferative stages, which define the number of Sertoli cells in adult stages, are thought to determine both testes size, sperm output and the number of germ cells in the adult testes [129, 142, 148]. During puberty the proliferative activity of Sertoli cells declines. At this point, Sertoli cells become elongated, with a large irregular and tripartite nucleolus, displaying abundant smooth and rough endoplasmic reticulum [149, 150].

Ever since fetal life, Sertoli cells are known to influence testes development, therefore actively determining male phenotype. These cells play a central role as drivers of the signaling machinery of testes development [6]. This undeniable importance of Sertoli cells in testes development is highlighted by a number of supporting evidence. These include the fact that they were shown to be critical for maintaining the differentiated phenotype of peritubular myoid cells in prepubertal life, for ensuring the maintenance of ALC progenitor population in the postnatal testes, and for guaranteeing normal ALC numbers [151]. Moreover, the role of Sertoli cells in germ cell differentiation and survival is highlighted by the way through which their secretions, namely growth factors and hormones, regulate and determine the whole process [152]. Glial cell line-derived neurotrophic factor (GDNF), bone morphogenetic proteins (BMPs), stem cell factor (SCF) and retinoic acid [107, 153], have been specifically linked to the differentiation and survival of germ cells. In fact, a number of several other molecules produced by Sertoli cells influence germline development, including activin [154], androgen binding protein (ABP) [155], transferrin [156], glycoproteins [157], sulphoproteins [158] and PDGF and estrogen, which with TGF-β, were implicated in postnatal germ cell survival [159 - 161].

Regarding glycoproteins, Sertoli cell secretions include them in quantities that may account for up to 15% of total proteins produced by these cells [127]. Important proteins released by Sertoli cells have been thoroughly listed by Griswold and McLean [162], and information about their physiology allowed to divide them into groups. A first category includes transport and bioprotective glycoproteins abundantly secreted, and metal ion transport glycoproteins such as transferrin and ceruloplasmin. A second group includes various proteases and proteases inhibitors, essential for tissue remodeling events taking place during the movement of spermatocytes through the BTB and spermiation. A third category would include glycoproteins involved in the formation of the basement membrane between Sertoli peritubular cells. A final class includes low abundance regulatory proteins that act as growth factors, paracrine or endocrine factors [129, 162], which are important for germ cell development and survival. Sertoli cells were also reported to release bioactive peptides, like prodynorphin, myoinositol [163] and nutrients or metabolic intermediates [129, 162]. In fact, the metabolic cooperation between Sertoli and germ cells involves the transfer of metabolic products that may include amino acids, carbohydrates, lipids, vitamins, and metal ions [127], and this contribution is vital for germ cells to guarantee physiologically adequate levels of these compounds.

Sertoli Cell Metabolism

Unlike what takes place in the early stages of development, when germ cells use primarily glucose as energy source, spermatids display an unusual dependence on lactate, probably related with a lower glycolytic potential [164]. This important change in the type of substrate required for their energy metabolism implies a pronounced metabolic and enzyme machinery alterations, although spermatids keep containing all the enzymes of the glycolytic pathway [165]. However, mature spermatozoa recover the glycolytic activity, metabolizing fructose but also the glucose available in the luminal fluid [164].

Sertoli cells are able to metabolize different substrates (such as fatty acids and ketone bodies), although they preferentially and actively metabolize glucose [166]. Upon cell entry, glucose undergoes a series of multi-step reaction sequence in which the first rate-limiting step is the irreversible conversion of fructose-phosphate to fructose-1,6-bisphosphate, which is catalyzed by phospho-fructokinase (PFK) [167]. The activity of this enzyme represents a crucial regulatory point of Sertoli cell metabolism [168]. Pyruvate, the end-product of the glycolytic process, may follow three main destinies: it may be converted in alanine (by alanine aminotransferase), it may be included in the Krebs cycle, or it can be interconverted into lactate (by lactate dehydrogenase). The later path was shown to be the most prevalent in Sertoli cells [169]. Robinson and Fritz were the first to suggest the metabolic preferences of Sertoli cells, reporting that only a small fraction of the pyruvate produced by glycolysis would be used in the Krebs cycle, being preferentially converted to lactate. It was later specified that only 25% of the pyruvate produced from glucose metabolism would be oxidized in the Krebs cycle [170]. It is true that both glucose and lactate are present in the adluminal compartment, since Sertoli cells release both those substrates from specific membrane transporters [171, 172], but lactate was in fact shown to be metabolically crucial to developing germ cell fate [171, 173, 174].

The importance of lactate supplementation from Sertoli cells to germ cells has been documented for a long time [175 - 177]. For instance, it was shown that lactate (but not glucose) increased respiration parameters and protein and RNA synthesis in isolated spermatocytes and spermatids [175]. Moreover, lactate was also reported to play an important role in protein synthesis in germ cells [178, 179]. An anti-apoptotic action was also proposed for lactate on germ cells (mostly in spermatocytes and spermatids) [174]. Hence, even in conditions where extracellular glucose levels are scarce, Sertoli cells seem to be able to optimize glucose uptake in order to sustain lactate production [180].

Carbohydrate metabolism in Sertoli cells involves a number of transporters and enzymes which are susceptible of internal (or external) control. Mechanisms regulating lactate secretion by Sertoli cells include the transport of glucose through the plasma membrane, which is mediated by GLUTs, the interconversion between pyruvate and lactate, performed by lactate dehydrogenase, and the actual release of lactate, which depends on the action of transporters from the monocarboxylate transporter family (MCTs) [166]. In Sertoli cells, the rate-limiting step of this process of lactate production and export is thought to be the facilitated diffusion of glucose, performed by GLUTs [181]. Several GLUT isoforms (namely GLUT1, GLUT2 and GLUT3) have been identified in the plasma membrane of Sertoli cells [181 - 184], while GLUT8 expression is debatable with reports testifying its presence in prepubertal testes [182], while others claim that it is limited to spermatids and spermatozoa in the testes [185]. GLUT1 and GLUT3 have been suggested to be especially important in glucose transport at this level, playing a synergistic role in glucose uptake to assure lactate production [181, 186]. As for lactate dehydrogenase, it determines the balance of the interconversion between pyruvate and lactate, which in the case of Sertoli cells, should favor the production of the later. Finally, lactate supplementation to germ cells depends on the activity of MCTs, which assure the flow of the lactate produced by Sertoli cells to germ cells. The SLC16A family of MCTs comprises 14 members, of which only MCTs 1–4 perform lactate transport [187]. Specifically MCT1 and MCT4 were reported to be present in Sertoli cells [188]. MCT1 transporters have a higher affinity for lactate [189] and should also be important for the import of lactate by germ cells, which possess them [190]. MTC4 has a lower affinity for lactate and is mostly a lactate exporter [188, 191], thought to be a decisive player in Sertoli cell physiology [172, 186, 192, 193]. Therefore, MCT4 should be responsible for lactate export from Sertoli cells, while MCT1 (and also MCT2) should facilitate lactate import to germ cells [194].

Sertoli cell metabolism and, more particularly, lactate production are thought to be under the control of FSH [195], epidermal growth factor (EGF) [196], insulin and IGF1 [197], paracrine factor P-Mod-S [198], tri-iodothyronine [199], bFGF [200], cytokines (TNF, and interleukin-1: IL-1) [173], arachidonic acid [201], carnitine [202] and sex steroid hormones [192, 203]. Moreover, Sertoli cells should be able to adjust their metabolism, ensuring an adequate lactate concentration in the extracellular microenvironment surrounding germ cells, even in conditions when glucose levels are scarce [180]. Sertoli cells supposedly change their metabolism profile by activating specific signal transduction pathways, like the one involving AMP-activated protein kinase (AMPK), which is a key mediator of energy homeostasis in the cell [204]. A decrease in glucose medium levels was shown to promote activation of AMPK, increase of glucose uptake, and an increase in GLUT1 and a decrease in GLUT3 expression levels [180]. Adenosine may be a messenger from germ cells, resulting in activation of AMPK, promoting both lactate production and junctional integrity, therefore guaranteeing optimal microenvironment conditions for spermatogenesis [205]. In glucose-deprived conditions, lactate production may be guaranteed through glycogen metabolism. Glycogen was shown to play an important role in testicular development, and to be involved in the determination of germ cell survival [206]. In fact, the presence not only of glycogen but also of glycogen phosphorylase was reported in Sertoli cells [207, 208], and the availability of the machinery necessary to metabolize glycogen should be indicative of some importance of glycogen to Sertoli cells. However, the actual role of glycogen metabolism and the mechanisms underlying its influence in spermatogenesis remain unclear.

Although glucose represents a reliable energetic source for Sertoli cells, they have the machinery to use other substrates, namely amino acids, lipids and even glycogen, as we have discussed before, allowing the maintenance of the necessary ATP production even in the absence of the primary substrate [109, 170, 180, 207]. This is an important feature evidently exposing Sertoli cells metabolic plasticity, which allows them to better ensure not only their survival and function but also the nurturing of gem cells. Sertoli cells were in fact shown to display the ability to adapt their energy metabolism to the oxidative substrates available to sustain their role in spermatogenic energetic supply [209]. Glutamine and leucine oxidation were suggested to greatly contribute to Sertoli cell energetic pool [170]. Also alanine, valine and glycine have been reported to be oxidized in Sertoli cells, although the last was described as a poor energetic substrate [209]. Glucose levels may modulate the metabolism of these amino acids (namely alanine and leucine oxidation), via competition between acetyl-CoA from glucose with the acetyl-CoA resulting from amino acid metabolism [209]. Glutamine inhibits the oxidation of leucine, valine, and alanine without changing their conversion to lipids, although alanine incorporation into proteins was hampered [209]. Despite the aforementioned facts, the exact weight of the contribution of amino acid metabolism to Sertoli cell energetic balance and lactate production remains, however, unquantified. Moreover, although Sertoli cells display reduced capacity for its oxidation, glycine participates in crucial functions in Sertoli cells, being essential in the synthesis of proteins and phospholipids [209]. Creatine synthesized from glycine and arginine in Sertoli cells was suggested to be important in the nurturing of spermatogenic cells [210]. This meaningful intervention of glycine in Sertoli cell physiology highlights the fact that the role of amino acid metabolism in these cells surpasses the strict nutritional support.

Sertoli cells are also able to metabolize lipids, and the β-oxidation pathway is in fact effective for ATP production [109, 170]. Moreover, these cells are important for the conversion of essential fatty acids in testes, and the relevance of Sertoli cells in testicular lipid metabolism is highlighted by the fact that, upon injection of labeled fatty acids in testes, they are readily and preferentially taken up and metabolized by Sertoli cells [211]. Processes including endocytosis, degradation of residual bodies and phagocytosis of apoptotic spermatogenic cells are significant sources for Sertoli cell lipid recycling and metabolism [109]. The importance of lipid metabolism in Sertoli cells is emphasized by the reported presence of metabolic enzymes involved in the biosynthesis of n-6 polyunsaturated fatty acids [212 - 214], and the fact that inactivation of genes involved in lipid metabolism may compromise spermatogenesis [215].

Another interesting fact is the production of high acetate amounts by Sertoli cells [216]. The actual meaning of this significant acetate production remains unexplained, but it was suggested that it may be important for sustaining a high rate of lipid metabolism, namely lipid synthesis and remodeling, in developing germ cells [216, 217]. In this context, acetate, which can be converted to acetyl-CoA by acetyl-CoA synthase in the cytosol or in mitochondria [218], could be important for cholesterol synthesis and should play an essential role in lipid and phospholipid anabolism [219].

Another important function of Sertoli cells is the production and the control of the seminiferous tubular fluid composition. This extracellular fluid, which composes a favorable microenvironment for sustained spermatogenesis progress, is produced by Sertoli cells after they reach their mature state and the BTB is established [220, 221]. This structure is in fact critical for the maintenance of a very stable composition of the seminiferous fluid within its limits [222], minimizing solute exchanges that could be elicit unwanted property changes. Besides the role in the sustenance of germ cells, the seminiferous tubular fluid also participates in other important mechanisms, like the transport of secreted products and the movement of newly formed sperm towards the epididymis [223].

Despite their unquestionable importance in the nourishing of developing germ cells, the fact is that Sertoli cells perform an almost paradoxical role by also inducing and modulating apoptosis in those cells [193, 224, 225]. It is thought that only 25% of the theoretical number of spermatocytes arise from the primordial population of spermatogonia [226]. This represents essentially a regulatory process, since Sertoli cells can only support a limited number of developing germ cells at a given time, and the ratio of Sertoli to male germ cells must remain constant. Therefore an excess number of dependent cells must be eliminated in order to ensure that others reach full maturation [109, 227]. Non-viable germ cells must then be duly removed and degraded, and the phagocytic activity of Sertoli cells is in fact another important function of these cells [109, 228]. Selective phagocytosis of germ cells involves the recognition of specific markers on the plasmatic membrane of the residual bodies of those cells [107, 229 - 231]. Viable and degenerating germ cells are differentiated by specific antigenic determinants, which ultimately define their fate [232, 233].

Regulation/Modulation of Sertoli Cell Function

Regulation of the function and the dynamics of the proliferation and differentiation of Sertoli cells is a complex process achieved by a significant array of circulating and local hormones and growth factors. Imbalances in this tightly regulated balance may result in infertility conditions [143]. Sertoli cells have a unique profile of expressed hormone receptors and are the major functional targets for the hormonal control of spermatogenesis [234, 235]. Androgens, FSH, thyroid hormones, estrogens, insulin, melatonin, FGF, activin, retinoids, relaxin, carnitine, arachidonic acid, PModS and IL-1 are known regulators of Sertoli cell physiology.

FSH plays a pivotal role in the control of Sertoli cells proliferation during the postnatal proliferation period, determining male reproductive potential [236]. It is secreted by the pituitary gland as a response to the presence of gonadotropin releasing hormone (GnRH) [237]. Prolactin levels may modulate FSH secretion. Specifically, high prolactin levels were reported to inhibit FSH secretion, with possible undesirable consequences to male reproductive function [238]. FSH was suggested to act through activation of G-protein coupled receptors and β-arresti--dependent signaling [143, 239, 240]. FSH was described to enhance the glycolytic metabolism in Sertoli cells, increasing glucose uptake [241] and lactate production [173, 179], as well as stimulating lactate dehydrogenase activity [173]. It was also shown to impact lipid metabolism in these cells, increasing the incorporation of acetate into triglyceride and phospholipids [242]. A mechanism proposed for the action of FSH is an increase in the levels of phosphorylated protein kinase B (PKB-P), via a phosphatidylinositol 3-kinase (PI3K) dependent mechanism [243]. Stimulation of the production and secretion of inhibin B by Sertoli cells is another event influenced by FSH. Inhibin B plasma levels are used to evaluate Sertoli cell function during childhood, while in adulthood they reflect the presence of germ cells, therefore reporting the functional state of spermatogenesis [244, 245]. Finally, FSH also promotes the expression of other important proteins such as transferrin and androgen receptors [246, 247]. Spermatogenesis depends on the critical balance between intratesticular sex steroid hormones. Sertoli cells present nuclear specific androgen receptor expression patterns that are differently regulated according to the stage of the seminiferous epithelium cycle [248, 249]. Androgen receptors in Sertoli cells may be activated by testosterone [250], which is produced by Leydig cells (through a luteinizing hormone stimulus) [251], or by its derivative dihydrotestosterone, which is produced from testosterone in the prostate and is even biologically more active [252]. Testosterone was shown to modulate the fatty acid profile of cultured Sertoli cells by controlling the activity of fatty acid desaturases [253]. However, most of the effects of androgens are thought to be mediated by metabolites of testosterone, namely the aforementioned dihydrotestosterone. Dihydrotestosterone was reported to promote glucose consumption in Sertoli cells [203], and to impact lactate production and export [192, 203]. A dihydro-testosterone-promoted shift from lactate production as a final product to Krebs cycle may potentially compromise spermatogenesis [168].

Thyroid hormones are also thought to impact Sertoli cell metabolism, changing the expression of some proteins and factors [199, 254 - 256]. Thyroid hormone receptors were in fact identified in rat Sertoli cells [257], and the proliferation and differentiation of these cells is coincident with a marked peak in the plasma levels of triiodothyronine (T3) [258]. In addition, Sertoli cell T3 production arrest was reported to hinder proliferation and to induce differentiation of cultured neonatal rat Sertoli cells [259]. Insulin is another hormone involved in Sertoli cell regulation. Insulin receptors have been reported to be present in Sertoli cells [260], and insulin has been linked to altered consumption of glucose and lactate production [261, 262], altered DNA synthesis and protein expression (namely enzymes and transporters involved in the production and export of lactate) and glucose uptake (GLUT1 and GLUT3 modulation) [186]. Also, IGF-1 receptors are present in Sertoli cells and their inactivation was reported to decrease the number of viable Sertoli cells [263]. Melatonin receptors have also been identified in rat Sertoli cells [264], and this hormone was shown to increase glucose consumption in Sertoli cells, by modulation of GLUT1 expression, and to decrease lactate dehydrogenase levels and activity, which reflected in decreased lactate production [265].

Since they display both aromatase and estrogen receptors, Sertoli cells are not only able to produce estrogen, but also susceptible to estrogen modulation [266]. Estrogen was in fact shown to impact Sertoli cell differentiation and proliferation [145, 267]. Estradiol receptors and G protein-coupled estrogen receptor 1 (GPER) were shown to mediate rapid 17β-estradiol signalling in Sertoli cells [268]. Estradiol regulation of Sertoli cell function is probably enforced by modulation of transcriptional events that are important for cell function and gene expression, and which may impact normal testis development and function, and ultimately male fertility [268 - 270]. Estrogen-dependent receptor ERα signalling was reported to be determinant for germ cell viability, supposedly through support of the function of Sertoli cells [271].

Other than hormones, Sertoli cells are also susceptible to other stimuli and respond to a number of other testicular products and sub-products, which are able to elicit autocrine or paracrine responses. bFGF is a testicular germ cell product that was implicated in the control of Sertoli cells physiological processes [272]. It enhances glucose metabolism and lactate production in Sertoli cells, in a process that is thought to be mediated through up-regulation of GLUT1 and lactate dehydrogenase A transcript levels and may involve modulation of lactate dehydrogenase activity [171]. Additionally, bFGF inhibits steroidogenesis in Sertoli cells [273] and is also involved in the intercellular interplay between these and peritubular cells [274]. EGF is another factor that has been implicated in the regulation of Sertoli cell function. It was reported to be able to impact cell metabolism, by modulating the levels of lactate dehydrogenase A [275] and stimulating the production of lactate, at least in Sertoli cells from immature rats [196]. Another protein, activin A, seems to have an impact in Sertoli cell function. Its reduction during puberty has been suggested to promote the differentiation and maturation of Sertoli cells in this period [276]. Moreover, the balance between activin and inhibin (an endogenous antagonist) is thought to be essential for Sertoli cell differentiation [277]. Retinoid signaling pathways are also indispensable for Sertoli cell function and differentiation at puberty, although the mechanisms involved remain undisclosed [278 - 280]. Also relaxin receptors were reported to be present in the adult testes [281]. Relaxin is thought to play a role in Sertoli cell proliferation, in a process involving activation of a Gi protein [282].

Other modulators of Sertoli cell metabolism include L-carnitine (which alters the activity of lactate dehydrogenase, changing the production of lactate and pyruvate) [202] and arachidonic acid (which stimulates lactate production, and increases glucose uptake, lactate dehydrogenase activity and lactate dehydrogenase mRNA levels) [201]. PModS, produced by peritubular cells, stimulates Sertoli cell differentiation and inhibin secretion [55, 283, 284]. It also enhances Sertoli cell lactate production throughout pubertal development [198]. Finally, IL-1 was shown to modulate Sertoli cell metabolism by increasing lactate production and lactate dehydrogenase A expression [173, 285], and by raising glucose uptake (by modulating GLUT1 expression) [181].

Given their entangled physiology, Sertoli cells represent plausible targets for a wide range of toxic compounds. In fact, Sertoli cells were reported to be a susceptible target of toxicant-mediated reproductive dysfunction, namely resulting from the action of several endocrine disruptors and environmental pollutants [103]. Sertoli cell–cell and Sertoli–germ cell junctions and the associated actin cytoskeleton structures have been proposed to compose a relevant toxicant target

[103, 286, 287]. The cytoskeleton of Sertoli cells comprises three main components: actin, which is responsible for the establishment of microfilament network; tubulin, which comprises the microtubule cytoskeleton; and vimentin, which is also an intermediate filament component [288].

Other toxicity manifestations in Sertoli cells include different ultrastructural changes, such as chromatin condensation or vacuolization of the cytoplasm [289, 290], or interference with normal cell metabolism. Germ cell apoptosis, specifically affecting spermatocytes, is considered a hallmark of toxicant-induced injury towards Sertoli cell [120, 291]. In the case of heavy metals (such as cadmium or lead), their toxicity towards Sertoli cells is reflected in both morphological and biochemical alterations [292 - 294]. Toxicant-induced injury may compromise the supportive capacity of Sertoli cells, with consequences to germ cell that may include increased apoptosis [120]. Notably, pyruvate and/or lactate production was reported has being a key testicular metabolic process susceptible of being impacted by environmental factors targeting Sertoli cells [295]. That would be the case of some phthalate esters [296 - 298], m-dinitrobenzene (DNB) [299], nitrobenzene [300], gossypol [301], polychlorinated biphenyls (PBCs) [302] and metformin [193]. In these cases, the reported increase in lactate production upon toxicant exposure should reflect a stimulation of the glycolytic process and/or inhibition of the Krebs cycle and mitochondrial respiration. However, not all reproductive toxicants increase Sertoli cell lactate production. In fact, cisplatinum [303], dichlorodiphenyltrichloroethane (DDT) [304] and 2,4-dichlorophenoxyacetic (2,4-D) [305] are examples of toxicants reported to elicit decreases in lactate production.

Box 3.1 | Summary

- Spermatogenesis relies on the presence and cooperative action of a number of different, very specific cell types.
- Leydig cells are primarily recognized for their steroidogenic activity.
- Peritubular cells have an important structural role, but a relevant paracrine function has been progressively ascribed to these cells.
- Sertoli cells are mainly known for their structural role in the establishment of the blood-testis barrier, and for the active nurturing of germ cells.

CONCLUDING REMARKS

Leydig cells, peritubular myoid cells, and Sertoli cells, all are able to contribute in a fine, specific manner to the whole picture consubstantiating spermatogenesis. They are all very different either morphologically, or physiologically, and all these idiosyncrasies end up representing important characteristics supporting the spermatogenic process. Despite the added attention previously paid to ones with regard to the others, they are now all considered vital, each in its own way, to male human fertility, and they are all known to surpass the fulfilment of a mere structural job, even peritubular cells. It is clear that the dynamic interaction and inter-regulation between these cells is a very complex process, but it is also evident that it represents an important aspect involved in the support of competent testes function.

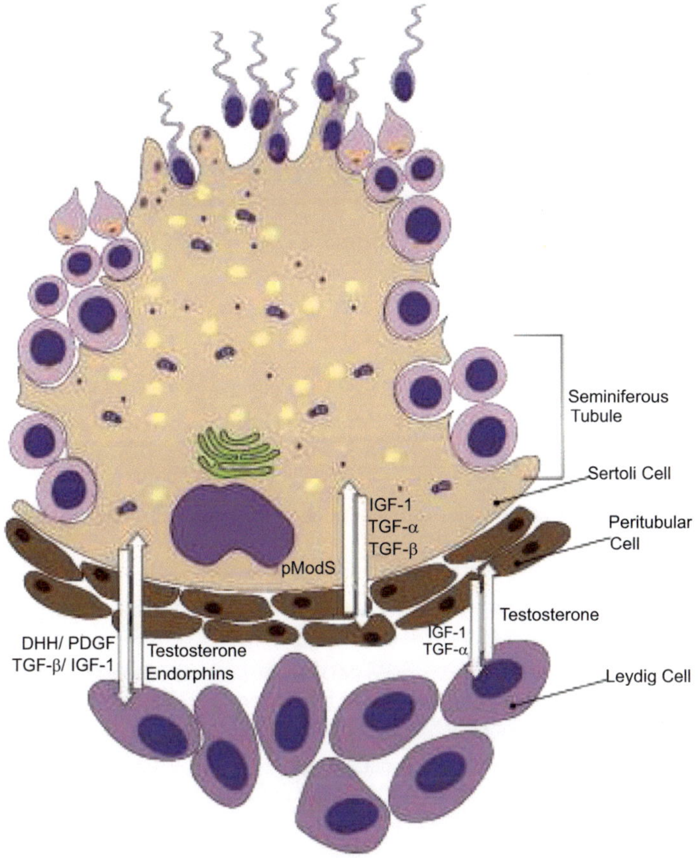

Fig. (3.2). Schematic diagram depicting the interplay and intermodulation taking place between Leydig, peritubular and Sertoli cells. Such interrelations involve both hormonal and paracrine regulation, and the reach of such interegulation is only starting to be grasped. Abbreviations: DHH: Desert hedgehog; IGF-1: insulin-like growth factor 1; PDGF: platelet-derived growth factor; PModS: peritubular factor that modulates Sertoli cell function; TGF: transforming growth factor.

The mechanisms underlying the interplay between these cell types, are just sparingly elucidated so far (a simple diagram portraying the more important known mechanisms is depicted in Fig. (**3.2**). The study of the mechanisms by which each of these cell types impact spermatogenesis and the full assessment of the importance of each of these cell types for testicular function and health could be inestimable. In fact, this knowledge could enable a much better understanding and, therefore, opposition of disease progression, and originate potential means to counteract infertility problems, or even hint putative targets susceptible of substantiating contraceptive strategies.

CONFLICT OF INTEREST

The authors confirm that they have no conflict of interest to declare for this publication.

ACKNOWLEDGEMENTS

This work was supported by the "Fundação para a Ciência e a Tecnologia"–FCT (PTDC/BBB-BQB/1368/20+14). UMIB is co-funded by FEDER *via* Programa Operacional Fatores de Competitividade-COMPETE/QREN & FSE and POPH funds (Pest-OE/SAU/UI0215/2014).

REFERENCES

[1] Leydig F. Zur anatomie der mannlichen geschlechtsorgane und analdrusen der saugethiere. 1850.

[2] Carreau S, de Vienne C, Galeraud-Denis I. Aromatase and estrogens in man reproduction: a review and latest advances. Adv Med Sci 2008; 53(2): 139-44. [http://dx.doi.org/10.2478/v10039-008-0022-z] [PMID: 18614433]

[3] Choi J, Smitz J. Luteinizing hormone and human chorionic gonadotropin: origins of difference. Mol Cell Endocrinol 2014; 383(1-2): 203-13. [http://dx.doi.org/10.1016/j.mce.2013.12.009] [PMID: 24365330]

[4] Dufau ML. The luteinizing hormone receptor. Annu Rev Physiol 1998; 60: 461-96. [http://dx.doi.org/10.1146/annurev.physiol.60.1.461] [PMID: 9558473]

[5] Sadate-Ngatchou PI, Pouchnik DJ, Griswold MD. Identification of testosterone-regulated genes in testes of hypogonadal mice using oligonucleotide microarray. Mol Endocrinol 2004; 18(2): 422-33. [http://dx.doi.org/10.1210/me.2003-0188] [PMID: 14605096]

[6] Svingen T, Koopman P. Building the mammalian testis: origins, differentiation, and assembly of the component cell populations. Genes Dev 2013; 27(22): 2409-26. [http://dx.doi.org/10.1101/gad.228080.113] [PMID: 24240231]

[7] Martin LJ. Cell interactions and genetic regulation that contribute to testicular Leydig cell development and differentiation. Mol Reprod Dev 2016; 83(6): 470-87. [http://dx.doi.org/10.1002/mrd.22648] [PMID: 27079813]

[8] OHara L, Smith LB. Androgen receptor roles in spermatogenesis and infertility. Best Pract Res Clin Endocrinol Metab 2015; 29(4): 595-605. [http://dx.doi.org/10.1016/j.beem.2015.04.006] [PMID: 26303086]

[9] Yao HH, Barsoum I. Fetal Leydig Cells. In: Payne AH, Hardy MP, Eds. The Leydig Cell in Health and Disease. Totowa, NJ: Humana Press 2007; pp. 47-54. [http://dx.doi.org/10.1007/978-1-59745-453-7_3]

[10] Wen Q, Cheng CY, Liu Y-X, Eds. Development, function and fate of fetal Leydig cells Semin Cell

Dev Biol. 2016; pp. 89-98.
[http://dx.doi.org/10.1016/j.semcdb.2016.03.003] [PMID: 26968934]

[11] Habert R, Lejeune H, Saez JM. Origin, differentiation and regulation of fetal and adult Leydig cells. Mol Cell Endocrinol 2001; 179(1-2): 47-74.
[http://dx.doi.org/10.1016/S0303-7207(01)00461-0] [PMID: 11420130]

[12] Mendis-Handagama SM, Ariyaratne HB. Differentiation of the adult Leydig cell population in the postnatal testis. Biol Reprod 2001; 65(3): 660-71.
[http://dx.doi.org/10.1095/biolreprod65.3.660] [PMID: 11514326]

[13] Haider SG. Cell biology of Leydig cells in the testis. Int Rev Cytol 2004; 233: 181-241.
[http://dx.doi.org/10.1016/S0074-7696(04)33005-6] [PMID: 15037365]

[14] Kuopio T, Paranko J, Pelliniemi LJ. Basement membrane and epithelial features of fetal-type Leydig cells in rat and human testis. Differentiation 1989; 40(3): 198-206.
[http://dx.doi.org/10.1111/j.1432-0436.1989.tb00599.x] [PMID: 2777005]

[15] Griswold SL, Behringer RR. Fetal Leydig cell origin and development. Sex Dev 2009; 3(1): 1-15.
[http://dx.doi.org/10.1159/000200077] [PMID: 19339813]

[16] Prince FP. The triphasic nature of Leydig cell development in humans, and comments on nomenclature. J Endocrinol 2001; 168(2): 213-6.
[http://dx.doi.org/10.1677/joe.0.1680213] [PMID: 11182757]

[17] Svechnikov K, Landreh L, Weisser J, *et al.* Origin, development and regulation of human Leydig cells. Horm Res Paediatr 2010; 73(2): 93-101.
[http://dx.doi.org/10.1159/000277141] [PMID: 20190545]

[18] Ge R-S, Hardy MP. Variation in the end products of androgen biosynthesis and metabolism during postnatal differentiation of rat Leydig cells. Endocrinology 1998; 139(9): 3787-95.
[PMID: 9724031]

[19] Benton L, Shan L-X, Hardy MP. Differentiation of adult Leydig cells. J Steroid Biochem Mol Biol 1995; 53(1-6): 61-8.
[http://dx.doi.org/10.1016/0960-0760(95)00022-R] [PMID: 7626518]

[20] Kilcoyne KR, Smith LB, Atanassova N, *et al.* Fetal programming of adult Leydig cell function by androgenic effects on stem/progenitor cells. Proc Natl Acad Sci USA 2014; 111(18): E1924-32.
[http://dx.doi.org/10.1073/pnas.1320735111] [PMID: 24753613]

[21] Walker WH. Testosterone signaling and the regulation of spermatogenesis. Spermatogenesis 2011; 1(2): 116-20.
[http://dx.doi.org/10.4161/spmg.1.2.16956] [PMID: 22319659]

[22] Orth JM. FSH-induced Sertoli cell proliferation in the developing rat is modified by β-endorphin produced in the testis. Endocrinology 1986; 119(4): 1876-8.
[http://dx.doi.org/10.1210/endo-119-4-1876] [PMID: 2944740]

[23] Boitani C, Farini D, Canipari R, Bardin CW. Estradiol and plasminogen activator secretion by cultured rat Sertoli cells in response to melanocyte-stimulating hormones. J Androl 1989; 10(3): 202-9.
[http://dx.doi.org/10.1002/j.1939-4640.1989.tb00087.x] [PMID: 2473057]

[24] Zimmermann S, Steding G, Emmen JM, *et al.* Targeted disruption of the Insl3 gene causes bilateral cryptorchidism. Mol Endocrinol 1999; 13(5): 681-91.
[http://dx.doi.org/10.1210/mend.13.5.0272] [PMID: 10319319]

[25] Li X, Wang Z, Jiang Z, *et al.* Regulation of seminiferous tubule-associated stem Leydig cells in adult rat testes. Proc Natl Acad Sci USA 2016; 113(10): 2666-71.
[http://dx.doi.org/10.1073/pnas.1519395113] [PMID: 26929346]

[26] Chen H, Hardy MP, Zirkin BR. Age-related decreases in Leydig cell testosterone production are not restored by exposure to LH *in vitro*. Endocrinology 2002; 143(5): 1637-42.
[http://dx.doi.org/10.1210/endo.143.5.8802] [PMID: 11956144]

[27] Ferrini RL, Barrett-Connor E. Sex hormones and age: a cross-sectional study of testosterone and estradiol and their bioavailable fractions in community-dwelling men. Am J Epidemiol 1998; 147(8): 750-4.
[http://dx.doi.org/10.1093/oxfordjournals.aje.a009519] [PMID: 9554416]

[28] Caires K, Broady J, McLean D. Maintaining the male germline: regulation of spermatogonial stem cells. J Endocrinol 2010; 205(2): 133-45.
[http://dx.doi.org/10.1677/JOE-09-0275] [PMID: 20147357]

[29] Beattie MC, Adekola L, Papadopoulos V, Chen H, Zirkin BR. Leydig cell aging and hypogonadism. Exp Gerontol 2015; 68: 87-91.
[http://dx.doi.org/10.1016/j.exger.2015.02.014] [PMID: 25700847]

[30] Luo L, Chen H, Zirkin BR. Are Leydig cell steroidogenic enzymes differentially regulated with aging? J Androl 1996; 17(5): 509-15.
[PMID: 8957694]

[31] Luo L, Chen H, Zirkin BR. Leydig cell aging: steroidogenic acute regulatory protein (StAR) and cholesterol side-chain cleavage enzyme. J Androl 2001; 22(1): 149-56.
[PMID: 11191081]

[32] Luo L, Chen H, Zirkin BR. Temporal relationships among testosterone production, steroidogenic acute regulatory protein (StAR), and P450 side-chain cleavage enzyme (P450scc) during Leydig cell aging. J Androl 2005; 26(1): 25-31.
[PMID: 15611563]

[33] Culty M, Luo L, Yao Z-X, Chen H, Papadopoulos V, Zirkin BR. Cholesterol transport, peripheral benzodiazepine receptor, and steroidogenesis in aging Leydig cells. J Androl 2002; 23(3): 439-47.
[PMID: 12002446]

[34] Maekawa M, Kamimura K, Nagano T. Peritubular myoid cells in the testis: their structure and function. Arch Histol Cytol 1996; 59(1): 1-13.
[http://dx.doi.org/10.1679/aohc.59.1] [PMID: 8727359]

[35] Mayerhofer A. Human testicular peritubular cells: more than meets the eye. Reproduction 2013; 145(5): R107-16.
[http://dx.doi.org/10.1530/REP-12-0497] [PMID: 23431272]

[36] Ross MH, Long IR. Contractile cells in human seminiferous tubules. Science 1966; 153(3741): 1271-3.
[http://dx.doi.org/10.1126/science.153.3741.1271] [PMID: 5918716]

[37] Skinner MK, Tung PS, Fritz IB. Cooperativity between Sertoli cells and testicular peritubular cells in the production and deposition of extracellular matrix components. J Cell Biol 1985; 100(6): 1941-7.
[http://dx.doi.org/10.1083/jcb.100.6.1941] [PMID: 3889013]

[38] Dym M, Fawcett DW. The blood-testis barrier in the rat and the physiological compartmentation of the seminiferous epithelium. Biol Reprod 1970; 3(3): 308-26.
[http://dx.doi.org/10.1093/biolreprod/3.3.308] [PMID: 4108372]

[39] Fawcett DW, Leak LV, Heidger PM Jr. Electron microscopic observations on the structural components of the blood-testis barrier. J Reprod Fertil Suppl 1970; 10: 105-22.
[PMID: 4951168]

[40] Davidoff MS, Breucker H, Holstein AF, Seidl K. Cellular architecture of the lamina propria of human seminiferous tubules. Cell Tissue Res 1990; 262(2): 253-61.
[http://dx.doi.org/10.1007/BF00309880] [PMID: 2076533]

[41] Holstein AF, Maekawa M, Nagano T, Davidoff MS. Myofibroblasts in the lamina propria of human semi-niferous tubules are dynamic structures of heterogeneous phenotype. Arch Histol Cytol 1996; 59(2): 109-25.
[http://dx.doi.org/10.1679/aohc.59.109] [PMID: 8790858]

[42] Tung PS, Skinner MK, Fritz IB. Cooperativity between Sertoli cells and peritubular myoid cells in the formation of the basal lamina in the seminiferous tubule. Ann N Y Acad Sci 1984; 438: 435-46.
[http://dx.doi.org/10.1111/j.1749-6632.1984.tb38304.x] [PMID: 6598327]

[43] Skinner MK, Fritz IB. Structural characterization of proteoglycans produced by testicular peritubular cells and Sertoli cells. J Biol Chem 1985; 260(21): 11874-83.
[PMID: 3930486]

[44] Albrecht M, Rämsch R, Köhn FM, Schwarzer JU, Mayerhofer A. Isolation and cultivation of human testicular peritubular cells: a new model for the investigation of fibrotic processes in the human testis and male infertility. J Clin Endocrinol Metab 2006; 91(5): 1956-60.
[http://dx.doi.org/10.1210/jc.2005-2169] [PMID: 16478819]

[45] Virtanen I, Kallajoki M, Närvänen O, *et al.* Peritubular myoid cells of human and rat testis are smooth muscle cells that contain desmin-type intermediate filaments. Anat Rec 1986; 215(1): 10-20.
[http://dx.doi.org/10.1002/ar.1092150103] [PMID: 3518542]

[46] Tung PS, Fritz IB. Characterization of rat testicular peritubular myoid cells in culture: alpha-smooth muscle isoactin is a specific differentiation marker. Biol Reprod 1990; 42(2): 351-65.
[http://dx.doi.org/10.1095/biolreprod42.2.351] [PMID: 2186815]

[47] Adam M, Schwarzer JU, Köhn FM, Strauss L, Poutanen M, Mayerhofer A. Mast cell tryptase stimulates production of decorin by human testicular peritubular cells: possible role of decorin in male infertility by interfering with growth factor signaling. Hum Reprod 2011; 26(10): 2613-25.
[http://dx.doi.org/10.1093/humrep/der245] [PMID: 21791437]

[48] Albrecht M. Insights into the nature of human testicular peritubular cells. Ann Anat 2009; 191(6): 532-40.
[http://dx.doi.org/10.1016/j.aanat.2009.08.002] [PMID: 19765961]

[49] Flenkenthaler F, Windschüttl S, Fröhlich T, Schwarzer JU, Mayerhofer A, Arnold GJ. Secretome analysis of testicular peritubular cells: a window into the human testicular microenvironment and the spermatogonial stem cell niche in man. J Proteome Res 2014; 13(3): 1259-69.
[http://dx.doi.org/10.1021/pr400769z] [PMID: 24422521]

[50] Welsh M, Moffat L, Belling K, *et al.* Androgen receptor signalling in peritubular myoid cells is essential for normal differentiation and function of adult Leydig cells. Int J Androl 2012; 35(1): 25-40.
[http://dx.doi.org/10.1111/j.1365-2605.2011.01150.x] [PMID: 21651570]

[51] Welsh M, Saunders PT, Atanassova N, Sharpe RM, Smith LB. Androgen action *via* testicular peritubular myoid cells is essential for male fertility. FASEB J 2009; 23(12): 4218-30.
[http://dx.doi.org/10.1096/fj.09-138347] [PMID: 19692648]

[52] Ailenberg M, Tung PS, Fritz IB. Transforming growth factor-beta elicits shape changes and increases contractility of testicular peritubular cells. Biol Reprod 1990; 42(3): 499-509.
[http://dx.doi.org/10.1095/biolreprod42.3.499] [PMID: 2160295]

[53] Skinner MK, Takacs K, Coffey RJ. Transforming growth factor-α gene expression and action in the seminiferous tubule: peritubular cell-Sertoli cell interactions. Endocrinology 1989; 124(2): 845-54.
[http://dx.doi.org/10.1210/endo-124-2-845] [PMID: 2463904]

[54] Tung PS, Fritz IB. Morphogenetic restructuring and formation of basement membranes by Sertoli cells and testis peritubular cells in co-culture: inhibition of the morphogenetic cascade by cyclic AMP derivatives and by blocking direct cell contact. Dev Biol 1987; 120(1): 139-53.
[http://dx.doi.org/10.1016/0012-1606(87)90112-6] [PMID: 2434375]

[55] Norton JN, Skinner MK. Regulation of Sertoli cell function and differentiation through the actions of a testicular paracrine factor P-Mod-S. Endocrinology 1989; 124(6): 2711-9.
[http://dx.doi.org/10.1210/endo-124-6-2711] [PMID: 2541997]

[56] Norton JN, Skinner MK. Regulation of Sertoli cell differentiation by the testicular paracrine factor PModS: potential role of immediate-early genes. Mol Endocrinol 1992; 6(12): 2018-26.
[PMID: 1491688]

[57] Norton JN, Vigne J-L, Skinner MK. Regulation of Sertoli cell differentiation by the testicular paracrine factor PModS: analysis of common signal transduction pathways. Endocrinology 1994; 134(1): 149-57.
[PMID: 7903930]

[58] Verhoeven G, Hoeben E, De Gendt K. Peritubular cell-Sertoli cell interactions: factors involved in PmodS activity. Andrologia 2000; 32(1): 42-5.
[PMID: 10702865]

[59] Skinner MK, Fritz IB. Testicular peritubular cells secrete a protein under androgen control that modulates Sertoli cell functions. Proc Natl Acad Sci USA 1985; 82(1): 114-8.
[http://dx.doi.org/10.1073/pnas.82.1.114] [PMID: 3855533]

[60] Hoeben E, Swinnen JV, Heyns W, Verhoeven G. Heregulins or neu differentiation factors and the interactions between peritubular myoid cells and Sertoli cells. Endocrinology 1999; 140(5): 2216-23.
[PMID: 10218974]

[61] Hoeben E, Deboel L, Rombauts L, Heyns W, Verhoeven G. Different cells and cell lines produce factors that modulate Sertoli cell function. Mol Cell Endocrinol 1994; 101(1-2): 263-75.
[http://dx.doi.org/10.1016/0303-7207(94)90243-7] [PMID: 9397961]

[62] Hoeben E. Local control of Sertoli cell function: Paracrine factors produced by peritubular myoid cells and cytokines. Coronet Books Incorporated 1997.

[63] Konrad L, Albrecht M, Renneberg H, Aum[UNKNOWN ENTITY &udie;]ller G. Transforming growth factor-β2 mediates mesenchymal-epithelial interactions of testicular somatic cells. Endocrinology 2000; 141: 3679-86.

[64] Welsh M, Moffat L, Belling K, *et al.* Androgen receptor signalling in peritubular myoid cells is essential for normal differentiation and function of adult Leydig cells. Int J Androl 2012; 35(1): 25-40.
[http://dx.doi.org/10.1111/j.1365-2605.2011.01150.x] [PMID: 21651570]

[65] Cailleau J, Vermeire S, Verhoeven G. Independent control of the production of insulin-like growth factor I and its binding protein by cultured testicular cells. Mol Cell Endocrinol 1990; 69(1): 79-89.
[http://dx.doi.org/10.1016/0303-7207(90)90091-L] [PMID: 2157618]

[66] Khan S, Teerds K, Dorrington J. Growth factor requirements for DNA synthesis by Leydig cells from the immature rat. Biol Reprod 1992; 46(3): 335-41.
[http://dx.doi.org/10.1095/biolreprod46.3.335] [PMID: 1617007]

[67] Mishra J, Gautam M, Dadhich R, Kowtharapu BS, Majumdar SS. Peritubular cells may modulate Leydig cell–mediated testosterone production through a nonclassic pathway. Fertil Steril 2012; 98: 1308-7.
[http://dx.doi.org/10.1016/j.fertnstert.2012.07.1124]

[68] Schell C, Albrecht M, Mayer C, Schwarzer JU, Frungieri MB, Mayerhofer A. Exploring human testicular peritubular cells: identification of secretory products and regulation by tumor necrosis factor-α. Endocrinology 2008; 149(4): 1678-86.
[http://dx.doi.org/10.1210/en.2007-1064] [PMID: 18187550]

[69] Spinnler K, Fröhlich T, Arnold GJ, Kunz L, Mayerhofer A. Human tryptase cleaves pro-nerve growth factor (pro-NGF): hints of local, mast cell-dependent regulation of NGF/pro-NGF action. J Biol Chem 2011; 286(36): 31707-13.
[http://dx.doi.org/10.1074/jbc.M111.233486] [PMID: 21768088]

[70] Spinnler K, Köhn FM, Schwarzer U, Mayerhofer A. Glial cell line-derived neurotrophic factor is constitutively produced by human testicular peritubular cells and may contribute to the spermatogonial stem cell niche in man. Hum Reprod 2010; 25(9): 2181-7. [http://dx.doi.org/10.1093/humrep/deq170] [PMID: 20601681]

[71] Landreh L, Spinnler K, Schubert K, *et al.* Human testicular peritubular cells host putative stem Leydig cells with steroidogenic capacity. J Clin Endocrinol Metab 2014; 99(7): E1227-35. [http://dx.doi.org/10.1210/jc.2013-4199] [PMID: 24684461]

[72] Oatley JM, Brinster RL. The germline stem cell niche unit in mammalian testes. Physiol Rev 2012; 92(2): 577-95. [http://dx.doi.org/10.1152/physrev.00025.2011] [PMID: 22535892]

[73] Windschüttl S, Kampfer C, Mayer C, *et al.* Human testicular peritubular cells secrete pigment epithelium-derived factor (PEDF), which may be responsible for the avascularity of the seminiferous tubules. Sci Rep 2015; 5: 12820. [http://dx.doi.org/10.1038/srep12820] [PMID: 26333415]

[74] Yoshida S, Sukeno M, Nabeshima Y. A vasculature-associated niche for undifferentiated spermatogonia in the mouse testis. Science 2007; 317(5845): 1722-6. [http://dx.doi.org/10.1126/science.1144885] [PMID: 17823316]

[75] Hargrove JL, MacIndoe JH, Ellis LC. Testicular contractile cells and sperm transport. Fertil Steril 1977; 28(11): 1146-57. [http://dx.doi.org/10.1016/S0015-0282(16)42909-2] [PMID: 562779]

[76] Kormano M, Hovatta O. Contractility and histochemistry of the myoid cell layer of the rat seminiferous tubules during postnatal development. Z Anat Entwicklungsgesch 1972; 137(3): 239-48. [http://dx.doi.org/10.1007/BF00519094] [PMID: 4344456]

[77] Rossi F, Ferraresi A, Romagni P, Silvestroni L, Santiemma V. Angiotensin II stimulates contraction and growth of testicular peritubular myoid cells *in vitro.* Endocrinology 2002; 143(8): 3096-104. [http://dx.doi.org/10.1210/endo.143.8.8955] [PMID: 12130575]

[78] Romano F, Gambara G, De Cesaris P, Ziparo E, Palombi F, Filippini A. Endothelin induces functional hypertrophy of peritubular smooth muscle cells. J Cell Physiol 2007; 212(1): 264-73. [http://dx.doi.org/10.1002/jcp.21028] [PMID: 17311294]

[79] Losinno AD, Morales A, Fernández D, Lopez LA. Peritubular myoid cells from rat seminiferous tubules contain actin and myosin filaments distributed in two independent layers. Biol Reprod 2012; 86(5): 150-, 1-8. [http://dx.doi.org/10.1095/biolreprod.111.095158] [PMID: 22357548]

[80] Romano F, Chiarenza C, Palombi F, *et al.* Platelet-derived growth factor-BB-induced hypertrophy of peritubular smooth muscle cells is mediated by activation of p38 MAP-kinase and of Rho-kinase. J Cell Physiol 2006; 207(1): 123-31. [http://dx.doi.org/10.1002/jcp.20554] [PMID: 16270352]

[81] Miyake K, Yamamoto M, Narita H, Hashimoto J, Mitsuya H. Evidence for contractility of the human seminiferous tubule confirmed by its response to noradrenaline and acetylcholine. Fertil Steril 1986; 46(4): 734-7. [http://dx.doi.org/10.1016/S0015-0282(16)49663-9] [PMID: 3758398]

[82] Tripiciano A, Filippini A, Ballarini F, Palombi F. Contractile response of peritubular myoid cells to prostaglandin F2α. Mol Cell Endocrinol 1998; 138(1-2): 143-50. [http://dx.doi.org/10.1016/S0303-7207(98)00010-0] [PMID: 9685223]

[83] Yamamoto M, Nagai T, Takaba H, Hashimoto J, Miyake K. *In-vitro* contractility of human seminiferous tubules in response to testosterone, dihydrotestosterone and estradiol. Urol Res 1989; 17(4): 265-8. [http://dx.doi.org/10.1007/BF00262608] [PMID: 2773191]

[84] Howl J, Rudge SA, Lavis RA, *et al.* Rat testicular myoid cells express vasopressin receptors: receptor structure, signal transduction, and developmental regulation. Endocrinology 1995; 136(5): 2206-13. [PMID: 7536665]

[85] Wartenberg H. Human testicular development and the role of the mesonephros in the origin of a dual Sertoli cell system. Andrologia 1978; 10(1): 1-21. [http://dx.doi.org/10.1111/j.1439-0272.1978.tb01306.x] [PMID: 629409]

[86] Combes AN, Wilhelm D, Davidson T, *et al.* Endothelial cell migration directs testis cord formation. Dev Biol 2009; 326(1): 112-20. [http://dx.doi.org/10.1016/j.ydbio.2008.10.040] [PMID: 19041858]

[87] Jeanes A, Wilhelm D, Wilson MJ, *et al.* Evaluation of candidate markers for the peritubular myoid cell lineage in the developing mouse testis. Reproduction 2005; 130(4): 509-16. [http://dx.doi.org/10.1530/rep.1.00718] [PMID: 16183868]

[88] Ostrer H, Huang HY, Masch RJ, Shapiro E. A cellular study of human testis development. Sex Dev 2007; 1(5): 286-92. [http://dx.doi.org/10.1159/000108930] [PMID: 18391539]

[89] Nurmio M, Kallio J, Adam M, Mayerhofer A, Toppari J, Jahnukainen K. Peritubular myoid cells have a role in postnatal testicular growth. Spermatogenesis 2012; 2(2): 79-87. [http://dx.doi.org/10.4161/spmg.20067] [PMID: 22670217]

[90] Schlatt S, Weinbauer GF, Arslan M, Nieschlag E. Appearance of α-smooth muscle actin in peritubular cells of monkey testes is induced by androgens, modulated by follicle-stimulating hormone, and maintained after hormonal withdrawal. J Androl 1993; 14(5): 340-50. [PMID: 8288489]

[91] Hovatta O. Effect of androgens and antiandrogens on the development of the myoid cells of the rat seminiferous tubules. Z Zellforsch Mikrosk Anat 1972; 131(3): 299-308. [http://dx.doi.org/10.1007/BF00582853] [PMID: 5074138]

[92] Palombi F, Farini D, Salanova M, de Grossi S, Stefanini M. Development and cytodifferentiation of peritubular myoid cells in the rat testis. Anat Rec 1992; 233(1): 32-40. [http://dx.doi.org/10.1002/ar.1092330106] [PMID: 1605376]

[93] O'Shaughnessy PJ, Ed. Hormonal control of germ cell development and spermatogenesis Seminars in cell & developmental biology. Elsevier 2014.

[94] Sandner F, Welter H, Schwarzer JU, Köhn FM, Urbanski HF, Mayerhofer A. Expression of the oestrogen receptor GPER by testicular peritubular cells is linked to sexual maturation and male fertility. Andrology 2014; 2(5): 695-701. [http://dx.doi.org/10.1111/j.2047-2927.2014.00243.x] [PMID: 25052196]

[95] Schell C, Albrecht M, Spillner S, *et al.* 15-Deoxy-delta 1214-prostaglandin-J2 induces hypertrophy and loss of contractility in human testicular peritubular cells: implications for human male fertility. Endocrinology 2010; 151(3): 1257-68. [http://dx.doi.org/10.1210/en.2009-1325] [PMID: 20133451]

[96] Welter H, Kampfer C, Lauf S, *et al.* Partial loss of contractile marker proteins in human testicular peritubular cells in infertility patients. Andrology 2013; 1(2): 318-24. [http://dx.doi.org/10.1111/j.2047-2927.2012.00030.x] [PMID: 23413143]

[97] Gülkesen KH, Erdoğru T, Sargin CF, Karpuzoğlu G. Expression of extracellular matrix proteins and vimentin in testes of azoospermic man: an immunohistochemical and morphometric study. Asian J Androl 2002; 4(1): 55-60. [PMID: 11907629]

[98] Haider SG, Talati J, Servos G. Ultrastructure of peritubular tissue in association with tubular hyalinization in human testis. Tissue Cell 1999; 31(1): 90-8. [http://dx.doi.org/10.1054/tice.1999.0005] [PMID: 10368990]

[99] Sherwood DR. Cell invasion through basement membranes: an anchor of understanding. Trends Cell Biol 2006; 16(5): 250-6.
[http://dx.doi.org/10.1016/j.tcb.2006.03.004] [PMID: 16580836]

[100] Díez-Torre A, Silván U, Moreno P, Gumucio J, Aréchaga J. Peritubular myoid cell-derived factors and its potential role in the progression of testicular germ cell tumours. Int J Androl 2011; 34(4 Pt 2): e252-64.
[http://dx.doi.org/10.1111/j.1365-2605.2011.01168.x] [PMID: 21623832]

[101] Sertoli E. Sulla struttura dei canalicoli seminiferi del testicolo studiata in rapporto allo sviluppo dei nemaspermi: 1. struttura dei canali seminiferi e sviluppo dei nemaspermi del ratto. V. Bona 1878.

[102] Bellvé AR. Purification, culture, and fractionation of spermatogenic cells. In: Wpmhs S, Ed. Guide to Techniques in Mouse Development. San Diego, USA: Academic Press 1993; pp. 84-113. [6]
[http://dx.doi.org/10.1016/0076-6879(93)25009-Q]

[103] Gao Y, Mruk DD, Cheng CY. Sertoli cells are the target of environmental toxicants in the testis - a mechanistic and therapeutic insight. Expert Opin Ther Targets 2015; 19(8): 1073-90.
[http://dx.doi.org/10.1517/14728222.2015.1039513] [PMID: 25913180]

[104] Byers S. A. HM, Djakiew D, Dym M. Growth and characterization of epidid ymal epithelial cells and Sertoli cells in dual environment culture chambers. J Androl 1986; 7: 59-68.
[http://dx.doi.org/10.1002/j.1939-4640.1986.tb00871.x] [PMID: 3944021]

[105] Janecki A, Jakubowiak A, Steinberger A. Regulation of transepithelial electrical resistance in two-compartment Sertoli cell cultures: *in vitro* model of the blood-testis barrier. Endocrinology 1991; 129(3): 1489-96.
[http://dx.doi.org/10.1210/endo-129-3-1489] [PMID: 1908377]

[106] Sheng C, Zheng Q, Wu J, *et al.* Direct reprogramming of Sertoli cells into multipotent neural stem cells by defined factors. Cell Res 2012; 22(1): 208-18.
[http://dx.doi.org/10.1038/cr.2011.175] [PMID: 22064700]

[107] Hai Y, Hou J, Liu Y, Eds. The roles and regulation of Sertoli cells in fate determinations of spermatogonial stem cells and spermatogenesis. Semin Cell Dev Biol. Elsevier 2014; 29: pp. 66-75.

[108] Griswold MD. The central role of Sertoli cells in spermatogenesis. Semin Cell Dev Biol 1998; 9(4): 411-6.
[http://dx.doi.org/10.1006/scdb.1998.0203] [PMID: 9813187]

[109] Xiong W, Wang H, Wu H, Chen Y, Han D. Apoptotic spermatogenic cells can be energy sources for Sertoli cells. Reproduction 2009; 137(3): 469-79.
[http://dx.doi.org/10.1530/REP-08-0343] [PMID: 19074501]

[110] Wong CH, Cheng CY. The blood testis barrier: Its biology, regulation, and physiological role in spermatogenesis. Curr Top Dev Biol. Academic Press 2005; pp. 263-96.

[111] Cheng CY, Mruk DD. The blood-testis barrier and its implications for male contraception. Pharmacol Rev 2012; 64(1): 16-64.
[http://dx.doi.org/10.1124/pr.110.002790] [PMID: 22039149]

[112] Kaur G, Thompson LA, Dufour JM, Eds. Sertoli cells–Immunological sentinels of spermatogenesis. Semin Cell Dev Biol. Elsevier 2014; pp. 36-44.

[113] Wong EWP, Mruk DD, Cheng CY. Biology and regulation of ectoplasmic specialization, an atypical adherens junction type, in the testis. Biochim Biophys Acta 2008; 1778: 692-708.
[http://dx.doi.org/10.1016/j.bbamem.2007.11.006]

[114] Morita K, Sasaki H, Fujimoto K, Furuse M, Tsukita S. Claudin-11/OSP-based tight junctions of myelin sheaths in brain and Sertoli cells in testis. J Cell Biol 1999; 145(3): 579-88.
[http://dx.doi.org/10.1083/jcb.145.3.579] [PMID: 10225958]

[115] Chung NP, Mruk D, Mo M-Y, Lee WM, Cheng CY. A 22-amino acid synthetic peptide corresponding to the second extracellular loop of rat occludin perturbs the blood-testis barrier and disrupts spermatogenesis reversibly *in vivo.* Biol Reprod 2001; 65(5): 1340-51. [http://dx.doi.org/10.1095/biolreprod65.5.1340] [PMID: 11673248]

[116] Cheng CY, Mruk DD. Cell junction dynamics in the testis: Sertoli-germ cell interactions and male contraceptive development. Physiol Rev 2002; 82(4): 825-74. [http://dx.doi.org/10.1152/physrev.00009.2002] [PMID: 12270945]

[117] Russell LD. The blood-testis barrier and its formation relative to spermatocyte maturation in the adult rat: a lanthanum tracer study. Anat Rec 1978; 190(1): 99-111. [http://dx.doi.org/10.1002/ar.1091900109] [PMID: 626419]

[118] Kahsai TZ, Enders GC, Gunwar S, *et al.* Seminiferous tubule basement membrane. Composition and organization of type IV collagen chains, and the linkage of α3(IV) and α5(IV) chains. J Biol Chem 1997; 272(27): 17023-32. [http://dx.doi.org/10.1074/jbc.272.27.17023] [PMID: 9202017]

[119] Hadley MA, Byers SW, Suárez-Quian CA, Kleinman HK, Dym M. Extracellular matrix regulates Sertoli cell differentiation, testicular cord formation, and germ cell development *in vitro.* J Cell Biol 1985; 101(4): 1511-22. [http://dx.doi.org/10.1083/jcb.101.4.1511] [PMID: 4044644]

[120] Murphy CJ, Richburg JH. Implications of Sertoli cell induced germ cell apoptosis to testicular pathology. Spermatogenesis 2015; 4(2): e979110. [http://dx.doi.org/10.4161/21565562.2014.979110] [PMID: 26413394]

[121] Weber JE, Russell LD, Wong V, Peterson RN. Three-dimensional reconstruction of a rat stage V Sertoli cell: II. Morphometry of SertoliSertoli and Sertoligerm-cell relationships. Am J Anat 1983; 167(2): 163-79. [http://dx.doi.org/10.1002/aja.1001670203] [PMID: 6613902]

[122] Russell L. Desmosome-like junctions between Sertoli and germ cells in the rat testis. Am J Anat 1977; 148(3): 301-12. [http://dx.doi.org/10.1002/aja.1001480302] [PMID: 857631]

[123] Russell L. Observations on rat Sertoli ectoplasmic (junctional) specializations in their association with germ cells of the rat testis. Tissue Cell 1977; 9(3): 475-98. [http://dx.doi.org/10.1016/0040-8166(77)90007-6] [PMID: 929577]

[124] Russell L, Clermont Y. Anchoring device between Sertoli cells and late spermatids in rat seminiferous tubules. Anat Rec 1976; 185(3): 259-78. [http://dx.doi.org/10.1002/ar.1091850302] [PMID: 937734]

[125] Vogl AW, Pfeiffer DC, Mulholland D, Kimel G, Guttman J. Unique and multifunctional adhesion junctions in the testis: ectoplasmic specializations. Arch Histol Cytol 2000; 63(1): 1-15. [http://dx.doi.org/10.1679/aohc.63.1] [PMID: 10770585]

[126] Kopera IA, Bilinska B, Cheng CY, Mruk DD. Sertoli-germ cell junctions in the testis: a review of recent data. Philos Trans R Soc Lond B Biol Sci 2010; 365(1546): 1593-605. [http://dx.doi.org/10.1098/rstb.2009.0251] [PMID: 20403872]

[127] Mruk DD, Cheng CY. Sertoli-Sertoli and Sertoli-germ cell interactions and their significance in germ cell movement in the seminiferous epithelium during spermatogenesis. Endocr Rev 2004; 25(5): 747-806. [http://dx.doi.org/10.1210/er.2003-0022] [PMID: 15466940]

[128] Russell LD, Tallon-Doran M, Weber JE, Wong V, Peterson RN. Three-dimensional reconstruction of a rat stage V Sertoli cell: III. A study of specific cellular relationships. Am J Anat 1983; 167(2): 181-92. [http://dx.doi.org/10.1002/aja.1001670204] [PMID: 6613903]

[129] Griswold MD. The central role of Sertoli cells in spermatogenesis. Semin Cell Dev Biol. London: Academic Press 1998; 9: pp. (4)411-6.
[http://dx.doi.org/10.1006/scdb.1998.0203]

[130] Cheng CY, Wong EW, Yan HH, Mruk DD. Regulation of spermatogenesis in the microenvironment of the seminiferous epithelium: new insights and advances. Mol Cell Endocrinol 2010; 315(1-2): 49-56.
[http://dx.doi.org/10.1016/j.mce.2009.08.004] [PMID: 19682538]

[131] Tarulli GA, Stanton PG, Lerchl A, Meachem SJ. Adult sertoli cells are not terminally differentiated in the Djungarian hamster: effect of FSH on proliferation and junction protein organization. Biol Reprod 2006; 74(5): 798-806.
[http://dx.doi.org/10.1095/biolreprod.105.050450] [PMID: 16407497]

[132] Tarulli GA, Stanton PG, Meachem SJ. Is the adult Sertoli cell terminally differentiated? Biol Reprod 2012; 87(1): 13, 1-11.
[http://dx.doi.org/10.1095/biolreprod.111.095091] [PMID: 22492971]

[133] Ahmed EA, Barten-van Rijbroek AD, Kal HB, *et al.* Proliferative activity *in vitro* and DNA repair indicate that adult mouse and human Sertoli cells are not terminally differentiated, quiescent cells. Biol Reprod 2009; 80(6): 1084-91.
[http://dx.doi.org/10.1095/biolreprod.108.071662] [PMID: 19164176]

[134] Chui K, Trivedi A, Cheng CY, *et al.* Characterization and functionality of proliferative human Sertoli cells. Cell Transplant 2011; 20(5): 619-35.
[http://dx.doi.org/10.3727/096368910X536563] [PMID: 21054948]

[135] Karl J, Capel B. Sertoli cells of the mouse testis originate from the coelomic epithelium. Dev Biol 1998; 203(2): 323-33.
[http://dx.doi.org/10.1006/dbio.1998.9068] [PMID: 9808783]

[136] Griswold MD. Interactions between germ cells and Sertoli cells in the testis. Biol Reprod 1995; 52(2): 211-6.
[http://dx.doi.org/10.1095/biolreprod52.2.211] [PMID: 7711190]

[137] Russo MA, Giustizieri ML, Favale A, *et al.* Spatiotemporal patterns of expression of neurotrophins and neurotrophin receptors in mice suggest functional roles in testicular and epididymal morphogenesis. Biol Reprod 1999; 61(4): 1123-32.
[http://dx.doi.org/10.1095/biolreprod61.4.1123] [PMID: 10491653]

[138] Cupp AS, Kim GH, Skinner MK. Expression and action of neurotropin-3 and nerve growth factor in embryonic and early postnatal rat testis development. Biol Reprod 2000; 63(6): 1617-28.
[http://dx.doi.org/10.1095/biolreprod63.6.1617] [PMID: 11090428]

[139] Gassei K, Ehmcke J, Schlatt S. Initiation of testicular tubulogenesis is controlled by neurotrophic tyrosine receptor kinases in a three-dimensional Sertoli cell aggregation assay. Reproduction 2008; 136(4): 459-69.
[http://dx.doi.org/10.1530/REP-08-0241] [PMID: 18660385]

[140] Levine E, Cupp AS, Skinner MK. Role of neurotropins in rat embryonic testis morphogenesis (cord formation). Biol Reprod 2000; 62(1): 132-42.
[http://dx.doi.org/10.1095/biolreprod62.1.132] [PMID: 10611077]

[141] Hiramatsu R, Harikae K, Tsunekawa N, Kurohmaru M, Matsuo I, Kanai Y. FGF signaling directs a center-to-pole expansion of tubulogenesis in mouse testis differentiation. Development 2010; 137(2): 303-12.
[http://dx.doi.org/10.1242/dev.040519] [PMID: 20040496]

[142] Sharpe RM, McKinnell C, Kivlin C, Fisher JS. Proliferation and functional maturation of Sertoli cells, and their relevance to disorders of testis function in adulthood. Reproduction 2003; 125(6): 769-84.
[http://dx.doi.org/10.1530/rep.0.1250769] [PMID: 12773099]

[143] Lucas TF, Nascimento AR, Pisolato R, Pimenta MT, Lazari MF, Porto CS. Receptors and signaling pathways involved in proliferation and differentiation of Sertoli cells. Spermatogenesis 2014; 4: e28138.
[http://dx.doi.org/10.4161/spmg.28138] [PMID: 25225624]

[144] Gondos B, Berndtson W. Postnatal and pubertal development. In: Russell LDaG MD, Ed. Clearwater, FL: Cache River Press 1993; pp. 115-54.

[145] ODonnell L, Robertson KM, Jones ME, Simpson ER. Estrogen and spermatogenesis. Endocr Rev 2001; 22(3): 289-318.
[PMID: 11399746]

[146] Bar-Shira Maymon B, Paz G, Elliott DJ, *et al.* Maturation phenotype of Sertoli cells in testicular biopsies of azoospermic men. Hum Reprod 2000; 15(7): 1537-42.
[http://dx.doi.org/10.1093/humrep/15.7.1537] [PMID: 10875862]

[147] Picut CA, Remick AK, de Rijk EP, Simons ML, Stump DG, Parker GA. Postnatal development of the testis in the rat: morphologic study and correlation of morphology to neuroendocrine parameters. Toxicol Pathol 2015; 43(3): 326-42.
[http://dx.doi.org/10.1177/0192623314547279] [PMID: 25217330]

[148] Orth JM, Gunsalus GL, Lamperti AA. Evidence from Sertoli cell-depleted rats indicates that spermatid number in adults depends on numbers of Sertoli cells produced during perinatal development. Endocrinology 1988; 122(3): 787-94.
[http://dx.doi.org/10.1210/endo-122-3-787] [PMID: 3125042]

[149] Nistal M, Abaurrea MA, Paniagua R. Morphological and histometric study on the human Sertoli cell from birth to the onset of puberty. J Anat 1982; 134(Pt 2): 351-63.
[PMID: 7076559]

[150] Paniagua R, Nistal M, Amat P, Rodríguez MC. Ultrastructural observations on nucleoli and related structures during human spermatogenesis. Anat Embryol (Berl) 1986; 174(3): 301-6.
[http://dx.doi.org/10.1007/BF00698780] [PMID: 3766986]

[151] Rebourcet D, OShaughnessy PJ, Pitetti J-L, *et al.* Sertoli cells control peritubular myoid cell fate and support adult Leydig cell development in the prepubertal testis. Development 2014; 141(10): 2139-49.
[http://dx.doi.org/10.1242/dev.107029] [PMID: 24803659]

[152] Skinner MK. Sertoli cell secreted regulatory factors. In: Biology SC, Ed. Skinner MKG, M D. San Diego, USA & London, UK: Elsevier Academic Press 2005; pp. 107-20.

[153] Jan SZ, Hamer G, Repping S, de Rooij DG, van Pelt AMM, Vormer TL. Molecular control of rodent spermatogenesis. Biochim Biophys Acta (BBA) - Molecular Basis of Disease 2012; 1822(12): 1838-50.
[http://dx.doi.org/10.1016/j.bbadis.2012.02.008]

[154] Meehan T, Schlatt S, OBryan MK, de Kretser DM, Loveland KL. Regulation of germ cell and Sertoli cell development by activin, follistatin, and FSH. Dev Biol 2000; 220(2): 225-37.
[http://dx.doi.org/10.1006/dbio.2000.9625] [PMID: 10753512]

[155] Fritz IB, Rommerts FG, Louis BG, Dorrington JH. Regulation by FSH and dibutyryl cyclic AMP of the formation of androgen-binding protein in Sertoli cell-enriched cultures. J Reprod Fertil 1976; 46(1): 17-24.
[http://dx.doi.org/10.1530/jrf.0.0460017] [PMID: 178864]

[156] Skinner MK, Griswold MD. Sertoli cells synthesize and secrete transferrin-like protein. J Biol Chem 1980; 255(20): 9523-5.
[PMID: 6776100]

[157] OBrien DA, Gabel CA, Eddy EM. Mouse Sertoli cells secrete mannose 6-phosphate containing glycoproteins that are endocytosed by spermatogenic cells. Biol Reprod 1993; 49(5): 1055-65.
[http://dx.doi.org/10.1095/biolreprod49.5.1055] [PMID: 8286571]

[158] Elkington JS, Fritz IB. Regulation of sulfoprotein synthesis by rat Sertoli cells in culture. Endocrinology 1980; 107(4): 970-6.
[http://dx.doi.org/10.1210/endo-107-4-970] [PMID: 6157522]

[159] Li H, Papadopoulos V, Vidic B, Dym M, Culty M. Regulation of rat testis gonocyte proliferation by platelet-derived growth factor and estradiol: identification of signaling mechanisms involved. Endocrinology 1997; 138(3): 1289-98.
[PMID: 9048638]

[160] Thuillier R, Wang Y, Culty M. Prenatal exposure to estrogenic compounds alters the expression pattern of platelet-derived growth factor receptors α and β in neonatal rat testis: identification of gonocytes as targets of estrogen exposure. Biol Reprod 2003; 68(3): 867-80.
[http://dx.doi.org/10.1095/biolreprod.102.009605] [PMID: 12604637]

[161] La Sala G, Farini D, De Felici M. Rapid estrogen signalling in mouse primordial germ cells. Exp Cell Res 2010; 316(10): 1716-27.
[http://dx.doi.org/10.1016/j.yexcr.2010.03.024] [PMID: 20380832]

[162] Griswold M, McLean D. The Sertoli cell. In: Neill JD, Ed. Knobil and Neill's physiology of reproduction. San Diego, USA: Elsevier 2006; pp. 949-75.
[http://dx.doi.org/10.1016/B978-012515400-0/50024-5]

[163] Robinson R, Fritz IB. Myoinositol biosynthesis by Sertoli cells, and levels of myoinositol biosynthetic enzymes in testis and epididymis. Can J Biochem 1979; 57(6): 962-7.
[http://dx.doi.org/10.1139/o79-117] [PMID: 224990]

[164] Bajpai M, Gupta G, Setty BS. Changes in carbohydrate metabolism of testicular germ cells during meiosis in the rat. Eur J Endocrinol 1998; 138(3): 322-7.
[http://dx.doi.org/10.1530/eje.0.1380322] [PMID: 9539308]

[165] Boussouar F, Benahmed M. Lactate and energy metabolism in male germ cells. Trends Endocrinol Metab 2004; 15(7): 345-50.
[http://dx.doi.org/10.1016/j.tem.2004.07.003] [PMID: 15350607]

[166] Rato L, Alves MG, Socorro S, Duarte AI, Cavaco JE, Oliveira PF. Metabolic regulation is important for spermatogenesis. Nat Rev Urol 2012; 9(6): 330-8.
[http://dx.doi.org/10.1038/nrurol.2012.77] [PMID: 22549313]

[167] Berg JM, Tymoczko JL, Stryer L. Section 16.1, Glycolysis Is an Energy-Conversion Pathway in Many Organisms. In: Berg JM, Tymoczko JL, Stryer L, Eds. Biochemistry. 5th ed., New York: W. H. Freeman 2002.

[168] Martins AD, Alves MG, Simões VL, *et al.* Control of Sertoli cell metabolism by sex steroid hormones is mediated through modulation in glycolysis-related transporters and enzymes. Cell Tissue Res 2013; 354(3): 861-8.
[http://dx.doi.org/10.1007/s00441-013-1722-7] [PMID: 24057877]

[169] Robinson R, Fritz IB. Metabolism of glucose by Sertoli cells in culture. Biol Reprod 1981; 24(5): 1032-41.
[http://dx.doi.org/10.1095/biolreprod24.5.1032] [PMID: 6268203]

[170] Grootegoed JA, Oonk RB, Jansen R, van der Molen HJ. Metabolism of radiolabelled energy-yielding substrates by rat Sertoli cells. J Reprod Fertil 1986; 77(1): 109-18.
[http://dx.doi.org/10.1530/jrf.0.0770109] [PMID: 3014133]

[171] Riera MF, Meroni SB, Schteingart HF, Pellizzari EH, Cigorraga SB. Regulation of lactate production and glucose transport as well as of glucose transporter 1 and lactate dehydrogenase A mRNA levels by basic fibroblast growth factor in rat Sertoli cells. J Endocrinol 2002; 173(2): 335-43.
[http://dx.doi.org/10.1677/joe.0.1730335] [PMID: 12010641]

[172] Brauchi S, Rauch MC, Alfaro IE, *et al.* Kinetics, molecular basis, and differentiation of L-lactate transport in spermatogenic cells. Am J Physiol Cell Physiol 2005; 288(3): C523-34.
[http://dx.doi.org/10.1152/ajpcell.00448.2003] [PMID: 15537707]

[173] Riera MF, Meroni SB, Gómez GE, Schteingart HF, Pellizzari EH, Cigorraga SB. Regulation of lactate production by FSH, iL1β, and TNFalpha in rat Sertoli cells. Gen Comp Endocrinol 2001; 122(1): 88-97.
[http://dx.doi.org/10.1006/gcen.2001.7619] [PMID: 11352557]

[174] Erkkilä K, Aito H, Aalto K, Pentikäinen V, Dunkel L. Lactate inhibits germ cell apoptosis in the human testis. Mol Hum Reprod 2002; 8(2): 109-17.
[http://dx.doi.org/10.1093/molehr/8.2.109] [PMID: 11818513]

[175] Jutte NH, Grootegoed JA, Rommerts FF, van der Molen HJ. Exogenous lactate is essential for metabolic activities in isolated rat spermatocytes and spermatids. J Reprod Fertil 1981; 62(2): 399-405.
[http://dx.doi.org/10.1530/jrf.0.0620399] [PMID: 7252921]

[176] Jutte NH, Jansen R, Grootegoed JA, Rommerts FF, Clausen OP, van der Molen HJ. Regulation of survival of rat pachytene spermatocytes by lactate supply from Sertoli cells. J Reprod Fertil 1982; 65(2): 431-8.
[http://dx.doi.org/10.1530/jrf.0.0650431] [PMID: 6808129]

[177] Mita M, Hall PF. Metabolism of round spermatids from rats: lactate as the preferred substrate. Biol Reprod 1982; 26(3): 445-55.
[http://dx.doi.org/10.1095/biolreprod26.3.445] [PMID: 7082719]

[178] Nakamura M, Hino A, Kato J. Stimulation of protein synthesis in round spermatids from rat testes by lactate. II. Role of adenosine triphosphate (ATP). J Biochem 1981; 90(4): 933-40.
[http://dx.doi.org/10.1093/oxfordjournals.jbchem.a133581] [PMID: 7309720]

[179] Jutte NH, Jansen R, Grootegoed JA, Rommerts FF, van der Molen HJ. FSH stimulation of the production of pyruvate and lactate by rat Sertoli cells may be involved in hormonal regulation of spermatogenesis. J Reprod Fertil 1983; 68(1): 219-26.
[http://dx.doi.org/10.1530/jrf.0.0680219] [PMID: 6302252]

[180] Riera MF, Galardo MN, Pellizzari EH, Meroni SB, Cigorraga SB. Molecular mechanisms involved in Sertoli cell adaptation to glucose deprivation. Am J Physiol Endocrinol Metab 2009; 297(4): E907-14.
[http://dx.doi.org/10.1152/ajpendo.00235.2009] [PMID: 19638510]

[181] Galardo MN, Riera MF, Pellizzari EH, *et al.* Regulation of expression of Sertoli cell glucose transporters 1 and 3 by FSH, IL1 β, and bFGF at two different time-points in pubertal development. Cell Tissue Res 2008; 334(2): 295-304.
[http://dx.doi.org/10.1007/s00441-008-0656-y] [PMID: 18802725]

[182] Carosa E, Radico C, Giansante N, *et al.* Ontogenetic profile and thyroid hormone regulation of type-1 and type-8 glucose transporters in rat Sertoli cells. Int J Androl 2005; 28(2): 99-106.
[http://dx.doi.org/10.1111/j.1365-2605.2005.00516.x] [PMID: 15811071]

[183] Kokk K, Veräjänkorva E, Wu XK, Tapfer H, Põldoja E, Pöllänen P. Immunohistochemical detection of glucose transporters class I subfamily in the mouse, rat and human testis. Medicina (Kaunas) 2004; 40(2): 156-60.
[PMID: 15007275]

[184] Angulo C, Castro MA, Rivas CI, *et al.* Molecular identification and functional characterization of the vitamin C transporters expressed by Sertoli cells. J Cell Physiol 2008; 217(3): 708-16.
[http://dx.doi.org/10.1002/jcp.21545] [PMID: 18668520]

[185] Gómez O, Romero A, Terrado J, Mesonero JE. Differential expression of glucose transporter GLUT8 during mouse spermatogenesis. Reproduction 2006; 131(1): 63-70.
[http://dx.doi.org/10.1530/rep.1.00750] [PMID: 16388010]

[186] Oliveira PF, Alves MG, Rato L, *et al.* Effect of insulin deprivation on metabolism and metabolism-associated gene transcript levels of *in vitro* cultured human Sertoli cells. Biochim Biophys Acta (BBA) - General Subjects 2012; 1820: 84-9.

[187] Adijanto J, Philp NJ. The SLC16A family of monocarboxylate transporters (MCTs)physiology and function in cellular metabolism, pH homeostasis, and fluid transport. Curr Top Membr 2012; 70: 275-311.
[http://dx.doi.org/10.1016/B978-0-12-394316-3.00009-0] [PMID: 23177990]

[188] Galardo MN, Riera MF, Pellizzari EH, Cigorraga SB, Meroni SB. The AMP-activated protein kinase activator, 5-aminoimidazole-4-carboxamide-1-b-D-ribonucleoside, regulates lactate production in rat Sertoli cells. J Mol Endocrinol 2007; 39(4): 279-88.
[http://dx.doi.org/10.1677/JME-07-0054] [PMID: 17909267]

[189] Draoui N, Feron O. Lactate shuttles at a glance: from physiological paradigms to anti-cancer treatments. Dis Model Mech 2011; 4(6): 727-32.
[http://dx.doi.org/10.1242/dmm.007724] [PMID: 22065843]

[190] Kishimoto A, Ishiguro-Oonuma T, Takahashi R, *et al.* Immunohistochemical localization of GLUT3, MCT1, and MCT2 in the testes of mice and rats: the use of different energy sources in spermatogenesis. Biomed Res 2015; 36(4): 225-34.
[http://dx.doi.org/10.2220/biomedres.36.225] [PMID: 26299481]

[191] Bonen A. The expression of lactate transporters (MCT1 and MCT4) in heart and muscle. Eur J Appl Physiol 2001; 86(1): 6-11.
[http://dx.doi.org/10.1007/s004210100516] [PMID: 11820324]

[192] Rato L, Alves MG, Socorro S, Carvalho RA, Cavaco JE, Oliveira PF. Metabolic modulation induced by oestradiol and DHT in immature rat Sertoli cells cultured *in vitro.* Biosci Rep 2012; 32(1): 61-9.
[http://dx.doi.org/10.1042/BSR20110030] [PMID: 21671886]

[193] Alves MG, Martins AD, Vaz CV, *et al.* Metformin and male reproduction: effects on Sertoli cell metabolism. Br J Pharmacol 2014; 171(4): 1033-42.
[http://dx.doi.org/10.1111/bph.12522] [PMID: 24261663]

[194] Halestrap AP, Price NT. The proton-linked monocarboxylate transporter (MCT) family: structure, function and regulation. Biochem J 1999; 343(Pt 2): 281-99.
[http://dx.doi.org/10.1042/bj3430281] [PMID: 10510291]

[195] Mita M, Price JM, Hall PF. Stimulation by follicle-stimulating hormone of synthesis of lactate by Sertoli cells from rat testis. Endocrinology 1982; 110(5): 1535-41.
[http://dx.doi.org/10.1210/endo-110-5-1535] [PMID: 6280966]

[196] Mallea LE, Machado AJ, Navaroli F, Rommerts FF. Epidermal growth factor stimulates lactate production and inhibits aromatization in cultured Sertoli cells from immature rats. Int J Androl 1986; 9(3): 201-8.
[http://dx.doi.org/10.1111/j.1365-2605.1986.tb00883.x] [PMID: 3100457]

[197] Oonk RB, Jansen R, Grootegoed JA. Differential effects of follicle-stimulating hormone, insulin, and insulin-like growth factor I on hexose uptake and lactate production by rat Sertoli cells. J Cell Physiol 1989; 139(1): 210-8.
[http://dx.doi.org/10.1002/jcp.1041390128] [PMID: 2496132]

[198] Mullaney BP, Rosselli M, Skinner MK. Developmental regulation of Sertoli cell lactate production by hormones and the testicular paracrine factor, PModS. Mol Cell Endocrinol 1994; 104(1): 67-73.
[http://dx.doi.org/10.1016/0303-7207(94)90052-3] [PMID: 7821707]

[199] Palmero S, Prati M, Bolla F, Fugassa E. Tri-iodothyronine directly affects rat Sertoli cell proliferation and differentiation. J Endocrinol 1995; 145(2): 355-62.
[http://dx.doi.org/10.1677/joe.0.1450355] [PMID: 7616169]

[200] Schteingart HF, Meroni SB, Cánepa DF, Pellizzari EH, Cigorraga SB. Effects of basic fibroblast growth factor and nerve growth factor on lactate production, gamma-glutamyl transpeptidase and aromatase activities in cultured Sertoli cells. Eur J Endocrinol 1999; 141(5): 539-45. [http://dx.doi.org/10.1530/eje.0.1410539] [PMID: 10576773]

[201] Meroni SB, Riera MF, Pellizzari EH, Schteingart HF, Cigorraga SB. Possible role of arachidonic acid in the regulation of lactate production in rat Sertoli cells. Int J Androl 2003; 26(5): 310-7. [http://dx.doi.org/10.1046/j.1365-2605.2003.00432.x] [PMID: 14511220]

[202] Palmero S, Bottazzi C, Costa M, Leone M, Fugassa E. Metabolic effects of L-carnitine on prepubertal rat Sertoli cells. Horm Metab Res 2000; 32(3): 87-90. [http://dx.doi.org/10.1055/s-2007-978596] [PMID: 10786925]

[203] Oliveira PF, Alves MG, Rato L, *et al.* Influence of 5α-dihydrotestosterone and 17β-estradiol on human Sertoli cells metabolism. Int J Androl 2011; 34(6 Pt 2): e612-20. [http://dx.doi.org/10.1111/j.1365-2605.2011.01205.x] [PMID: 21812787]

[204] Hardie DG. Minireview: the AMP-activated protein kinase cascade: the key sensor of cellular energy status. Endocrinology 2003; 144(12): 5179-83. [http://dx.doi.org/10.1210/en.2003-0982] [PMID: 12960015]

[205] Galardo MN, Riera MF, Pellizzari EH, *et al.* Adenosine regulates Sertoli cell function by activating AMPK. Mol Cell Endocrinol 2010; 330(1-2): 49-58. [http://dx.doi.org/10.1016/j.mce.2010.08.007] [PMID: 20723579]

[206] Villarroel-Espíndola F, Maldonado R, Mancilla H, *et al.* Muscle glycogen synthase isoform is responsible for testicular glycogen synthesis: glycogen overproduction induces apoptosis in male germ cells. J Cell Biochem 2013; 114(7): 1653-64. [http://dx.doi.org/10.1002/jcb.24507] [PMID: 23386391]

[207] Leiderman B, Mancini RE. Glycogen content in the rat testis from postnatal to adult ages. Endocrinology 1969; 85(3): 607-9. [http://dx.doi.org/10.1210/endo-85-3-607] [PMID: 4307365]

[208] Slaughter GR, Means AR. Follicle-stimulating hormone activation of glycogen phosphorylase in the Sertoli cell-enriched rat testis. Endocrinology 1983; 113(4): 1476-85. [http://dx.doi.org/10.1210/endo-113-4-1476] [PMID: 6193956]

[209] Kaiser GR, Monteiro SC, Gelain DP, Souza LF, Perry ML, Bernard EA. Metabolism of amino acids by cultured rat Sertoli cells. Metabolism 2005; 54(4): 515-21. [http://dx.doi.org/10.1016/j.metabol.2004.11.005] [PMID: 15798960]

[210] Moore NP, Gray TJ, Timbrell JA. Creatine metabolism in the seminiferous epithelium of rats. I. Creatine synthesis by isolated and cultured cells. J Reprod Fertil 1998; 112(2): 325-30. [http://dx.doi.org/10.1530/jrf.0.1120325] [PMID: 9640271]

[211] Beckman JK, Coniglio JG. The metabolism of polyunsaturated fatty acids in rat Sertoli and germinal cells. Lipids 1980; 15(6): 389-94. [http://dx.doi.org/10.1007/BF02534061] [PMID: 7401936]

[212] Coniglio JG, Sharp J. Biosynthesis of [14C]arachidonic acid from [14C]linoleate in primary cultures of rat Sertoli cells. Lipids 1989; 24(1): 84-5. [http://dx.doi.org/10.1007/BF02535270] [PMID: 2501611]

[213] Huynh S, Oulhaj H, Bocquet J, Nouvelot A. Metabolic utilization of linoleate and α-linolenate in cultured Sertoli cells. Comp Biochem Physiol B 1991; 99(2): 265-70. [http://dx.doi.org/10.1016/0305-0491(91)90039-G] [PMID: 1684926]

[214] Oulhaj H, Huynh S, Nouvelot A. The biosynthesis of polyunsaturated fatty acids by rat sertoli cells. Comp Biochem Physiol B 1992; 102(4): 897-904. [http://dx.doi.org/10.1016/0305-0491(92)90099-D] [PMID: 1356704]

[215] Chung S, Wang SP, Pan L, Mitchell G, Trasler J, Hermo L. Infertility and testicular defects in hormone-sensitive lipase-deficient mice. Endocrinology 2001; 142(10): 4272-81. [http://dx.doi.org/10.1210/endo.142.10.8424] [PMID: 11564684]

[216] Alves MG, Socorro S, Silva J, *et al. In vitro* cultured human Sertoli cells secrete high amounts of acetate that is stimulated by 17β-estradiol and suppressed by insulin deprivation. Biochim Biophys Acta (BBA)-Molecular Cell Research 2012; 1823: 1389-94.

[217] Bajpai M, Gupta G, Jain SK, Setty BS. Lipid metabolising enzymes in isolated rat testicular germ cells and changes associated with meiosis. Andrologia 1998; 30(6): 311-5. [http://dx.doi.org/10.1111/j.1439-0272.1998.tb01176.x] [PMID: 9835944]

[218] Howard BV, Howard WJ, Bailey JM. Acetyl coenzyme A synthetase and the regulation of lipid synthesis from acetate in cultured cells. J Biol Chem 1974; 249(24): 7912-21. [PMID: 4473453]

[219] Baenke F, Peck B, Miess H, Schulze A. Hooked on fat: the role of lipid synthesis in cancer metabolism and tumour development. Dis Model Mech 2013; 6(6): 1353-63. [http://dx.doi.org/10.1242/dmm.011338] [PMID: 24203995]

[220] Jegou B, Le Gac F, de Kretser DM. Seminiferous tubule fluid and interstitial fluid production. I. Effects of age and hormonal regulation in immature rats. Biol Reprod 1982; 27(3): 590-5. [http://dx.doi.org/10.1095/biolreprod27.3.590] [PMID: 6814545]

[221] Jégou B, Le Gac F, Irby DC, de Kretser DM. Studies on seminiferous tubule fluid production in the adult rat: effect of hypophysectomy and treatment with FSH, LH and testosterone. Int J Androl 1983; 6(3): 249-60. [http://dx.doi.org/10.1111/j.1365-2605.1983.tb00539.x] [PMID: 6411627]

[222] Koskimies AI, Kormano M. The proteins in fluids from the seminiferous tubules and rete testis of the rat. J Reprod Fertil 1973; 34(3): 433-4. [http://dx.doi.org/10.1530/jrf.0.0340433] [PMID: 4795263]

[223] Rato L, Socorro S, Cavaco JE, Oliveira PF. Tubular fluid secretion in the seminiferous epithelium: ion transporters and aquaporins in Sertoli cells. J Membr Biol 2010; 236(2): 215-24. [http://dx.doi.org/10.1007/s00232-010-9294-x] [PMID: 20697886]

[224] Barone F, Aguanno S, DAgostino A. Modulation of MAA-induced apoptosis in male germ cells: role of Sertoli cell P/Q-type calcium channels. Reprod Biol Endocrinol 2005; 3: 13. [http://dx.doi.org/10.1186/1477-7827-3-13] [PMID: 15840169]

[225] Print CG, Loveland KL. Germ cell suicide: new insights into apoptosis during spermatogenesis. BioEssays 2000; 22(5): 423-30. [http://dx.doi.org/10.1002/(SICI)1521-1878(200005)22:5<423::AID-BIES4>3.0.CO;2-0] [PMID: 10797482]

[226] Huckins C. The morphology and kinetics of spermatogonial degeneration in normal adult rats: an analysis using a simplified classification of the germinal epithelium. Anat Rec 1978; 190(4): 905-26. [http://dx.doi.org/10.1002/ar.1091900410] [PMID: 637327]

[227] Miething A. Germ-cell death during prespermatogenesis in the testis of the golden hamster. Cell Tissue Res 1992; 267(3): 583-90. [http://dx.doi.org/10.1007/BF00319381] [PMID: 1571969]

[228] Chemes H. The phagocytic function of Sertoli cells: a morphological, biochemical, and endocrinological study of lysosomes and acid phosphatase localization in the rat testis. Endocrinology 1986; 119(4): 1673-81. [http://dx.doi.org/10.1210/endo-119-4-1673] [PMID: 3757907]

[229] Morales C, Clermont Y, Hermo L. Nature and function of endocytosis in Sertoli cells of the rat. Am J Anat 1985; 173(3): 203-17. [http://dx.doi.org/10.1002/aja.1001730305] [PMID: 20726121]

[230] Morales C, Clermont Y, Nadler NJ. Cyclic endocytic activity and kinetics of lysosomes in Sertoli cells of the rat: a morphometric analysis. Biol Reprod 1986; 34(1): 207-18. [http://dx.doi.org/10.1095/biolreprod34.1.207] [PMID: 3955137]

[231] Clermont Y, Morales C, Hermo L. Endocytic activities of Sertoli cells in the rat. Ann N Y Acad Sci 1987; 513: 1-15. [http://dx.doi.org/10.1111/j.1749-6632.1987.tb24994.x] [PMID: 3328532]

[232] Bellvé AR, Moss SB. Monoclonal antibodies as probes of reproductive mechanisms. Biol Reprod 1983; 28(1): 1-26. [http://dx.doi.org/10.1095/biolreprod28.1.1] [PMID: 6338940]

[233] Millette CF, Bellvé AR. Selective partitioning of plasma membrane antigens during mouse spermatogenesis. Dev Biol 1980; 79(2): 309-24. [http://dx.doi.org/10.1016/0012-1606(80)90118-9] [PMID: 7000579]

[234] Alves MG, Rato L, Carvalho RA, Moreira PI, Socorro S, Oliveira PF. Hormonal control of Sertoli cell metabolism regulates spermatogenesis. Cell Mol Life Sci 2013; 70(5): 777-93. [http://dx.doi.org/10.1007/s00018-012-1079-1] [PMID: 23011766]

[235] Hansson V, Purvis K, Ritzen E, French FS, Eds. Hormonal regulation of Sertoli cell function in the rat Annales de Biologie Animale Biochimie Biophysique. EDP Sciences 1978.

[236] Grigorova M, Punab M, Zilaitienė B, *et al.* Genetically determined dosage of follicle-stimulating hormone (FSH) affects male reproductive parameters. J Clin Endocrinol Metab 2011; 96(9): E1534-41. [http://dx.doi.org/10.1210/jc.2011-0632] [PMID: 21733993]

[237] Nett TM, Turzillo AM, Baratta M, Rispoli LA. Pituitary effects of steroid hormones on secretion of follicle-stimulating hormone and luteinizing hormone. Domest Anim Endocrinol 2002; 23(1-2): 33-42. [http://dx.doi.org/10.1016/S0739-7240(02)00143-1] [PMID: 12142224]

[238] Weber RF, Ooms MP, Vreeburg JT. Effects of a prolactin- and adrenocorticotropin-secreting tumor on gonadotropin levels and accessory sex organ weights in adult male rats: a possible role of the adrenals. Endocrinology 1982; 111(2): 412-7. [http://dx.doi.org/10.1210/endo-111-2-412] [PMID: 6284478]

[239] McLachlan RI, ODonnell L, Meachem SJ, *et al.* Identification of specific sites of hormonal regulation in spermatogenesis in rats, monkeys, and man. Recent Prog Horm Res 2002; 57: 149-79. [http://dx.doi.org/10.1210/rp.57.1.149] [PMID: 12017541]

[240] Marion S, Kara E, Crepieux P, *et al.* G protein-coupled receptor kinase 2 and β-arrestins are recruited to FSH receptor in stimulated rat primary Sertoli cells. J Endocrinol 2006; 190(2): 341-50. [http://dx.doi.org/10.1677/joe.1.06857] [PMID: 16899567]

[241] Hall PF, Mita M. Influence of follicle-stimulating hormone on glucose transport by cultured Sertoli cells. Biol Reprod 1984; 31(5): 863-9. [http://dx.doi.org/10.1095/biolreprod31.5.863] [PMID: 6097313]

[242] Guma FC, Wagner M, Martini LH, Bernard EA. Effect of FSH and insulin on lipogenesis in cultures of Sertoli cells from immature rats. Braz J Med Biol Res 1997; 30(5): 591-7. [http://dx.doi.org/10.1590/S0100-879X1997000500004] [PMID: 9283625]

[243] Meroni SB, Riera MF, Pellizzari EH, Cigorraga SB. Regulation of rat Sertoli cell function by FSH: possible role of phosphatidylinositol 3-kinase/protein kinase B pathway. J Endocrinol 2002; 174(2): 195-204. [http://dx.doi.org/10.1677/joe.0.1740195] [PMID: 12176658]

[244] de Kretser DM, Buzzard JJ, Okuma Y, *et al.* The role of activin, follistatin and inhibin in testicular physiology. Mol Cell Endocrinol 2004; 225(1-2): 57-64. [http://dx.doi.org/10.1016/j.mce.2004.07.008] [PMID: 15451568]

[245] Grinspon RP, Loreti N, Braslavsky D, *et al.* Sertoli cell markers in the diagnosis of paediatric male hypogonadism. J Pediatr Endocrinol Metab 2012; 25(1-2): 3-11.
[http://dx.doi.org/10.1515/jpem-2011-0453] [PMID: 22570945]

[246] Suire S, Fontaine I, Guillou F. Follicle stimulating hormone (FSH) stimulates transferrin gene transcription in rat Sertoli cells: cis and trans-acting elements involved in FSH action *via* cyclic adenosine 3,5-monophosphate on the transferrin gene. Mol Endocrinol 1995; 9(6): 756-66.
[PMID: 8592521]

[247] Verhoeven G, Cailleau J. Follicle-stimulating hormone and androgens increase the concentration of the androgen receptor in Sertoli cells. Endocrinology 1988; 122(4): 1541-50.
[http://dx.doi.org/10.1210/endo-122-4-1541] [PMID: 2831032]

[248] Bremner WJ, Millar MR, Sharpe RM, Saunders PT. Immunohistochemical localization of androgen receptors in the rat testis: evidence for stage-dependent expression and regulation by androgens. Endocrinology 1994; 135(3): 1227-34.
[PMID: 8070367]

[249] Zhou Q, Nie R, Prins GS, Saunders PT, Katzenellenbogen BS, Hess RA. Localization of androgen and estrogen receptors in adult male mouse reproductive tract. J Androl 2002; 23(6): 870-81.
[PMID: 12399534]

[250] Lindzey J, Kumar MV, Grossman M, Young C, Tindall DJ. Molecular mechanisms of androgen action. Vitam Horm 1994; 49: 383-432.
[http://dx.doi.org/10.1016/S0083-6729(08)61151-6] [PMID: 7810074]

[251] Mendis-Handagama SM. Luteinizing hormone on Leydig cell structure and function. Histol Histopathol 1997; 12(3): 869-82.
[PMID: 9225169]

[252] Dohle GR, Smit M, Weber RF. Androgens and male fertility. World J Urol 2003; 21(5): 341-5.
[http://dx.doi.org/10.1007/s00345-003-0365-9] [PMID: 14566423]

[253] Hurtado de Catalfo GE, de Gómez Dumm IN. Influence of testosterone on polyunsaturated fatty acid biosynthesis in Sertoli cells in culture. Cell Biochem Funct 2005; 23(3): 175-80.
[http://dx.doi.org/10.1002/cbf.1135] [PMID: 15376235]

[254] van Haaster LH, de Jong FH, Docter R, de Rooij DG. High neonatal triiodothyronine levels reduce the period of Sertoli cell proliferation and accelerate tubular lumen formation in the rat testis, and increase serum inhibin levels. Endocrinology 1993; 133(2): 755-60.
[PMID: 8344214]

[255] Fugassa E, Palmero S, Gallo G. Triiodothyronine decreases the production of androgen binding protein by rat Sertoli cells. Biochem Biophys Res Commun 1987; 143(1): 241-7.
[http://dx.doi.org/10.1016/0006-291X(87)90656-5] [PMID: 3827920]

[256] Palmero S, Prati M, Barreca A, Minuto F, Giordano G, Fugassa E. Thyroid hormone stimulates the production of insulin-like growth factor I (IGF-I) by immature rat Sertoli cells. Mol Cell Endocrinol 1990; 68(1): 61-5.
[http://dx.doi.org/10.1016/0303-7207(90)90170-D] [PMID: 2303160]

[257] Palmero S, Maggiani S, Fugassa E. Nuclear triiodothyronine receptors in rat Sertoli cells. Mol Cell Endocrinol 1988; 58(2-3): 253-6.
[http://dx.doi.org/10.1016/0303-7207(88)90161-X] [PMID: 3208996]

[258] Hadj-Sahraoui N, Seugnet I, Ghorbel MT, Demeneix B. Hypothyroidism prolongs mitotic activity in the post-natal mouse brain. Neurosci Lett 2000; 280(2): 79-82.
[http://dx.doi.org/10.1016/S0304-3940(00)00768-0] [PMID: 10686382]

[259] Cooke PS, Zhao Y-D, Bunick D. Triiodothyronine inhibits proliferation and stimulates differentiation of cultured neonatal Sertoli cells: possible mechanism for increased adult testis weight and sperm production induced by neonatal goitrogen treatment. Biol Reprod 1994; 51(5): 1000-5. [http://dx.doi.org/10.1095/biolreprod51.5.1000] [PMID: 7531505]

[260] Oonk RB, Grootegoed JA. Identification of insulin receptors on rat Sertoli cells. Mol Cell Endocrinol 1987; 49(1): 51-62. [http://dx.doi.org/10.1016/0303-7207(87)90063-3] [PMID: 3549388]

[261] Oonk RB, Grootegoed JA, van der Molen HJ. Comparison of the effects of insulin and follitropin on glucose metabolism by Sertoli cells from immature rats. Mol Cell Endocrinol 1985; 42(1): 39-48. [http://dx.doi.org/10.1016/0303-7207(85)90005-X] [PMID: 3928417]

[262] Borland K, Mita M, Oppenheimer CL, *et al.* The actions of insulin-like growth factors I and II on cultured Sertoli cells. Endocrinology 1984; 114(1): 240-6. [http://dx.doi.org/10.1210/endo-114-1-240] [PMID: 6360662]

[263] Froment P, Vigier M, Nègre D, *et al.* Inactivation of the IGF-I receptor gene in primary Sertoli cells highlights the autocrine effects of IGF-I. J Endocrinol 2007; 194(3): 557-68. [http://dx.doi.org/10.1677/JOE-07-0258] [PMID: 17761895]

[264] Yang W-C, Tang K-Q, Fu C-Z, Riaz H, Zhang Q, Zan L-S. Melatonin regulates the development and function of bovine Sertoli cells *via* its receptors MT1 and MT2. Anim Reprod Sci 2014; 147(1-2): 10-6. [http://dx.doi.org/10.1016/j.anireprosci.2014.03.017] [PMID: 24768045]

[265] Rocha CS, Martins AD, Rato L, Silva BM, Oliveira PF, Alves MG. Melatonin alters the glycolytic profile of Sertoli cells: implications for male fertility. Mol Hum Reprod 2014; 20(11): 1067-76. [http://dx.doi.org/10.1093/molehr/gau080] [PMID: 25205674]

[266] Smith LB, Walker WH, O'Donnell L. Hormonal regulation of spermatogenesis through Sertoli cells by androgens and estrogens. Sertoli Cell Biology 2014; p. 175.

[267] Lucas TF, Siu ER, Esteves CA, *et al.* 17beta-estradiol induces the translocation of the estrogen receptors ESR1 and ESR2 to the cell membrane, MAPK3/1 phosphorylation and proliferation of cultured immature rat Sertoli cells. Biol Reprod 2008; 78(1): 101-14. [http://dx.doi.org/10.1095/biolreprod.107.063909] [PMID: 17928626]

[268] Lucas TF, Pimenta MT, Pisolato R, Lazari MF, Porto CS. 17β-estradiol signaling and regulation of Sertoli cell function. Spermatogenesis 2011; 1(4): 318-24. [http://dx.doi.org/10.4161/spmg.1.4.18903] [PMID: 22332115]

[269] Kumar N, Srivastava S, Burek M, Förster CY, Roy P. Assessment of estradiol-induced gene regulation and proliferation in an immortalized mouse immature Sertoli cell line. Life Sci 2016; 148: 268-78. [http://dx.doi.org/10.1016/j.lfs.2016.01.027] [PMID: 26784849]

[270] Lazari MF, Lucas TF, Yasuhara F, *et al.* Estrogen receptors and function in the male reproductive system. Arq Bras Endocrinol Metabol 2009; 53(8): 923-33. [PMID: 20126844]

[271] Sinkevicius KW, Laine M, Lotan TL, Woloszyn K, Richburg JH, Greene GL. Estrogen-dependent and -independent estrogen receptor-alpha signaling separately regulate male fertility. Endocrinology 2009; 150(6): 2898-905. [http://dx.doi.org/10.1210/en.2008-1016] [PMID: 19264877]

[272] Han IS, Sylvester SR, Kim KH, *et al.* Basic fibroblast growth factor is a testicular germ cell product which may regulate Sertoli cell function. Mol Endocrinol 1993; 7(7): 889-97. [PMID: 8413313]

[273] Brucato S, Bocquet J, Villers C. Cell surface heparan sulfate proteoglycans: target and partners of the basic fibroblast growth factor in rat Sertoli cells. Eur J Biochem 2002; 269(2): 502-11. [http://dx.doi.org/10.1046/j.0014-2956.2001.02672.x] [PMID: 11856308]

[274] El Ramy R, Verot A, Mazaud S, Odet F, Magre S, Le Magueresse-Battistoni B. Fibroblast growth factor (FGF) 2 and FGF9 mediate mesenchymal-epithelial interactions of peritubular and Sertoli cells in the rat testis. J Endocrinol 2005; 187(1): 135-47.
[http://dx.doi.org/10.1677/joe.1.06146] [PMID: 16214949]

[275] Boussouar F, Benahmed M. Epidermal growth factor regulates glucose metabolism through lactate dehydrogenase A messenger ribonucleic acid expression in cultured porcine Sertoli cells. Biol Reprod 1999; 61(4): 1139-45.
[http://dx.doi.org/10.1095/biolreprod61.4.1139] [PMID: 10491655]

[276] Mithraprabhu S, Mendis S, Meachem SJ, *et al.* Activin bioactivity affects germ cell differentiation in the postnatal mouse testis *in vivo.* Biol Reprod 2010; 82(5): 980-90.
[http://dx.doi.org/10.1095/biolreprod.109.079855] [PMID: 20130270]

[277] Tanimoto Y, Tanimoto K, Sugiyama F, *et al.* Male sterility in transgenic mice expressing activin betaA subunit gene in testis. Biochem Biophys Res Commun 1999; 259(3): 699-705.
[http://dx.doi.org/10.1006/bbrc.1999.0833] [PMID: 10364482]

[278] Hasegawa K, Saga Y. Retinoic acid signaling in Sertoli cells regulates organization of the blood-testis barrier through cyclical changes in gene expression. Development 2012; 139(23): 4347-55.
[http://dx.doi.org/10.1242/dev.080119] [PMID: 23095883]

[279] Sugimoto R, Nabeshima Y, Yoshida S. Retinoic acid metabolism links the periodical differentiation of germ cells with the cycle of Sertoli cells in mouse seminiferous epithelium. Mech Dev 2012; 128(11-12): 610-24.
[http://dx.doi.org/10.1016/j.mod.2011.12.003] [PMID: 22200512]

[280] Vernet N, Dennefeld C, Guillou F, Chambon P, Ghyselinck NB, Mark M. Prepubertal testis development relies on retinoic acid but not rexinoid receptors in Sertoli cells. EMBO J 2006; 25(24): 5816-25.
[http://dx.doi.org/10.1038/sj.emboj.7601447] [PMID: 17124491]

[281] Cardoso LC, Nascimento AR, Royer C, Porto CS, Lazari MF. Locally produced relaxin may affect testis and vas deferens function in rats. Reproduction 2010; 139(1): 185-96.
[http://dx.doi.org/10.1530/REP-09-0146] [PMID: 19812235]

[282] Nascimento AR, Pimenta MT, Lucas TF, Royer C, Porto CS, Lazari MF. Intracellular signaling pathways involved in the relaxin-induced proliferation of rat Sertoli cells. Eur J Pharmacol 2012; 691(1-3): 283-91.
[http://dx.doi.org/10.1016/j.ejphar.2012.07.021] [PMID: 22819701]

[283] Skinner MK, McLachlan RI, Bremner WJ. Stimulation of Sertoli cell inhibin secretion by the testicular paracrine factor PModS. Mol Cell Endocrinol 1989; 66(2): 239-49.
[http://dx.doi.org/10.1016/0303-7207(89)90036-1] [PMID: 2515083]

[284] Rosselli M, Skinner MK. Developmental regulation of Sertoli cell aromatase activity and plasminogen activator production by hormones, retinoids and the testicular paracrine factor, PModS. Biol Reprod 1992; 46(4): 586-94.
[http://dx.doi.org/10.1095/biolreprod46.4.586] [PMID: 1576255]

[285] Nehar D, Mauduit C, Boussouar F, Benahmed M. Interleukin 1α stimulates lactate dehydrogenase A expression and lactate production in cultured porcine sertoli cells. Biol Reprod 1998; 59(6): 1425-32.
[http://dx.doi.org/10.1095/biolreprod59.6.1425] [PMID: 9828188]

[286] Xiao X, Mruk DD, Tang EI, *et al.* Environmental toxicants perturb human Sertoli cell adhesive function *via* changes in F-actin organization mediated by actin regulatory proteins. Hum Reprod 2014; 29(6): 1279-91.
[http://dx.doi.org/10.1093/humrep/deu011] [PMID: 24532171]

[287] Zheng W, Pan S, Wang G, *et al.* Zearalenone impairs the male reproductive system functions *via* inducing structural and functional alterations of sertoli cells. Environ Toxicol Pharmacol 2016; 42: 146-55.
[http://dx.doi.org/10.1016/j.etap.2016.01.013] [PMID: 26851377]

[288] Vogl AW, Vaid KS, Guttman JA. The sertoli cell cytoskeleton. In: Cheng CY, Ed. Molecular Mechanisms in Spermatogenesis. New York, NY: Springer New York 2008; pp. 186-211.

[289] Foster PM, Foster JR, Cook MW, Thomas LV, Gangolli SD. Changes in ultrastructure and cytochemical localization of zinc in rat testis following the administration of di-n-pentyl phthalate. Toxicol Appl Pharmacol 1982; 63(1): 120-32.
[http://dx.doi.org/10.1016/0041-008X(82)90031-X] [PMID: 7071867]

[290] Raychoudhury SS, Blake CA, Millette CF. Toxic effects of octylphenol on cultured rat spermatogenic cells and Sertoli cells. Toxicol Appl Pharmacol 1999; 157(3): 192-202.
[http://dx.doi.org/10.1006/taap.1999.8664] [PMID: 10373403]

[291] Boekelheide K. Mechanisms of toxic damage to spermatogenesis. JNCI Monographs 2005; 2005: 6-8.
[http://dx.doi.org/10.1093/jncimonographs/lgi006]

[292] Adhikari N, Sinha N, Saxena DK. Effect of lead on Sertoli-germ cell coculture of rat. Toxicol Lett 2000; 116(1-2): 45-9.
[http://dx.doi.org/10.1016/S0378-4274(00)00199-5] [PMID: 10906421]

[293] Hew KW, Heath GL, Jiwa AH, Welsh MJ. Cadmium *in vivo* causes disruption of tight junction-associated microfilaments in rat Sertoli cells. Biol Reprod 1993; 49(4): 840-9.
[http://dx.doi.org/10.1095/biolreprod49.4.840] [PMID: 8218650]

[294] Janecki A, Jakubowiak A, Steinberger A. Effect of cadmium chloride on transepithelial electrical resistance of Sertoli cell monolayers in two-compartment culturesa new model for toxicological investigations of the blood-testis barrier *in vitro.* Toxicol Appl Pharmacol 1992; 112(1): 51-7.
[http://dx.doi.org/10.1016/0041-008X(92)90278-Z] [PMID: 1733048]

[295] Guerrero-Bosagna C, Savenkova M, Haque MM, Nilsson E, Skinner MK. Environmentally induced epigenetic transgenerational inheritance of altered Sertoli cell transcriptome and epigenome: molecular etiology of male infertility. PLoS One 2013; 8(3): e59922.
[http://dx.doi.org/10.1371/journal.pone.0059922] [PMID: 23555832]

[296] Chapin RE, Gray TJ, Phelps JL, Dutton SL. The effects of mono-(2-ethylhexyl)-phthalate on rat Sertoli cell-enriched primary cultures. Toxicol Appl Pharmacol 1988; 92(3): 467-79.
[http://dx.doi.org/10.1016/0041-008X(88)90186-X] [PMID: 3353991]

[297] Moss EJ, Cook MW, Thomas LV, Gray TJ. The effect of mono-(2-ethylhexyl) phthalate and other phthalate esters on lactate production by Sertoli cells *in vitro.* Toxicol Lett 1988; 40(1): 77-84.
[http://dx.doi.org/10.1016/0378-4274(88)90185-3] [PMID: 3341051]

[298] Thysen B, Morris PL, Gatz M, Bloch E. The effect of mono(2-ethylhexyl) phthalate on Sertoli cell transferrin secretion *in vitro.* Toxicol Appl Pharmacol 1990; 106(1): 154-7.
[http://dx.doi.org/10.1016/0041-008X(90)90115-B] [PMID: 2123578]

[299] Williams J, Foster PM. The production of lactate and pyruvate as sensitive indices of altered rat Sertoli cell function *in vitro* following the addition of various testicular toxicants. Toxicol Appl Pharmacol 1988; 94(1): 160-70.
[http://dx.doi.org/10.1016/0041-008X(88)90346-8] [PMID: 3131928]

[300] Allenby G, Sharpe RM, Foster PM. Changes in Sertoli cell function *in vitro* induced by nitrobenzene. Fundam Appl Toxicol 1990; 14(2): 364-75.
[http://dx.doi.org/10.1016/0272-0590(90)90216-7] [PMID: 2108073]

[301] Monsees TK, Winterstein U, Schill WB, Miska W. Influence of gossypol on the secretory function of cultured rat sertoli cells. Toxicon 1998; 36(5): 813-6.
[http://dx.doi.org/10.1016/S0041-0101(97)00162-1] [PMID: 9655644]

[302] Raychoudhury SS, Flowers AF, Millette CF, Finlay MF. Toxic effects of polychlorinated biphenyls on cultured rat Sertoli cells. J Androl 2000; 21(6): 964-73.
[PMID: 11105924]

[303] Huang HF, Pogach LM, Nathan E, Giglio W. Acute and chronic effects of cisplatinum upon testicular function in the rat. J Androl 1990; 11(5): 436-45.
[PMID: 2254177]

[304] Monsees TK, Franz M, Gebhardt S, Winterstein U, Schill WB, Hayatpour J. Sertoli cells as a target for reproductive hazards. Andrologia 2000; 32(4-5): 239-46.
[http://dx.doi.org/10.1046/j.1439-0272.2000.00391.x] [PMID: 11021515]

[305] Alves MG, Neuhaus-Oliveira A, Moreira PI, Socorro S, Oliveira PF. Exposure to 2,4-dichlorophenoxyacetic acid alters glucose metabolism in immature rat Sertoli cells. Reprod Toxicol 2013; 38: 81-8.
[http://dx.doi.org/10.1016/j.reprotox.2013.03.005] [PMID: 23538319]

CHAPTER 4

Basic Aspects of Spermatogenesis

Bernardo C. Rodrigues[1,2,*] and **Mário Sousa**[2,3]

[1] *Health Sciences Research Center, University of Beira Interior, Rua Marquês d'Ávila e Bolama, 6201-001, Covilhã, Portugal*

[2] *Department of Microscopy, Laboratory of Cell Biology, Institute of Biomedical Sciences Abel Salazar and Unit for Multidisciplinary Research in Biomedicine, University of Porto, Rua de Jorge Viterbo Ferreira, 4050-313, Porto, Portugal*

[3] *Centre for Reproductive Genetics Prof. Alberto Barros (CGR), Av. Bessa. 4100-012 Porto, Portugal*

Abstract: In what male reproduction is concerned, postnatal testis development comprises five sequencial stages: neonatal, infantile, juvenile, peripubertal and late pubertal. Each of these stages is associated with several regulation factors that may directly or indirectly affect them. After full testis differentiation, the individual is ready to commit to spermatogenesis. Spermatogenesis is a highly complex process that aims to produce spermatozoa through three consecutive steps (mitosis, meiosis and spermiogenesis) that culminate in spermiation. All these checkpoints have an intrinsic relationship with the cycle of the seminiferous epithelium, which allows their deeper understanding and integration. Given all the participants involved in spermatogenic cycle, it can be easily realized that there is a need for a controlled environment that maintains its correct development. This is achieved through the interconnected role of hormonal and paracrine/autocrine regulation factors. Each of them target a specific variety of somatic and germ cells, balancing their response in accordance with testis needs. Attention has also been given to the factors that control the genetic environment. In fact, male fertility is associated with a unique and indispensable set of genes, which are naturally influenced by several protein families with transcriptional and/or translational approaches. With this information in mind, the present chapter aims to discuss the most relevant research on the mechanisms involved in the basis of spermatogenesis.

Keywords: Autocrine Regulation, Cycle of the Seminiferous Epithelium, Hormonal Regulation, Male Fertility, Meiosis, Mitosis, Paracrine Regulation, Phases of Spermatogenesis, Postnatal Testis, Regulation of Spermatogenesis, Spermatogenesis, Spermiation, Spermiogenesis, Testis Development, Transcriptional Regulation, Translational Regulation.

* **Corresponding author Bernardo C. Rodrigues:** Av. Infante D. Henrique 6200-506 Covilhã, Portugal; Tel: +351 275 329 002; Fax:+351 275 329 099; E-mail: bernardorodrigues.biomedical@gmail.com

Marco G. Alves and Pedro F. Oliveira (Eds.)

INTRODUCTION

Male fertility is a highly complex concept that involves an evolutionary process, initiating in the embryo and finishing in the adult individual. There are countless moments in which an impairment can occur, so it is pivotal to understand and describe in detail all the hallmarks that contribute to offspring's maintenance.

Mammalian species do not have a fully differentiated and mature sexual organ at birth. In addition, postnatal testis development involves the proliferation and differentiation of somatic and germ cells through five sequential periods: neonatal, infantile, juvenile, peripubertal and late pubertal. Each of these stages is associated with several regulation factors that may directly or indirectly affect them. Any disturbance in these regulators, as seen in some animal models, results in sexual disruption and, in most cases, infertility.

After full differentiation of the testis, male mammals are ready to develop one of the most important biological processes of cellular transformation: spermatogenesis. This event starts at puberty and continues throughout the entire humans' life, with a well-defined goal: the production of spermatozoa, one of the most specialized and capacitated haploid cells. This mechanism involves three consecutive fully characterized steps. Firstly, mitosis, which is associated with the proliferation and differentiation of spermatogonia. Then, meiosis, which represents the reduction of the number of chromosomes (from diploid to haploid). Finally, spermiogenesis, that transforms round spermatids into highly structured spermatozoa. It also must be highlighted the vital role of spermiation, which allows spermatozoa to be released into the lumen of the seminiferous tubule. All these periods have an intrinsic relationship with the cycle of the seminiferous epithelium, which allows their deeper understanding and integration.

With all the participants involved in the spermatogenic cycle, it can be realized that there is a need for a controlled environment that maintain not only the correct growth and differentiation of germ cells, but also the proliferation and function of the somatic ones. This happens through the interconnected role of hormonal and paracrine/autocrine regulation factors. Concerning the hormonal control, the participation of the hypothalamus and pituitary is unquestionable. The hypothalamic secretion of gonadotropin-releasing hormone stimulates the gonadotroph cells in the anterior pituitary that consequently secrete two gonadotrophins, luteinizing hormone and follicle-stimulating hormone. These, latter then, act directly on the testis to stimulate somatic cell function. In the paracrine/autocrine pathway, local metabolites, growth factors and cytokines have been shown to complement the mechanisms under hormonal control. Each of factors target a specific variety of somatic and germ cells, balancing their response in accordance with testis' needs.

Researchers have been giving attention not only to the hormonal and paracrine/autocrine regulation of spermatogenesis, but also to the factors that control the genetic environment. This is because male fertility is associated with a unique set of genes, known as chauvinist genes, which are stimulated by germ cells and encode a set of proteins that are essential for the correct interplay seen in the seminiferous epithelium. The process of gene expression is naturally influenced by several protein families with transcriptional and/or translational approaches.

The present chapter aims to discuss the most relevant findings concerning the mechanisms involved in the basis of spermatogenesis, focusing not only in the regulation of postnatal testis development, but also in the complex and structured mechanisms that occur throughout the spermatogenic cycle.

FACTORS THAT REGULATE POSTNATAL TESTIS DEVELOPMENT

At birth, human testis consist of sex cords with interstitial tissue in between, enclosed in a capsule. The cords, which give rise to the seminiferous tubules where the spermatozoa are formed, contain gonocytes, precursors of the germ cells, and the undifferentiated cells, precursors of the Sertoli cells. The interstitial tissue contains fetal-type Leydig cells.

During postnatal testis development, five time periods are recognized in male mammals. These stages include the neonatal, infantile, juvenile, peripubertal and late pubertal periods [1]. In rat, the neonatal period (postnatal days, PNDs 0–7) is the time of transition from fetal gonocytes to mitotically active spermatogonia, high rate of Sertoli cells mitosis and maturation and replacement of fetal Leydig cells by progenitor Leydig cells. The infantile period (PNDs 8–20) is the time when Sertoli cells cease to divide, the tubules start to segregate into stages and spermatocyte development occurs. The juvenile period (PNDs 21–32) is characterized by maintenance of the first wave of spermatogenesis to round spermatids and dramatic increase in tubular diameter. During the peripubertal period (PNDs 33–55) there is active spermiogenesis, as tubular diameter continues to expand and spermatids develop. During the late pubertal period (PNDs 56–70) there is continued growth of the testis and morphological features, consistent with the appearance of a normal adult testis [2]. Along this process, there are innumerous regulators identified as pivotal to the correct development of postnatal testis. The following information synthetize some of that elements.

Follicle-Stimulating Hormone (FSH)

FSH is a gonadotropin synthesized and secreted by the anterior pituitary gland. This hormone was shown to have some crucial function on testis development, mainly due to its influence in Sertoli cells during perinatal period [3]. FSH induces androgen receptors (AR) expression on Sertoli cells, which begins by PNDs 4 to 6 in the rat [4, 5] and reaches a density maximum at PNDs 10 to 15 [6]. During the late infantile period, serum FSH levels decline, due to the continually rising levels of inhibin, reaching a nadir by PND 18. Then, serum FSH levels increase again throughout the juvenile period, reaching a peak at PND 26 [7]. This peak is known to be critical for the final maturation, function and survival of Leydig cells, as shown by FSH-receptor (FSH-R) ablation studies [8, 9].

To enable comprehensive analysis on the impact of FSH on Sertoli and germ cell development, this gonadotropin was suppressed in Sprague–Dawley rats. Acute suppression of FSH resulted in decreased testis weights in 9 and 18 PND rats, which was attributed to the decreased Sertoli cell population at PND 9 and a decreased germ cell population in PND 18. These data demonstrated that FSH differentially affects Sertoli and germ cells in an age-dependent manner, promoting Sertoli cell mitosis at day 9, and supporting germ cell viability at day 18 [10]. Concomitant studies showed that high serum FSH levels during postnatal period are very important to facilitate germ cell transition from gonocyte to spermatogonia [11]. Finally, a recent new investigation defended that FSH treatment increase length of the seminiferous cords and testicular weight by increasing first the early proliferation of peritubular cells and later also the proliferation of the Sertoli cells [12].

Luteinizing Hormone (LH)

LH is a gonadotropin produced in the anterior pituitary gland. It acts through LH-receptor (LH-R) which is mainly expressed in Leydig cells [13]. LH-R knockout (KO) mice models frequently show normal sexual development until birth, but postnatally their testicular growth and descent as well as external genital and accessory sex organ maturation are blocked [14]. This sugests that LH/LH-R signaling is not essential for fetal testis development, but it is very important after male birth [15]. Complementing this information, studies using a similar model showed that, after birth, LH-R null mice contained the same number of Sertoli cells, spermatogonia, and early spermatocytes as wild-type siblings, but contained smaller and less Leydig cells [16]. This information allowed further studies to focus in understanding how LH could contribute to postnatal Leydig cell development.

Differentiation of the Leydig cell population starts in rodent testes around the second postnatal week [17]. This developmental process consists of multiple steps, in which undifferentiated mesenchymal precursor cells are transformed into mature adult Leydig cells with steroidogenic potential. Evidence from several lines of investigations showed that LH is not required at the onset of Leydig cell differentiation, although it is essential to induce the steroidogenic function in the later stages of Leydig cell lineage. In fact, at the time of mesenchymal cell proliferation and differentiation into Leydig cell progenitors, the serum LH level is quite low and it does not begin to rise until much later [7]. Complementing information focusing toward the end of the juvenile period showed that LH rising levels are very important in the later stages in the lineage, i.e., proliferation of progenitors and their differentiation until mature adult Leydig cells [17]. In conclusion, LH action is not essential for the differentiation and function of mouse fetal Leydig cells and mesenchymal cells after birth, but it is crucial in the later stages of Leydig cells maturation. It should also be highlighted the major role of LH as an indirect regulator of testosterone postnatal functions.

Testosterone

Testosterone, an androgen, is a steroid hormone that in the testis is produced by Leydig cells, as a consequence of LH stimulation. Its action is mediated by AR, which are expressed in Leydig, Sertoli and peritubular cells [18]. It is well established that androgens play the central role in masculinization of the reproductive tract and genitalia during the sexual differentiation process in the male. More specifically, it was shown that they play an essential role in the morphological and functional differentiation of the somatic testicular cells, prior to the onset of spermatogenic activity.

As previously mentioned, Leydig cells differentiation process is known to be under the strict control of LH. Additionally, some studies demonstrated that exogenous administration of testosterone increases AR expression on these cells, identifying testosterone as an important collaborator of LH in the process [19].

Concurrently to what happens with Leydig cells, Sertoli cells also have to undergo a maturation process during postnatal period, where they lose the ability to proliferate and switch-on various functions that are essential for the support of germ cells during spermatogenesis [5]. There are several lines of evidence that point to a role for androgens in these events. Such a role seems intrinsically logical when considering that maturation and acquisition of full androgen responsiveness are prerequisites for Sertoli cells to support full spermatogenesis in adulthood [20]. Recent data consolidated this information, showing that AR-null mice present reduced Sertoli cell number at birth and that these numbers remain significantly lower than normal up to adulthood. This result highlighted the role of testosterone in Sertoli cell proliferation during fetal and early neonatal life, in the regulation of late stages of Sertoli cell proliferation and in the requirement for specific transcript expression during prepubertal development [21].

Further studies using seminiferous tubules of prepubertal rats grown under the influence of testosterone concluded that this steroid hormone also contributes to the maturation and functioning of peritubular cells [22]. In fact, newborn mouse testis implanted in hypophysectomized hosts and treated with testosterone exhibited some of the changes observed during normal peritubular cell development [23]. However, the failure of testosterone alone to induce normal maturation of the peritubular tissue suggested that other pituitary hormones may also be required.

Finally, it can also be pointed out that testosterone accelerates the development of the seminiferous tubules lumen of the rat, which is consistent with the reports about the differentiation of the various cell types comprising the tubule [24].

Activin A and Inhibin B

Activin A and inhibin B are two closely related protein complexes and members of the transforming growth factor (TGF)-β superfamily. They were initially identified by their ability to regulate FSH secretion at the pituitary, showing opposite biological effects. Activin A concentration significantly declines between PNDs 0 and 1 in male mice, concomitantly with the start of gonocyte proliferation [25]. Subsequently, its level raises to peak at PND 3, after which the first spermatogonial stem cells appear. These observations suggest a dual role of activin A: first, as an inducer of mitotic arrest and then, as an inducer of mitotic proliferation of gonocytes [26]. Activin A also has a mitogenic action on Sertoli cells, evident from the observations of delayed fertility in male mice, smaller testis size and reduced sperm output following deletion of the activin type II receptor [27]. Inhibin B is produced by Sertoli cells and Leydig cells in the adult [28]. Total testicular levels in mice raise from PND 0 to a peak at PND 4, which reflects a period of Sertoli cells proliferation that culminates in the formation of a stable, non-mitotic Sertoli cells population. Thus, inhibin B is suggested to play a critical role in the modulation of activin-induced Sertoli cells proliferation. Studies in men and adolescent boys with Klinefelter syndrome, which have low levels of inhibin B, showed normal testis histology in infancy, but later degeneration of the germ cell tissue [29].

Hepatocyte Growth Factor (HGF)

HGF is one of the growth factors regulating mammalian testicular development.

The multiple actions of HGF are transduced by its receptor, c-met, a transmembrane glycoprotein detectable in peritubular cells and Sertoli cells isolated from pubertal animals [30]. Interestingly, c-met expressing Sertoli cells cultured on reconstituted basement membrane, reorganize into cord-like structures [30], demonstrating that the system is functionally active and is involved in testis development and function. This finding illustrates a role for HGF in the regulation of germ cells that are differentiating during the same period and also in lumen formation in the tubules.

Thyroid Hormone (TH)

Although the main role of TH is to stimulate the oxidative metabolism in many tissues in the body, recent findings provide clear evidence that 3,5,3'-triiodothyronine (T3) is an important regulator of neonatal testis development. It is established that T3 control Sertoli cells and Leydig cells proliferation and differentiation during testicular development in rat and other mammal species [31, 32]. This is effected through TH receptors (TRα1 and TRβ1), present in human and rat testis from neonatal to adult life [33]. The TRα1 expression was found to be maximal in late fetal and early neonatal life and restricted to Sertoli cells, suggesting these as the main target cells for T3 action in testis. Nevertheless, other TR isoforms, including TRβ1, are also found in Leydig cells, peritubular cells, and germ cells [34 - 36]. T3 is responsible for neonatal Sertoli cells to differentiate from a mitogenic to a non-mitogenic/secretory state, characteristic of more mature animals. In fact, transient neonatal hypothyroidism results in an increase in adult testis weight and daily sperm production in rats. This increase results from prolonged Sertoli cells mitogenesis, leading to increased adult Sertoli cells populations [37, 38]. Other studies showed that hypothyroidism increases germ cell degeneration and blocks the progression of germ cells after the spermatid stage [39, 40], an effect that reflects impaired Sertoli cells function. Concomitantly, transient juvenile hyperthyroidism results in an early cessation of Sertoli cells proliferation and in a strong stimulatory effect on their maturation, decreasing testis size and sperm production [41, 42]. Subsequent studies have demonstrated a similar behavior for Leydig cells. It is known that neonatal hypothyroidism induces mitogenic effects by arresting Leydig cells differentiation and allowing continuous proliferation of precursor mesenchymal cells that accumulate in the interstitium [43]. Conversely, hyperthyroidism was shown to stimulate the differentiation of mesenchymal cells into progenitor Leydig cells and the increase of mesenchymal cells number produced in prepubertal rat testis.

SRY-Related Box (SOX) Family

Members of the SOX family are proteins that have been conserved during the evolution of vertebrates, having a role as transcription factors. As well as playing an important role during fetal development, they have also been identified in various postnatal tissues. Much remains unknown about the role of these transcription factors after birth. One of the most studied SOX members is *Sox9* . Previous findings have established that *Sox9* expression is tightly associated with Sertoli cells development and its expression remains exclusively in Sertoli cells after testis cord formation [44]. A conditional KO model with *Sox9* inactivation at embryonic days, after the sex determination stage, only leads to late-onset sterility, showing that mutant male mice have normal embryonic and early postnatal development and are initially fertile, but become sterile at 5 to 6 months [45]. This provides evidence that the protein is dispensable for embryonic testis differentiation, but essential for maintaining the proper postnatal reproductive ability.

Anti-Müllerian Hormone (AMH)

AMH is a protein with a well-known impact on male reproductive development, highlighted by its important role inhibiting the development of the Müllerian ducts in the male embryo. Mice AMH expression is elevated in Sertoli cells before pubertal onset, until 6th PND, drop significantly from 7th to 13th PND and reach levels near its lowest limit of detection from day 15 onwards [46]. It shows some important functions in postnatal mouse testis, like in Leydig cells steroidogenesis [47] and maturation of gonocytes to spermatogonia [48]. A possible involvement of AMH in Leydig cells development was also revealed. Transgenic mice that chronically overexpress human AMH have undescended testes, are incompletely masculinized externally, and rapidly become infertile [49].

Estrogens

The effects of estrogens are mediated primarily by nuclear estrogen receptors (ERs), ERα and ERβ, which are both expressed in testicular cells of several species [50]. While both ERα and ERβ were identified in Leydig cells, spermatocytes and round spermatids, only ERβ was found in Sertoli cells and spermatogonia [18, 51, 52]. The absence of mature Leydig cells in testes of rats who received a single injection of 17β-estradiol (E2) at PND 5 [53] suggested that Leydig cells development is sensitive to estrogens. In fact, testicular estrogen levels decline during the period between 10th and 21st PND [54], which correspond with the onset of precursor cell differentiation into progenitors and then to the early adult Leydig cells. Some studies with ERα KO models also pointed out a parallel increase in testosterone production during this period [55]. Further investigation showed that mice inactivation of ERβ gene induce a 50% increase in the number of gonocytes observed, due to an increase in the proliferation and a decrease in the apoptosis of these cells [56]. These data clearly show that endogenous estrogens inhibit testicular development and control steroidogenesis during neonatal life.

Insulin-Like Growth Factor (IGF)-1

IGF-1 is a protein belonging to the insulin-like growth factor family, which is characterized by high sequence similarity to insulin. It is proved that IGF-1 has stimulatory effects on Leydig cells differentiation. Studies provided clear evidence that testosterone production is significantly reduced in IGF1-null mice and this deficiency is associated with a significant developmental delay in Leydig cells and altered LH-stimulated androgen secretion *in vitro* [57]. It is also known that the administration of IGF-I increases testicular LH receptors and LH-stimulated biosynthesis of androgens from immature type Leydig cells in mice characterized by low circulatory growth hormone and testosterone levels, delayed puberty, and poor response to exogenous gonadotropins [58].

PHASES OF SPERMATOGENESIS

Spermatogenesis typically defines a complex biological process of cellular transformation that starts at puberty and continues throughout the entire humans' life. It represents the differentiation of diploid cells (spermatogonia), into haploid cells (spermatozoa), over an extended period of time. This is a well-balanced mechanism subdivided into three consecutive steps, described below and summarized in Fig. (**4.1**). It starts with the proliferation and differentiation of spermatogonia by the process of mitosis. Then, it is followed by the reduction of the chromosome number from diploid to haploid, by the process of meiosis. Finally, it ends with the transformation of round spermatids into the complex structure of the spermatozoon, by the process of spermiogenesis. The following text synthetizes each one of these periods in detail.

Mitosis

The mitotic stage is a precise sequence of divisions that involves the proliferation and maintenance of spermatogonia, the most immature germ cell. The self-renewal capacity of spermatogonia allows not only the production of stem cells that remain along the base of the seminiferous tubule, but also the differentiation in a one-way tract to spermatozoa. The number of spermatogonial types that have been identified varies amongst the different mammalian species. In humans, A pale, A dark and B spermatogonial forms can be distinguished [59]. The identification of the actual mechanism of spermatogonial restoration still remains a matter of debate.

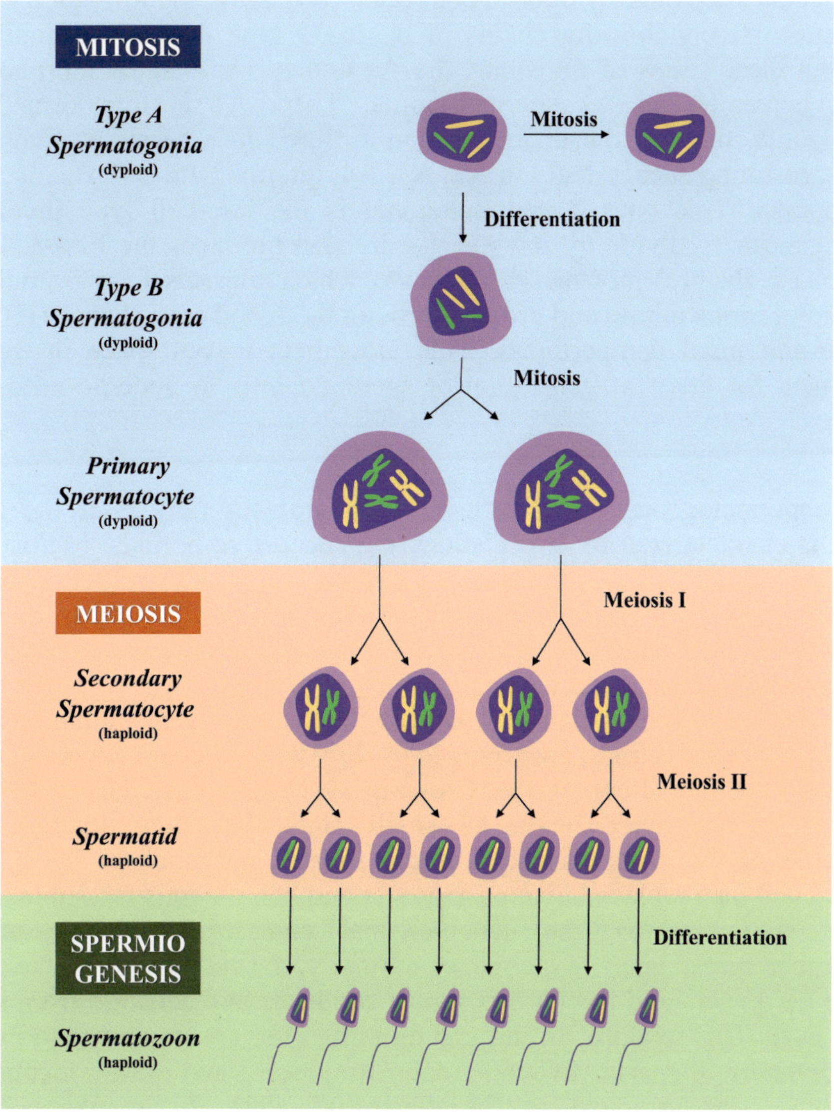

Fig. (4.1). Schematic representation of the stages of spermatogenesis. In the mitotic phase, spermatogonia undergo either self-renewal or differentiation, with both processes involving successive mitotic divisions. In turn, type B spermatogonia differentiate into primary spermatocytes that enter meiosis. The first meiotic division originates secondary spermatocytes. These cells enter a second meiotic division and produce two spermatids genetically unique. Spermatids undergo morphological changes, associated with spermiogenesis, and highly differentiated spermatozoa are produced.

During the mitotic process, the undifferentiated type A spermatogonia divides, originating two new single cells (As) or a paired spermatogonia (Ap). The Ap was titled that way because, in the mechanism of mitosis, the two newly formed spermatogonia keep their cytoplasm connected [60]. After the formation of Ap, it divides successively forming chains of up to 32 type A spermatogonia (Aa). Continuing these series of divisions, the Aa undergo associated morphological changes, becoming an A1 spermatogonia. Then, A1 is transformed in B spermatogonia, through the differentiation suffered in a series of five mitotic divisions, resulting successively in A2, A3, A4, intermediate and, finally, type B spermatogonia. This type B spermatogonia is the last cell type involved in spermatogenesis to divide by mitosis. Its division produces the first cell of the meiotic phase, the preleptotene spermatocyte, which migrates away from the base of the seminiferous tubule and crosses through the blood-testis barrier (BTB), to enter the adluminal compartment. This movement leaves space in the basal compartment for the next generation of spermatogonia to undergo mitosis.

Meiosis

Pursuing spermatogenesis, preleptotene spermatocytes (2n) enter the meiotic phase. It is characterized by two distinct and successive periods: Meiosis I and Meiosis II, both including prophase, metaphase, anaphase, and telophase. The Prophase I of the first meiotic division may last for nearly three weeks and is subdivided in five stages: leptotene, zygotene, pachytene, diplotene and diakinesis. During the leptotene stage, the chromosomes begin to condense and become structured in long filaments. During the zygotene stage, the homologous chromosomes, called tetrads, are arranged linearly by a process known as synapsis and form synaptonemal complexes. Crossing over takes place during this phase. Pachytene spermatocytes begin as small cells, but their nuclei enlarge significantly as the chromosomes become shorter and thicken. Synapses are completed and then replaced by crossing-over and homologous recombination. In diplotene spermatocytes, the synaptonemal complexes dissolve and the chromosomes spread apart in the nucleus. Finally, during diakinesis, the nuclear envelope disappears and the chromosomes condense and separate from sites of crossing over. This random sorting and crossing over are important to maintain genetic diversity in sperm [61 - 63]. After prophase I and during metaphase I, chromosomes are arranged in the equatorial plate. In anaphase I, each chromosome consists of two chromatids migrating to opposite poles. Finally, in telophase I, cell division occurs with the formation of secondary spermatocytes with half the number of chromosomes of spermatogenesis. After the first meiotic division, each daughter cell contains only one partner of the homologous chromosome pairs, being called secondary spermatocyte (n), but the DNA is double (2n), because of the presence of sister chromatids.

The second meiotic division lasts a short period of time. It is during this period that each secondary spermatocyte produces two spermatids (n) genetically unique, with a haploid number of single chromosomes. At the end of telophase of Meiosis II, the spermatids do not completely separate but remain interconnected for synchronous development. It can be postulated that each primary spermatocyte can theoretically give origin to four spermatids, although fewer actually do, as the complexity of meiosis is associated with a loss of some germ cells. To originate spermatozoa, these spermatids undergo a complete process of differentiation, known as spermiogenesis.

Spermiogenesis

Spermiogenesis is the third and final stage of spermatogenesis. It is a series of differentiation events that induce morphological transformations, turning spherical haploid spermatids into elongated, highly condensed and mature spermatozoa. Based on the biogenesis of individual sperm accessory structures and on the progression of sperm nuclear condensation, spermiogenesis can be divided into distinct steps, identified by arabic numerals. Individual authors distinguish up to 19 steps in rats, 16 steps in mice, 14 steps in primates, 12 steps in carnivores and 6 steps in humans [64]. The following information is mostly based on studies focused on mouse models.

In step 1 spermatids, the nucleus condenses and migrates to the periphery of the cell. In this premature point of spermiogenesis, spermatids present a perinuclear Golgi apparatus region without an acrosome vesicle or granule. In the following steps 2 and 3, there is a marked development of the Golgi apparatus, which will be important to produce vesicles and granules containing the enzymatic components of the acrosomic system that will later surround the developing spermatozoon nucleus. The hydrolytic enzymes contained in the acrosomic system are required for sperm-egg interaction and fertilization. Between steps 4 and 8, the acrosomic granule caps the nuclear surface, becoming thinner and flattened [65]. In late step 8, the nuclei begin to change their shape, elongating. It is worth to mention that during the elongation period, there is an active transcription of several mRNAs, which are kept in a translationally repressed state. They are required later in spermiogenesis, when nuclear elongation ceases all transcriptional activity [66]. Steps 9 to 14 involve the migration of the acrosomal system over the ventral surface of the elongating spermatid nucleus. These spermatid steps also involve sperm head shaping and nuclear hypercondensation. This is achieved by the replacement of histones with transitional proteins (highly basic and small lysine-arginine-rich proteins), that help in the transformation of the nucleosomal chromatin into smooth condensed chromatin fibers [67]. These transitional proteins are later replaced by protamines, the key sperm nuclear proteins [68]. Concomitantly, the spermatid centrosome, composed by two perpendicularly apposed centrioles and a halo of microtubule-nucleating pericentriolar material, is reduced to a single, proximal centriole, embedded in a dense mass of capitulum [69]. This is achieved by the degradation of the distal centriole, which contributes for the growth of the axoneme. The axoneme consists on a series of equally spaced doublet microtubules surrounding two single central microtubules, being very important for the development of the flagella. During spermiogenesis, this structure becomes lodged at the acrosomal pole of the nucleus, forming the neck of the spermatozoon. Later, during the formation of the tail, the axoneme is modified by the development of a series of nine electron-dense fibers, named the outer dense fibers, in the region of the midpiece of the spermatozoon and distally by the formation of the fibrous sheath in the region of the major piece. It must be highlighted that the central filamentous core composing the midpiece is coated by a spiral structure that results from the fusion of individual mitochondria. The local presence of these organelles is vital for ATP production and, consequently, for flagellar movement [62]. ATP is obtained through glucose and fructose oxidative phosphorylation, so any alteration in the ability of spermatozoa to metabolize these substrates and produce ATP compromises sperm quality and thus, male fertility [70]. The final maturation steps 15 and 16 show only a few changes in nuclear and acrosomal migration. The nucleus continues to condense and the acrosome matures into a thin structure that projects at the apex, but covers nearly all the nucleus, except for that portion connected to the tail [71].

Spermiation

Spermiation is one of the fundamental steps in the development of mature and fertile spermatozoa. Because there is no consensus on the inclusion or not of spermiation as the final stage of spermatogenesis [61, 62, 72], we approach it as an independent event.

Spermiation is initiated after spermiogenesis, when the majority of late spermatids align along the luminal edge at the beginning of stage VII in rats and mice. It is the process by which mature spermatids are released from the support of Sertoli cells, into the lumen of the seminiferous tubule. It involves several interconnected hallmarks: extension of the spermatid into the tubule lumen; removal of specialized adhesion junctions, including the ectoplasmic specialization (ES); formation and degradation of tubulobulbar complexes (TBCs); retraction of the Sertoli cell cytoplasm from around the spermatid and, finally, the disengagement of the spermatid into the tubule lumen.

Before spermiation starts, the elongated spermatids, formed during spermiogenesis, are engulfed in Sertoli cell crypts. To be released, they must firstly be translocated to the luminal edge of the epithelium. This transport is facilitated by the Sertoli cell cytoskeleton and, more importantly, by the ES junctional plaque [73, 74]. ES is established between Sertoli cell cytoplasm and round spermatids and remains associated with elongating spermatids until the beginning of spermiation [75]. It is comprised of hexagonally-packed actin filaments sandwiched between the Sertoli cell membrane and the underlying endoplasmic reticulum [76]. Besides effectively translocating the spermatid to the luminal edge, ES is also involved in the stabilization of intercellular adhesion junctions [77]. After the translocation process, specialized structures called TBCs form between the spermatid and the Sertoli cell. These structures first appear as a bristle coated pit containing clathrin, a protein involved in endocytosis and in TBCs formation [78]. Then, TBCs elongate into the classic structure, including a tubular region surrounded by actin, a bulbous portion surrounded by endoplasmic reticulum, and a clathrin-coated tip. TBCs formation was found to be associated with areas where ES is absent, which is consistent with the proposition that TBCs main function is the ES disassembly [79]. TBCs also have been proposed to play a key role in final sperm head/acrosome remodelling and in the reduction of the spermatid cytoplasm volume [80, 81]. After TBCs formation, there is a change in the connection between spermatids and the Sertoli cells. The spermatid head and the flagella are pushed out into the tubule lumen, in a way that Sertoli cell cytoplasm only contacts a small portion of the spermatid head. In the other hand, the spermatid cytoplasm remains attached to the Sertoli cell so by the end of stage VII, it is located below the level of the spermatid head and becomes more condensed. Spermiation ends when the spermatids disengage from the Sertoli cell and are released into the lumen of the seminiferous tubule, whereupon they are referred to as spermatozoa. The excess of the spermatid's cytoplasm condenses to form the residual body that undergoes phagocytosis by Sertoli cells [82, 83].

Spermatogenesis and the Cycle of the Seminiferous Epithelium

As previously mentioned, during spermiogenesis, germ cells undergo changes through 6, 16 and 19 steps in humans, mice and rats, respectively, before transforming into spermatozoa. These germ cells are restricted to spatial units of the seminiferous epithelium, referred as stages and designated by roman numerals. Several steps occur together to form a stage, and several stages are necessary to form a mature spermatozoon from an immature stem cell. The cycle of the seminiferous epithelium refers to the synchronous evolution of one stage of spermatogenesis to the next or a complete and ordered series of cell stages, which occur at a given segment of a seminiferous epithelium over time. Similarly to what happens with the steps, the division of the stages of the seminiferous epithelium is different for each specie (I–VI, I–XII and I–XIV in human, mouse and rat, respectively).

There are several causes, both intrinsic and extrinsic, for the germ cells to be arranged in distinct stages. In fact, cellular associations suggesting specific stages have been found as early as 10th PND [84], which is about the same time that AR begin to be expressed in early Sertoli cells, showing that these cells regulate the formation of stages. Concomitantly, investigations using vitamin A deficient rats showed an arrest of spermatogenesis, with type A1 spermatogonia differentiation inhibited [85, 86]. Thus, in this model, it appears that the regulation involves both Sertoli and germ cell responses to vitamin A. In fact, a retinoic acid receptor KO (RARα-/-) mouse model further revealed that vitamin A may be involved in the initial establishment of stages and their long-term regulation, which also appears to be stage-specific [87]. There are also numerous studies showing stage specific expression of proteins and dependences upon androgens and FSH, with these factors having a greater influence just before spermiation in stage VIII [88 - 91].

With respect to mice, it has been reported that steps 1–8 spermatids are present at the stages I–VIII of the seminiferous epithelial cycle, and the initial elongating spermatids (step 9 spermatids) are visible at stage IX. During stages VII–VIII, adhesive connections between Sertoli cells and spermatids are remodeled as these last ones start to elongate. At this stage of development, desmosome-based connections between Sertoli cells and the less mature germ cells are replaced by the stronger ES adhesion complexes, which are specific for elongated spermatids. Subsequent steps of elongation are established during stages X–XII and the mature step 16 spermatids are finally released into the lumen during spermiation at stage VIII [62]. Spermatozoa then continues its maturation through the rete testis, efferent ducts and epididymis, before becoming totally fertile in the female reproductive tract.

REGULATION OF SPERMATOGENESIS CYCLE

The complexity of the spermatogenic event exposes many hallmark mechanisms in which an impairment can occur. Thus, there is an increased necessity to maintain not only the proper growth and differentiation of germ cells, but also the proliferation and function of the somatic cells in the seminiferous epithelium. This regulation is achieved mainly through the action of two endocrine factors, LH and FSH, which are components of the hypothalamic-pituitary gonadal (HPG) axis. Additionally, there are also evidence that support the need for the secretion of local factors (paracrine and autocrine) by Sertoli cells, Leydig cells, peritubular cells and germ cells.

Hormonal Regulators

Within the HPG axis, neurons of the hypothalamus produce the decapeptide gonadotropin-releasing hormone (GnRH) that enters the hypothalamic-pituitary portal system. It is characteristically secreted in a pulsatile mode and it stimulates the gonadotroph cells in the anterior pituitary expressing the GnRH receptors. The gonadotroph cells consequently secrete two gonadotrophins, FSH and LH, which act directly on the testis to stimulate the distinct somatic cells that support spermatogenesis.

FSH

FSH action is mediated by its receptor, FSH-R, which is exclusively expressed in Sertoli cells [92]. There are several studies highlighting the relevance of FSH in the maintenance of the spermatogenic event. Its role starts during the prepubertal period, in which FSH influences Sertoli cells proliferation. Given the fact that Sertoli cells population determines, in a direct way, the number of germ cells undergoing spermatogenesis at a given time [88], one can conclude that FSH contributes to the regulation of germ cell number in the adult individual. This concept is corroborated by targeted mutations in the murine FSH-R, which led to dramatically reduced testes weight (due to reduced Sertoli cell population) and epididymal spermatozoa numbers [93 - 95]. Nevertheless, the animals maintained normal sexual development illustrating that, in rodents, the absence of FSH only affects spermatogenesis quantitatively. Furthermore, studies with FSH-R KO mice and FSH KO mice also presented a significant increase in germ cell death [96, 97], suggesting that this gonadotropin acts also as a germ cell apoptosis suppressor [98, 99]. While it is clear that FSH is involved at multiple stages of spermatogenesis by promoting germ cell survival and differentiation up to round spermatids, it should be noted that spermatid elongation cannot be restored by FSH, illustrating the need for additional factors at more advanced stages [100, 101]. Finally, FSH was also shown to be important in regulating spermiation process. Studies using gonadotropin suppression, resulted in spermiation failure, in which spermatids are not released, but instead are retained and phagocytosed by the Sertoli cell [102, 103]. That spermiation failure is caused by a dysfunction in the final disengagement of spermatids from the Sertoli cell [104].

LH

LH induces the production of testosterone by Leydig cells through LH-receptor (LH-R) [13]. Since these cells are located in the testicular interstitial space, testosterone needs to diffuse into the seminiferous tubules in order to exert its biological activity. The control of this hormone synthesis is suggested to be the only vital function of LH within the adult testis.

Testosterone

Testosterone is one of the most important regulators of spermatogenesis and its testicular levels in men and rodents are 25 to 125-fold higher than those observed in serum [105]. Testosterone action is mediated by AR, which are expressed in Leydig, Sertoli and peritubular cells [18]. This distribution provides evidence that this hormone does not act directly in germ cells, but indirectly through somatic cells. Studies about testosterone withdrawal from rat testes showed increased germ cell apoptosis, namely spermatogonia and spermatocytes [106 - 108]. These data suggest that testosterone in some way may function as a cell survival factor, protecting germ cells from apoptotic death. Concomitantly, mice in which AR from Sertoli cells were lost (SCARKO mice) showed a spermatogenic arrest at the late spermatocyte stage [109, 110], indicating that cell autonomous action of the AR in Sertoli cells is an absolute requirement for androgens to maintain complete spermatogenesis. Other studies focusing in the absence of testosterone showed that there is a loss of pachytene spermatocytes and round spermatids between stages VII–VIII [111 - 113], which are known to be particularly sensitive to androgen withdrawal [114]. Recent data indicates that this germ cell loss is due to a failure of Sertoli cells to produce N-cadherin [115]. This adhesion molecule is part of the ES that develops between Sertoli cells and round spermatids at the onset of the elongation process. In the absence of testosterone, this junction is disrupted, leading to the loss of spermatid adhesion and causing their premature release [116]. Alongside, some studies pointed out that testosterone suppression induces the phagocytosis of elongated spermatozoa that fail to disengage from Sertoli cells, revealing that androgens also have a role in spermiation [114]. With that in mind, it was found that testosterone loss causes overexpression of certain proteins, namely SPARC (secreted protein acidic and rich in cysteine), that modules focal adhesions; CTGF (connective tissue growth factor), that modulates adhesion and interacts with integrins that form contacts with elongated spermatids; and LGALS1 (beta-galactoside-binding protein), that surrounds spermatids during spermiation and can modulate integrin-mediated adhesion and signaling [117]. It is also worth mentioning that while androgens have a positive regulatory influence on differentiating germ cells, there is a well-established negative effect of androgens on the differentiation of spermatogonial stem cells [118].

The apparent different roles interplayed by FSH and testosterone make it understandable to think that they act independently and with different goals. However, these hormones have cooperative and synergistic effects, promoting maximal quantitative spermatogenic output [119]. FSH and testosterone cooperativity is apparent in that they act at different phases of spermatogenesis. For example and as previously mentioned, FSH is involved in increasing the number of spermatogonia available, whereas testosterone is involved in spermatid maturation. Other reports identified the ability of either hormone to stimulate or maintain spermatogenesis when even low levels of the other are present [120]. In particular, there appears to be a strong case for a potentiating effect of FSH on androgen action [121]. Another major site of androgen and FSH cooperativity is the prevention of apoptosis of germ cell, particularly of spermatocytes and round spermatids. Germ cell survival during gonadotropin withdrawal could be maintained by either hormone alone, but the combination of both androgens and FSH had a synergistic effect [122]. Spermiation also seems to be supported by both FSH and Testosterone. When either androgen or FSH was suppressed in adult rats, Sertoli cells failed to release approximately 10% of elongated spermatids. However, the suppression of both hormones in combination had a much bigger impact in which 50% of the spermatids failed to be released [103]. Taken together, it seems likely that androgen and FSH regulate distinct and overlapping functions in Sertoli cells which cooperate to support different aspects of germ cell development.

Estrogens

Although estrogens are frequently labeled as the female hormones, E2 plays an important role in the maintenance of male fertility [50]. This is evident from the presence of ER in the seminiferous epithelium. As previously described in this chapter, while both ERα and ERβ were identified in Leydig cells, spermatocytes and round spermatids, only ERβ was found in Sertoli cells and spermatogonia [18, 51, 52]. In fact, male mice lacking ERα are infertile, exhibiting severe impairment of spermatogenesis and dramatically decreased epididymal sperm counts [123]. Subsequent studies demonstrated that the diameter of the seminiferous tubules is increased and the architecture of the germinal epithelium is disrupted in those animals. The underlying cause for this spermatogenic defect is the reduced fluid resorption in the efferent ducts, causing back pressure in the testis and dilution of the sperm travelling to the epididymis [124]. Hence, it has been suggested that a key function of E2 in the male reproductive tract is the regulation of luminal fluid reabsorption in the rete testis and efferent ducts. Further investigation about E2 exogenous treatment and ER agonists treatment showed decreased sperm counts [125, 126]. An elegant investigation tried to identify the mechanisms involved in these results [127]. It showed that, in one hand, administration of ERα agonist caused an arrest in differentiation of round spermatids into elongated spermatids, mainly due to down-regulation of genes involved in spermiogenesis: Transition Protein 1 (TNP1) and 2 (TNP2), and Protamine (PRM1). In the other hand, administration of ERβ agonist caused a spermiation failure and spermatocyte apoptosis [127], which was corroborated by E2 treatment studies [125, 128]. The observed spermiation failure was attributed to defects in TBCs formation [129] and the increase in spermatocyte apoptosis was attributed to an increase in oxidative stress [130]. Yet, there are some studies identifying E2 as a survival factor on germ cells [131, 132]. With that in mind, it is worth mentioning that E2 effects, inhibiting or promoting apoptosis, may strictly depend on the hormonal levels [133].

Paracrine and Autocrine Regulators

Beyond the hormonal factors, there is increasing evidence that a multiplicity of metabolites, growth factors and cytokines are involved in local control mechanisms that influence spermatogenesis. Some are briefly discussed in the next paragraphs.

Metabolites and Associated Factors

Pyruvate, acetate and lactate are metabolic precursors produced by Sertoli cells and required for germ cell metabolism, as will be discussed in the following chapters. These metabolites are important not only for ATP production, but also for the differentiation and survival of developing germ cells [134]. Moreover, Sertoli cells also abundantly produce transferrin, ceruloplasmin and the androgen binding protein (ABP). The first two have an important role in iron and copper transport into germ cells, respectively. ABP is thought to regulate spermatogenesis by maintaining high androgen levels in the testis and epididymis [135, 136]. Testicular ABP production is known to be influenced by testosterone and FSH, since gonadotrophin deficiency lowers ABP content [137, 138]. In fact, testosterone levels and AR expression are maximal prior to the onset of spermatid elongation (stages VII-VIII) and ABP levels are highest during the final stages of spermatid maturation (stages VIII-XI) in the rodent testis [19]. The presence of ABP in Sertoli cell processes that surround the elongated spermatids has suggested that its high affinity for androgens contributes to the generation of high androgen concentrations in the vicinity of certain meiotic germ cells [139]. Other studies involving mice overexpressing ABP exhibited reduced fertility and focal spermatogenic dysfunction, suggesting that elevated levels of this binding protein might capture and prevent androgens from acting on germ cells [140].

Growth Factors

Activin and inhibin are two closely related protein complexes expressed and secreted by the testis. They are produced in Sertoli cells [141] and due to their structural homology to TGF-β, both have been implicated in the regulation of germ cell proliferation and differentiation. It is known that activin can stimulate spermatogonial proliferation *in vivo* and *in vitro* [142]. In contrast, testicular administration of inhibin results in a significant reduction in spermatogonial numbers in the testes of adult mice and chinese hamsters [143]. The action of these growth factors is also related with the regulation of the HPG axis. Inhibin feeds back upon the pituitary to specifically inhibit FSH release. In addition, it can also restrict FSH action at the testicular level, interfering with FSH binding to FSH-R [144]. As it could be expected and in an opposite way, there is a stimulatory effect of activin on FSH secretion and on circulating FSH concentrations [145].

TGF-α and TGF-β are glycoproteins that play distinctively important roles in spermatogenesis, being expressed in somatic and germ cells. Both of these factors have been reported to regulate BTB dynamics, due to their effects on the expression levels of tight junctions and adherent junctions' integral membrane proteins [146]. In particular, TGF-α stimulates the proliferation of peritubular and Leydig cells, and influences the production of lactate, estrogen and transferrin by Sertoli cells [147 - 149]. It was shown that the amount of TGF-α produced by Sertoli cells significantly declines during the assembly of the BTB *in vitro*, illustrating that this growth factor can, in fact, modulate Sertoli cells function [150]. Concerning TGF-β, this growth factor has been purified from medium collected from cultured Sertoli cells, suggesting these cells as a sources of TGF-β in the testis [151]. TGF-β has three mammalian isoforms (TGF-β1, TGF-β2, and TGF-β3) that act as inhibitors of cell proliferation and facilitate cellular differentiation in a wide variety of cells. All cell types in the testis have been shown to contain type I and II TGF-β receptors [152, 153]. In addition, several studies have suggested that TGF-β influences Leydig cells proliferation and steroidogenesis, Sertoli cells aromatase activity and lactate production [154 - 156].

The family of fibroblast growth factors (FGFs) includes a set of structurally related peptides that act as growth and differentiating factors for a wide variety of cells and tissues. *In vitro* studies have suggested that FGFs may regulate testosterone biosynthesis and proliferation of the immature Sertoli cells [157]. Early postnatal actions of FGFs also showed potential indirect effects on gonocyte proliferation [158]. FGF2, also known as bFGF, is the most studied FGFs' member and it has a proven impact in the testis. It is secreted by Sertoli cells [159] and acts through its receptor (FGF-R type 1), present in Sertoli, Leydig, peritubular cells and, to a lesser extent, in germ cells [160]. Recently, it has been demonstrated that FGF2 is essential for the proliferation and maintenance of spermatogonial stem cells [161, 162].

Besides the role of IGFs in postnatal testis development, these growth factors also have an important role in spermatogenesis regulation. More specifically, IGF-I and IGF-II were shown to interfere in somatic and germ cells development and function. IGF-I is secreted by Leydig cells and Sertoli cells [163, 164], while its receptors have been identified in all testicular somatic cells [165], in secondary spermatocytes and early spermatids [164]. *In vitro* studies have demonstrated that administration of IGF-I to cultured immature Leydig cells resulted in a stimulation of LH binding and testosterone biosynthesis [166, 167]. IGF-I also exerts a priming effect on the capacity of the Sertoli cells to respond to FSH [168, 169]. IGF-II and its receptor are known to be expressed both in Sertoli and germ cells [170] and it has been shown to mediate Sertoli cell-spermatogenic cell interactions. IGF-II can also modulate gene expression in the spermatogenic cells [171, 172].

Cytokines

Cytokines are small secretory proteins that, in the testes, are mainly secreted by Sertoli cells, Leydig cells and testicular immune cells [173]. Although they are classically defined as growth factors involved in immune cell communication, cytokines also influence other events, triggering cell proliferation and differentiation [19]. Interleukin (IL)-1α has been pointed out as a pivotal regulator of spermatogenesis. It directly influences transferrin expression and lactate production by Sertoli cells [174, 175], as well as its prepubertal proliferation [176]. Interestingly, Sertoli cells also express an antagonist form of IL-1α, termed IL-1RA [177]. These positive and negative acting forms of IL-1α are proposed to regulate cellular interactions between Sertoli cells and germ cells. Other studies suggested a role for IL-1α in DNA synthesis by spermatogonia and meiotic cells in the rat testis, whereas mice lacking IL-1 type-1 receptor were fully fertile [178]. IL-6 is also produced by Sertoli cells in response to the autocrine action of IL-1α [179, 180]. This cytokine seems to have a role in the modulation of the BTB dynamics, inhibiting meiotic DNA synthesis during the spermatogenic cycle and influencing the secretion of transferrin and inhibin B by Sertoli cells [181, 182].

The stem cell factor (SCF), also known as c-kit ligand, is another cytokine that has been demonstrated to play an important role in the development of the testis. It is only produced by Sertoli cells (following FSH stimulation) [183] and acts, through its receptor, c-kit, which is present in spermatogonia and in preleptotene spermatocytes [184, 185]. Mutant mice lacking either c-kit or SCF are sterile and their gonads lack germ cells [186]. Data showed that the interaction of SCF with its receptor stimulates spermatogonia survival, proliferation and differentiation [187, 188]. It also has been reported that Sertoli cells from mice mutant for the SCF are unable to bind spermatocytes [189], illustrating that the c-kit and SCF also mediate cellular adhesion between these two cell types.

TRANSCRIPTIONAL AND TRANSLATIONAL CONTROL DURING SPERMATOGENESIS

Endocrine, paracrine and autocrine regulation are essential for seminiferous epithelium functional and structural maintenance and thus for a proper germ cell development. However, these are not the only paths described as pivotal to spermatogenesis, since genetics also plays an important role. Indeed, germ cells seem to stimulate a unique set of genes known as chauvinists that encode proteins crucial for seminiferous tubules structure and function. The process of gene expression is naturally influenced by a well-orchestrated regulatory environment, through transcriptional and translational factors.

Transcriptional Factors (DNA-binding Proteins)

Stage-specific gene expression and transcriptional activity in germ cells are two processes directly dependent on specialized regulation factors. The action of these transcription factors is achieved by binding to characteristic promoter motifs in the DNA sequence, upstream of the protein coding region, thereby inducing changes in chromatin structure and modulating the activity of the transcriptional machinery.

Zinc-finger Family

The Zinc-Finger family is the largest class of transcription factors in higher eukaryotes. Several of its members are expressed in the testis. Two of these factors, Wilms' Tumor (WT1) and Promyelocytic Leukemia Zinc Factor (PLZF), have been shown to have important roles on spermatogenesis.

Wt1 gene encodes its respective transcription factor, which has a critical role in embryonic development of the gonads [190]. Using a tissue-specific RNA interference approach that disrupts the expression of WT1 in adult testes, it was shown that WT1 absence is associated with a decrease in male mice fertility. Indeed, those animal presented an increase in germ cell apoptosis, reduced sperm count, reduced sperm motility and loss of adherent junctions between Sertoli cells and spermatids [191]. Further analysis on those testes showed that integrin cytoplasmic domain associated protein 1α (ICAP1-α) and epidermal growth factor receptor pathway substrate 8 (EPS8) expression was altered. These are signaling molecules important to the junction formation, so the disruption of this adherent junction may be the causal event that led to the other phenotypic alterations in these mice.

PLZF, also known as zinc-finger protein 145, is a protein exclusively expressed in a subset of spermatogonia that exhibit stem-cell like properties in postnatal and adult testes. The co-expression of this transcription factor with OCT-4, a protein used as a marker for undifferentiated cells, further enhanced this role already described. Plzf-mutant mice were found to exhibit a deficit in spermatogonia that progressively worsened as the animals aged, without any effect on Sertoli cells [192, 193]. This deficit was described to the loss of self-renewal activity of spermatogonia, leading to increased apoptosis.

Heat Shock Transcriptions Factors (HSFs)

HSFs belong to a family that is generally known for its role in fighting cellular stress situations, activating genes in response to heat shock. *Hsf2* is amongst the primary vertebrate HSF proteins. Several studies pointed out the pivotal role of this factor during reproductive mammalian development processes, including in embryogenesis and spermatogenesis [194, 195].

Hsf2 mRNA expression in testes is cell and stage specific. In adult mice, *Hsf2* is abundantly expressed in the nuclei of early pachytene spermatocytes and round spermatids [196]. Ablation of *Hsf2* on male mice caused subfertility, a marked reduction in testis and epididymis size, a severe reduction in sperm counts and a loss of pachytene spermatocytes (via apoptosis) [194]. These observations suggest that *Hsf2* promotes the survival of meiotic germ cells and/or their differentiation into spermatids. *Hsf2*-mutant mice also exhibit pronounced DNA fragmentation and altered levels of chromatin-packing proteins in epididymal spermatozoa, pointing out that *Hsf2* is also a participant on the chromatin reorganization events that occur during late stages of spermatogenesis [197]. In fact, it was demonstrated that the constitutive *Hsf2* DNA-binding activity present in testis is involved in the regulation of spontaneous expression of *Hsp70.2*, a testis-specific member of the *Hsp70* gene family [198]. HSP70.2 is a TNP chaperone, tightly associated with major spermatid DNA-packaging proteins, TNP1 and TNP2 [199].

Basic-domain-leucine-zipper (b-zip) Family

Members of the b-zip family that are expressed in the testes include cAMP response element modulator (CREM), cAMP response element binding protein (CREB), and activating transcription factor 1 (ATF1). CREM and CREB can bind as homo and heterodimers to a regulatory palindromic DNA sequence, the cAMP response element (CRE), which is found in the promoter regions of cAMP responsive genes.

Several studies indicated that CREM participates in developmental specific regulation of post-meiotic genes during spermiogenesis. Although levels of CREM in the pre-pubertal testis are very low, an essential, developmentally regulated switch in CREM expression occurs at puberty, at which time levels of CREM increase dramatically into adulthood [200]. Many isoforms of CREM are generated by alternative splicing, being some of them transcriptional activators and others repressors. While only CREM repressor isoforms are observed in pre-meiotic germ cells, from the pachytene spermatocyte stage onwards there is a remarkable switch from repressor mRNAs to activating mRNAs [201]. This switch in CREM function is intimately directed and modulated by the HPT axis, namely FSH [202]. A very important activator isoform in the testis is CREM-T, which plays a key role in late stages of spermatogenesis. The activation of CREM-T requires the association of a coactivator known as activator of CREM in testes (ACT) [203], which shows similar developmental expression pattern as CREM-T [204]. ACT displays intrinsic transactivation potential, capable of converting CREM-T into an activator isoform, leading to its activation in a phosphorylation-independent manner [205]. Experimental studies showed that *Crem-T* KO mice are sterile due to arrest of spermatogenesis at the round spermatid stage [206, 207]. Infertility in these mice is attributable to the lack of expression of key postmeiotic genes required for germ cell-differentiation. In *Crem*-null mice these genes fail to be expressed resulting in arrested germ cell differentiation and eventually in spermatocytes apoptosis [206]. Concomitantly, only CREM repressor isoforms were detected in several infertile patients with impaired spermatogenesis [208, 209].

The specific role of CREB in the testes is still elusive. However and similarly to CREM, many CREB isoforms are generated by alternative splicing in the testicular tissue. Studies using *Creb* KO mice failed to provide relevant information concerning its involvement on spermatogenesis. Animals carrying mutations in all CREB isoforms exhibited severe developmental disorders and died shortly after birth [210]. Adult animals with Sertoli cells expressing a negative form of CREB showed an increased germ-cell apoptosis and a dramatic reduction of round spermatids [211].

Homeobox Family

Homeobox family includes a wide variety of subfamilies, in which reproductive homeobox X-linked (*Rhox*) gene cluster is included. In adult and postnatal mice, *Rhox* genes are preferentially expressed in male reproductive tissues, and thus they are likely to encode a large family of homeodomain transcription factors committed to the regulation of reproductive functions. Within this subgroup, *Rhox5* is one of the well-studied members. It is worth mentioning that this was the first transcription factor gene shown to be dependent on testosterone or LH to be expressed [212]. Inactivation of *Rhox5* lead to mice subfertility, with increased male germ cell apoptosis, decreased sperm cell count and impaired sperm motility

[213]. Although these effects are focused on germ cells, *RHOX5* is exclusively expressed in Sertoli cells within postnatal and adult testis [212]. This supports the hypothesis that *RHOX5* regulates the expression of important Sertoli cell genes that, consequently, modulate germ cell survival. Another Sertoli-specific member of this family is *Rhox8*. Studies about *Rhox8* ablation had similar results to that obtained with *Rhox5*-null mice [214]. However, it should be highlighted that although *Rhox5* expression is androgen-dependent, *Rhox8* expression is androgen-independent, suggesting that the two sinnergize through different steps of spermatogenesis.

Translational Factors (RNA-binding Proteins)

The relevance of transcriptional factors in spermatogenesis is unquestionable. Nevertheless, several studies proved that translational factors can also have impact in spermatogenesis in a post-transcriptional mode, being many of them highly or uniquely expressed in germ cells. More than 700 mRNAs are translationally regulated in the developing testes, which highlights the extensive role of these RNA-binding proteins.

DEAD-box Family of RNA Helicases

DEAD-box RNA helicases are multi-functional proteins known to regulate a variety of events, including translation. One of the most important members of this family is Gonadotrophin-regulated testicular RNA helicase (GRTH), an enzyme that is essential for spermatogenesis progress, being express in meiotic spermatocytes, spermatids and Leydig cells [215]. It is the only member of this family known to have functions at the meiotic and haploid stages of mammalian spermatogenesis [216]. Studies targeting the disruption of *Grth* in mice caused male infertility, with animals exhibiting azoospermia, increased apoptosis of spermatocytes, arrest of spermatogenesis at step 8 of round spermatids and failure to elongate degeneration of germ cells [217]. More recent studies pointed out that GRTH promotes survival of spermatocytes by regulating apoptotic pathways. It was described that deletion of GRTH reduces the levels of anti-apoptotic proteins and elevates the levels of pro-apoptotic proteins in germ cells [218]. GRTH specifically was shown to bind the mRNAs of those proteins, supporting its direct role in their biogenesis and regulation. Although there was disruption of the expression of these proteins in *Grth*-null mice, the levels of their RNA transcripts were unaltered, suggesting that GRTH only affects translation.

Signal Transduction and Activation of RNA (STAR) Family

The STAR family is an emerging class of evolutionary conserved RNA-binding proteins. It is characterized by a large heterogeneous nuclear ribonucleoprotein K homology domain, embedded in a region that confers specificity for RNA binding. This extended RNA binding domain is called GSG, from the names of STAR proteins of three different organisms (GRP33/SAM68/GLD-1).

SAM68 has been suggested to affect cell proliferation and survival during spermatogenesis. It is a ubiquitously expressed factor that regulates many steps of RNA metabolism, including translation. The protein accumulates in germ cells approaching the meiotic divisions and it is maintained in haploid round spermatids, suggesting a role in those cells [219]. The establishment of a *Sam68* KO mouse model has revealed that this protein is essential for male fertility. Adult *Sam68*-null males have seminiferous tubules largely devoid of round and elongated spermatids [220]. Although the precise developmental stage of the intervention of SAM68 was not determined, it was described to occur when germ cells complete meiosis and differentiate into round spermatids. Accompanying this loss of spermatids, there was also an increase in postnatal germ cell apoptosis and various aberrations in elongated spermatids. Taken together, these results indicate that SAM68 plays an important role in germ cell differentiation.

Y-box Family

Y-box proteins represent a family of nucleic acid-binding proteins comprising a domain termed the cold-shock domain, which contains sequences that are over 40% identical to the small bacterial cold shock proteins. Y-box proteins were originally identified as DNA-binding proteins, but it was discovered later that these proteins are also RNA-binding proteins that first interact with mRNAs when they are transcribed in the nucleus. Many Y-box proteins then travel with mRNAs to the cytoplasm, where they regulate their fate. Some highlight has been given to mouse Y-box protein 2 (MSY2), namely in concerning its role in spermatogenesis. In fact, *Msy2*-null mice were shown to be sterile [221], presenting an abnormally high number of apoptotic meiotic spermatocytes, which lead to a massive loss of step 8/9 spermatids. These animals also presented misshapen and multi-nucleated spermatids and lacking spermatozoa in the epididymis [222]. It has been suggested that MSY2 is responsible for the control of *Prm1* and *Tnp2* genes, which are crucial for the structural reorganization of spermatid chromatin during the final stages of spermatogenesis. The loss of expression of these genes is likely to contribute to the nuclear condensation defects that occur in *Msy2*-null late stage spermatids.

Heterogeneous Nuclear Ribonuclear Protein (hnRNP) Family

hnRNPs is a family of RNA-binding proteins that coat newly synthesized RNAs and participate in a wide variety of events, including mRNA splicing, nuclear mRNA export, and translation. Deleted in Azoospermia Associated Protein 1

(DAZAP1) is one of the most important members of this family. Mammalian DAZAP1 is widely expressed in adults, especially in testes [223]. In germ cells, DAZAP1 is found in the nucleus from mid-pachytene spermatocytes to round spermatids, and relocates to the cytoplasm in elongating spermatids [224]. As with other hnRNPs, DAZAP1 binds newly synthesized transcripts and, through processes of splicing, export and translation, controls the expression of specific messengers. *Dazap1*-mutant mice were shown to be infertile, exhibiting testes with significantly increased numbers of apoptotic male germ cells, an accumulation of post-pachytene spermatocytes and a complete absence of post meiotic germ cells [225]. A potential explanation for this role in mRNA translation was initially suggested by the association of DAZAP1 with the DAZ family of proteins [226], which activates the translation of specific mRNAs in germ cells.

P-element-induced Wimpy Testis (PIWI) Family

The PIWI family is another class of translational control factors, composed of four proteins in humans (HIWI, HIWI2, HIWI3 and HILI) and three in mice (MIWI, MIWI2 and MILI) [227]. These proteins bind to PIWI-interacting (pi)RNAs, a subclass of germ cell specific small RNAs, regulating their activity [228]. The three murine PIWI proteins were already identified in testis and were shown to be expressed during spermatogenesis, pointing out their requirement for male fertility [229, 230]. Both *Miwi* and *Mili* are expressed in spermatocytes and neither is expressed in somatic cells. In addition, *Mili* is also expressed in spermatogonia [230]. *Mili* expression persists until the formation of postmeiotic spermatids [231, 232]. *Miwi* and *Miwi2* expression is far more restricted, being *Miwi* expressed in meiotic germ cells [233], and Miwi2 in gonocytes until shortly after birth [234]. Studies with *Miwi2* mutant mice displayed predominant arrest at the leptotene stage of meiosis [229]. The mutant spermatogenic cells show defects in double stranded DNA break repair, consistent with a role in proper meiotic recombination [229, 231]. Similarly, *Mili*-null mice are blocked at the zygotene or early pachytene stages of meiotic prophase [231]. Interestingly, MIWI appears to control the progression of spermiogenesis together with CREM [235]. MIWI and CREM do not regulate each other's expression. However, MIWI complexes with and stabilizes mRNA transcripts from CREM-dependent target genes including ACT, whose function was previously reported in this chapter. Interestingly, as in *Crem*-null mice, there is a spermiogenic arrest at the round spermatid stage in *Miwi*-null mice [235]. Thus, MIWI and CREM pathways act together to initiate spermiogenesis. Finally, it is important to emphasize that one investigation identified estrogen as a pivotal inhibitor of MILI and MIWI activity, highlighting the relevance of hormonal control in this process [236].

Box 4.1 | Summary

- Postnatal testicular development depends in a wide range of regulators, such as follicle-stimulating hormone, luteinizing hormone, testosterone, activin A, inhibin B, hepatocyte growth factor, thyroid hormone, SRY-related box family, anti-Müllerian hormone, estrogen and insulin-like growth factor-1.
- Spermatogenesis is a well-balanced mechanism that can be subdivided into three consecutive steps: 1) Mitosis, associated with the proliferation and differentiation of spermatogonia; 2) Meiosis, the reduction of the chromosome number from diploid to haploid; 3) Spermiogenesis, the transformation of round spermatids into the complex structure of the spermatozoon.
- Spermiation is a vital process that allows the release of mature spermatozoa into the seminiferous tubule lumen.
- Stages of seminiferous epithelium are key spatial divisions that allow the organization of the different germ cell steps in their associative environment.
- Spermatogenic process is regulated in a hormonal way by the hypothalamus-pituitary gonadal axis, represented by their secretions: gonadotrophin-releasing hormone, luteinizing hormone, follicle-stimulating hormone, testosterone and estrogen.
- Spermatogenesis is also regulated in a paracrine/autocrine way by the local secretion of metabolites, growth factors and cytokines.
- The genetic environment associated with spermatogenesis involves the action of transcriptional regulators, like Zinc-Finger family, Heat Shock transcriptional factors, Basic-Domain-Leucine-Zipper family and Homeobox family.
- The action of translational regulators, like DEAD-box family of RNA helicases, Signal Transduction and Activation of RNA family, Y-box family, Heterogeneous nuclear ribonuclear protein family and P-element-induced wimpy testis family on the spermatogenic event should be highlighted.

CONCLUDING REMARKS

Every newborn can be seen not only as a symbol of an evolutionary theory, but also as a key to species maintenance. That is a key reason to address all the features that make our reproduction so unique. For male mammals, testes development starts in the embryonic phase and extends to the postnatal period, being involved in a series of sequential events that prepare the gonads for the reproductive activity. This highlights the role of key factors, such as FSH, LH, testosterone, activin A, inhibin B, HGF, TH, SOX family, AMH, Estrogens and IGF-1. Each one of these act in an interdependent manner, controlling the rate of proliferation, differentiation and function of Sertoli, Leydig, peritubular and germ cells in a way that, entering puberty, the individual is ready to fully commit to spermatogenesis.

Spermatogenesis is the crucial mechanism responsible for male fertility. It involves the coordination of somatic cells with a well-defined objective: helping germ cells to undergo from stem cell spermatogonia to the most differentiated and complex haploid cells in the body, the spermatozoa. This happens through a series of three main periods (Mitosis, Meiosis and Spermiogenesis) that culminate in the release of mature spermatozoa at the time of spermiation. Along this process, the seminiferous epithelium is organized in stages, in association with different steps of germ cell development.

The regulation of the spermatogenic cycle involves hormonal and paracrine/autocrine factors. From the hormonal point of view, it must be highlighted the extreme important of the HPG axis, represented by its secretion products: GnRH, produced in the hypothalamus; LH and FSH, produced in the pituitary; testosterone and estrogens, produced in the testis. In a paracrine/ autocrine point of view, it has been shown that metabolites, growth factors and cytokines synergize to control the spermatogenic process. Each of these factors have specific roles affecting some of the germ and somatic cells in precise time periods. In addition, there is a pivotal role for nucleic acids, the basis of our genetic information, in this regulatory path. As any other process in human body, spermatogenesis involves a specific set of genes that encode several essential proteins for this event. These genes are under the strict control of some transcriptional and translational regulatory protein families that can act as DNA-binding or RNA-binding proteins, respectively.

In conclusion, it is of major importance to known the regulatory mechanisms underlying spermatogenesis to fully understand male reproduction. This chapter presented the most relevant information available on this subject. However, there is yet much to be investigated about how this complex and perfect-needed system occurs. When we do it, maybe we will be able to avert some of the most common dysfunctions associated with male fertility.

CONFLICT OF INTEREST

The authors confirm that they have no conflict of interest to declare for this publication.

ACKNOWLEDGEMENT

This work was supported by the "Fundação para a Ciência e a Tecnologia"–FCT

(PTDC/BBB-BQB/1368/2014) and CICS (UID/Multi/00709/2013).

REFERENCES

[1] Ojeda SR, Advis JP, Andrews WW, Eds. Neuroendocrine control of the onset of puberty in the rat. Federation proceedings 1980.

[2] Picut CA, Remick AK, de Rijk EP, Simons ML, Stump DG, Parker GA. Postnatal development of the testis in the rat: morphologic study and correlation of morphology to neuroendocrine parameters. Toxicol Pathol 2015; 43(3): 326-42.
[http://dx.doi.org/10.1177/0192623314547279] [PMID: 25217330]

[3] Baker PJ, OShaughnessy PJ. Role of gonadotrophins in regulating numbers of Leydig and Sertoli cells during fetal and postnatal development in mice. Reproduction 2001; 122(2): 227-34.
[http://dx.doi.org/10.1530/rep.0.1220227] [PMID: 11467973]

[4] Bremner WJ, Millar MR, Sharpe RM, Saunders PT. Immunohistochemical localization of androgen receptors in the rat testis: evidence for stage-dependent expression and regulation by androgens. Endocrinology 1994; 135(3): 1227-34.
[http://dx.doi.org/10.1210/endo.135.3.8070367] [PMID: 8070367]

[5] Sharpe RM, McKinnell C, Kivlin C, Fisher JS. Proliferation and functional maturation of Sertoli cells, and their relevance to disorders of testis function in adulthood. Reproduction 2003; 125(6): 769-84.
[http://dx.doi.org/10.1530/rep.0.1250769] [PMID: 12773099]

[6] Ketelslegers JM, Hetzel WD, Sherins RJ, Catt KJ. Developmental changes in testicular gonadotropin receptors: plasma gonadotropins and plasma testosterone in the rat. Endocrinology 1978; 103(1): 212-22.
[http://dx.doi.org/10.1210/endo-103-1-212] [PMID: 217637]

[7] Lee VW, de Kretser DM, Hudson B, Wang C. Variations in serum FSH, LH and testosterone levels in male rats from birth to sexual maturity. J Reprod Fertil 1975; 42(1): 121-6.
[http://dx.doi.org/10.1530/jrf.0.0420121] [PMID: 1110463]

[8] Baker PJ, Pakarinen P, Huhtaniemi IT, *et al.* Failure of normal Leydig cell development in follicle-stimulating hormone (FSH) receptor-deficient mice, but not FSHbeta-deficient mice: role for constitutive FSH receptor activity. Endocrinology 2003; 144(1): 138-45.
[http://dx.doi.org/10.1210/en.2002-220637] [PMID: 12488339]

[9] OShaughnessy PJ, Monteiro A, Abel M. Testicular development in mice lacking receptors for follicle stimulating hormone and androgen. PLoS One 2012; 7(4): e35136.
[http://dx.doi.org/10.1371/journal.pone.0035136] [PMID: 22514715]

[10] Meachem SJ, Ruwanpura SM, Ziolkowski J, Ague JM, Skinner MK, Loveland KL. Developmentally distinct *in vivo* effects of FSH on proliferation and apoptosis during testis maturation. J Endocrinol 2005; 186(3): 429-46.
[http://dx.doi.org/10.1677/joe.1.06121] [PMID: 16135663]

[11] Rossi P, Dolci S. Paracrine mechanisms involved in the control of early stages of mammalian spermatogenesis. Front Endocrinol. 2013; 4: 181.
[http://dx.doi.org/10.3389/fendo.2013.00181]]

[12] Nurmio M, Kallio J, Adam M, Mayerhofer A, Toppari J, Jahnukainen K. Peritubular myoid cells have a role in postnatal testicular growth. Spermatogenesis 2012; 2(2): 79-87.
[http://dx.doi.org/10.4161/spmg.20067] [PMID: 22670217]

[13] Eblen A, Bao S, Lei ZM, Nakajima ST, Rao CV. The presence of functional luteinizing hormone/chorionic gonadotropin receptors in human sperm. J Clin Endocrinol Metab 2001; 86(6): 2643-8.
[http://dx.doi.org/10.1210/jcem.86.6.7533] [PMID: 11397866]

[14] Zhang F-P, Poutanen M, Wilbertz J, Huhtaniemi I. Normal prenatal but arrested postnatal sexual development of luteinizing hormone receptor knockout (LuRKO) mice. Mol Endocrinol 2001; 15(1): 172-83.
[http://dx.doi.org/10.1210/mend.15.1.0582] [PMID: 11145748]

[15] Zhang FP, Pakarainen T, Zhu F, Poutanen M, Huhtaniemi I. Molecular characterization of postnatal development of testicular steroidogenesis in luteinizing hormone receptor knockout mice. Endocrinology 2004; 145(3): 1453-63.
[http://dx.doi.org/10.1210/en.2003-1049] [PMID: 14645113]

[16] Lei ZM, Mishra S, Ponnuru P, Li X, Yang ZW, Rao CV. Testicular phenotype in luteinizing hormone receptor knockout animals and the effect of testosterone replacement therapy. Biol Reprod 2004; 71(5): 1605-13.
[http://dx.doi.org/10.1095/biolreprod.104.031161] [PMID: 15253923]

[17] Mendis-Handagama SM, Ariyaratne HB. Differentiation of the adult Leydig cell population in the postnatal testis. Biol Reprod 2001; 65(3): 660-71.
[http://dx.doi.org/10.1095/biolreprod65.3.660] [PMID: 11514326]

[18] Zhou Q, Nie R, Prins GS, Saunders PT, Katzenellenbogen BS, Hess RA. Localization of androgen and estrogen receptors in adult male mouse reproductive tract. J Androl 2002; 23(6): 870-81.
[PMID: 12399534]

[19] Weinbauer GF, Wessels J. Paracrine control of spermatogenesis. Andrologia 1999; 31(5): 249-62.
[http://dx.doi.org/10.1046/j.1439-0272.1999.00295.x] [PMID: 10526633]

[20] Hill CM, Anway MD, Zirkin BR, Brown TR. Intratesticular androgen levels, androgen receptor localization, and androgen receptor expression in adult rat Sertoli cells. Biol Reprod 2004; 71(4): 1348-58.
[http://dx.doi.org/10.1095/biolreprod.104.029249] [PMID: 15215201]

[21] Johnston H, Baker PJ, Abel M, *et al.* Regulation of Sertoli cell number and activity by follicle-stimulating hormone and androgen during postnatal development in the mouse. Endocrinology 2004; 145(1): 318-29.
[http://dx.doi.org/10.1210/en.2003-1055] [PMID: 14551232]

[22] Hovatta O. Effect of androgens and antiandrogens on the development of the myoid cells of the rat seminiferous tubules. Z Zellforsch Mikrosk Anat 1972; 131(3): 299-308.
[http://dx.doi.org/10.1007/BF00582853] [PMID: 5074138]

[23] Bressler RS, Ross MH. Differentiation of peritubular myoid cells of the testis: effects of intratesticular implantation of newborn mouse testes into normal and hypophysectomized adults. Biol Reprod 1972; 6(1): 148-59.
[http://dx.doi.org/10.1093/biolreprod/6.1.148] [PMID: 5014041]

[24] Bressler RS, Lustbader IJ. Effect of testosterone on development of the lumen in seminiferous tubules of the rat. Andrologia 1978; 10(4): 291-8.
[http://dx.doi.org/10.1111/j.1439-0272.1978.tb03035.x] [PMID: 717808]

[25] Barakat B, OConnor AE, Gold E, de Kretser DM, Loveland KL. Inhibin, activin, follistatin and FSH serum levels and testicular production are highly modulated during the first spermatogenic wave in mice. Reproduction 2008; 136(3): 345-59.
[http://dx.doi.org/10.1530/REP-08-0140] [PMID: 18515316]

[26] Meehan T, Schlatt S, OBryan MK, de Kretser DM, Loveland KL. Regulation of germ cell and Sertoli cell development by activin, follistatin, and FSH. Dev Biol 2000; 220(2): 225-37.
[http://dx.doi.org/10.1006/dbio.2000.9625] [PMID: 10753512]

[27] Matzuk MM, Kumar TR, Bradley A. Different phenotypes for mice deficient in either activins or activin receptor type II. Nature 1995; 374(6520): 356-60.
[http://dx.doi.org/10.1038/374356a0] [PMID: 7885474]

[28] de Kretser DM, Loveland KL, Meehan T, OBryan MK, Phillips DJ, Wreford NG. Inhibins, activins and follistatin: actions on the testis. Mol Cell Endocrinol 2001; 180(1-2): 87-92. [http://dx.doi.org/10.1016/S0303-7207(01)00502-0] [PMID: 11451576]

[29] Müller J, Skakkebaek NE, Ratcliffe SG. Quantified testicular histology in boys with sex chromosome abnormalities. Int J Androl 1995; 18(2): 57-62. [http://dx.doi.org/10.1111/j.1365-2605.1995.tb00386.x] [PMID: 7665210]

[30] Catizone A, Ricci G, Galdieri M. Expression and functional role of hepatocyte growth factor receptor (C-MET) during postnatal rat testis development. Endocrinology 2001; 142(5): 1828-34. [http://dx.doi.org/10.1210/endo.142.5.8172] [PMID: 11316747]

[31] Holsberger DR, Cooke PS. Understanding the role of thyroid hormone in Sertoli cell development: a mechanistic hypothesis. Cell Tissue Res 2005; 322(1): 133-40. [http://dx.doi.org/10.1007/s00441-005-1082-z] [PMID: 15856309]

[32] Mendis-Handagama SM, Siril Ariyaratne HB. Leydig cells, thyroid hormones and steroidogenesis. Indian J Exp Biol 2005; 43(11): 939-62. [PMID: 16313060]

[33] Wagner MS, Wajner SM, Maia AL. The role of thyroid hormone in testicular development and function. J Endocrinol 2008; 199(3): 351-65. [http://dx.doi.org/10.1677/JOE-08-0218] [PMID: 18728126]

[34] Buzzard JJ, Morrison JR, OBryan MK, Song Q, Wreford NG. Developmental expression of thyroid hormone receptors in the rat testis. Biol Reprod 2000; 62(3): 664-9. [http://dx.doi.org/10.1095/biolreprod62.3.664] [PMID: 10684808]

[35] Canale D, Agostini M, Giorgilli G, *et al.* Thyroid hormone receptors in neonatal, prepubertal, and adult rat testis. J Androl 2001; 22(2): 284-8. [PMID: 11229803]

[36] Jannini EA, Crescenzi A, Rucci N, *et al.* Ontogenetic pattern of thyroid hormone receptor expression in the human testis. J Clin Endocrinol Metab 2000; 85(9): 3453-7. [http://dx.doi.org/10.1210/jcem.85.9.6803] [PMID: 10999848]

[37] Cooke PS, Hess RA, Porcelli J, Meisami E. Increased sperm production in adult rats after transient neonatal hypothyroidism. Endocrinology 1991; 129(1): 244-8. [http://dx.doi.org/10.1210/endo-129-1-244] [PMID: 2055187]

[38] Cooke PS, Meisami E. Early hypothyroidism in rats causes increased adult testis and reproductive organ size but does not change testosterone levels. Endocrinology 1991; 129(1): 237-43. [http://dx.doi.org/10.1210/endo-129-1-237] [PMID: 2055186]

[39] Francavilla S, Cordeschi G, Properzi G, *et al.* Effect of thyroid hormone on the pre- and post-natal development of the rat testis. J Endocrinol 1991; 129(1): 35-42. [http://dx.doi.org/10.1677/joe.0.1290035] [PMID: 1903146]

[40] De França LR, Hess RA, Cooke PS, Russell LD. Neonatal hypothyroidism causes delayed Sertoli cell maturation in rats treated with propylthiouracil: evidence that the Sertoli cell controls testis growth. Anat Rec 1995; 242(1): 57-69. [http://dx.doi.org/10.1002/ar.1092420108] [PMID: 7604982]

[41] van Haaster LH, de Jong FH, Docter R, de Rooij DG. High neonatal triiodothyronine levels reduce the period of Sertoli cell proliferation and accelerate tubular lumen formation in the rat testis, and increase serum inhibin levels. Endocrinology 1993; 133(2): 755-60. [http://dx.doi.org/10.1210/endo.133.2.8344214] [PMID: 8344214]

[42] Palmero S, Prati M, Bolla F, Fugassa E. Tri-iodothyronine directly affects rat Sertoli cell proliferation and differentiation. J Endocrinol 1995; 145(2): 355-62. [http://dx.doi.org/10.1677/joe.0.1450355] [PMID: 7616169]

[43] Teerds KJ, de Rooij DG, de Jong FH, van Haaster LH. Development of the adult-type Leydig cell population in the rat is affected by neonatal thyroid hormone levels. Biol Reprod 1998; 59(2): 344-50. [http://dx.doi.org/10.1095/biolreprod59.2.344] [PMID: 9687306]

[44] Morais da Silva S, Hacker A, Harley V, Goodfellow P, Swain A, Lovell-Badge R. *Sox9* expression during gonadal development implies a conserved role for the gene in testis differentiation in mammals and birds. Nat Genet 1996; 14(1): 62-8. [http://dx.doi.org/10.1038/ng0996-62] [PMID: 8782821]

[45] Barrionuevo F, Georg I, Scherthan H, *et al.* Testis cord differentiation after the sex determination stage is independent of *Sox9* but fails in the combined absence of *Sox9* and Sox8. Dev Biol 2009; 327(2): 301-12. [http://dx.doi.org/10.1016/j.ydbio.2008.12.011] [PMID: 19124014]

[46] Al-Attar L, Noël K, Dutertre M, *et al.* Hormonal and cellular regulation of Sertoli cell anti-Müllerian hormone production in the postnatal mouse. J Clin Invest 1997; 100(6): 1335-43. [http://dx.doi.org/10.1172/JCI119653] [PMID: 9294098]

[47] Racine C, Rey R, Forest MG, *et al.* Receptors for anti-müllerian hormone on Leydig cells are responsible for its effects on steroidogenesis and cell differentiation. Proc Natl Acad Sci USA 1998; 95(2): 594-9. [http://dx.doi.org/10.1073/pnas.95.2.594] [PMID: 9435237]

[48] Josso N. Antimüllerian hormone: new perspectives for a sexist molecule. Endocr Rev 1986; 7(4): 421-33. [http://dx.doi.org/10.1210/edrv-7-4-421] [PMID: 3536462]

[49] Behringer RR, Cate RL, Froelick GJ, Palmiter RD, Brinster RL. Abnormal sexual development in transgenic mice chronically expressing müllerian inhibiting substance. Nature 1990; 345(6271): 167-70. [http://dx.doi.org/10.1038/345167a0] [PMID: 2336108]

[50] Carreau S, Hess RA. Oestrogens and spermatogenesis. Philos Trans R Soc Lond B Biol Sci 2010; 365(1546): 1517-35. [http://dx.doi.org/10.1098/rstb.2009.0235] [PMID: 20403867]

[51] Bois C, Delalande C, Nurmio M, *et al.* Age- and cell-related gene expression of aromatase and estrogen receptors in the rat testis. J Mol Endocrinol 2010; 45(3): 147-59. [http://dx.doi.org/10.1677/JME-10-0041] [PMID: 20554652]

[52] van Pelt AM, de Rooij DG, van der Burg B, van der Saag PT. Gustafsson J-Ak, Kuiper GG. Ontogeny of Estrogen Receptor-β Expression in Rat Testis. Endocrinology 1999; 140: 478-83. [http://dx.doi.org/10.1210/endo.140.1.6438] [PMID: 9886860]

[53] Dhar JD, Setty BS. Epididymal response to exogenous testosterone in rats sterilized neonatally by estrogen. Endokrinologie 1976; 68(1): 14-21. [PMID: 1001264]

[54] Tsai-Morris C-H, Aquilano DR, Dufau ML. Cellular localization of rat testicular aromatase activity during development. Endocrinology 1985; 116(1): 38-46. [http://dx.doi.org/10.1210/endo-116-1-38] [PMID: 2981072]

[55] Delbès G, Levacher C, Duquenne C, Racine C, Pakarinen P, Habert R. Endogenous estrogens inhibit mouse fetal Leydig cell development *via* estrogen receptor α. Endocrinology 2005; 146(5): 2454-61. [http://dx.doi.org/10.1210/en.2004-1540] [PMID: 15661855]

[56] Delbès G, Levacher C, Pairault C, *et al.* Estrogen receptor β-mediated inhibition of male germ cell line development in mice by endogenous estrogens during perinatal life. Endocrinology 2004; 145(7): 3395-403. [http://dx.doi.org/10.1210/en.2003-1479] [PMID: 15044378]

[57] Baker J, Hardy MP, Zhou J, *et al.* Effects of an Igfl gene null mutation on mouse reproduction. Mol Endocrinol 1996; 10(7): 903-18.
[http://dx.doi.org/10.1210/mend.10.7.8813730] [PMID: 8813730]

[58] Chatelain PG, Sanchez P, Saez JM. Growth hormone and insulin-like growth factor I treatment increase testicular luteinizing hormone receptors and steroidogenic responsiveness of growth hormone deficient dwarf mice. Endocrinology 1991; 128(4): 1857-62.
[http://dx.doi.org/10.1210/endo-128-4-1857] [PMID: 2004605]

[59] Waheeb R, Hofmann MC. Human spermatogonial stem cells: a possible origin for spermatocytic seminoma. Int J Androl 2011; 34(4 Pt 2): e296-305.
[http://dx.doi.org/10.1111/j.1365-2605.2011.01199.x] [PMID: 21790653]

[60] Roosen-Runge EC. Kinetics of spermatogenesis in mammals. Ann N Y Acad Sci 1952; 55(4): 574-84.
[http://dx.doi.org/10.1111/j.1749-6632.1952.tb26577.x] [PMID: 13139145]

[61] Sharma R, Agarwal A. Spermatogenesis: an overview Sperm Chromatin. Springer 2011; pp. 19-44.
[http://dx.doi.org/10.1007/978-1-4419-6857-9_2]

[62] Oliveira PF, Alves MG. Sertoli Cell Metabolism and Spermatogenesis. Springer 2015; pp. 15-24.
[http://dx.doi.org/10.1007/978-3-319-19791-3_3]

[63] Kasuga H, Aigaki T, Osanai M. Spermatogenesis, Overview. Reproduction 1999; 21: 199-221.

[64] de Jonge CJ, Barratt C. The sperm cell: production, maturation, fertilization, regeneration. Cambridge University Press 2006; pp. 1-40.
[http://dx.doi.org/10.1017/CBO9780511545115]

[65] Moreno RD, Ramalho-Santos J, Sutovsky P, Chan EK, Schatten G. Vesicular traffic and golgi apparatus dynamics during mammalian spermatogenesis: implications for acrosome architecture. Biol Reprod 2000; 63(1): 89-98.
[http://dx.doi.org/10.1095/biolreprod63.1.89] [PMID: 10859246]

[66] Rathke C, Baarends WM, Awe S, Renkawitz-Pohl R. Chromatin dynamics during spermiogenesis. Biochimica et Biophysica Acta (BBA)-Gene Regulatory Mechanisms. 2014; 1839: 155-68.
[http://dx.doi.org/10.1016/j.bbagrm.2013.08.004] [PMID: 24091090]

[67] Hecht NB. Molecular mechanisms of male germ cell differentiation. BioEssays 1998; 20(7): 555-61.
[http://dx.doi.org/10.1002/(SICI)1521-1878(199807)20:7<555::AID-BIES6>3.0.CO;2-J] [PMID: 9723004]

[68] Meistrich ML, Mohapatra B, Shirley CR, Zhao M. Roles of transition nuclear proteins in spermiogenesis. Chromosoma 2003; 111(8): 483-8.
[http://dx.doi.org/10.1007/s00412-002-0227-z] [PMID: 12743712]

[69] Sutovsky P, Manandhar G, Schatten G. Biogenesis of the centrosome during mammalian gametogenesis and fertilization. Protoplasma 1999; 206: 249-62.
[http://dx.doi.org/10.1007/BF01288213]

[70] Lin C-Y, Hung PH, VandeVoort CA, Miller MG. 1H NMR to investigate metabolism and energy supply in rhesus macaque sperm. Reprod Toxicol 2009; 28(1): 75-80.
[http://dx.doi.org/10.1016/j.reprotox.2009.03.005] [PMID: 19490998]

[71] Russell LD, Ettlin RA, Sinha-Hikim AP, Clegg ED. Histological and histopathological evaluation of the testis. Int J Androl 1990; 16: 1-286.
[http://dx.doi.org/10.1111/j.1365-2605.1993.tb01156.x]

[72] Sutovsky P, Manandhar G. Mammalian spermatogenesis and sperm structure: anatomical and compartmental analysis. The Sperm Cell: Production, Maturation, Fertilization, Regeneration 2006; 1-30.
[http://dx.doi.org/10.1017/CBO9780511545115.002]

[73] Guttman JA, Kimel GH, Vogl AW. Dynein and plus-end microtubule-dependent motors are associated with specialized Sertoli cell junction plaques (ectoplasmic specializations). J Cell Sci 2000; 113(Pt 12): 2167-76.
[PMID: 10825290]

[74] Russell LD, Saxena NK, Turner TT. Cytoskeletal involvement in spermiation and sperm transport. Tissue Cell 1989; 21(3): 361-79.
[http://dx.doi.org/10.1016/0040-8166(89)90051-7] [PMID: 2479117]

[75] Russell L. Observations on rat Sertoli ectoplasmic (junctional) specializations in their association with germ cells of the rat testis. Tissue Cell 1977; 9(3): 475-98.
[http://dx.doi.org/10.1016/0040-8166(77)90007-6] [PMID: 929577]

[76] Wong EW, Mruk DD, Cheng CY. Biology and regulation of ectoplasmic specialization, an atypical adherens junction type, in the testis. Biochimica et Biophysica Acta 2008; 1778: 692-708.
[http://dx.doi.org/10.1016/j.bbamem.2007.11.006] [PMID: 18068662]

[77] Vogl AW, Pfeiffer DC, Mulholland D, Kimel G, Guttman J. Unique and multifunctional adhesion junctions in the testis: ectoplasmic specializations. Arch Histol Cytol 2000; 63(1): 1-15.
[http://dx.doi.org/10.1679/aohc.63.1] [PMID: 10770585]

[78] Young JS, Guttman JA, Vaid KS, Shahinian H, Vogl AW. Cortactin (CTTN), N-WASP (WASL), and clathrin (CLTC) are present at podosome-like tubulobulbar complexes in the rat testis. Biol Reprod 2009; 80(1): 153-61.
[http://dx.doi.org/10.1095/biolreprod.108.070615] [PMID: 18799755]

[79] Young JS, Guttman JA, Vaid KS, Vogl AW. Tubulobulbar complexes are intercellular podosome-like structures that internalize intact intercellular junctions during epithelial remodeling events in the rat testis. Biol Reprod 2009; 80(1): 162-74.
[http://dx.doi.org/10.1095/biolreprod.108.070623] [PMID: 18799754]

[80] Sprando RL, Russell LD. Comparative study of cytoplasmic elimination in spermatids of selected mammalian species. Am J Anat 1987; 178(1): 72-80.
[http://dx.doi.org/10.1002/aja.1001780109] [PMID: 3825964]

[81] Vogl AW, Young JS, Du M. New insights into roles of tubulobulbar complexes in sperm release and turnover of blood-testis barrier. Int Rev Cell Mol Biol 2013; 303: 319-55.
[http://dx.doi.org/10.1016/B978-0-12-407697-6.00008-8] [PMID: 23445814]

[82] Hess RA, Miller LA, Kirby JD, Margoliash E, Goldberg E. Immunoelectron microscopic localization of testicular and somatic cytochromes c in the seminiferous epithelium of the rat. Biol Reprod 1993; 48(6): 1299-308.
[http://dx.doi.org/10.1095/biolreprod48.6.1299] [PMID: 8391332]

[83] de França LR, Ye SJ, Ying L, Sandberg M, Russell LD. Morphometry of rat germ cells during spermatogenesis. Anat Rec 1995; 241(2): 181-204.
[http://dx.doi.org/10.1002/ar.1092410206] [PMID: 7710135]

[84] Kluin PM, Kramer MF, de Rooij DG. Spermatogenesis in the immature mouse proceeds faster than in the adult. Int J Androl 1982; 5(3): 282-94.
[http://dx.doi.org/10.1111/j.1365-2605.1982.tb00257.x] [PMID: 7118267]

[85] Ismail N, Morales C, Clermont Y. Role of spermatogonia in the stage-synchronization of the seminiferous epithelium in vitamin-A-deficient rats. Am J Anat 1990; 188(1): 57-63.
[http://dx.doi.org/10.1002/aja.1001880107] [PMID: 2346119]

[86] Ismail N, Morales CR. Effects of vitamin A deficiency on the inter-Sertoli cell tight junctions and on the germ cell population. Microsc Res Tech 1992; 20(1): 43-9.
[http://dx.doi.org/10.1002/jemt.1070200106] [PMID: 1611150]

[87] Chung SS, Sung W, Wang X, Wolgemuth DJ. Retinoic acid receptor α is required for synchronization of spermatogenic cycles and its absence results in progressive breakdown of the spermatogenic process. Dev Dyn 2004; 230(4): 754-66.
[http://dx.doi.org/10.1002/dvdy.20083] [PMID: 15254909]

[88] Sharpe RM. Regulation of spermatogenesis. Physiol Rep 1994; 1: 1363-434.

[89] Vihko KK, Toppari J, Parvinen M. Stage-specific regulation of plasminogen activator secretion in the rat seminiferous epithelium. Endocrinology 1987; 120(1): 142-5.
[http://dx.doi.org/10.1210/endo-120-1-142] [PMID: 3023024]

[90] Xu J, Beyer AR, Walker WH, McGee EA. Developmental and stage-specific expression of Smad2 and Smad3 in rat testis. J Androl 2003; 24(2): 192-200.
[http://dx.doi.org/10.1002/j.1939-4640.2003.tb02662.x] [PMID: 12634305]

[91] Zhang YQ, He XZ, Zhang JS, Wang RA, Zhou J, Xu RJ. Stage-specific localization of transforming growth factor beta1 and beta3 and their receptors during spermatogenesis in men. Asian J Androl 2004; 6(2): 105-9.
[PMID: 15154083]

[92] Rannikki AS, Zhang F-P, Huhtaniemi IT. Ontogeny of follicle-stimulating hormone receptor gene expression in the rat testis and ovary. Mol Cell Endocrinol 1995; 107(2): 199-208.
[http://dx.doi.org/10.1016/0303-7207(94)03444-X] [PMID: 7768331]

[93] Dierich A, Sairam MR, Monaco L, *et al.* Impairing follicle-stimulating hormone (FSH) signaling *in vivo*: targeted disruption of the FSH receptor leads to aberrant gametogenesis and hormonal imbalance. Proc Natl Acad Sci USA 1998; 95(23): 13612-7.
[http://dx.doi.org/10.1073/pnas.95.23.13612] [PMID: 9811848]

[94] Abel MH, Wootton AN, Wilkins V, Huhtaniemi I, Knight PG, Charlton HM. The effect of a null mutation in the follicle-stimulating hormone receptor gene on mouse reproduction. Endocrinology 2000; 141(5): 1795-803.
[http://dx.doi.org/10.1210/endo.141.5.7456] [PMID: 10803590]

[95] Siegel ET, Kim H-G, Nishimoto HK, Layman LC. The molecular basis of impaired follicle-stimulating hormone action: evidence from human mutations and mouse models. Reprod Sci 2013; 20(3): 211-33.
[http://dx.doi.org/10.1177/1933719112461184] [PMID: 23184658]

[96] Abel MH, Baker PJ, Charlton HM, *et al.* Spermatogenesis and sertoli cell activity in mice lacking sertoli cell receptors for follicle-stimulating hormone and androgen. Endocrinology 2008; 149(7): 3279-85.
[http://dx.doi.org/10.1210/en.2008-0086] [PMID: 18403489]

[97] Wreford NG, Rajendra Kumar T, Matzuk MM, De Kretser DM. Analysis of the Testicular Phenotype of the Follicle-Stimulating Hormone β-Subunit Knockout and the Activin Type II Receptor Knockout Mice by Stereological Analysis. Endocrinology 2001; 142: 2916-20.
[http://dx.doi.org/10.1210/endo.142.7.8230] [PMID: 11416011]

[98] Ruwanpura SM, McLachlan RI, Stanton PG, Loveland KL, Meachem SJ. Pathways involved in testicular germ cell apoptosis in immature rats after FSH suppression. J Endocrinol 2008; 197(1): 35-43.
[http://dx.doi.org/10.1677/JOE-07-0637] [PMID: 18372230]

[99] Henriksén K, Kangasniemi M, Parvinen M, Kaipia A, Hakovirta H. *In vitro*, follicle-stimulating hormone prevents apoptosis and stimulates deoxyribonucleic acid synthesis in the rat seminiferous epithelium in a stage-specific fashion. Endocrinology 1996; 137(5): 2141-9.
[http://dx.doi.org/10.1210/endo.137.5.8612559] [PMID: 8612559]

[100] Sinha-Hikim AP, Swerdloff RS. Temporal and stage-specific changes in spermatogenesis of rat after gonadotropin deprivation by a potent gonadotropin-releasing hormone antagonist treatment. Endocrinology 1993; 133(5): 2161-70.
[http://dx.doi.org/10.1210/endo.133.5.8404667] [PMID: 8404667]

[101] Bartlett JM, Weinbauer GF, Nieschlag E. Differential effects of FSH and testosterone on the maintenance of spermatogenesis in the adult hypophysectomized rat. J Endocrinol 1989; 121(1): 49-58.
[http://dx.doi.org/10.1677/joe.0.1210049] [PMID: 2497224]

[102] Russell LD. The perils of sperm release let my children go. Int J Androl 1991; 14(5): 307-11.
[http://dx.doi.org/10.1111/j.1365-2605.1991.tb01097.x] [PMID: 1794915]

[103] Saito K, ODonnell L, McLachlan RI, Robertson DM. Spermiation failure is a major contributor to early spermatogenic suppression caused by hormone withdrawal in adult rats. Endocrinology 2000; 141(8): 2779-85.
[http://dx.doi.org/10.1210/endo.141.8.7628] [PMID: 10919263]

[104] Beardsley A, ODonnell L. Characterization of normal spermiation and spermiation failure induced by hormone suppression in adult rats. Biol Reprod 2003; 68(4): 1299-307.
[http://dx.doi.org/10.1095/biolreprod.102.009811] [PMID: 12606480]

[105] Rato L, Alves MG, Dias TR, *et al.* High-energy diets may induce a pre-diabetic state altering testicular glycolytic metabolic profile and male reproductive parameters. Andrology 2013; 1(3): 495-504.
[http://dx.doi.org/10.1111/j.2047-2927.2013.00071.x] [PMID: 23495257]

[106] Hikim AP, Wang C, Leung A, Swerdloff RS. Involvement of apoptosis in the induction of germ cell degeneration in adult rats after gonadotropin-releasing hormone antagonist treatment. Endocrinology 1995; 136(6): 2770-5.
[http://dx.doi.org/10.1210/endo.136.6.7750502] [PMID: 7750502]

[107] ODonnell L, Narula A, Balourdos G, *et al.* Impairment of spermatogonial development and spermiation after testosterone-induced gonadotropin suppression in adult monkeys (Macaca fascicularis). J Clin Endocrinol Metab 2001; 86(4): 1814-22.
[http://dx.doi.org/10.1210/jcem.86.4.7400] [PMID: 11297623]

[108] Tapanainen JS, Tilly JL, Vihko KK, Hsueh AJ. Hormonal control of apoptotic cell death in the testis: gonadotropins and androgens as testicular cell survival factors. Mol Endocrinol 1993; 7(5): 643-50.
[http://dx.doi.org/10.1210/mend.7.5.8316250] [PMID: 8316250]

[109] De Gendt K, Swinnen JV, Saunders PT, *et al.* A Sertoli cell-selective knockout of the androgen receptor causes spermatogenic arrest in meiosis. Proc Natl Acad Sci USA 2004; 101(5): 1327-32.
[http://dx.doi.org/10.1073/pnas.0308114100] [PMID: 14745012]

[110] Tsai MY, Yeh SD, Wang RS, *et al.* Differential effects of spermatogenesis and fertility in mice lacking androgen receptor in individual testis cells. Proc Natl Acad Sci USA 2006; 103(50): 18975-80.
[http://dx.doi.org/10.1073/pnas.0608565103] [PMID: 17142319]

[111] Pakarainen T, Zhang F-P, Mäkelä S, Poutanen M, Huhtaniemi I. Testosterone replacement therapy induces spermatogenesis and partially restores fertility in luteinizing hormone receptor knockout mice. Endocrinology 2005; 146(2): 596-606.
[http://dx.doi.org/10.1210/en.2004-0913] [PMID: 15514086]

[112] Sun Y-T, Irby DC, Robertson DM, de Kretser DM. The effects of exogenously administered testosterone on spermatogenesis in intact and hypophysectomized rats. Endocrinology 1989; 125(2): 1000-10.
[http://dx.doi.org/10.1210/endo-125-2-1000] [PMID: 2502373]

[113] Awoniyi CA, Sprando RL, Santulli R, Chandrashekar V, Ewing LL, Zirkin BR. Restoration of spermatogenesis by exogenously administered testosterone in rats made azoospermic by hypophysectomy or withdrawal of luteinizing hormone alone. Endocrinology 1990; 127(1): 177-84. [http://dx.doi.org/10.1210/endo-127-1-177] [PMID: 2113863]

[114] Kerr JB, Millar M, Maddocks S, Sharpe RM. Stage-dependent changes in spermatogenesis and Sertoli cells in relation to the onset of spermatogenic failure following withdrawal of testosterone. Anat Rec 1993; 235(4): 547-59. [http://dx.doi.org/10.1002/ar.1092350407] [PMID: 8385423]

[115] Perryman KJ, Stanton PG, Loveland KL, McLachlan RI, Robertson DM. Hormonal dependency of neural cadherin in the binding of round spermatids to Sertoli cells *in vitro*. Endocrinology 1996; 137(9): 3877-83. [http://dx.doi.org/10.1210/endo.137.9.8756560] [PMID: 8756560]

[116] Muffly KE, Nazian SJ, Cameron DF. Effects of follicle-stimulating hormone on the junction-related Sertoli cell cytoskeleton and daily sperm production in testosterone-treated hypophysectomized rats. Biol Reprod 1994; 51(1): 158-66. [http://dx.doi.org/10.1095/biolreprod51.1.158] [PMID: 7918871]

[117] ODonnell L, Pratis K, Wagenfeld A, *et al.* Transcriptional profiling of the hormone-responsive stages of spermatogenesis reveals cell-, stage-, and hormone-specific events. Endocrinology 2009; 150(11): 5074-84. [http://dx.doi.org/10.1210/en.2009-0755] [PMID: 19797402]

[118] Meistrich ML. Hormonal stimulation of the recovery of spermatogenesis following chemo- or radiotherapy. Review article. APMIS 1998; 106(1): 37-45. [http://dx.doi.org/10.1111/j.1699-0463.1998.tb01317.x] [PMID: 9524560]

[119] Ruwanpura SM, McLachlan RI, Meachem SJ. Hormonal regulation of male germ cell development. J Endocrinol 2010; 205(2): 117-31. [http://dx.doi.org/10.1677/JOE-10-0025] [PMID: 20144980]

[120] Meachem SJ, Wreford NG, Stanton PG, Robertson DM, McLachlan RI. Follicle-stimulating hormone is required for the initial phase of spermatogenic restoration in adult rats following gonadotropin suppression. J Androl 1998; 19(6): 725-35. [PMID: 9876024]

[121] O'Donnell L, Meachem SJ, Stanton PG, McLachlan RI. Endocrine regulation of spermatogenesis. Knobil and Neill's physiology of reproduction 2006; 1: 1017-70. [http://dx.doi.org/10.1016/B978-012515400-0/50026-9]

[122] El Shennawy A, Gates RJ, Russell LD. Hormonal regulation of spermatogenesis in the hypophysectomized rat: cell viability after hormonal replacement in adults after intermediate periods of hypophysectomy. J Androl 1998; 19(3): 320-34. [PMID: 9639049]

[123] Eddy EM, Washburn TF, Bunch DO, *et al.* Targeted disruption of the estrogen receptor gene in male mice causes alteration of spermatogenesis and infertility. Endocrinology 1996; 137(11): 4796-805. [http://dx.doi.org/10.1210/endo.137.11.8895349] [PMID: 8895349]

[124] Hess RA, Bunick D, Lee K-H, *et al.* A role for oestrogens in the male reproductive system. Obstet Gynecol Surv 1998; 53: 359-60. [http://dx.doi.org/10.1097/00006254-199806000-00017] [PMID: 9393999]

[125] DSouza R, Gill-Sharma MK, Pathak S, Kedia N, Kumar R, Balasinor N. Effect of high intratesticular estrogen on the seminiferous epithelium in adult male rats. Mol Cell Endocrinol 2005; 241(1-2): 41-8. [http://dx.doi.org/10.1016/j.mce.2005.04.011] [PMID: 15936871]

[126] Dumasia K, Kumar A, Kadam L, Balasinor NH. Effect of estrogen receptor-subtype-specific ligands on fertility in adult male rats. J Endocrinol 2015; 225(3): 169-80. [http://dx.doi.org/10.1530/JOE-15-0045] [PMID: 25869617]

[127] Dumasia K, Kumar A, Deshpande S, Sonawane S, Balasinor NH. Differential roles of estrogen receptors, ESR1 and ESR2, in adult rat spermatogenesis. Mol Cell Endocrinol 2016; 428: 89-100. [http://dx.doi.org/10.1016/j.mce.2016.03.024] [PMID: 27004961]

[128] Blanco-Rodríguez J, Martínez-García C. Apoptosis pattern elicited by oestradiol treatment of the seminiferous epithelium of the adult rat. J Reprod Fertil 1997; 110(1): 61-70. [http://dx.doi.org/10.1530/jrf.0.1100061] [PMID: 9227358]

[129] D'Souza R, Pathak S, Upadhyay R, *et al.* Disruption of tubulobulbar complex by high intratesticular estrogens leading to failed spermiation. Endocrinology 2009; 150(4): 1861-9. [http://dx.doi.org/10.1210/en.2008-1232] [PMID: 19095743]

[130] Mishra DP, Shaha C. Estrogen-induced spermatogenic cell apoptosis occurs *via* the mitochondrial pathway: role of superoxide and nitric oxide. J Biol Chem 2005; 280(7): 6181-96. [http://dx.doi.org/10.1074/jbc.M405970200] [PMID: 15545282]

[131] Pentikäinen V, Erkkilä K, Suomalainen L, Parvinen M, Dunkel L. Estradiol acts as a germ cell survival factor in the human testis *in vitro*. J Clin Endocrinol Metab 2000; 85(5): 2057-67. [http://dx.doi.org/10.1210/jcem.85.5.6600] [PMID: 10843196]

[132] Robertson KM, ODonnell L, Jones ME, *et al.* Impairment of spermatogenesis in mice lacking a functional aromatase (cyp 19) gene. Proc Natl Acad Sci USA 1999; 96(14): 7986-91. [http://dx.doi.org/10.1073/pnas.96.14.7986] [PMID: 10393934]

[133] Correia S, Cardoso HJ, Cavaco JE, Socorro S. Oestrogens as apoptosis regulators in mammalian testis: angels or devils? Expert Rev Mol Med 2015; 17: e2. [http://dx.doi.org/10.1017/erm.2014.25] [PMID: 26258687]

[134] Boussouar F, Benahmed M. Lactate and energy metabolism in male germ cells. Trends Endocrinol Metab 2004; 15(7): 345-50. [http://dx.doi.org/10.1016/j.tem.2004.07.003] [PMID: 15350607]

[135] Le Magueresse B, Pineau C, Guillou F, Jégou B. Influence of germ cells upon transferrin secretion by rat Sertoli cells *in vitro*. J Endocrinol 1988; 118(3): R13-6. [http://dx.doi.org/10.1677/joe.0.118R013] [PMID: 3183569]

[136] Sylvester SR. Secretion of transport and binding proteins. Florida: The Sertoli Cell, Cache River Press Clarwater 1993; pp. 201-16.

[137] Danzo BJ, Pavlou SN, Anthony HL. Hormonal regulation of androgen-binding protein in the rat. Endocrinology 1990; 127(6): 2829-38. [http://dx.doi.org/10.1210/endo-127-6-2829] [PMID: 2123442]

[138] Huang HF, Pogach LM, Nathan E, Giglio W, Seebode JJ. Synergistic effects of follicle-stimulating hormone and testosterone on the maintenance of spermiogenesis in hypophysectomized rats: relationship with the androgen-binding protein status. Endocrinology 1991; 128(6): 3152-61. [http://dx.doi.org/10.1210/endo-128-6-3152] [PMID: 1903701]

[139] Martin-du Pan RC, Campana A. Physiopathology of spermatogenic arrest. Fertil Steril 1993; 60(6): 937-46. [http://dx.doi.org/10.1016/S0015-0282(16)56388-2] [PMID: 8243695]

[140] Larriba S, Esteban C, Toràn N, *et al.* Androgen binding protein is tissue-specifically expressed and biologically active in transgenic mice. J Steroid Biochem Mol Biol 1995; 53(1-6): 573-8. [http://dx.doi.org/10.1016/0960-0760(95)00103-7] [PMID: 7626512]

[141] Steinberger A, Steinberger E. Secretion of an FSH-inhibiting factor by cultured Sertoli cells. Endocrinology 1976; 99(3): 918-21.
[http://dx.doi.org/10.1210/endo-99-3-918] [PMID: 954678]

[142] Mather JP, Attie KM, Woodruff TK, Rice GC, Phillips DM. Activin stimulates spermatogonial proliferation in germ-Sertoli cell cocultures from immature rat testis. Endocrinology 1990; 127(6): 3206-14.
[http://dx.doi.org/10.1210/endo-127-6-3206] [PMID: 2249646]

[143] van Dissel-Emiliani FM, Grootenhuis AJ, de Jong FH, de Rooij DG. Inhibin reduces spermatogonial numbers in testes of adult mice and Chinese hamsters. Endocrinology 1989; 125(4): 1899-903.
[http://dx.doi.org/10.1210/endo-125-4-1898] [PMID: 2791973]

[144] Vijayalakshmi S, Bandivdekar AH, Joshi LR, Moodbidri SB, Sheth AR. Isolation and characterization of ovine testicular and ovarian inhibin. Arch Androl 1980; 5(2): 179-88.
[http://dx.doi.org/10.3109/01485018008986313] [PMID: 6775607]

[145] Ling N, Ying S-Y, Ueno N, *et al.* Pituitary FSH Is Released by a Heterodimer of the [beta]-Subunits from the Two Forms of Inhibin. Obstet Gynecol Surv 1987; 42: 109-11.
[http://dx.doi.org/10.1097/00006254-198702000-00015] [PMID: 3086749]

[146] Wong CH, Cheng CY. The blood-testis barrier: its biology, regulation, and physiological role in spermatogenesis. Curr Top Dev Biol 2005; 71: 263-96.
[http://dx.doi.org/10.1016/S0070-2153(05)71008-5] [PMID: 16344108]

[147] Mallea LE, Machado AJ, Navaroli F, Rommerts FF. Epidermal growth factor stimulates lactate production and inhibits aromatization in cultured Sertoli cells from immature rats. Int J Androl 1986; 9(3): 201-8.
[http://dx.doi.org/10.1111/j.1365-2605.1986.tb00883.x] [PMID: 3100457]

[148] Onoda M, Suarez-Quian CA. Modulation of transferrin secretion by epidermal growth factor in immature rat Sertoli cells *in vitro*. J Reprod Fertil 1994; 100(2): 541-50.
[http://dx.doi.org/10.1530/jrf.0.1000541] [PMID: 8021875]

[149] Skinner MK, Takacs K, Coffey RJ. Transforming growth factor-alpha gene expression and action in the seminiferous tubule: peritubular cell-Sertoli cell interactions. Endocrinology 1989; 124(2): 845-54.
[http://dx.doi.org/10.1210/endo-124-2-845] [PMID: 2463904]

[150] Siu MK, Lee WM, Cheng CY. The interplay of collagen IV, tumor necrosis factor-α, gelatinase B (matrix metalloprotease-9), and tissue inhibitor of metalloproteases-1 in the basal lamina regulates Sertoli cell-tight junction dynamics in the rat testis. Endocrinology 2003; 144(1): 371-87.
[http://dx.doi.org/10.1210/en.2002-220786] [PMID: 12488366]

[151] Skinner MK, Moses HL. Transforming growth factor beta gene expression and action in the seminiferous tubule: peritubular cell-Sertoli cell interactions. Mol Endocrinol 1989; 3(4): 625-34.
[http://dx.doi.org/10.1210/mend-3-4-625] [PMID: 2725526]

[152] Le Magueresse-Battistoni B, Morera A-M, Goddard I, Benahmed M. Expression of mRNAs for transforming growth factor-beta receptors in the rat testis. Endocrinology 1995; 136(6): 2788-91.
[http://dx.doi.org/10.1210/endo.136.6.7750505] [PMID: 7750505]

[153] Olaso R, Pairault C, Habert R. Expression of type I and II receptors for transforming growth factor β in the adult rat testis. Histochem Cell Biol 1998; 110(6): 613-8.
[http://dx.doi.org/10.1007/s004180050324] [PMID: 9860260]

[154] Gonzalez CR, Calandra RS, Gonzalez-Calvar SI. Testicular expression of the TGF-B1 system and the control of Leydig cell proliferation. Adv Biosci Biotechnol 2013; 4: 1-7.
[http://dx.doi.org/10.4236/abb.2013.410A4001] [PMID: 24883227]

[155] Morera AM, Cochet C, Keramidas M, Chauvin MA, de Peretti E, Benahmed M. Direct regulating effects of transforming growth factor β on the Leydig cell steroidogenesis in primary culture. J Steroid Biochem 1988; 30(1-6): 443-7.
[http://dx.doi.org/10.1016/0022-4731(88)90139-2] [PMID: 3164434]

[156] Morera AM, Esposito G, Ghiglieri C, Chauvin MA, Hartmann DJ, Benahmed M. Transforming growth factor beta 1 inhibits gonadotropin action in cultured porcine Sertoli cells. Endocrinology 1992; 130(2): 831-6.
[http://dx.doi.org/10.1210/endo.130.2.1370796] [PMID: 1370796]

[157] Sordoillet C, Chauvin MA, Revol A, Morera AM, Benahmed M. Fibroblast growth factor is a regulator of testosterone secretion in cultured immature Leydig cells. Mol Cell Endocrinol 1988; 58(2-3): 283-6.
[http://dx.doi.org/10.1016/0303-7207(88)90166-9] [PMID: 3208997]

[158] Van Dissel-Emiliani FM, De Boer-Brouwer M, De Rooij DG. Effect of fibroblast growth factor-2 on Sertoli cells and gonocytes in coculture during the perinatal period. Endocrinology 1996; 137(2): 647-54.
[http://dx.doi.org/10.1210/endo.137.2.8593814] [PMID: 8593814]

[159] Mullaney BP, Skinner MK. Basic fibroblast growth factor (bFGF) gene expression and protein production during pubertal development of the seminiferous tubule: follicle-stimulating hormone-induced Sertoli cell bFGF expression. Endocrinology 1992; 131(6): 2928-34.
[http://dx.doi.org/10.1210/endo.131.6.1446630] [PMID: 1446630]

[160] Le Magueresse-Battistoni B, Wolff J, Morera A-M, Benahmed M. Fibroblast growth factor receptor type 1 expression during rat testicular development and its regulation in cultured Sertoli cells. Endocrinology 1994; 135(6): 2404-11.
[http://dx.doi.org/10.1210/endo.135.6.7988424] [PMID: 7988424]

[161] Ebata KT, Yeh JR, Zhang X, Nagano MC. Soluble growth factors stimulate spermatogonial stem cell divisions that maintain a stem cell pool and produce progenitors *in vitro*. Exp Cell Res 2011; 317(10): 1319-29.
[http://dx.doi.org/10.1016/j.yexcr.2011.03.013] [PMID: 21420950]

[162] Zhang Y, Wang S, Wang X, Liao S, Wu Y, Han C. Endogenously produced FGF2 is essential for the survival and proliferation of cultured mouse spermatogonial stem cells. Cell Res 2012; 22(4): 773-6.
[http://dx.doi.org/10.1038/cr.2012.17] [PMID: 22290421]

[163] Handelsman DJ, Spaliviero JA, Scott CD, Baxter RC. Identification of insulin-like growth factor-I and its receptors in the rat testis. Acta Endocrinol 1985; 109(4): 543-9.
[http://dx.doi.org/10.1530/acta.0.1090543] [PMID: 2994333]

[164] Vannelli BG, Barni T, Orlando C, Natali A, Serio M, Balboni GC. Insulin-like growth factor-I (IGF-I) and IGF-I receptor in human testis: an immunohistochemical study. Fertil Steril 1988; 49(4): 666-9.
[http://dx.doi.org/10.1016/S0015-0282(16)59837-9] [PMID: 2965033]

[165] Cailleau J, Vermeire S, Verhoeven G. Independent control of the production of insulin-like growth factor I and its binding protein by cultured testicular cells. Mol Cell Endocrinol 1990; 69(1): 79-89.
[http://dx.doi.org/10.1016/0303-7207(90)90091-L] [PMID: 2157618]

[166] Benahmed M, Morera AM, Chauvin MC, de Peretti E. Somatomedin C/insulin-like growth factor 1 as a possible intratesticular regulator of Leydig cell activity. Mol Cell Endocrinol 1987; 50(1-2): 69-77.
[http://dx.doi.org/10.1016/0303-7207(87)90078-5] [PMID: 2953635]

[167] Morera AM, Chauvin MA, de Peretti E, Binoux M, Benahmed M. Somatomedin C/insulin-like growth factor 1: an intratesticular differentiative factor of Leydig cells? Horm Res 1987; 28(1): 50-7.
[http://dx.doi.org/10.1159/000180925] [PMID: 3447942]

[168] Rappaport MS, Smith EP. Insulin-like growth factor I inhibits aromatization induced by follicle-stimulating hormone in rat sertoli cell culture. Biol Reprod 1996; 54(2): 446-52. [http://dx.doi.org/10.1095/biolreprod54.2.446] [PMID: 8788198]

[169] Khan SA, Ndjountche L, Pratchard L, Spicer LJ, Davis JS. Follicle-stimulating hormone amplifies insulin-like growth factor I-mediated activation of AKT/protein kinase B signaling in immature rat Sertoli cells. Endocrinology 2002; 143(6): 2259-67. [http://dx.doi.org/10.1210/endo.143.6.8838] [PMID: 12021190]

[170] OBrien DA, Welch JE, Fulcher KD, Eddy EM. Expression of mannose 6-phosphate receptor messenger ribonucleic acids in mouse spermatogenic and Sertoli cells. Biol Reprod 1994; 50(2): 429-35. [http://dx.doi.org/10.1095/biolreprod50.2.429] [PMID: 8142560]

[171] Perrot V, Funkenstein B. Cellular distribution of insulin-like growth factor II (IGF-II) mRNA and hormonal regulation of IGF-I and IGF-II mRNA expression in rainbow trout testis (Oncorhynchus mykiss). Fish Physiol Biochem 1999; 20: 219-29. [http://dx.doi.org/10.1023/A:1007735314871]

[172] Tsuruta JK, OBrien DA. Sertoli cell-spermatogenic cell interaction: the insulin-like growth factor-II/cation-independent mannose 6-phosphate receptor mediates changes in spermatogenic cell gene expression in mice. Biol Reprod 1995; 53(6): 1454-64. [http://dx.doi.org/10.1095/biolreprod53.6.1454] [PMID: 8562703]

[173] Meinhardt A, Hedger MP. Immunological, paracrine and endocrine aspects of testicular immune privilege. Mol Cell Endocrinol 2011; 335(1): 60-8. [http://dx.doi.org/10.1016/j.mce.2010.03.022] [PMID: 20363290]

[174] Huleihel M, Lunenfeld E. Involvement of intratesticular IL-1 system in the regulation of Sertoli cell functions. Mol Cell Endocrinol 2002; 187(1-2): 125-32. [http://dx.doi.org/10.1016/S0303-7207(01)00690-6] [PMID: 11988319]

[175] Nehar D, Mauduit C, Boussouar F, Benahmed M. Interleukin 1α stimulates lactate dehydrogenase A expression and lactate production in cultured porcine sertoli cells. Biol Reprod 1998; 59(6): 1425-32. [http://dx.doi.org/10.1095/biolreprod59.6.1425] [PMID: 9828188]

[176] Petersen C, Boitani C, Fröysa B, Söder O. Interleukin-1 is a potent growth factor for immature rat sertoli cells. Mol Cell Endocrinol 2002; 186(1): 37-47. [http://dx.doi.org/10.1016/S0303-7207(01)00680-3] [PMID: 11850120]

[177] Zeyse D, Lunenfeld E, Beck M, Prinsloo I, Huleihel M. Interleukin-1 receptor antagonist is produced by sertoli cells *in vitro*. Endocrinology 2000; 141(4): 1521-7. [http://dx.doi.org/10.1210/endo.141.4.7401] [PMID: 10746659]

[178] Cohen PE, Pollard JW. Normal sexual function in male mice lacking a functional type I interleukin-1 (IL-1) receptor. Endocrinology 1998; 139(2): 815-8. [http://dx.doi.org/10.1210/endo.139.2.5914] [PMID: 9449661]

[179] Syed V, Stéphan JP, Gérard N, *et al.* Residual bodies activate Sertoli cell interleukin-1 alpha (IL-1 alpha) release, which triggers IL-6 production by an autocrine mechanism, through the lipoxygenase pathway. Endocrinology 1995; 136(7): 3070-8. [http://dx.doi.org/10.1210/endo.136.7.7789334] [PMID: 7789334]

[180] Okuda Y, Bardin CW, Hodgskin LR, Morris PL. Interleukins-1 alpha and -1 beta regulate interleukin-6 expression in Leydig and Sertoli cells. Recent Prog Horm Res 1995; 50: 367-72. [PMID: 7740168]

[181] Zhang H, Yin Y, Wang G, Liu Z, Liu L, Sun F. Interleukin-6 disrupts blood-testis barrier through inhibiting protein degradation or activating phosphorylated ERK in Sertoli cells. 2014. Report No.: 4

[182] Boockfor FR, Schwarz LK. Effects of interleukin-6, interleukin-2, and tumor necrosis factor α on transferrin release from Sertoli cells in culture. Endocrinology 1991; 129(1): 256-62. [http://dx.doi.org/10.1210/endo-129-1-256] [PMID: 1905226]

[183] Rossi P, Albanesi C, Grimaldi P, Geremia R. Expression of the mRNA for the ligand of c-kit in mouse Sertoli cells. Biochem Biophys Res Commun 1991; 176(2): 910-4. [http://dx.doi.org/10.1016/S0006-291X(05)80272-4] [PMID: 1709019]

[184] Manova K, Nocka K, Besmer P, Bachvarova RF. Gonadal expression of c-kit encoded at the W locus of the mouse. Development 1990; 110(4): 1057-69. [PMID: 1712701]

[185] Yoshinaga K, Nishikawa S, Ogawa M, *et al.* Role of c-kit in mouse spermatogenesis: identification of spermatogonia as a specific site of c-kit expression and function. Development 1991; 113(2): 689-99. [PMID: 1723681]

[186] Munsie M, Schlatt S, deKretser DM, Loveland KL. Expression of stem cell factor in the postnatal rat testis. Mol Reprod Dev 1997; 47(1): 19-25. [http://dx.doi.org/10.1002/(SICI)1098-2795(199705)47:1<19::AID-MRD3>3.0.CO;2-T] [PMID: 9110310]

[187] Tajima Y, Sawada K, Morimoto T, Nishimune Y. Switching of mouse spermatogonial proliferation from the c-kit receptor-independent type to the receptor-dependent type during differentiation. J Reprod Fertil 1994; 102(1): 117-22. [http://dx.doi.org/10.1530/jrf.0.1020117] [PMID: 7528277]

[188] Allard EK, Blanchard KT, Boekelheide K. Exogenous stem cell factor (SCF) compensates for altered endogenous SCF expression in 2,5-hexanedione-induced testicular atrophy in rats. Biol Reprod 1996; 55(1): 185-93. [http://dx.doi.org/10.1095/biolreprod55.1.185] [PMID: 8793074]

[189] Marziali G, Lazzaro D, Sorrentino V. Binding of germ cells to mutant Sld Sertoli cells is defective and is rescued by expression of the transmembrane form of the c-kit ligand. Dev Biol 1993; 157(1): 182-90. [http://dx.doi.org/10.1006/dbio.1993.1122] [PMID: 7683283]

[190] Park SY, Jameson JL. Minireview: transcriptional regulation of gonadal development and differentiation. Endocrinology 2005; 146(3): 1035-42. [http://dx.doi.org/10.1210/en.2004-1454] [PMID: 15604204]

[191] Rao MK, Pham J, Imam JS, *et al.* Tissue-specific RNAi reveals that WT1 expression in nurse cells controls germ cell survival and spermatogenesis. Genes Dev 2006; 20(2): 147-52. [http://dx.doi.org/10.1101/gad1367806] [PMID: 16418481]

[192] Buaas FW, Kirsh AL, Sharma M, *et al.* Plzf is required in adult male germ cells for stem cell self-renewal. Nat Genet 2004; 36(6): 647-52. [http://dx.doi.org/10.1038/ng1366] [PMID: 15156142]

[193] Costoya JA, Hobbs RM, Barna M, *et al.* Essential role of Plzf in maintenance of spermatogonial stem cells. Nat Genet 2004; 36(6): 653-9. [http://dx.doi.org/10.1038/ng1367] [PMID: 15156143]

[194] Wang G, Zhang J, Moskophidis D, Mivechi NF. Targeted disruption of the heat shock transcription factor (hsf)-2 gene results in increased embryonic lethality, neuronal defects, and reduced spermatogenesis. Genesis 2003; 36(1): 48-61. [http://dx.doi.org/10.1002/gene.10200] [PMID: 12748967]

[195] Wang G, Ying Z, Jin X, *et al.* Essential requirement for both hsf1 and *Hsf2* transcriptional activity in spermatogenesis and male fertility. Genesis 2004; 38(2): 66-80. [http://dx.doi.org/10.1002/gene.20005] [PMID: 14994269]

[196] Alastalo T-P, Lönnström M, Leppä S, *et al.* Stage-specific expression and cellular localization of the heat shock factor 2 isoforms in the rat seminiferous epithelium. Exp Cell Res 1998; 240(1): 16-27. [http://dx.doi.org/10.1006/excr.1997.3926] [PMID: 9570917]

[197] Åkerfelt M, Henriksson E, Laiho A, *et al.* Promoter ChIP-chip analysis in mouse testis reveals Y chromosome occupancy by *Hsf2* . Proc Natl Acad Sci USA 2008; 105(32): 11224-9. [http://dx.doi.org/10.1073/pnas.0800620105] [PMID: 18682557]

[198] Sarge KD, Park-Sarge O-K, Kirby JD, Mayo KE, Morimoto RI. Expression of heat shock factor 2 in mouse testis: potential role as a regulator of heat-shock protein gene expression during spermatogenesis. Biol Reprod 1994; 50(6): 1334-43. [http://dx.doi.org/10.1095/biolreprod50.6.1334] [PMID: 8080921]

[199] Govin J, Caron C, Escoffier E, *et al.* Post-meiotic shifts in HSPA2/HSP70.2 chaperone activity during mouse spermatogenesis. J Biol Chem 2006; 281(49): 37888-92. [http://dx.doi.org/10.1074/jbc.M608147200] [PMID: 17035236]

[200] Hogeveen KN, Sassone-Corsi P. Regulation of gene expression in post-meiotic male germ cells: CREM-signalling pathways and male fertility. Hum Fertil (Camb) 2006; 9(2): 73-9. [http://dx.doi.org/10.1080/14647270500463400] [PMID: 16825108]

[201] Foulkes NS, Mellström B, Benusiglio E, Sassone-Corsi P. Developmental switch of CREM function during spermatogenesis: from antagonist to activator. 1992; 355: 80-4. [http://dx.doi.org/10.1038/355080a0] [PMID: 1370576]

[202] Foulkes NS, Schlotter F, Pévet P, Sassone-Corsi P. Pituitary hormone FSH directs the CREM functional switch during spermatogenesis. Nature 1993; 362(6417): 264-7. [http://dx.doi.org/10.1038/362264a0] [PMID: 7681549]

[203] Fimia GM, De Cesare D, Sassone-Corsi P. A family of LIM-only transcriptional coactivators: tissue-specific expression and selective activation of CREB and CREM. Mol Cell Biol 2000; 20(22): 8613-22. [http://dx.doi.org/10.1128/MCB.20.22.8613-8622.2000] [PMID: 11046156]

[204] De Cesare D, Fimia GM, Sassone-Corsi P. Signaling routes to CREM and CREB: plasticity in transcriptional activation. Trends Biochem Sci 1999; 24(7): 281-5. [http://dx.doi.org/10.1016/S0968-0004(99)01414-0] [PMID: 10390618]

[205] Fimia GM, De Cesare D, Sassone-Corsi P. CBP-independent activation of CREM and CREB by the LIM-only protein ACT. Nature 1999; 398(6723): 165-9. [http://dx.doi.org/10.1038/18237] [PMID: 10086359]

[206] Nantel F, Monaco L, Foulkes NS, *et al.* Spermiogenesis deficiency and germ-cell apoptosis in CREM-mutant mice. Nature 1996; 380(6570): 159-62. [http://dx.doi.org/10.1038/380159a0] [PMID: 8600390]

[207] Blendy JA, Kaestner KH, Weinbauer GF, Nieschlag E, Schütz G. Severe impairment of spermatogenesis in mice lacking the CREM gene. Nature 1996; 380(6570): 162-5. [http://dx.doi.org/10.1038/380162a0] [PMID: 8600391]

[208] Palermo I, Arcidiacono G, Barone N, *et al.* Normal expression of isoforms activating cyclic adenosine monophosphate responsive element modulator in patients with spermatid maturation arrest. Fertil Steril 2004; 82 (Suppl. 3): 1072-6. [http://dx.doi.org/10.1016/j.fertnstert.2004.05.077] [PMID: 15474076]

[209] Peri A, Krausz C, Cioppi F, *et al.* Cyclic adenosine 3,5-monophosphate-responsive element modulator gene expression in germ cells of normo- and oligoazoospermic men. J Clin Endocrinol Metab 1998; 83(10): 3722-6. [http://dx.doi.org/10.1210/jcem.83.10.5211] [PMID: 9768690]

[210] Rudolph D, Tafuri A, Gass P, Hämmerling GJ, Arnold B, Schütz G. Impaired fetal T cell development and perinatal lethality in mice lacking the cAMP response element binding protein. Proc Natl Acad Sci USA 1998; 95(8): 4481-6.
[http://dx.doi.org/10.1073/pnas.95.8.4481] [PMID: 9539763]

[211] Scobey MJ, Bertera S, Somers JP, Watkins SC, Zeleznik AJ, Walker WH. Delivery of a Cyclic Adenosine 3′, 5′-Monophosphate Response Element-Binding Protein (CREB) Mutant to Seminiferous Tubules Results in Impaired Spermatogenesis. Endocrinology 2001; 142: 948-54.
[http://dx.doi.org/10.1210/endo.142.2.7948] [PMID: 11159868]

[212] Lindsey JS, Wilkinson MF. Pem: a testosterone- and LH-regulated homeobox gene expressed in mouse Sertoli cells and epididymis. Dev Biol 1996; 179(2): 471-84.
[http://dx.doi.org/10.1006/dbio.1996.0276] [PMID: 8903361]

[213] Maclean JA II, Chen MA, Wayne CM, *et al. Rhox*: a new homeobox gene cluster. Cell 2005; 120(3): 369-82.
[http://dx.doi.org/10.1016/j.cell.2004.12.022] [PMID: 15707895]

[214] Welborn JP, Davis MG, Ebers SD, *et al. Rhox8* Ablation in the Sertoli Cells Using a Tissue-Specific RNAi Approach Results in Impaired Male Fertility in Mice. Biol Reprod 2015; 93(1): 8.
[http://dx.doi.org/10.1095/biolreprod.114.124834] [PMID: 25972016]

[215] Tsai-Morris CH, Sheng Y, Gutti R, Li J, Pickel J, Dufau ML. Gonadotropin-regulated testicular RNA helicase (GRTH/DDX25) gene: cell-specific expression and transcriptional regulation by androgen in transgenic mouse testis. J Cell Biochem 2010; 109(6): 1142-7.
[http://dx.doi.org/10.1002/jcb.22493] [PMID: 20108248]

[216] Tanaka SS, Toyooka Y, Akasu R, *et al.* The mouse homolog of Drosophila Vasa is required for the development of male germ cells. Genes Dev 2000; 14(7): 841-53.
[PMID: 10766740]

[217] Tsai-Morris C-H, Sheng Y, Lee E, Lei K-J, Dufau ML. Gonadotropin-regulated testicular RNA helicase (GRTH/Ddx25) is essential for spermatid development and completion of spermatogenesis. Proc Natl Acad Sci USA 2004; 101(17): 6373-8.
[http://dx.doi.org/10.1073/pnas.0401855101] [PMID: 15096601]

[218] Gutti RK, Tsai-Morris C-H, Dufau ML. Gonadotropin-regulated testicular helicase (DDX25), an essential regulator of spermatogenesis, prevents testicular germ cell apoptosis. J Biol Chem 2008; 283(25): 17055-64.
[http://dx.doi.org/10.1074/jbc.M708449200] [PMID: 18430733]

[219] Paronetto MP, Zalfa F, Botti F, Geremia R, Bagni C, Sette C. The nuclear RNA-binding protein Sam68 translocates to the cytoplasm and associates with the polysomes in mouse spermatocytes. Mol Biol Cell 2006; 17(1): 14-24.
[http://dx.doi.org/10.1091/mbc.E05-06-0548] [PMID: 16221888]

[220] Paronetto MP, Messina V, Bianchi E, *et al.* Sam68 regulates translation of target mRNAs in male germ cells, necessary for mouse spermatogenesis. J Cell Biol 2009; 185(2): 235-49.
[http://dx.doi.org/10.1083/jcb.200811138] [PMID: 19380878]

[221] Yang J, Medvedev S, Yu J, *et al.* Absence of the DNA-/RNA-binding protein MSY2 results in male and female infertility. Proc Natl Acad Sci USA 2005; 102(16): 5755-60.
[http://dx.doi.org/10.1073/pnas.0408718102] [PMID: 15824319]

[222] Yang J, Morales CR, Medvedev S, Schultz RM, Hecht NB. In the absence of the mouse DNA/RNA-binding protein MSY2, messenger RNA instability leads to spermatogenic arrest. Biol Reprod 2007; 76(1): 48-54.
[http://dx.doi.org/10.1095/biolreprod.106.055095] [PMID: 17035640]

[223] Kurihara Y, Watanabe H, Kawaguchi A, *et al.* Dynamic changes in intranuclear and subcellular localizations of mouse Prrp/DAZAP1 during spermatogenesis: the necessity of the C-terminal proline-rich region for nuclear import and localization. Arch Histol Cytol 2004; 67(4): 325-33. [http://dx.doi.org/10.1679/aohc.67.325] [PMID: 15700540]

[224] Vera Y, Dai T, Hikim AP, *et al.* Deleted in azoospermia associated protein 1 shuttles between nucleus and cytoplasm during normal germ cell maturation. J Androl 2002; 23(5): 622-8. [PMID: 12185095]

[225] Hsu LC, Chen H-Y, Lin Y-W, *et al.* DAZAP1, an hnRNP protein, is required for normal growth and spermatogenesis in mice. RNA 2008; 14(9): 1814-22. [http://dx.doi.org/10.1261/rna.1152808] [PMID: 18669443]

[226] Tsui S, Dai T, Roettger S, Schempp W, Salido EC, Yen PH. Identification of two novel proteins that interact with germ-cell-specific RNA-binding proteins DAZ and DAZL1. Genomics 2000; 65(3): 266-73. [http://dx.doi.org/10.1006/geno.2000.6169] [PMID: 10857750]

[227] Peters L, Meister G. Argonaute proteins: mediators of RNA silencing. Mol Cell 2007; 26(5): 611-23. [http://dx.doi.org/10.1016/j.molcel.2007.05.001] [PMID: 17560368]

[228] Grivna ST, Beyret E, Wang Z, Lin H. A novel class of small RNAs in mouse spermatogenic cells. Genes Dev 2006; 20(13): 1709-14. [http://dx.doi.org/10.1101/gad.1434406] [PMID: 16766680]

[229] Carmell MA, Girard A, van de Kant HJ, *et al.* MIWI2 is essential for spermatogenesis and repression of transposons in the mouse male germline. Dev Cell 2007; 12(4): 503-14. [http://dx.doi.org/10.1016/j.devcel.2007.03.001] [PMID: 17395546]

[230] Kuramochi-Miyagawa S, Kimura T, Yomogida K, *et al.* Two mouse piwi-related genes: miwi and mili. Mech Dev 2001; 108(1-2): 121-33. [http://dx.doi.org/10.1016/S0925-4773(01)00499-3] [PMID: 11578866]

[231] Kuramochi-Miyagawa S, Kimura T, Ijiri TW, *et al.* Mili, a mammalian member of piwi family gene, is essential for spermatogenesis. Development 2004; 131(4): 839-49. [http://dx.doi.org/10.1242/dev.00973] [PMID: 14736746]

[232] Unhavaithaya Y, Hao Y, Beyret E, *et al.* MILI, a PIWI-interacting RNA-binding protein, is required for germ line stem cell self-renewal and appears to positively regulate translation. J Biol Chem 2009; 284(10): 6507-19. [http://dx.doi.org/10.1074/jbc.M809104200] [PMID: 19114715]

[233] Kojima K, Kuramochi-Miyagawa S, Chuma S, *et al.* Associations between PIWI proteins and TDRD1/MTR-1 are critical for integrated subcellular localization in murine male germ cells. Genes Cells 2009; 14(10): 1155-65. [http://dx.doi.org/10.1111/j.1365-2443.2009.01342.x] [PMID: 19735482]

[234] Kuramochi-Miyagawa S, Watanabe T, Gotoh K, *et al.* DNA methylation of retrotransposon genes is regulated by Piwi family members MILI and MIWI2 in murine fetal testes. Genes Dev 2008; 22(7): 908-17. [http://dx.doi.org/10.1101/gad.1640708] [PMID: 18381894]

[235] Deng W, Lin H. miwi, a murine homolog of piwi, encodes a cytoplasmic protein essential for spermatogenesis. Dev Cell 2002; 2(6): 819-30. [http://dx.doi.org/10.1016/S1534-5807(02)00165-X] [PMID: 12062093]

[236] Pan Y, Hu M, Liang H, Wang JJ, Tang LJ. The expression of the PIWI family members miwi and mili in mice testis is negatively affected by estrogen. Cell Tissue Res 2012; 350(1): 177-81. [http://dx.doi.org/10.1007/s00441-012-1447-z] [PMID: 22628161]

CHAPTER 5

Hormonal Control of Male Reproductive Function

Maria J. Meneses[1,2] and **Ana D. Martins**[1,*]

[1] *Department of Microscopy, Laboratory of Cell Biology, Institute of Biomedical Sciences Abel Salazar (ICBAS) and Unit for Multidisciplinary Research in Biomedicine (UMIB), University of Porto, 4050-313 Porto, Portugal*

[2] *ProRegeM PhD Program, CEDOC – Chronic Diseases Research Center and NOVA Medical School, New University of Lisbon, 1150-082 Lisboa, Portugal*

Abstract: Hormones are key regulators of the reproductive system. These signaling molecules are transported in the blood stream to reach target organs in order to regulate physiologic processes and their function. The most relevant hormones for male reproductive system are those involved in the hypothalamus-pituitary-gonads axis. Through several stimuli, anterior pituitary produces luteinizing hormone and follicle-stimulating hormone that act on testicular cells modulating both steroidogenesis and spermatogenesis. In fact, steroidogenesis, namely the production of testosterone, is crucial for the normal occurrence of spermatogenesis and for feedback actions to the pituitary and hypothalamus. However, spermatogenesis and Sertoli cells are also important to the regulation of this axis through the production of activin and inhibin B that, along with testosterone, also transmit feedback to the brain. Interestingly, in the last years, new intervenient have appeared in the regulation of male reproductive function with the discovery that adipose tissue is an endocrine organ and thus also produces hormones that may be important for this process. Along with the latter, gut hormones, which are related with the nutrient homeostasis, also modulate the function of testicular cells. In some cases, this interaction was only found due to metabolic disorders, like hyper- or hypothyroidism, obesity or diabetes mellitus. Herein, we propose to discuss the action and function of these hormones that interact with male reproductive system.

Keywords: Adipokines, Androgens, Estrogens, Follicle stimulating hormone, Ghrelin, Glucagon like peptide-1, Gonadotropin-releasing hormone, Hormonal control, Hormones, Luteinizing hormone, Obestatin, Resistin, Testosterone, Thyroid hormones, 5α-dihydrotestosterone.

INTRODUCTION

Reproduction is a key process for the survival of a specie thus being subjected to a

* **Corresponding author Ana D. Martins:** Department of Microscopy, Laboratory of Cell Biology, Institute of Biomedical Sciences Abel Salazar (ICBAS), Rua de Jorge Viterbo Ferreira, Nº 228, 4050-313 Porto, Portugal; Tel: +351 220 428 000; E-mail: anacdmartins@gmail.com

tight control. The main players in this regulation are hormones which act as dynamic signaling molecules that modulate several events such as gene transcription and translation, directly influencing the reproductive phenotype. The most known hormones are those who belong to the hypothalamic-pituitary gonadal (HPG) axis. In males, the latter is based on the interaction between the hypothalamus, pituitary and the testes [1]. In brief, gonadotropin releasing hormone (GnRH) is synthesized by the hypothalamus, which will stimulate the pituitary to produce gonadotropins: the luteinizing hormone (LH) and the follicle-stimulating hormone (FSH). LH binds to membrane receptors on Leydig cells and stimulates testosterone production while FSH binds to membrane receptors on Sertoli cells, stimulating among other events, the production/secretion of 17β-estradiol, activin and inhibin B [2]. The 17β-estradiol acts on Leydig cells in order to inhibit the production of testosterone [3]; and while, activin produce a positive feedback [4] and inhibin B and 17β-estradiol produces a negative feedback on pituitary [4 - 7].

Over the last few years, other intervenient in the control of male reproductive function have been unveiled. In fact, male fertility is also dependent on overall metabolic and energetic homeostasis [8]. Although testicular metabolism was overlooked during several decades, the adequate overall body metabolic functioning and particularly in testicular cells is crucial for the normal occurrence of spermatogenesis. As nowadays this is a hot research field, other hormones associated with all body metabolic regulation were found to influence male reproductive function [9]. In fact, insulin, which is linked with glucose homeostasis is now known as an important regulator of spermatogenesis [10] (see Chapter 12). Similarly, gut hormones have been described as important regulators of male reproductive potential, besides its well-known role in controlling feeding/fasting status [11]. Moreover, as adipose tissue was recognized as an endocrine organ, the hormones that it produces, the adipokines, were also reported to interact with several other body systems, namely the reproductive system. Thyroid hormones (THs) are also known to influence the reproductive function of males [12]. In fact, they are so important for the modulation of male reproductive potential, that any fluctuation in thyroid hormone levels, either hypo- or hyperthyroidism may lead to impaired spermatogenesis. During this chapter, we will discuss the most relevant hormones and pathways that interact with male reproductive system.

THE HYPOTHALAMIC-PITUITARY-GONADAL (HPG) AXIS

The HPG axis is formed by the hypothalamus, pituitary, and gonads (testes in the male) (Fig. **5.1**). This axis is the key hormonal control system that modulates spermatogenesis and all the events occurring on the male reproductive tract. The hypothalamus synthesizes and releases neuro-hormones, namely GnRH [1]. The mammalian GnRH is a peptide hormone synthesized and released from GnRH-producing neurons within the arcuate nucleus of the hypothalamus [13]. Still, this secretion is not uniform during life, and changes happen during sexual development [14] (see Chapter 6). GnRH-producing neurons have an intrinsic pulse-generating ability leading to a pulsatile release of GnRH [15]. This pulsatile frequency and the concentration of GnRH influences the subsequent release of LH and FSH [16] having a crucial role in maintaining a normal steroidogenesis and gametogenesis. After its secretion, GnRH enters to the hypothalamic-pituitary portal system and bind to GnRH cell membrane receptors (GnRHR) on gonadotropic cells. These cells are located in the adenohypophysis, which represents 80% of the pituitary gland. The GnRHR is a transmembrane protein and its levels are regulated by GnRH. In fact, GnRHR levels increase when endogenous GnRH is increased. However, a continuous exposure to GnRH leads to desensitization causing a GnRHR downregulation [17]. When GnRHR is activated, it triggers several signal transduction pathways that lead to the release of the gonadotropins LH and FSH [18].

As GnRH, these gonadotropins are released in a pulsatile manner. However, while slower GnRH pulses lead to FSH synthesis, faster pulses favor LH synthesis and release [19]. An increase in the amplitude of LH pulses marks the beginning of puberty and the reactivation of reproductive axis, stimulating the secretion of gonadal sex steroid hormones. As puberty progresses, testosterone starts to control GnRH release, maintaining the frequency of LH pulses [20]. The major androgen produced in the testes is testosterone, a key regulator of spermatogenesis. This hormone is produced by Leydig cells in response to LH and targets Sertoli cells (Fig. **5.1**) that have androgens receptors (ARs) located in the nucleus and cytoplasm [21 - 23]. The other pituitary hormone secreted in response to GnRH is FSH that binds to G-protein coupled receptors, exclusively located in Sertoli cells [2] (Fig. **5.1**).

The activation of FSH receptor results in an increase of cyclic AMP signaling pathway, leading to increased levels of phosphorylated protein kinase B (PKB-P) through a phosphatidylinositol 3-kinase (PI3K)-dependent mechanism [24] and to the production and secretion of inhibin B by Sertoli cells. Inhibin B is a member of the transforming growth factor β family of proteins and its co-receptor betaglycan bind to the activin type II receptor, blocking its association with activin. Therefore, it selectively inhibits FSH biosynthesis and secretion through a negative feedback controlled by GnRH [25] without affecting LH secretion [26] (Fig. **5.1**). Inhibin is a dimer composed by an α subunit and either a βA- or a βB-subunit. In contrast, activin, a dimer composed of two identical inhibin β subunits, plays a positive feedback to the anterior pituitary and stimulates FSH release [27,

28] (Fig. **5.1**). In brief, activin binds to serine-threonine kinase membrane receptors on pituitary gonadotroph cells. This leads to the release of FSH and to the transcriptional activation of FSHB and GnRHR, genes encoding for the β subunit of FSH and the receptor of GnRH. Therefore, the number of GnRHR on the cell membrane upsurges thus increasing the expression of the gene that codifies for LH (LHB) and LH secretion in response to GnRH.

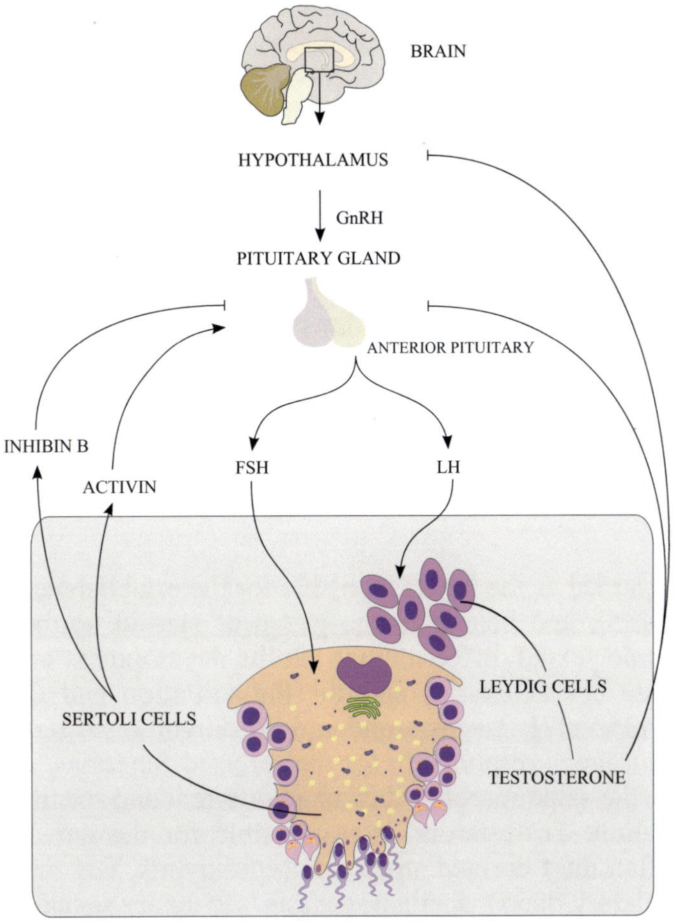

Fig. (5.1). Schematic illustration of the hypothalamic-pituitary-gonadal axis. GnRH released by the hypothalamus stimulates the synthesis and release of the gonadotrophins FSH and LH by the anterior pituitary. These gonadotrophins are transported to the testis where FSH stimulates inhibin production by Sertoli cells. Inhibin has a negative feedback effect on the pituitary release of FSH. Sertoli cells may also secrete activin to increase FSH secretion. LH stimulates testosterone production by the Leydig cells. After entering the circulation, testosterone is transported to the hypothalamus and exerts a negative feedback effect on hypothalamic GnRH release and has a direct negative effect on the release of FSH and LH by the pituitary. Abbreviations: FSH, follicle-stimulating hormone; GnRH, gonadotropin-releasing hormone; LH, luteinizing hormone.

Growth Hormone

Growth hormone (GH) is a hormone produced by the somatotropic cells of the anterior pituitary in response to hypothalamic growth hormone releasing hormone [29]. GH exerts its functions, namely in steroidogenesis, gametogenesis, and gonadal differentiation, through its receptor, growth hormone receptor (GHR). In fact, GH is thought to play an important role in testicular differentiation and development for several reasons. First, a lack of GH secretion in adult rats results in a delay in testes growth and in the differentiation of the germ cells [30]. Moreover, administration of GH blockers stops the differentiation of the Wolffian duct in male fetal mice, whereas GH administration in female fetuses stabilizes the Wolffian duct [31]. GH also has a role after birth, namely in gametogenesis. Sperm motility, concentration and morphology are reduced in GH-deficient animals but restored upon GH administration [32, 33] illustrating the relevance of GH to those mechanisms although they remain to be unveiled. However, it is known that GH binds GHRs on Sertoli cells and increases the synthesis and/or modification of proteins such as insulin-like growth factor 1 (IGF-1), IGF-binding proteins, that mediate the stimulatory effects of GH on spermatogenesis. In what concerns to steroidogenesis, it is primarily regulated by LH. However, GH binds Leydig GHRs, activates second messengers, and stimulates the activity of several steroidogenic enzymes directly and by increasing LH receptor abundance [34].

ANDROGENS

Androgens are regarded as the key responsible for the establishment of the sexual male phenotype [35], and belong to the group of steroid hormones. They are essential in the male sexual differentiation, in the development and maintenance of secondary male characteristics and for the initiation and development of spermatogenesis [35 - 37]. Testosterone and 5α-dihydrotestosterone (DHT) are the two major androgens responsible for the referred functions. Although these androgens bind to the same receptor, they have different and specific roles in male sexual differentiation. Testosterone is responsible for the development of the embryonic Wolffian duct derived structures (epididymis, *vas deferens*, seminal vesicles and ejaculatory ducts), spermatogenesis, secondary sexual characteristics, such as muscle development, voice deepening, and axillary and pubic hair growth [38, 39]. On the other side, DHT, a metabolite of testosterone, plays a crucial role in prostate development and growth, development of external genitalia and male patterns of facial and body hair growth or male-pattern baldness [39, 40].

Cholesterol is the precursor for the synthesis of steroids hormones. The testes have the ability to convert this organic molecule to androgens. The steroidogenic acute regulatory protein (StAR) transports cholesterol to the inner membrane of mitochondria, making this a limiting step during steroidogenesis [41]. Inside the mitochondria, the side chain cleavage system comprised of CYP11A1, ferrodoxin and ferrodoxin-reductase are responsible for the conversion of cholesterol to pregnenolone. It is then translocated from the mitochondria and transported to the smooth endoplasmic reticulum, where it is converted into testosterone and finally secreted by the Leydig cell [42]. Once on the circulation this hormone exerts a negative feedback com hypothalamus (Fig. **5.1**) [43].

The action of testosterone and DHT is mediated by the AR, a member of the nuclear receptor superfamily [44, 45]. Although the complete structure of AR is not fully elucidated, it is known that AR is structurally divided into functional domains: an N-terminal domain (NTD), a DNA binding domain (DBD), a C-terminal ligand binding domain (LBD), and a minor hinge region between DBD and LBD. A huge part of AR transcriptional activity is mediated by NTD which is the most active co-regulator interaction surface. The interaction of DHT and testosterone with AR is different. DHT has a two-fold higher affinity to the AR than testosterone. However, the dissociation of testosterone to the receptor is five-fold slower than DHT [39].

ESTROGENS

The connection between male function and estrogens has been under discussion for a long time. Nowadays it is widely accepted that estrogens have an important role in the development and maintenance of male fertility [46, 47]. In fact, estrogens are produced in the testis, being immature Sertoli cells the major source of estrogens during pre-puberty, while in adult life the major producer of estrogens is the Leydig cell [48, 49]. One of the main targets for estrogens is the Leydig cell, inhibiting the production of testosterone [50]. In the 30's it was described that C19 androgens could be directly transformed in C18 phenolic estrogens. Later, the enzyme responsible for this reversible reaction was described and named aromatase or cytochrome P450 aromatase (P450arom) [51]. This enzyme belongs to the cytochrome P450 superfamily [52] and is composed by two polypeptides, a specific P450arom encoded by the CYP19 gene and a ubiquitous NADPH cytochrome P450 reductase. Besides to be expressed in Sertoli and Leydig cell, the aromatase is also expressed by germ cells [53, 54]. The aromatization of androgens in order to synthesize estrogens englobes three reactions: sequential hydroxylation on the C19 methyl group and demethylation that lead to the removal of C19 as formic acid and the aromatization of the steroid A-ring, a characteristic of C18 estrogens [55]. Dehydroepiandrosterone, testosterone and androstenedione are the main aromatase substrates. In human male reproductive tract, Leydig [56, 57] and Sertoli cells [57, 58] are reported as estrogens producers. The 17β-estradiol produced by these cells has a negative feedback on pituitary [6].

The biological effects of testicular estrogens are mediated by estrogen receptors (ERs). Estrogens diffuse in the cell and bind to nuclear ERs, forming an estrogen-ER complex, modulating transcriptional target genes. In testicular cells, estrogens are important on male gamete maturation and three ERs known to mediate estrogen effects are present in these cells: ERα [59], ERβ [60] and G-protei--coupled estrogen receptor 1 (GPER) [61]. ERα and ERβ are nuclear receptors (NRs) of a family of ligand-modulated transcription factors [62 - 64]. The expression of ERα and ERβ is now globally accepted in the testicular tissue. The full-length ERα (66 kDa) and one isoform lacking the exon 1 (46 kDa) were found in immature male germ cells, and the 46 kDa isoform was observed in spermatozoa. ERα can also be found in Leydig cells [65, 66] and in the cells of the epithelium of efferent ductus, the region linking rete testis to the head of the epididymis [66 - 68]. The expression of this receptor was also found in spermatocytes, spermatids and spermatozoa [46, 54, 69, 70]. As concerning Erβ, two proteins, which correspond to a long (60 kDa) and short (50 kDa) forms of ERβ were identified in germ cells [71]. The expression of ERβ has also been described in Leydig [72], Sertoli [73] and peritubular cells [72, 73]

GPER, also known as G-protein coupled receptor 30, is an orphan G-protein coupled receptor with seven transmembrane domains [74]. A study performed in 2000 found that rapid 17β-estradiol-mediated activation of extracellular signal-regulated kinases (ERKs) was dependent on GPER, being the most recent known ER [61]. It is located on cell surface and is both, structurally and genetically distinct of ERα and ERβ. It is responsible for a quick activation of different pathways, leading to the rapid phosphorylation of the mitogen-activated protein kinases ERK1/2 [61, 75], stimulation of adenylyl cyclase [76, 77], PI3K signaling pathways activation and mobilization of intracellular calcium stores [78]. The expression of GPER was demonstrated in male reproductive tract, namely in Sertoli cells, diploid germ cells, epididymis, vas deferens, seminal vesicles and prostate (for review [79]). However, GPER is not present in haploid germ cells [80].

INSULIN

Insulin is a peptide hormone secreted by pancreatic β cells located in the islets of Langerhans [81]. Since its discovery, insulin has been considered a key circulating signal for energy homeostasis. In fact, this peptide has a crucial role in the physiological maintenance of blood glucose levels, and its dysregulation may lead to the onset of several metabolic disorders (see Chapter 12). Due to its importance, the exocytosis of insulin from β cells is a tightly regulated process.

The effects of insulin on peripheral tissues, and specially on male reproductive system, are mediated by the insulin receptor, which is widely expressed in testicular tissue, more specifically in Sertoli, Leydig and peritubular cells [82, 83]. When insulin binds to its receptor, the latter is phosphorylated and some effector proteins, namely PI3K are recruited and activate several signaling pathways [84]. These are involved in different cellular processes, such as metabolism, differentiation and proliferation [85]. Although the specific molecular mechanisms remain to be unveiled, it is known that insulin affects male reproductive function at multiple levels. In fact, besides energy homeostasis (see Chapter 12), insulin is necessary for testicular embryonic development [86]. When the family of insulin receptor tyrosine kinase are absent, XY mice develop ovaries and a female phenotype, indicating that insulin signaling pathway is required for male embryonic development [86].

In addition, ablation of insulin receptor leads to a decrease in both testes size and sperm production due to reduced proliferation rate of immature Sertoli cells during late embryonic period [87]. HPG axis functioning is also modulated by insulin. GnRH secretion is sensitive to metabolic signals and pathological situations that lead to hypoinsulinemia or hyperinsulinemia which are commonly linked with disturbed GnRH/LH pulses [88]. Indeed, exogenous insulin administration was found to increase LH that in turn promotes testosterone synthesis in Leydig cells [89]. In sum, besides energy homeostasis, insulin modulates the male reproductive system in several ways, even before birth. However, some of the mechanisms that lead to these effects remain to be unveiled.

THYROID HORMONES

Thyroid hormones (THs) are crucial for the homeostasis maintenance of some processes, particularly the control of body overall metabolism, protein synthesis, fat metabolism, neural development, normal growth and maturation of bones, as well as renal and cardiovascular functions [90, 91]. The thyroid gland synthetizes THs through iodination of tyrosine residues of the glycoprotein thyroglobulin [92, 93]. The hypothalamus and pituitary gland are the major controllers of THs production. Neurons in the paraventricular nucleus inside the hypothalamus secrete thyrotropin-releasing hormone that stimulates the pituitary gland, via a G-protein-coupled receptor, to secrete thyrotropin/thyroid-stimulating hormone (TSH). In turn, TSH binds to thyroid follicular cell basolateral membrane, which express a G-protein-coupled TSH receptor [94]. The prohormone thyroxine

(3,3',5,5'-tetraiodothyronine or T4) is the main product of the thyroid gland, but it has low biological activity. Through the intracellular removal of an iodine atom from the outer-ring of T4, 3,30,5-triiodothyronine (T3), the biologically active hormone is originated. The iodine uptake is regulated by TSH and is mediated by the sodium/iodide symporter. T3 has 100-fold higher affinity to thyroid hormone receptor (THR) than T4 [95, 96], so the reaction catalyzed by type 1 and type 2 iodothyronine deiodinases is essential. After its biosynthesis, THs enter the blood stream and bind to plasma thyroid hormone binding proteins in order to be distributed, since they are hydrophobic. However, THs need transporters to cross cell membranes and reach target cells, being monocarboxylate transporter 8 the most important transporter to perform that duty [97].

The effects of THs are mediated by a nuclear THR that belongs to the superfamily of NRs, and modulates gene transcription in response to hormone binding. Recognizing specific nucleotide sequences, the nuclear response elements, THRs bind to the promoter region of target genes and recruit co-activators or co-repressor proteins [62, 98, 99]. In human Sertoli cells, THRα1 and THRα2 have already been described [100]. In rat Sertoli cells, T3 suppresses the expression of immature Sertoli cell markers [101, 102]. On the other hand, hypothyroidism extends the expression of these markers in neonatal rats [101], showing a role of T3 in the maturation of Sertoli cells. Moreover, T3 regulates gap junctions between Sertoli cells through an increase of connexin 43 levels, a gap junction protein [103]. THs are also very important for Leydig cells. Indeed, after elimination of Leydig cells population in rats, T3 treated rats have a faster and bigger recovery of Leydig cells population when compared to controls with normal concentrations of THs [104]. Moreover, THs also influence steroidogenesis, increasing the production of testosterone [105, 106]. During germ cell development, THRα is expressed in type B spermatogonia and THRβ1 is expressed in intermediate type spermatogonia [12], suggesting a role for THs in sustaining different populations of germ cells. Along the male reproductive tract, THRα1 and THRβ1 are also expressed in the epididymis [107].

GUT HORMONES

Ghrelin

Ghrelin, as well as obestatin, is a gastrointestinal hormone obtained by post-translational processing of its precursor, preproghrelin [108]. Preproghrelin is composed by a 23 amino acids signal peptide and by proghrelin, a 94 amino acids peptide [109]. Ghrelin is a 28 amino acids segment of proghrelin, which is also composed by a carboxy-terminal peptide, the C-ghrelin [110 - 112]. Besides ghrelin, the proghrelin can be also processed to obestatin [113]. Ghrelin is subjected to posttranslational modifications comprising the acylation of the hydroxyl group of the Ser3 [114]. This acylation is required to activate the ghrelin receptor, also known as growth hormone secretagogue receptor (GHS-R), and to mediate its effects on GH secretion and food intake [115]. However, acylated ghrelin represents less than 10% of the circulating ghrelin [111, 116, 117]. Nevertheless, it has been hypothesized that desacylated ghrelin has a role in modulating the effects of acylated ghrelin.

The effects of ghrelin in the reproductive axis have been discussed for several years, and some studies suggest that this hormone is an important modulator of male reproductive function at different levels. Firstly, this hormone acts on the HPG axis, inhibiting the secretion of GnRH, LH and FSH [118 - 121] and stimulating the secretion of prolactin [122]. Moreover, in male rats it has the capacity to delay puberty onset [123] and downregulate Kiss1 [124], which encodes for a protein that stimulates the secretion of GnRH. The presence of GHS-R has been demonstrated in human germ cells, pachytene spermatocytes [125], Leydig [125] and Sertoli cells [11, 125]. Moreover, ghrelin has been detected in Sertoli and Leydig cells [125]. Additionally, in cases of varicocele, obstructive azoospermia or normozoospermia the serum levels of testosterone are inversely correlated with ghrelin levels, suggesting an effect on spermatogenesis [126]. In normal fed rats, ghrelin decreases testicular mass, but does not alter testosterone levels, while in food restricted rats, ghrelin decreases testosterone plasma levels [127]. An in vitro study, using adult rat testicular tissue, demonstrated that ghrelin inhibits human chorionic gonadotropin- and cAMP-stimulated testosterone secretion [128]. This inhibitory effect of ghrelin is associated with a decrease in human chorionic gonadotropin-stimulated expression of mRNAs encoding StAR, and P450 cholesterol side-chain cleavage, 3β-hydroxy steroid dehydrogenase, and 17β-hydroxy steroid dehydrogenase type III enzymes [128]. There are also evidence that ghrelin affects the development and maintenance of testicular cells. In fact, ghrelin has an inhibitory action in stem cell factor mRNA expression, a crucial signal for the development of Leydig cell and germ cells production [125, 129].

Therefore, the effect of ghrelin on stem cell factor expression may disturb spermatogenesis and Leydig cell proliferation. More recently, the effects of ghrelin in cultured Sertoli cell suggested this hormone as an energy status sensor for the male reproductive system. Moreover, there is an inverse association of this hormone with the production of lactate, thus controlling the nutritional support of spermatogenesis [11]. Hence, ghrelin acts as a regulator of testicular development and function, as this hormone modulates Leydig cells development and function and Sertoli cell metabolism.

Obestatin

Obestatin is a peptide with 23 amino acids that was discovered approximately ten years ago due to bioinformatic studies. It was found that it is a result of the carboxy-terminal part of proghrelin, the same prepropeptide from which ghrelin derives [113]. Obestatin was purified for the first time from rat stomach mucosa. Since then, it was already identified in several tissues and cell types, namely gastric mucosa, duodenum, colon, pancreas, spleen, mammary glands and in Leydig cells [130]. However, in human tissues, the information about the distribution of this peptide is scarce [131].

In order to maintain its regular conformation, obestatin has a post-translational amide modification on the C-terminal. Moreover, it is known that it is a circulating peptide with a pulsatile secretion [132]. However, its secretion has no effects on the expression profile of other hormones, namely GH, leptin and corticosterone [133, 134]. Nevertheless, obestatin enhances testosterone production by Leydig cells [135]. In fact, obestatin expression is present in human Sertoli and Leydig cells, rete testis, efferent ducts, *vas deferens* and seminal vesicles [136]. Although obestatin was firstly associated as the ligand for the G-protein coupled receptor 39, this fact was later excluded due to subsequent studies. Nowadays, it is proposed that obestatin binds to glucagon-like peptide 1 receptor (GLP-1R) [137], although more studies are needed to confirm this hypothesis.

Glucagon-Like Peptide-1

Secreted mainly from entero endocrine L-cells in the epithelium of the distal ileum and colon, but also from cells in the pancreas, and in the central nervous system [138], glucagon-like peptide 1 (GLP-1) belongs to gastrointestinal peptide hormone incretin family [139 - 141]. GLP-1 has several effects on pancreatic β cells, such as stimulation of glucose-induced secretion of insulin and β cell neogenesis, besides inhibiting β cell apoptosis. Moreover, GLP-1 delays gastric emptying and increases peripheral glucose disposal [142, 143]. Furthermore, as GLP-1 can cross the blood-brain barrier [144], it acts in the brain in order to enhance satiety. GLP-1 binds to its receptor, GLP-1R, a member of a glucagon receptor family of G protein-coupled receptors [145], which is widely expressed in the pancreatic islets, heart, brain, kidney and stomach [146 - 151]. The human GLP-1R has an N-terminal extracellular domain and some glycosylation sites, essential for the coupling of GLP-1 and for the successful trafficking and processing of the receptor [152 - 154].

GLP-1 was identified in 1981 in the translational products of mRNAs isolated from the pancreatic islets of anglerfish being the second incretin to be discovered

[155, 156]. GLP-1 is part of the product of proglucagon gene, and has approximately 50% of homology to glucagon [157]. In the circulation, there are two types of bioactive GLP-1 being GLP-17-36 amide, which corresponds to proglucagon 78–107 with its C-terminal Arg amidated, the most common circulating form in humans [158, 159]. However, the half-life of this hormone is very short, since it is cleared by the kidney and inactivated by the ubiquitous proteolytic enzyme dipeptidyl peptidase-4, which cleaves two amino acids from the n-terminus of GLP-1 [160].

Although it is known that GLP-1 has a key role in maintaining glucose and nutrient homeostasis, little is known about the effects of GLP-1 in male reproductive function. However, GLP-1 has several effects in the central nervous system that may impair HPG axis. Moreover, the administration of GLP-1 in healthy men result in a decrease of testosterone production independent of LH levels, illustrating a role of GLP-1 in steroidogenesis [161]. In addition, GLP-1 seems to have a role in puberty onset, since it alters the secretion of hypothalamic GnRH [162]. The same study showed, through a knockout mouse model of GLP-1 receptor, that even though the levels of gonadal sex steroids were normal, the males have decreased gonadal weight [162]. Although more studies are needed to unveil the mechanisms by which GLP-1 affects male reproductive function, it is already clear that this hormone may modulate it in several ways.

ADIPOKINES

Leptin

Leptin is a 16 kDa adipocyte-derived protein encoded by the obese (ob) gene [163]. Besides adipocytes, leptin is locally produced in other tissues, such as ovary, skeletal muscle and stomach [164, 165]. This may suggest pleiotropic effects of leptin on several biological functions. In fact, leptin plays a key role in appetite modulation, but was also reported it has a role in immune and gonadal functions and stress responses [166 - 168]. As leptin is mostly produced in white adipose tissue, its concentration in the blood stream is positively correlated with the amount of fat mass of an individual.

After being secreted by adipocytes, leptin circulates in the bloodstream bound to a circulating isoform of LepR. Then, it surpasses the blood-brain barrier via the short leptin receptor isoform to the hypothalamus [169]. Here, leptin binds to its receptor (LepR) on neurons producing anorexigenic proopiomelanocortin (POMC) and Agouti-related protein (AgRP) within the arcuate nucleus. When leptin binds to LepR, signal transducer and activator of transcription 3 is activated, which will then bind to pomc and agrp promoters, activating the first and inactivating the second one [170]. Besides, leptin also activates PI3K, which in turn induces the synthesis of PIP3. The accumulation of the latter leads to 3-phosphoinositide-dependent protein kinase 1 and protein kinase B activation resulting in the inactivation forkhead box protein O1 that functions as inhibitor of POMC expression and activator of AgRP [171]. This will then suppress energy intake and stimulate energy expenditure. Consequently, leptin is known as the satiety hormone.

As leptin has a key role in the regulation of nutrient homeostasis, this hormone also impacts male reproductive function, mainly through its neuroendocrine effects. In fact, leptin deficiency leads to pubertal failure and infertility (see Chapter 6) [172]. On the other hand, in obese men, the increased concentration of leptin inhibits testosterone production by Leydig cells, impairing spermatogenesis [173]. This effect may be due to the capacity of leptin to decrease testicular expression levels of StAR and cholesterol side-chain cleavage enzyme, upstream elements of the steroidogenic pathway, in a dose-dependent manner [174]. Moreover, leptin was found to regulate estrogen synthesis through modulation of aromatase namely in the prostate [175]. In addition, leptin also causes alterations in testicular physiology. Hyperleptinemia causes a decrease in the number of spermatocytes and sperm resulting in a decrease in the diameter of the seminiferous tubules. Likewise, the number of Leydig cells is also decreased as well as testis weight [176]. In what concerns to Sertoli cells, it was recently found that leptin modulates the nutritional support of spermatogenesis [168]. Furthermore, leptin crosses blood-testis barrier [177] and its levels in the seminal plasma are inversely correlated with normal sperm parameters [178]. Nonetheless, it is reported that leptin has no effects on motility, capacitation and acrosome reaction of human spermatozoa [179].

Resistin

Resistin is known as an adipocyte-derived signaling molecule as it was firstly identified in adipose tissue of obese mice. However, although human adipocytes produce resistin, it is not the major source of this molecule [180]. In fact, it is also expressed in the muscle, pancreatic cells and macrophages. As shown by its name, resistin is resistant to the action of insulin, thus being implicated in obesity and type 2 diabetes mellitus [181]. Indeed, resistin circulating levels are increased in obese individuals [182]. Moreover, the synthesis and release of this adipokine is stimulated by several factors, namely inflammatory processes, hyperglycemia and action of gonadal hormones [182]. Although the mechanism of resistin action remains to be unveiled, some facts about its role in the male reproductive tract are already known. Indeed, resistin is expressed in both Leydig and Sertoli cells in adult rodents [183]. Moreover, as resistin stimulates Leydig cells survival and proliferation, these cells may auto-regulate their proliferation in an autocrine or paracrine manner [184]. However, these effects are controversial since other authors have shown that changes in the levels of this hormone had no effect on male fertility. This led to the hypothesis that these results might be a synergistic effect with other adipose tissue derived hormones. Moreover, as rodent and human resistin have differences at protein and genomic levels, it is even more difficult to translate the results obtained in studies with rodents [185].

CONCLUDING REMARKS

Reproductive function, as well as the development of secondary sexual characteristics, is highly regulated. In fact, normal testicular function is dependent upon the action of hormones through both endocrine and paracrine pathways. As discussed, HPG axis is the major intervenient known to affect and control male reproduction. The key roles played by the hormones of this axis in the regulation of steroidogenesis and spermatogenesis are known for several decades. Androgens, which exert feedback actions on the hypothalamus and anterior pituitary, also have a crucial role for spermatogenesis. These hormones may also be converted into estrogens, which have been acquiring attention since they were also found to have a key role in male reproduction. However, some new intervenient have been discovered in the last few years. The drastic increase of metabolic disorders, and its association with the decrease in fertility rates, has brought attention to this topic and its related hormones are also on spotlight. In fact, these may be one of the missing links between the disease and the already known consequence of impaired reproductive function in males.

Box 5.1 | Summary

- Male reproductive function is highly regulated by hormones, signaling molecules secreted by glands directly into the blood stream, which transports them to target organs and tissues to exert their function;
- Hypothalamic–pituitary–gonadal axis represents the interaction between hypothalamus, pituitary and gonads. Testicular functions are controlled by a master switch, the GnRH pulse generator and feedback systems: LH-testosterone and FSH-inhibin.
- Thyroid hormones interfere in testicular development and steroidogenesis.
- Feeding status and overall homeostasis is important for spermatogenesis. Hormones related with the latter, namely gut hormones and adipokines, modulate male reproductive function.

CONFLICT OF INTEREST

The authors confirm that they have no conflict of interest to declare for this publication.

ACKNOWLEDGEMENTS

This work was supported by the "Fundação para a Ciência e a Tecnologia"–FCT (PTDC/BIM-MET/4712/2014), UMIB (PEst-OE/SAU/UI0215/2014. Ana D. Martins (SFRH/BD/108726/2015) and Maria J. Meneses (PD/BD/114256/2016) were also funded by FCT.

REFERENCES

[1] Seeburg PH, Mason AJ, Stewart TA, Nikolics K. The mammalian GnRH gene and its pivotal role in reproduction. Recent Prog Horm Res 1987; 43: 69-98. [http://dx.doi.org/10.1016/B978-0-12-571143-2.50008-3] [PMID: 3306841]

[2] McLachlan RI, ODonnell L, Meachem SJ, *et al.* Identification of specific sites of hormonal regulation in spermatogenesis in rats, monkeys, and man. Recent Prog Horm Res 2002; 57: 149-79. [http://dx.doi.org/10.1210/rp.57.1.149] [PMID: 12017541]

[3] Bartke A, Williams KI, Dalterio S. Effects of estrogens on testicular testosterone production *in vitro.* Biol Reprod 1977; 17(5): 645-9. [http://dx.doi.org/10.1095/biolreprod17.5.645] [PMID: 597532]

[4] Muttukrishna S, Knight PG. Inverse effects of activin and inhibin on the synthesis and secretion of FSH and LH by ovine pituitary cells *in vitro.* J Mol Endocrinol 1991; 6(2): 171-8. [http://dx.doi.org/10.1677/jme.0.0060171] [PMID: 1904234]

[5] Rochira V, Zirilli L, Genazzani AD, *et al.* Hypothalamic-pituitary-gonadal axis in two men with aromatase deficiency: evidence that circulating estrogens are required at the hypothalamic level for the integrity of gonadotropin negative feedback. Eur J Endocrinol 2006; 155(4): 513-22. [http://dx.doi.org/10.1530/eje.1.02254] [PMID: 16990650]

[6] Dumasia K, Kumar A, Kadam L, Balasinor NH. Effect of estrogen receptor-subtype-specific ligands on fertility in adult male rats. J Endocrinol 2015; 225(3): 169-80. [http://dx.doi.org/10.1530/JOE-15-0045] [PMID: 25869617]

[7] DSouza R, Gill-Sharma MK, Pathak S, Kedia N, Kumar R, Balasinor N. Effect of high intratesticular estrogen on the seminiferous epithelium in adult male rats. Mol Cell Endocrinol 2005; 241(1-2): 41-8. [http://dx.doi.org/10.1016/j.mce.2005.04.011] [PMID: 15936871]

[8] Oliveira PF, Alves MG, Rato L, *et al.* Effect of insulin deprivation on metabolism and metabolism-associated gene transcript levels of in vitro cultured human Sertoli cells. BBA - Gen Subjects 2012; 1820: 84-9.

[9] Rato L, Meneses MJ, Silva BM, Sousa M, Alves MG, Oliveira PF. New insights on hormones and factors that modulate Sertoli cell metabolism. Histol Histopathol 2016; 31(5): 499-513. [http://dx.doi.org/10.14670/HH-11-717] [PMID: 26711246]

[10] Meneses MJ, Silva BM, Sousa M, Sá R, Oliveira PF, Alves MG. Antidiabetic Drugs: Mechanisms of Action and Potential Outcomes on Cellular Metabolism. Curr Pharm Des 2015; 21(25): 3606-20. [http://dx.doi.org/10.2174/1381612821666150710145753] [PMID: 26166608]

[11] Martins AD, Sá R, Monteiro MP, *et al.* Ghrelin acts as energy status sensor of male reproduction by modulating Sertoli cells glycolytic metabolism and mitochondrial bioenergetics. Mol Cell Endocrinol 2016; 434: 199-209.

[http://dx.doi.org/10.1016/j.mce.2016.07.008] [PMID: 27392494]

[12] Buzzard JJ, Morrison JR, OBryan MK, Song Q, Wreford NG. Developmental expression of thyroid hormone receptors in the rat testis. Biol Reprod 2000; 62(3): 664-9. [http://dx.doi.org/10.1095/biolreprod62.3.664] [PMID: 10684808]

[13] Bouligand J, Ghervan C, Guiochon-Mantel A, Young J. Hypogonadotropic hypogonadism and GNRH1 mutations in mice and humans. Front Horm Res. 2003; 39: pp. 111-20. [http://dx.doi.org/10.1159/000312697] [PMID: 20389089]

[14] Cimino I, Casoni F, Liu X, *et al.* Novel role for anti-Müllerian hormone in the regulation of GnRH neuron excitability and hormone secretion. Nat Commun 2016; 7: 10055. [http://dx.doi.org/10.1038/ncomms10055] [PMID: 26753790]

[15] Funabashi T, Daikoku S, Shinohara K, Kimura F. Pulsatile gonadotropin-releasing hormone (GnRH) secretion is an inherent function of GnRH neurons, as revealed by the culture of medial olfactory placode obtained from embryonic rats. Neuroendocrinology 2000; 71(2): 138-44. [http://dx.doi.org/10.1159/000054529] [PMID: 10686527]

[16] Thackray VG, Mellon PL, Coss D. Hormones in synergy: regulation of the pituitary gonadotropin genes. Mol Cell Endocrinol 2010; 314(2): 192-203. [http://dx.doi.org/10.1016/j.mce.2009.09.003] [PMID: 19747958]

[17] Katt JA, Duncan JA, Herbon L, Barkan A, Marshall JC. The frequency of gonadotropin-releasing hormone stimulation determines the number of pituitary gonadotropin-releasing hormone receptors. Endocrinology 1985; 116(5): 2113-5. [http://dx.doi.org/10.1210/endo-116-5-2113] [PMID: 2985372]

[18] Millar RP, Lu Z-L, Pawson AJ, Flanagan CA, Morgan K, Maudsley SR. Gonadotropin-releasing hormone receptors. Endocr Rev 2004; 25(2): 235-75. [http://dx.doi.org/10.1210/er.2003-0002] [PMID: 15082521]

[19] Burger LL, Dalkin AC, Aylor KW, Haisenleder DJ, Marshall JC. GnRH pulse frequency modulation of gonadotropin subunit gene transcription in normal gonadotropes-assessment by primary transcript assay provides evidence for roles of GnRH and follistatin. Endocrinology 2002; 143(9): 3243-9. [http://dx.doi.org/10.1210/en.2002-220216] [PMID: 12193535]

[20] Boyar RM, Rosenfeld RS, Kapen S, *et al.* Human puberty. Simultaneous augmented secretion of luteinizing hormone and testosterone during sleep. J Clin Invest 1974; 54(3): 609-18. [http://dx.doi.org/10.1172/JCI107798] [PMID: 4852310]

[21] OHara L, Smith LB. Androgen receptor roles in spermatogenesis and infertility. Best Pract Res Clin Endocrinol Metab 2015; 29(4): 595-605. [http://dx.doi.org/10.1016/j.beem.2015.04.006] [PMID: 26303086]

[22] Aquila S, De Amicis F. Steroid receptors and their ligands: effects on male gamete functions. Exp Cell Res 2014; 328(2): 303-13. [http://dx.doi.org/10.1016/j.yexcr.2014.07.015] [PMID: 25062984]

[23] Wang RS, Yeh S, Chen LM, *et al.* Androgen receptor in sertoli cell is essential for germ cell nursery and junctional complex formation in mouse testes. Endocrinology 2006; 147(12): 5624-33. [http://dx.doi.org/10.1210/en.2006-0138] [PMID: 16973730]

[24] Meroni SB, Riera MF, Pellizzari EH, Cigorraga SB. Regulation of rat Sertoli cell function by FSH: possible role of phosphatidylinositol 3-kinase/protein kinase B pathway. J Endocrinol 2002; 174(2): 195-204. [http://dx.doi.org/10.1677/joe.0.1740195] [PMID: 12176658]

[25] Griswold MD. The central role of Sertoli cells in spermatogenesis. Semin Cell Dev Biol 1998; 9(4): 411-6. [http://dx.doi.org/10.1006/scdb.1998.0203] [PMID: 9813187]

[26] Childs GV, Miller BT, Miller WL. Differential effects of inhibin on gonadotropin stores and gonadotropin-releasing hormone binding to pituitary cells from cycling female rats. Endocrinology 1997; 138(4): 1577-84.
[http://dx.doi.org/10.1210/endo.138.4.5090] [PMID: 9075718]

[27] Vale W, Rivier J, Vaughan J, *et al.* Purification and characterization of an FSH releasing protein from porcine ovarian follicular fluid. Nature 1986; 321(6072): 776-9.
[http://dx.doi.org/10.1038/321776a0] [PMID: 3012369]

[28] Ling N, Ying SY, Ueno N, *et al.* Pituitary FSH is released by a heterodimer of the beta-subunits from the two forms of inhibin. Nature 1986; 321(6072): 779-82.
[http://dx.doi.org/10.1038/321779a0] [PMID: 3086749]

[29] Gunawardane K, Krarup Hansen T, Sandahl Christiansen J, Lunde Jorgensen JO. Normal Physiology of Growth Hormone in Adults. 2000.
[PMID: 25905284]

[30] Arsenijevic Y, Wehrenberg WB, Conz A, Eshkol A, Sizonenko PC, Aubert ML. Growth hormone (GH) deprivation induced by passive immunization against rat GH-releasing factor delays sexual maturation in the male rat. Endocrinology 1989; 124(6): 3050-9.
[http://dx.doi.org/10.1210/endo-124-6-3050] [PMID: 2498066]

[31] Nguyen AP, Chandorkar A, Gupta C. The role of growth hormone in fetal mouse reproductive tract differentiation. Endocrinology 1996; 137(9): 3659-66.
[http://dx.doi.org/10.1210/endo.137.9.8756530] [PMID: 8756530]

[32] Gravance CG, Breier BH, Vickers MH, Casey PJ. Impaired sperm characteristics in postpubertal growth-hormone-deficient dwarf (dw/dw) rats. Anim Reprod Sci 1997; 49(1): 71-6.
[http://dx.doi.org/10.1016/S0378-4320(97)00019-5] [PMID: 9458951]

[33] Breier BH, Vickers MH, Gravance CG, Casey PJ. Growth hormone (GH) therapy markedly increases the motility of spermatozoa and the concentration of insulin-like growth factor-I in seminal vesicle fluid in the male GH-deficient dwarf rat. Endocrinology 1996; 137(9): 4061-4.
[http://dx.doi.org/10.1210/endo.137.9.8756586] [PMID: 8756586]

[34] Bex F, Bartke A, Goldman BD, Dalterio S. Prolactin, growth hormone, luteinizing hormone receptors, and seasonal changes in testicular activity in the golden hamster. Endocrinology 1978; 103(6): 2069-80.
[http://dx.doi.org/10.1210/endo-103-6-2069] [PMID: 218802]

[35] McKeown M. Sex determination and differentiation. Dev Genet 1994; 15(3): 201-4.
[http://dx.doi.org/10.1002/dvg.1020150302] [PMID: 8062454]

[36] Alves MG, Rato L, Carvalho RA, Moreira PI, Socorro S, Oliveira PF. Hormonal control of Sertoli cell metabolism regulates spermatogenesis. Cell Mol Life Sci 2013; 70(5): 777-93.
[http://dx.doi.org/10.1007/s00018-012-1079-1] [PMID: 23011766]

[37] Verhoeven G, Willems A, Denolet E, Swinnen JV, De Gendt K. Androgens and spermatogenesis: lessons from transgenic mouse models. Philos Trans R Soc Lond B Biol Sci 2010; 365(1546): 1537-56.
[http://dx.doi.org/10.1098/rstb.2009.0117] [PMID: 20403868]

[38] Randall VA. Role of 5 alpha-reductase in health and disease. Baillieres Clin Endocrinol Metab 1994; 8(2): 405-31.
[http://dx.doi.org/10.1016/S0950-351X(05)80259-9] [PMID: 8092979]

[39] Grino PB, Griffin JE, Wilson JD. Testosterone at high concentrations interacts with the human androgen receptor similarly to dihydrotestosterone. Endocrinology 1990; 126(2): 1165-72.
[http://dx.doi.org/10.1210/endo-126-2-1165] [PMID: 2298157]

[40] Wilson JD, Griffin JE, Russell DW. Steroid 5 alpha-reductase 2 deficiency. Endocr Rev 1993; 14(5): 577-93.
[http://dx.doi.org/10.1210/edrv-14-5-577] [PMID: 8262007]

[41] Manna PR, Stetson CL, Slominski AT, Pruitt K. Role of the steroidogenic acute regulatory protein in health and disease. Endocrine 2016; 51(1): 7-21.
[http://dx.doi.org/10.1007/s12020-015-0715-6] [PMID: 26271515]

[42] Wing TY, Ewing LL, Zirkin BR. Effects of luteinizing hormone withdrawal on Leydig cell smooth endoplasmic reticulum and steroidogenic reactions which convert pregnenolone to testosterone. Endocrinology 1984; 115(6): 2290-6.
[http://dx.doi.org/10.1210/endo-115-6-2290] [PMID: 6499769]

[43] Veldhuis JD, Iranmanesh A, Mulligan T. Age and testosterone feedback jointly control the dose-dependent actions of gonadotropin-releasing hormone in healthy men. J Clin Endocrinol Metab 2005; 90(1): 302-9.
[http://dx.doi.org/10.1210/jc.2004-1313] [PMID: 15494457]

[44] Chang CS, Kokontis J, Liao ST. Molecular cloning of human and rat complementary DNA encoding androgen receptors. Science 1988; 240(4850): 324-6.
[http://dx.doi.org/10.1126/science.3353726] [PMID: 3353726]

[45] Lubahn DB, Joseph DR, Sullivan PM, Willard HF, French FS, Wilson EM. Cloning of human androgen receptor complementary DNA and localization to the X chromosome. Science 1988; 240(4850): 327-30.
[http://dx.doi.org/10.1126/science.3353727] [PMID: 3353727]

[46] Carreau S, de Vienne C, Galeraud-Denis I. Aromatase and estrogens in man reproduction: a review and latest advances. Adv Med Sci 2008; 53(2): 139-44.
[http://dx.doi.org/10.2478/v10039-008-0022-z] [PMID: 18614433]

[47] Nilsson S, Mäkelä S, Treuter E, *et al.* Mechanisms of estrogen action. Physiol Rev 2001; 81(4): 1535-65.
[PMID: 11581496]

[48] Carreau S. Germ cells: a new source of estrogens in the male gonad. Mol Cell Endocrinol 2001; 178(1-2): 65-72.
[http://dx.doi.org/10.1016/S0303-7207(01)00411-7] [PMID: 11403896]

[49] Abney TO. The potential roles of estrogens in regulating Leydig cell development and function: a review. Steroids 1999; 64(9): 610-7.
[http://dx.doi.org/10.1016/S0039-128X(99)00041-0] [PMID: 10503717]

[50] ODonnell L, Robertson KM, Jones ME, Simpson ER. Estrogen and spermatogenesis. Endocr Rev 2001; 22(3): 289-318.
[http://dx.doi.org/10.1210/edrv.22.3.0431] [PMID: 11399746]

[51] Steinach E, Kun H. Transformation of male sex hormones into a substance with the action of a female hormone. Lancet 1937; 230: 845.
[http://dx.doi.org/10.1016/S0140-6736(00)88745-0]

[52] Nelson DR, Kamataki T, Waxman DJ, *et al.* The P450 superfamily: update on new sequences, gene mapping, accession numbers, early trivial names of enzymes, and nomenclature. DNA Cell Biol 1993; 12(1): 1-51.
[http://dx.doi.org/10.1089/dna.1993.12.1] [PMID: 7678494]

[53] Lambard S, Silandre D, Delalande C, Denis-Galeraud I, Bourguiba S, Carreau S. Aromatase in testis: expression and role in male reproduction. J Steroid Biochem Mol Biol 2005; 95(1-5): 63-9.
[http://dx.doi.org/10.1016/j.jsbmb.2005.04.020] [PMID: 16019206]

[54] Carreau S, Bourguiba S, Lambard S, Galeraud-Denis I, Genissel C, Levallet J. Reproductive system: aromatase and estrogens. Mol Cell Endocrinol 2002; 193(1-2): 137-43. [http://dx.doi.org/10.1016/S0303-7207(02)00107-7] [PMID: 12161013]

[55] Simpson E, Santen RJ. Celebrating 75 years of oestradiol. J Mol Endocrinol 2015; 55(3): T1-T20. [http://dx.doi.org/10.1530/JME-15-0128] [PMID: 26438567]

[56] Payne AH, Kelch RP, Musich SS, Halpern ME. Intratesticular site of aromatization in the human. J Clin Endocrinol Metab 1976; 42(6): 1081-7. [http://dx.doi.org/10.1210/jcem-42-6-1081] [PMID: 932173]

[57] Carreau S. The testicular aromatase: from gene to physiological role. Reprod Biol 2002; 2(1): 5-12. [PMID: 14666158]

[58] Foucault P, Carreau S, Kuczynski W, Guillaumin JM, Bardos P, Drosdowsky MA. Human Sertoli cells *in vitro*. Lactate, estradiol-17 beta and transferrin production. J Androl 1992; 13(5): 361-7. [http://dx.doi.org/10.1002/j.1939-4640.1992.tb03325.x] [PMID: 1429217]

[59] Green S, Walter P, Kumar V, *et al.* Human oestrogen receptor cDNA: sequence, expression and homology to v-erb-A. Nature 1986; 320(6058): 134-9. [http://dx.doi.org/10.1038/320134a0] [PMID: 3754034]

[60] Kuiper GG, Enmark E, Pelto-Huikko M, Nilsson S, Gustafsson JA. Cloning of a novel receptor expressed in rat prostate and ovary. Proc Natl Acad Sci USA 1996; 93(12): 5925-30. [http://dx.doi.org/10.1073/pnas.93.12.5925] [PMID: 8650195]

[61] Filardo EJ, Quinn JA, Bland KI, Frackelton AR Jr. Estrogen-induced activation of Erk-1 and Erk-2 requires the G protein-coupled receptor homolog, GPR30, and occurs *via* trans-activation of the epidermal growth factor receptor through release of HB-EGF. Mol Endocrinol 2000; 14(10): 1649-60. [http://dx.doi.org/10.1210/mend.14.10.0532] [PMID: 11043579]

[62] Evans RM. The steroid and thyroid hormone receptor superfamily. Science 1988; 240(4854): 889-95. [http://dx.doi.org/10.1126/science.3283939] [PMID: 3283939]

[63] Escriva H, Bertrand S, Laudet V. The evolution of the nuclear receptor superfamily. Essays Biochem 2004; 40: 11-26. [http://dx.doi.org/10.1042/bse0400011] [PMID: 15242336]

[64] Laudet V, Hänni C, Coll J, Catzeflis F, Stéhelin D. Evolution of the nuclear receptor gene superfamily. EMBO J 1992; 11(3): 1003-13. [PMID: 1312460]

[65] Eisenhauer KM, McCue PM, Nayden DK, Osawa Y, Roser JF. Localization of aromatase in equine Leydig cells. Domest Anim Endocrinol 1994; 11(3): 291-8. [http://dx.doi.org/10.1016/0739-7240(94)90020-5] [PMID: 7956176]

[66] Saunders PT, Millar MR, Macpherson S, *et al.* ERbeta1 and the ERbeta2 splice variant (ERbetacx/beta2) are expressed in distinct cell populations in the adult human testis. J Clin Endocrinol Metab 2002; 87(6): 2706-15. [http://dx.doi.org/10.1210/jcem.87.6.8619] [PMID: 12050238]

[67] Hess RA. The efferent ductules: structure and functions. In: Robaire B, Hinton BT, Eds. The epididymis: from molecules to clinical practice: a comprehensive survey of the efferent ducts, the epididymis and the vas deferens. Boston, MA: Springer, US 2002; pp. 49-80.

[68] Hess RA, Bunick D, Lubahn DB, Zhou Q, Bouma J. Morphologic changes in efferent ductules and epididymis in estrogen receptor-alpha knockout mice. J Androl 2000; 21(1): 107-21. [http://dx.doi.org/10.1002/j.1939-4640.2000.tb03282.x] [PMID: 10670526]

[69] Pentikäinen V, Erkkilä K, Suomalainen L, Parvinen M, Dunkel L. Estradiol acts as a germ cell survival factor in the human testis *in vitro*. J Clin Endocrinol Metab 2000; 85(5): 2057-67. [http://dx.doi.org/10.1210/jcem.85.5.6600] [PMID: 10843196]

[70] Carreau S, Lambard S, Delalande C, Denis-Galeraud I, Bilinska B, Bourguiba S. Aromatase expression and role of estrogens in male gonad : a review. Reprod Biol Endocrinol 2003; 1: 35. [http://dx.doi.org/10.1186/1477-7827-1-35] [PMID: 12747806]

[71] Lambard S, Galeraud-Denis I, Saunders PT, Carreau S. Human immature germ cells and ejaculated spermatozoa contain aromatase and oestrogen receptors. J Mol Endocrinol 2004; 32(1): 279-89. [http://dx.doi.org/10.1677/jme.0.0320279] [PMID: 14766008]

[72] Pelletier G, El-Alfy M. Immunocytochemical localization of estrogen receptors alpha and beta in the human reproductive organs. J Clin Endocrinol Metab 2000; 85(12): 4835-40. [http://dx.doi.org/10.1210/jcem.85.12.7029] [PMID: 11134151]

[73] Saunders PT, Sharpe RM, Williams K, *et al.* Differential expression of oestrogen receptor alpha and beta proteins in the testes and male reproductive system of human and non-human primates. Mol Hum Reprod 2001; 7(3): 227-36. [http://dx.doi.org/10.1093/molehr/7.3.227] [PMID: 11228242]

[74] Carmeci C, Thompson DA, Ring HZ, Francke U, Weigel RJ. Identification of a gene (GPR30) with homology to the G-protein-coupled receptor superfamily associated with estrogen receptor expression in breast cancer. Genomics 1997; 45(3): 607-17. [http://dx.doi.org/10.1006/geno.1997.4972] [PMID: 9367686]

[75] Lappano R, De Marco P, De Francesco EM, Chimento A, Pezzi V, Maggiolini M. Cross-talk between GPER and growth factor signaling. J Steroid Biochem Mol Biol 2013; 137: 50-6. [http://dx.doi.org/10.1016/j.jsbmb.2013.03.005] [PMID: 23542661]

[76] Filardo EJ, Quinn JA, Frackelton AR Jr, Bland KI. Estrogen action *via* the G protein-coupled receptor, GPR30: stimulation of adenylyl cyclase and cAMP-mediated attenuation of the epidermal growth factor receptor-to-MAPK signaling axis. Mol Endocrinol 2002; 16(1): 70-84. [http://dx.doi.org/10.1210/mend.16.1.0758] [PMID: 11773440]

[77] Thomas P, Pang Y, Filardo EJ, Dong J. Identity of an estrogen membrane receptor coupled to a G protein in human breast cancer cells. Endocrinology 2005; 146(2): 624-32. [http://dx.doi.org/10.1210/en.2004-1064] [PMID: 15539556]

[78] Revankar CM, Cimino DF, Sklar LA, Arterburn JB, Prossnitz ER. A transmembrane intracellular estrogen receptor mediates rapid cell signaling. Science 2005; 307(5715): 1625-30. [http://dx.doi.org/10.1126/science.1106943] [PMID: 15705806]

[79] Solakidi S, Psarra AM, Nikolaropoulos S, Sekeris CE. Estrogen receptors alpha and beta (ERalpha and ERbeta) and androgen receptor (AR) in human sperm: localization of ERbeta and AR in mitochondria of the midpiece. Hum Reprod 2005; 20(12): 3481-7. [http://dx.doi.org/10.1093/humrep/dei267] [PMID: 16123086]

[80] Oliveira PF, Alves MG, Martins AD, *et al.* Expression pattern of G protein-coupled receptor 30 in human seminiferous tubular cells. Gen Comp Endocrinol 2014; 201: 16-20. [http://dx.doi.org/10.1016/j.ygcen.2014.02.022] [PMID: 24681226]

[81] Strachan MW, Frier BM. History, normal physiology, and production of insulin insulin therapy. Springer 2013; pp. 1-8. [http://dx.doi.org/10.1007/978-1-4471-4760-2_1]

[82] Ballester J, Muñoz MC, Domínguez J, Rigau T, Guinovart JJ, Rodríguez-Gil JE. Insulin-dependent diabetes affects testicular function by FSH- and LH-linked mechanisms. J Androl 2004; 25(5): 706-19. [http://dx.doi.org/10.1002/j.1939-4640.2004.tb02845.x] [PMID: 15292100]

[83] Oonk RB, Grootegoed JA. Identification of insulin receptors on rat Sertoli cells. Mol Cell Endocrinol 1987; 49(1): 51-62. [http://dx.doi.org/10.1016/0303-7207(87)90063-3] [PMID: 3549388]

[84] Tatulian SA. Structural dynamics of insulin receptor and transmembrane signaling. Biochemistry 2015; 54(36): 5523-32.
[http://dx.doi.org/10.1021/acs.biochem.5b00805] [PMID: 26322622]

[85] Liang J, Slingerland JM. Multiple roles of the PI3K/PKB (Akt) pathway in cell cycle progression. Cell Cycle 2003; 2(4): 339-45.
[http://dx.doi.org/10.4161/cc.2.4.433] [PMID: 12851486]

[86] Nef S, Verma-Kurvari S, Merenmies J, *et al.* Testis determination requires insulin receptor family function in mice. Nature 2003; 426(6964): 291-5.
[http://dx.doi.org/10.1038/nature02059] [PMID: 14628051]

[87] Pitetti JL, Calvel P, Zimmermann C, *et al.* An essential role for insulin and IGF1 receptors in regulating sertoli cell proliferation, testis size, and FSH action in mice. Mol Endocrinol 2013; 27(5): 814-27.
[http://dx.doi.org/10.1210/me.2012-1258] [PMID: 23518924]

[88] Bucholtz DC, Chiesa A, Pappano WN, *et al.* Regulation of pulsatile luteinizing hormone secretion by insulin in the diabetic male lamb. Biol Reprod 2000; 62(5): 1248-55.
[http://dx.doi.org/10.1095/biolreprod62.5.1248] [PMID: 10775173]

[89] Schoeller EL, Albanna G, Frolova AI, Moley KH. Insulin rescues impaired spermatogenesis *via* the hypothalamic-pituitary-gonadal axis in Akita diabetic mice and restores male fertility. Diabetes 2012; 61(7): 1869-78.
[http://dx.doi.org/10.2337/db11-1527] [PMID: 22522616]

[90] Yen PM, Ando S, Feng X, Liu Y, Maruvada P, Xia X. Thyroid hormone action at the cellular, genomic and target gene levels. Mol Cell Endocrinol 2006; 246(1-2): 121-7.
[http://dx.doi.org/10.1016/j.mce.2005.11.030] [PMID: 16442701]

[91] Tata JR. Amphibian metamorphosis as a model for the developmental actions of thyroid hormone. Mol Cell Endocrinol 2006; 246(1-2): 10-20.
[http://dx.doi.org/10.1016/j.mce.2005.11.024] [PMID: 16413959]

[92] Zimmermann MB. Iodine deficiency. Endocr Rev 2009; 30(4): 376-408.
[http://dx.doi.org/10.1210/er.2009-0011] [PMID: 19460960]

[93] Rubio IG, Medeiros-Neto G. Mutations of the thyroglobulin gene and its relevance to thyroid disorders. Curr Opin Endocrinol Diabetes Obes 2009; 16(5): 373-8.
[http://dx.doi.org/10.1097/MED.0b013e32832ff218] [PMID: 19633549]

[94] Chiamolera MI, Wondisford FE. Minireview: Thyrotropin-releasing hormone and the thyroid hormone feedback mechanism. Endocrinology 2009; 150(3): 1091-6.
[http://dx.doi.org/10.1210/en.2008-1795] [PMID: 19179434]

[95] Cheng SY, Leonard JL, Davis PJ. Molecular aspects of thyroid hormone actions. Endocr Rev 2010; 31(2): 139-70.
[http://dx.doi.org/10.1210/er.2009-0007] [PMID: 20051527]

[96] Brent GA. Mechanisms of thyroid hormone action. J Clin Invest 2012; 122(9): 3035-43.
[http://dx.doi.org/10.1172/JCI60047] [PMID: 22945636]

[97] Bernal J, Guadaño-Ferraz A, Morte B. Thyroid hormone transportersfunctions and clinical implications. Nat Rev Endocrinol 2015; 11(7): 406-17.
[http://dx.doi.org/10.1038/nrendo.2015.66] [PMID: 25942657]

[98] Nagy L, Schwabe JW. Mechanism of the nuclear receptor molecular switch. Trends Biochem Sci 2004; 29(6): 317-24.
[http://dx.doi.org/10.1016/j.tibs.2004.04.006] [PMID: 15276186]

[99] Yen PM. Physiological and molecular basis of thyroid hormone action. Physiol Rev 2001; 81(3): 1097-142.
[PMID: 11427693]

[100] Jannini EA, Crescenzi A, Rucci N, *et al.* Ontogenetic pattern of thyroid hormone receptor expression in the human testis. J Clin Endocrinol Metab 2000; 85(9): 3453-7.
[http://dx.doi.org/10.1210/jcem.85.9.6803] [PMID: 10999848]

[101] Bunick D, Kirby J, Hess RA, Cooke PS. Developmental expression of testis messenger ribonucleic acids in the rat following propylthiouracil-induced neonatal hypothyroidism. Biol Reprod 1994; 51(4): 706-13.
[http://dx.doi.org/10.1095/biolreprod51.4.706] [PMID: 7819453]

[102] Catalano S, Pezzi V, Chimento A, *et al.* Triiodothyronine decreases the activity of the proximal promoter (PII) of the aromatase gene in the mouse Sertoli cell line, TM4. Mol Endocrinol 2003; 17(5): 923-34.
[http://dx.doi.org/10.1210/me.2002-0102] [PMID: 12586841]

[103] Gilleron J, Nebout M, Scarabelli L, *et al.* A potential novel mechanism involving connexin 43 gap junction for control of sertoli cell proliferation by thyroid hormones. J Cell Physiol 2006; 209(1): 153-61.
[http://dx.doi.org/10.1002/jcp.20716] [PMID: 16823880]

[104] Ariyaratne HB, Mills N, Mason JI, Mendis-Handagama SM. Effects of thyroid hormone on Leydig cell regeneration in the adult rat following ethane dimethane sulphonate treatment. Biol Reprod 2000; 63(4): 1115-23.
[http://dx.doi.org/10.1095/biolreprod63.4.1115] [PMID: 10993834]

[105] Maran RR, Arunakaran J, Aruldhas MM. T3 directly stimulates basal and modulates LH induced testosterone and oestradiol production by rat Leydig cells *in vitro*. Endocr J 2000; 47(4): 417-28.
[http://dx.doi.org/10.1507/endocrj.47.417] [PMID: 11075722]

[106] Jana NR, Halder S, Bhattacharya S. Thyroid hormone induces a 52 kDa soluble protein in goat testis Leydig cell which stimulates androgen release. Biochim Biophys Acta 1996; 1292(2): 209-14.
[http://dx.doi.org/10.1016/0167-4838(95)00193-X] [PMID: 8597565]

[107] De Paul AL, Mukdsi JH, Pellizas CG, *et al.* Thyroid hormone receptor alpha 1-beta 1 expression in epididymal epithelium from euthyroid and hypothyroid rats. Histochem Cell Biol 2008; 129(5): 631-42.
[http://dx.doi.org/10.1007/s00418-008-0397-8] [PMID: 18299881]

[108] Gualillo O, Lago F, Casanueva FF, Dieguez C. One ancestor, several peptides post-translational modifications of preproghrelin generate several peptides with antithetical effects. Mol Cell Endocrinol 2006; 256(1-2): 1-8.
[http://dx.doi.org/10.1016/j.mce.2006.05.007] [PMID: 16828223]

[109] Korbonits M, Goldstone AP, Gueorguiev M, Grossman AB. Ghrelina hormone with multiple functions. Front Neuroendocrinol 2004; 25(1): 27-68.
[http://dx.doi.org/10.1016/j.yfrne.2004.03.002] [PMID: 15183037]

[110] Seim I, Collet C, Herington AC, Chopin LK. Revised genomic structure of the human ghrelin gene and identification of novel exons, alternative splice variants and natural antisense transcripts. BMC Genomics 2007; 8: 298.
[http://dx.doi.org/10.1186/1471-2164-8-298] [PMID: 17727735]

[111] Pemberton C, Wimalasena P, Yandle T, Soule S, Richards M. C-terminal pro-ghrelin peptides are present in the human circulation. Biochem Biophys Res Commun 2003; 310(2): 567-73.
[http://dx.doi.org/10.1016/j.bbrc.2003.09.045] [PMID: 14521948]

[112] Bang AS, Soule SG, Yandle TG, Richards AM, Pemberton CJ. Characterisation of proghrelin peptides in mammalian tissue and plasma. J Endocrinol 2007; 192(2): 313-23.
[http://dx.doi.org/10.1677/JOE-06-0021] [PMID: 17283231]

[113] Zhang JV, Ren PG, Avsian-Kretchmer O, *et al.* Obestatin, a peptide encoded by the ghrelin gene, opposes ghrelins effects on food intake. Science 2005; 310(5750): 996-9.
[http://dx.doi.org/10.1126/science.1117255] [PMID: 16284174]

[114] Kojima M, Hosoda H, Date Y, Nakazato M, Matsuo H, Kangawa K. Ghrelin is a growth-hormon--releasing acylated peptide from stomach. Nature 1999; 402(6762): 656-60.
[http://dx.doi.org/10.1038/45230] [PMID: 10604470]

[115] Tolle V, Zizzari P, Tomasetto C, Rio MC, Epelbaum J, Bluet-Pajot MT. *In vivo* and *in vitro* effects of ghrelin/motilin-related peptide on growth hormone secretion in the rat. Neuroendocrinology 2001; 73(1): 54-61.
[http://dx.doi.org/10.1159/000054620] [PMID: 11174017]

[116] Patterson M, Murphy KG, le Roux CW, Ghatei MA, Bloom SR. Characterization of ghrelin-like immunoreactivity in human plasma. J Clin Endocrinol Metab 2005; 90(4): 2205-11.
[http://dx.doi.org/10.1210/jc.2004-1641] [PMID: 15657369]

[117] Hosoda H, Doi K, Nagaya N, *et al.* Optimum collection and storage conditions for ghrelin measurements: octanoyl modification of ghrelin is rapidly hydrolyzed to desacyl ghrelin in blood samples. Clin Chem 2004; 50(6): 1077-80.
[http://dx.doi.org/10.1373/clinchem.2003.025841] [PMID: 15161728]

[118] Fernandez-Fernandez R, Martini AC, Navarro VM, *et al.* Novel signals for the integration of energy balance and reproduction. Mol Cell Endocrinol 2006; 254-255: 127-32.
[http://dx.doi.org/10.1016/j.mce.2006.04.026] [PMID: 16759792]

[119] Lebrethon MC, Aganina A, Fournier M, Gérard A, Parent AS, Bourguignon JP. Effects of *in vivo* and *in vitro* administration of ghrelin, leptin and neuropeptide mediators on pulsatile gonadotrophin-releasing hormone secretion from male rat hypothalamus before and after puberty. J Neuroendocrinol 2007; 19(3): 181-8.
[http://dx.doi.org/10.1111/j.1365-2826.2006.01518.x] [PMID: 17280591]

[120] Lanfranco F, Bonelli L, Baldi M, Me E, Broglio F, Ghigo E. Acylated ghrelin inhibits spontaneous luteinizing hormone pulsatility and responsiveness to naloxone but not that to gonadotropin-releasing hormone in young men: evidence for a central inhibitory action of ghrelin on the gonadal axis. J Clin Endocrinol Metab 2008; 93(9): 3633-9.
[http://dx.doi.org/10.1210/jc.2008-0049] [PMID: 18559917]

[121] Vulliémoz NR, Xiao E, Xia-Zhang L, Rivier J, Ferin M. Astressin B, a nonselective corticotropin-releasing hormone receptor antagonist, prevents the inhibitory effect of ghrelin on luteinizing hormone pulse frequency in the ovariectomized rhesus monkey. Endocrinology 2008; 149(3): 869-74.
[http://dx.doi.org/10.1210/en.2007-1350] [PMID: 18063681]

[122] Benso A, Calvi E, Gramaglia E, *et al.* Other than growth hormone neuroendocrine actions of ghrelin. Endocr Dev 2013; 25: 59-68.
[http://dx.doi.org/10.1159/000346054] [PMID: 23652392]

[123] Fernández-Fernández R, Tena-Sempere M, Navarro VM, *et al.* Effects of ghrelin upon gonadotropin-releasing hormone and gonadotropin secretion in adult female rats: *in vivo* and *in vitro* studies. Neuroendocrinology 2005; 82(5-6): 245-55.
[http://dx.doi.org/10.1159/000092753] [PMID: 16721030]

[124] Forbes S, Li XF, Kinsey-Jones J, OByrne K. Effects of ghrelin on Kisspeptin mRNA expression in the hypothalamic medial preoptic area and pulsatile luteinising hormone secretion in the female rat. Neurosci Lett 2009; 460(2): 143-7.
[http://dx.doi.org/10.1016/j.neulet.2009.05.060] [PMID: 19477231]

[125] Gaytan F, Barreiro ML, Caminos JE, *et al.* Expression of ghrelin and its functional receptor, the type 1a growth hormone secretagogue receptor, in normal human testis and testicular tumors. J Clin Endocrinol Metab 2004; 89(1): 400-9.
[http://dx.doi.org/10.1210/jc.2003-031375] [PMID: 14715878]

[126] Ishikawa T, Fujioka H, Ishimura T, Takenaka A, Fujisawa M. Ghrelin expression in human testis and serum testosterone level. J Androl 2007; 28(2): 320-4.
[http://dx.doi.org/10.2164/jandrol.106.000810] [PMID: 17079741]

[127] Sirotkin AV, Chrenková M, Nitrayová S, *et al.* Effects of chronic food restriction and treatments with leptin or ghrelin on different reproductive parameters of male rats. Peptides 2008; 29(8): 1362-8.
[http://dx.doi.org/10.1016/j.peptides.2008.03.011] [PMID: 18455268]

[128] Tena-Sempere M, Barreiro ML, Gonzalez LC, *et al.* Novel expression and functional role of ghrelin in rat testis. Endocrinology 2002; 143: 717-25.
[http://dx.doi.org/10.1210/endo.143.2.8646]

[129] Hakovirta H, Yan W, Kaleva M, *et al.* Function of stem cell factor as a survival factor of spermatogonia and localization of messenger ribonucleic acid in the rat seminiferous epithelium. Endocrinology 1999; 140: 1492-8.
[http://dx.doi.org/10.1210/endo.140.3.6589] [PMID: 10067878]

[130] Dun SL, Brailoiu GC, Brailoiu E, Yang J, Chang JK, Dun NJ. Distribution and biological activity of obestatin in the rat. J Endocrinol 2006; 191(2): 481-9.
[http://dx.doi.org/10.1677/joe.1.06944] [PMID: 17088418]

[131] Grönberg M, Tsolakis AV, Magnusson L, Janson ET, Saras J. Distribution of obestatin and ghrelin in human tissues: immunoreactive cells in the gastrointestinal tract, pancreas, and mammary glands. J Histochem Cytochem 2008; 56(9): 793-801.
[http://dx.doi.org/10.1369/jhc.2008.951145] [PMID: 18474938]

[132] Zizzari P, Longchamps R, Epelbaum J, Bluet-Pajot MT. Obestatin partially affects ghrelin stimulation of food intake and growth hormone secretion in rodents. Endocrinology 2007; 148(4): 1648-53.
[http://dx.doi.org/10.1210/en.2006-1231] [PMID: 17204551]

[133] Bresciani E, Rapetti D, Donà F, *et al.* Obestatin inhibits feeding but does not modulate GH and corticosterone secretion in the rat. J Endocrinol Invest 2006; 29(8): RC16-8.
[http://dx.doi.org/10.1007/BF03344175] [PMID: 17033254]

[134] Nogueiras R, Pfluger P, Tovar S, *et al.* Effects of obestatin on energy balance and growth hormone secretion in rodents. Endocrinology 2007; 148(1): 21-6.
[http://dx.doi.org/10.1210/en.2006-0915] [PMID: 17008393]

[135] Yamamoto D, Ikeshita N, Daito R, *et al.* Neither intravenous nor intracerebroventricular administration of obestatin affects the secretion of GH, PRL, TSH and ACTH in rats. Regul Pept 2007; 138(2-3): 141-4.
[http://dx.doi.org/10.1016/j.regpep.2006.09.001] [PMID: 17055593]

[136] Moretti E, Vindigni C, Tripodi SA, *et al.* Immunolocalisation of ghrelin and obestatin in human testis, seminal vesicles, prostate and spermatozoa. Andrologia 2014; 46(9): 979-85.
[http://dx.doi.org/10.1111/and.12183] [PMID: 24147986]

[137] Granata R, Gallo D, Luque RM, *et al.* Obestatin regulates adipocyte function and protects against diet-induced insulin resistance and inflammation. FASEB J 2012; 26(8): 3393-411.
[http://dx.doi.org/10.1096/fj.11-201343] [PMID: 22601779]

[138] Han VK, Hynes MA, Jin C, Towle AC, Lauder JM, Lund PK. Cellular localization of proglucagon/glucagon-like peptide I messenger RNAs in rat brain. J Neurosci Res 1986; 16(1): 97-107.
[http://dx.doi.org/10.1002/jnr.490160110] [PMID: 2427741]

[139] Creutzfeldt W. The incretin concept today. Diabetologia 1979; 16(2): 75-85. [http://dx.doi.org/10.1007/BF01225454] [PMID: 32119]

[140] Baggio LL, Drucker DJ. Biology of incretins: GLP-1 and GIP. Gastroenterology 2007; 132(6): 2131-57. [http://dx.doi.org/10.1053/j.gastro.2007.03.054] [PMID: 17498508]

[141] Campbell JE, Drucker DJ. Pharmacology, physiology, and mechanisms of incretin hormone action. Cell Metab 2013; 17(6): 819-37. [http://dx.doi.org/10.1016/j.cmet.2013.04.008] [PMID: 23684623]

[142] Nadkarni P, Chepurny OG, Holz GG. Regulation of glucose homeostasis by GLP-1. Prog Mol Biol Transl Sci 2014; 121: 23-65. [http://dx.doi.org/10.1016/B978-0-12-800101-1.00002-8] [PMID: 24373234]

[143] Drucker DJ. The biology of incretin hormones. Cell Metab 2006; 3(3): 153-65. [http://dx.doi.org/10.1016/j.cmet.2006.01.004] [PMID: 16517403]

[144] Flint A, Raben A, Astrup A, Holst JJ. Glucagon-like peptide 1 promotes satiety and suppresses energy intake in humans. J Clin Invest 1998; 101(3): 515-20. [http://dx.doi.org/10.1172/JCI990] [PMID: 9449682]

[145] Mayo KE, Miller LJ, Bataille D, *et al.* International Union of Pharmacology. XXXV. The glucagon receptor family. Pharmacol Rev 2003; 55(1): 167-94. [http://dx.doi.org/10.1124/pr.55.1.6] [PMID: 12615957]

[146] Alvarez E, Martínez MD, Roncero I, *et al.* The expression of GLP-1 receptor mRNA and protein allows the effect of GLP-1 on glucose metabolism in the human hypothalamus and brainstem. J Neurochem 2005; 92(4): 798-806. [http://dx.doi.org/10.1111/j.1471-4159.2004.02914.x] [PMID: 15686481]

[147] Bullock BP, Heller RS, Habener JF. Tissue distribution of messenger ribonucleic acid encoding the rat glucagon-like peptide-1 receptor. Endocrinology 1996; 137(7): 2968-78. [http://dx.doi.org/10.1210/endo.137.7.8770921] [PMID: 8770921]

[148] Campos RV, Lee YC, Drucker DJ. Divergent tissue-specific and developmental expression of receptors for glucagon and glucagon-like peptide-1 in the mouse. Endocrinology 1994; 134(5): 2156-64. [http://dx.doi.org/10.1210/endo.134.5.8156917] [PMID: 8156917]

[149] Wei Y, Mojsov S. Tissue-specific expression of the human receptor for glucagon-like peptide-I: brain, heart and pancreatic forms have the same deduced amino acid sequences. FEBS Lett 1995; 358(3): 219-24. [http://dx.doi.org/10.1016/0014-5793(94)01430-9] [PMID: 7843404]

[150] Wei Y, Mojsov S. Distribution of GLP-1 and PACAP receptors in human tissues. Acta Physiol Scand 1996; 157(3): 355-7. [http://dx.doi.org/10.1046/j.1365-201X.1996.42256000.x] [PMID: 8830893]

[151] Schmidtler J, Dehne K, Allescher HD, *et al.* Rat parietal cell receptors for GLP-1-(7-36) amide: northern blot, cross-linking, and radioligand binding. Am J Physiol 1994; 267(3 Pt 1): G423-32. [PMID: 7943240]

[152] Thorens B. Expression cloning of the pancreatic beta cell receptor for the gluco-incretin hormone glucagon-like peptide 1. Proc Natl Acad Sci USA 1992; 89(18): 8641-5. [http://dx.doi.org/10.1073/pnas.89.18.8641] [PMID: 1326760]

[153] Dillon JS, Tanizawa Y, Wheeler MB, *et al.* Cloning and functional expression of the human glucagon-like peptide-1 (GLP-1) receptor. Endocrinology 1993; 133(4): 1907-10. [http://dx.doi.org/10.1210/endo.133.4.8404634] [PMID: 8404634]

[154] Graziano MP, Hey PJ, Borkowski D, Chicchi GG, Strader CD. Cloning and functional expression of a human glucagon-like peptide-1 receptor. Biochem Biophys Res Commun 1993; 196(1): 141-6. [http://dx.doi.org/10.1006/bbrc.1993.2226] [PMID: 8216285]

[155] Lund PK, Goodman RH, Habener JF. Pancreatic pre-proglucagons are encoded by two separate mRNAs. J Biol Chem 1981; 256(13): 6515-8. [PMID: 6165720]

[156] Shields D, Warren TG, Roth SE, Brenner MJ. Cell-free synthesis and processing of multiple precursors to glucagon. Nature 1981; 289(5797): 511-4. [http://dx.doi.org/10.1038/289511a0] [PMID: 6110189]

[157] Bell GI, Sanchez-Pescador R, Laybourn PJ, Najarian RC. Exon duplication and divergence in the human preproglucagon gene. Nature 1983; 304(5924): 368-71. [http://dx.doi.org/10.1038/304368a0] [PMID: 6877358]

[158] Holst JJ, Orskov C, Nielsen OV, Schwartz TW. Truncated glucagon-like peptide I, an insulin-releasing hormone from the distal gut. FEBS Lett 1987; 211(2): 169-74. [http://dx.doi.org/10.1016/0014-5793(87)81430-8] [PMID: 3542566]

[159] Orskov C, Holst JJ, Nielsen OV. Effect of truncated glucagon-like peptide-1 [proglucagon-(78107) amide] on endocrine secretion from pig pancreas, antrum, and nonantral stomach. Endocrinology 1988; 123(4): 2009-13. [http://dx.doi.org/10.1210/endo-123-4-2009] [PMID: 2901341]

[160] Deacon CF, Johnsen AH, Holst JJ. Degradation of glucagon-like peptide-1 by human plasma *in vitro* yields an N-terminally truncated peptide that is a major endogenous metabolite *in vivo*. J Clin Endocrinol Metab 1995; 80(3): 952-7. [http://dx.doi.org/10.1210/jcem.80.3.7883856] [PMID: 7883856]

[161] Jeibmann A, Zahedi S, Simoni M, Nieschlag E, Byrne MM. Glucagon-like peptide-1 reduces the pulsatile component of testosterone secretion in healthy males. Eur J Clin Invest 2005; 35(9): 565-72. [http://dx.doi.org/10.1111/j.1365-2362.2005.01542.x] [PMID: 16128863]

[162] MacLusky NJ, Cook S, Scrocchi L, *et al.* Neuroendocrine function and response to stress in mice with complete disruption of glucagon-like peptide-1 receptor signaling. Endocrinology 2000; 141(2): 752-62. [http://dx.doi.org/10.1210/endo.141.2.7326] [PMID: 10650957]

[163] Campfield LA, Smith FJ, Burn P. The OB protein (leptin) pathwaya link between adipose tissue mass and central neural networks. Horm Metab Res 1996; 28(12): 619-32. [http://dx.doi.org/10.1055/s-2007-979867] [PMID: 9013731]

[164] Bado A, Levasseur S, Attoub S, *et al.* The stomach is a source of leptin. Nature 1998; 394(6695): 790-3. [http://dx.doi.org/10.1038/29547] [PMID: 9723619]

[165] Cioffi JA, Van Blerkom J, Antczak M, Shafer A, Wittmer S, Snodgrass HR. The expression of leptin and its receptors in pre-ovulatory human follicles. Mol Hum Reprod 1997; 3(6): 467-72. [http://dx.doi.org/10.1093/molehr/3.6.467] [PMID: 9239734]

[166] Roubos EW, Dahmen M, Kozicz T, Xu L. Leptin and the hypothalamo-pituitary-adrenal stress axis. Gen Comp Endocrinol 2012; 177(1): 28-36. [http://dx.doi.org/10.1016/j.ygcen.2012.01.009] [PMID: 22293575]

[167] Matarese G, Moschos S, Mantzoros CS. Leptin in immunology. J Immunol 2005; 174(6): 3137-42. [http://dx.doi.org/10.4049/jimmunol.174.6.3137] [PMID: 15749839]

[168] Martins AD, Moreira AC, Sa R, *et al.* Leptin modulates human Sertoli cells acetate production and glycolytic profile: a novel mechanism of obesity-induced male infertility? [http://dx.doi.org/10.1016/j.bbadis.2015.06.005] [PMID: 26071642]

[169] Bjorbaek C, Elmquist JK, Michl P, *et al.* Expression of leptin receptor isoforms in rat brain microvessels. Endocrinology 1998; 139: 3485-91.
[http://dx.doi.org/10.1210/endo.139.8.6154] [PMID: 9681499]

[170] Ernst MB, Wunderlich CM, Hess S, *et al.* Enhanced Stat3 activation in POMC neurons provokes negative feedback inhibition of leptin and insulin signaling in obesity. J Neurosci 2009; 29(37): 11582-93.
[http://dx.doi.org/10.1523/JNEUROSCI.5712-08.2009] [PMID: 19759305]

[171] Belgardt BF, Husch A, Rother E, *et al.* PDK1 deficiency in POMC-expressing cells reveals FOXO1-dependent and -independent pathways in control of energy homeostasis and stress response. Cell Metab 2008; 7(4): 291-301.
[http://dx.doi.org/10.1016/j.cmet.2008.01.006] [PMID: 18396135]

[172] Urbanski HF. Leptin and puberty. Trends Endocrinol Metab 2001; 12(10): 428-9.
[http://dx.doi.org/10.1016/S1043-2760(01)00505-7] [PMID: 11701332]

[173] Goulis DG, Tarlatzis BC. Metabolic syndrome and reproduction: I. testicular function. Gynecol Endocrinol 2008; 24(1): 33-9.
[http://dx.doi.org/10.1080/09513590701582273] [PMID: 18224542]

[174] Tena-Sempere M, Manna PR, Zhang FP, *et al.* Molecular mechanisms of leptin action in adult rat testis: potential targets for leptin-induced inhibition of steroidogenesis and pattern of leptin receptor messenger ribonucleic acid expression. J Endocrinol 2001; 170(2): 413-23.
[http://dx.doi.org/10.1677/joe.0.1700413] [PMID: 11479137]

[175] Alves-Pereira JL, Colli S, Marques DS, Sampaio FJ, Ramos CF. Molecular and morphometric analysis of the rat ventral prostate injected with leptin. Regul Pept 2012; 176(1-3): 6-12.
[http://dx.doi.org/10.1016/j.regpep.2012.02.002] [PMID: 22387703]

[176] Yuan M, Huang G, Li J, *et al.* Hyperleptinemia directly affects testicular maturation at different sexual stages in mice, and suppressor of cytokine signaling 3 is involved in this process. Reprod Biol Endocrinol 2014; 12: 15.
[http://dx.doi.org/10.1186/1477-7827-12-15] [PMID: 24502529]

[177] Banks WA, McLay RN, Kastin AJ, Sarmiento U, Scully S. Passage of leptin across the blood-testis barrier. Am J Physiol 1999; 276(6 Pt 1): E1099-104.
[PMID: 10362623]

[178] Hofny ER, Ali ME, Abdel-Hafez HZ, *et al.* Semen parameters and hormonal profile in obese fertile and infertile males. Fertil Steril 2010; 94(2): 581-4.
[http://dx.doi.org/10.1016/j.fertnstert.2009.03.085] [PMID: 19423100]

[179] Li HW, Chiu PC, Cheung MP, Yeung WS, O WS. Effect of leptin on motility, capacitation and acrosome reaction of human spermatozoa. Int J Androl 2009; 32(6): 687-94.
[http://dx.doi.org/10.1111/j.1365-2605.2008.00931.x] [PMID: 19076257]

[180] Fain JN, Cheema PS, Bahouth SW, Lloyd Hiler M. Resistin release by human adipose tissue explants in primary culture. Biochem Biophys Res Commun 2003; 300(3): 674-8.
[http://dx.doi.org/10.1016/S0006-291X(02)02864-4] [PMID: 12507502]

[181] Silha JV, Krsek M, Skrha JV, Sucharda P, Nyomba BL, Murphy LJ. Plasma resistin, adiponectin and leptin levels in lean and obese subjects: correlations with insulin resistance. Eur J Endocrinol 2003; 149(4): 331-5.
[http://dx.doi.org/10.1530/eje.0.1490331] [PMID: 14514348]

[182] Steppan CM, Bailey ST, Bhat S, *et al.* The hormone resistin links obesity to diabetes. Nature 2001; 409(6818): 307-12.
[http://dx.doi.org/10.1038/35053000] [PMID: 11201732]

[183] Nogueiras R, Barreiro ML, Caminos JE, *et al.* Novel expression of resistin in rat testis: functional role and regulation by nutritional status and hormonal factors. J Cell Sci 2004; 117(Pt 15): 3247-57. [http://dx.doi.org/10.1242/jcs.01196] [PMID: 15226398]

[184] Jean S, Landry D, Daigle M, Martin LJ. Influence of the adipose derived hormone resistin on signal transducer and activator of transcription factors, steroidogenesis and proliferation of Leydig cells. Asian Pac J Reprod 2012; 1: 1-6. [http://dx.doi.org/10.1016/S2305-0500(13)60038-X]

[185] Yang R-Z, Huang Q, Xu A, *et al.* Comparative studies of resistin expression and phylogenomics in human and mouse. Biochem Biophys Res Commun 2003; 310(3): 927-35. [http://dx.doi.org/10.1016/j.bbrc.2003.09.093] [PMID: 14550293]

CHAPTER 6

Male Puberty: A Triggered Biochemical Event towards Sexual Maturation

Ana D. Martins and **João P. Monteiro***

Department of Microscopy, Laboratory of Cell Biology, Institute of Biomedical Sciences Abel Salazar (ICBAS) and Unit for Multidisciplinary Research in Biomedicine (UMIB), University of Porto, 4050-313 Porto, Portugal

Abstract: The finding of a concise definition for puberty has proved to be a difficult task for the scientific community and it remains an intense matter of discussion. Nowadays, there is consensus that puberty is a dynamic process influenced by many factors. In this chapter, we will discuss some of the most relevant biochemical markers of puberty and briefly emphasize their relevance in the development and onset of puberty. We will expose the neuroendocrine control that lies behind this very complex hormonally-dependent process. In addition, since puberty is definitely not experienced in the same way by all individuals, we will also discuss genetic, metabolic and nutritional factors as key modulators for the control of puberty onset. The final section of this chapter is dedicated to a brief overview on puberty-associated disorders, pinpointing the clinical features that should be taken into consideration and the deleterious signals that may occur until sexual maturation is achieved.

Keywords: Anti-müllerian hormone, GABA, Glutamate, Growth Hormone, Insulin Growth Factor Binding Protein-3, Insulin Growth Factor-1, Kisspeptin, Leptin, Melatonin, Tanner Stages.

INTRODUCTION

Over time, the establishment of a definitive definition for puberty by the scientific community has proved to be a real challenge, consistently wrapped in interesting debate. If one takes a look into the definition present in dictionaries, it always points to something along the lines of: "the period in people's lives when they develop from a child into an adult, because of changes in their body that make them able to have children". This definition, requires significant further clarification and is rather simple but is globally accepted by both law and scientific communities. In a more detailed definition, we can define puberty as a period in which we attain secondary sexual characteristics and develop a repro-

* **Corresponding author João P. Monteiro:** Rua de Jorge Viterbo Ferreira, 4050-313, Porto, Portugal; Tel: +351 220 428 000; E-mail: jpspmonteiro@yahoo.com

ductive capacity. Yet, as a very complex event, puberty is not a single and immediate episode since it requires a whole set of processes, not only physical but also psychological that occur in human body during a specific life phase. There are many physical manifestations of puberty in males, including the increase of testis; development of pubic, axillary and facial hair; accelerated body growth; increased muscle strength, among others. In addition, psychological changes may also occur to an extent that is dependent on the individual. Recent studies provided compelling evidence that puberty onset is not only the product of spontaneous body changes but also of hormonal and biochemical-mediated events. The entire environment surrounding the child, from the place of birth, to their nutritional status and their genetic heritage, are all suggested to influence not only puberty but particularly its onset. Physical changes can be observed as a result of differentiation and growth, which in the human case may be more visible during the last phase of growth. In fact, puberty is characterized by a cascade of morphological, physiological, psychosocial, cognitive, emotional and behavioral adjustments associated with the increased gonadal and, in some cases, adrenal activity. The beginning of puberty and its duration is determined by two main physiological processes: the gonadarche and the adrenarche. The gonadarche involves the maturation and enlargement of the gonads, along with increased secretion of sex steroids and, consequently, the initiation of spermatogenesis. The adrenarche encloses the maturation of the adrenal cortex and consequent increase in the secretion of adrenal androgens. The physical manifestations of adrenarche, known as pubarche, embrace the appearance of pubic and axillary hair, acne and adult apocrine odor. Interestingly, the absence of adrenarche does not inhibit fertility, neither influences the timing of gonadarche. In sum, puberty comprises many biological changes, some of which are physically observed while others are discrete and can only be biochemically understood.

BIOLOGY OF PUBERTY

Growth and physical maturation during puberty enclose a wide range of cellular and somatic changes. Evaluation of growth is traditionally based on the assessment of height, but changes in body proportions and composition are also important elements to be taken into consideration. Puberty is characterized by increased growth rate and the appearance of somatic sexual differences. The beginning of puberty is expected to take place at the biological age of 13 in boys [1]. The testis of pre-pubertal boys display a very active and marked hormonal profile [2 - 4]. Testis growth is already visible during childhood, and they increase their volume between the 9 to 13 years until they reach the adult volume [5, 6], mainly due to changes in the seminiferous tubules, during the gonadarche. Leydig cells in the testis of pre-pubertal boys are relatively scarce, although recognizable [7 - 9]. In the beginning of puberty, the number of germ cells exponentially increases, leading to a rise in the seminiferous tubule diameter and testicular growth. However, the seminiferous tubule length and Sertoli cell numbers remain relatively constant [4, 10]. At the beginning of puberty, Sertoli cells form the blood-testis barrier, the secretion of seminiferous fluid starts, and the lumen is formed in the seminiferous tubules, resulting in increased diameter [11]. Germ cell population raises, as they are first disposed around the base of Sertoli cells, and then move towards the center of the tubules, according to their maturation stage. FSH was shown to be at least in part responsible for the population of Sertoli cells in rats in a post-natal phase [12, 13]. In addition, FSH receptors increase in Sertoli cells and maximal FSH sensitivity is achieved, along with a very high metabolic activity [14] associated with the many functions of these cells, including aromatase activity and secretion of estrogen and anti-müllerian hormone (AMH). The first indicator of pubertal maturation of seminiferous tubules occurs at the peak of spermatogonial multiplication, and involves the entrance of spermatocytes in meiosis [3]. For a period of 2-4 years, meiotic spermatocytes/spermatids are continuously produced and degraded, gradually progressing in the maturation course while reducing germ cell degradation, leading to an increase in spermatogenic ratios [4], and ultimately to accomplished fertility [4]. The increase in testicular testosterone is due to an early activation of Leydig cell precursors, which respond to LH stimulation [15 - 17]. During pre-puberty, the increase of pulsatile LH levels activates the steroidogenically competent Leydig cell precursors first. At this point, immature Leydig cells and their precursors are abundant [4]. The rise in testosterone concentration in the testis precedes the pronounced growth of seminiferous tubules and the development of secondary sexual characteristics [15, 16]. Therefore, it promotes the increase of seminiferous tubule diameter and testicular volume, as well as spermatogenic development [3].

The five stages defined by Tanner and colleagues [18] for the development of secondary sexual characteristics are nowadays most frequently used to define physical development in developing individuals. Tanner stages go from stage 1 (pre-pubertal) to stage 5 (post-pubertal), and their definition takes into account different physical parameters, such as the growth of pubic hair, genital development and height spurt in boys. Tanner stage 1 represents a pre-pubertal stage and stage 5 is attained at complete development, while stages 2-4 are intermediate stages of development. Tanner stage 3 is reached at mid-puberty and is related with the surge in gonadal hormones (testosterone). Tanner stages are a good external indicator physical sexual development, although they are far from capturing all features related to and leading to biological maturity [19].

NEUROENDOCRINE CONTROL OF PUBERTY

Puberty is a complex process, resulting from coordinated neuroendocrine mechanisms, and involving the activation and maturation of the hypothalamus - pituitary- gonadal axis (HPG) [20, 21] in a tightly regulated process by a complex network of excitatory and inhibitory factors. The onset of puberty relies on a functional HPG axis which is active in embryonic and early postnatal stages but it is silenced during childhood. Though the exact mechanisms remain a matter of intense research and debate, reactivation of GnRH secretion stimulates the secretion of LH and FSH that control and activate the production of gonadal sex steroids. Genetic and environmental factors are also known to be responsible for observed variations in the timing of puberty to each individual [22, 23].

Box 6.1 | Summary

- Puberty onset is linked to significant gonadotropin-releasing hormone (GnRH) pulsing, which precedes an increase in sex hormone levels (namely luteinizing hormone - LH, and follicle-stimulating hormone - FSH), which will in turn determine pre-pubertal and pubertal changes.
- Some factors/neurotransmitters that were described to be involved in pubertal neurocircuitry, modulating hormone release, include kisspeptin, glutamate, GABA, catecholamines, neuropeptide Y (NPY), opioid peptides, melatonin and growth hormone.
- Hormones related to food intake and satiety sensation, namely ghrelin and leptin, were also shown to impact puberty, more specifically the puberty onset.
- Factors like insulin growth factor-1 (IGF-1), anti-müllerian hormone (AMH) and insulin-like factor 3 (INSL3) are also involved in puberty and may serve as prospective markers during puberty progression.
- Other than genetic determination, puberty may also be determined by multiple external factors, including at least the nutritional status, health condition and geographic constraints.

The neuroendocrine control of puberty depends on an elaborated neuronal network involving cooperative action of several neural, hormonal and environmental regulatory signals, progressing at different levels in the HPG axis (summarized in Box **6.1**). LH and FSH levels are the responsible for pre-pubertal and pubertal changes. LH levels, in human males, increase immediately after birth [24], then decline within 6 months and continue relatively low until the beginning of puberty. On the other hand, FSH levels are elevated 3 months after birth, and then decrease [25]. The GnRH neurosecretory system enters a quiescent stage, at the age of 4-6 months, until the beginning of puberty [26, 27]. Before puberty, FSH and LH levels are low, pulsatile and a little higher at night than in the morning [28 - 30]. Previous to the physical signs of puberty manifestation, the levels of FSH and LH rise, and the pulses become more distinct, as the release of gonadotropins starts [29, 30]. In the testes, there is initiation of testosterone secretion, among other steroids, like dihydrotestosterone, androstenedione, and estradiol. At the ages between 10 and 17 years old, the levels of plasmatic testosterone widely increase [5]. This growth in testosterone levels is associated with the increase in LH secretion during sleep (Fig. **6.1**).

The secretory activity of GnRH neurons is controlled by neurocircuitry regulation. This neurocircuitry is responsible for the increase in GnRH secretion, which does not occur until the beginning of puberty, due to immaturity of the circuit [31, 32] (Fig. **6.1**). The neuronal mechanisms that control GnRH neuron activity include synaptic input from other neurons, which may be excitatory, inhibitory, or both, depending on the physiological conditions.

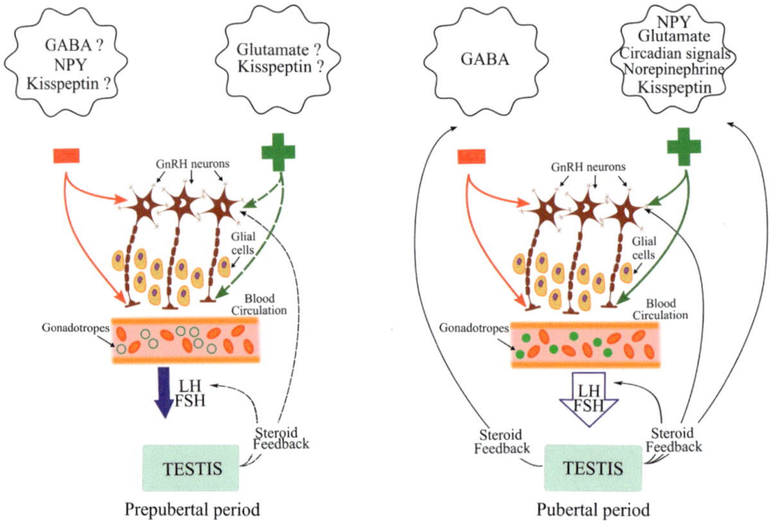

Fig. (6.1). Schematic diagram of probable mechanisms involved in the neuroendocrine control of puberty onset. A gonadal-steroid feedback is operating in pre-pubertal and pubertal period. There is a relationship between neurotransmitters and neuropeptides that control GnRH release which seems to be a key event for puberty onset. During pre-pubertal period, a GABA inhibition on GnRH neurons appears to keep GnRH release low. At puberty onset, a decreased in GABA concentration allows excitatory kisspeptinergic and glutamatergic input to GnRH neurons to become dominant. This leads to an increase in GnRH release, responsible for the cascade of events that triggers puberty. However, those mechanisms remain not fully understood as it has been described that metabolic and circadian signals also have an important role in puberty. During the puberty period, the kisspeptin, NPY, norepinephrine and glutamate and GABA signals, stimulatory and inhibitory respectively, begin or strengthen the participation in GnRH release. During pubertal period, gonadal steroids are as well involved in the formation of an adult pattern to GnRH release. Abbreviations: FSH: follicle-stimulating hormone; GnRH: gonadotropin-releasing hormone; LH: luteinizing hormone; NPY: neuropeptide Y.

One of the systems that controls the secretion of GnRH is the kisspeptin-GPR54. Kisspeptins are encoded by the Kiss1 gene and work through the GPR54 (also called kisspeptin receptor or Kiss1R) [33 - 35]. The receptor belongs to the family of G-protein coupled seven-transmembrane receptors, and its ligand is a peptide derivate from metastasis suppressor gene KiSS-1 [36 - 38]. Human kisspeptin is translated to preprokisspeptin (Kisspeptin-145), and then cleaved at the site next to dibasic residues by subtilisin-like convertase. Finally, the C-terminal-RFG is amidated by carboxypeptidase, like in GnRH peptides processing [36]. Interestingly, infusions of kisspeptin are known to transiently increase LH secretion. Afterwards, LH decreases to basal levels [39, 40], due to the effect of GnRH. This implies kisspeptin as responsible for pulsatile GnRH and LH secretion providing clear evidence that this system is involved in the reactivation of gonadotropin secretion at the puberty onset [41, 42] (Fig. **6.1**).

In the hypothalamus, the major excitatory amino acid neurotransmitter is glutamate [43, 44]. Glutamate has two types of receptors: the metabotropic and the ionotropic, and both are present in the hypothalamus [45, 46] (Fig. **6.1**). The metabotropic receptors are big monomeric transmembrane proteins, holding seven-transmembrane domains, and initiate intracellular signaling through G protein coupling [47, 48]. The ionotropic receptors are ligand-gated cation channels that mediate fast excitatory postsynaptic potentials [49]. The activation of these receptors functions as a stimulation to GnRH/LH secretion in adults [50]. Thus, the synthesis of glutamate and its availability is crucial for the stimulation of GnRH release and consequently for the control of puberty onset (Fig. **6.1**). For instance, it was shown that in developmental rat hypothalamus, glutamine is responsible for a dose-dependent release of GnRH [51], due to the formed glutamate. This dose-dependent mechanism clearly highlights the relevance of glutamate to puberty onset.

The inhibitory role of GABA before puberty is not yet clear (Fig. **6.1**), since mutations in GABA-related human genes do not imply an abnormal puberty [52]. Still, there are findings indicating an important role for GABA in puberty onset. GABA is present in the hypothalamus and is the dominant inhibitory neurotransmitter [53] (Fig. **6.1**). Glutamate is the GABA precursor through a decarboxylation reaction, catalyzed by glutamic acid decarboxylase (GAD). GABA is stored in vesicles and is released in the presence of extracellular Ca2+ by exocytosis [54]. In Rhesus monkeys, GABA levels are higher in pre-puberty, then in mid-puberty [55, 56]. Also in pre-pubertal monkeys, infusions of antisense oligodeoxynucleotides for GAD67 and GAD65 mRNAs into the stalk-median eminence (SME) increased GnRH release [57, 58], probably due to a reduction in the synthesis and release of GABA [55, 57]. In the prepubertal period, the low levels of LHRH release are consequence of dominant inhibitory mechanism of GABA (Fig. **6.1**), and the subtraction of this inhibition may trigger an increase in LHRH release and the onset of puberty [56].

Weiner and Ganong [59] were the first to describe the effects of catecholamines in the puberty of female rats. Catecholamines are organic compounds that contain a catechol nucleus (a benzene ring with two adjacent hydroxyl substituents) and an amine group. In a physiological context, when referring to catecholamines, it implies 3,4-dihydrophenylethylamine (known as dopamine) and its metabolic products, noradrenaline and adrenaline. In brief, the synthesis of catecholamines is carried out from L-tyrosine that serves as a precursor and can cross the blood-brain barrier. Its synthesis follows a series of chemical reactions that end-up in the formation of products with a high relevance for neuronal physiology and also in puberty [60]. Adrenergic neurons have been implicated in the pulsatile release of GnRH and consequently LH release (Fig. **6.1**). In rodents, the inhibition of norepinephrine synthesis, with bis-(4-methyl-1-homopiperazinil-thiocarbonil) disulfide, suppresses the post castration-induced LH release, while the inhibition with α-methyl-paratyrosine suppresses post castration-induced LH release only in juvenile rats [61]. This illustrates that catecholamines may also be a factor triggering puberty in males.

One of the main peptides found in the central nervous system is the neuropeptide Y (NPY). This peptide has 36-amino acids and is one of the most studied in the context of neuroendocrine function [62]. The receptor for this peptide belongs to the family of G-protein coupled receptors and has at least 6 receptor subtypes (Y1-6) [63]. In rat, the presence of NPY in the hypothalamus increases before the birth and during development, reaching its maximum near the puberty of the individual [64, 65]. In pre-pubertal male monkeys, intraventricular injection of a NPY antagonist, blocking the Y1 receptor, stimulated LH release [66] illustrating the relevance for the control of circulating LH. Nevertheless, the most important role for NPY seems to be either acting as a restraint to puberty onset by increasing GnRH [66] or enabling pubertal progression by serving as a stimulatory signal [31] (Fig. **6.1**), though the role for each of these mechanisms and their mode of action remain unclear.

There is also clear evidence that opioid peptides suppress LH release [67, 68], suggesting a possible role for these peptides in puberty. Endogenous opioid peptides are small molecules produced in several parts of the body, including in the CNS and in glands such as the pituitary or the adrenal glands. They can function as hormones and as neuromodulators. These peptides can complement the inhibitory role of GABA before puberty by providing homeostatic counterbalance to the cascade of excitatory events that are responsible for the pubertal increase in GnRH (for review [69]). However, the opioid peptides are not described to play a role in restraining the initiation of puberty and thus, their possible role in this process is speculative and remains controversial. This is due to the complexity of the opioid system which may employ different opioid peptides and receptors, in addition to distinct opioid-producing neuronal subsets. Each may have a separate contribution or not contribution at all. Thus, it is very difficult to assess the extent of opioid system in the restraining of puberty initiation.

Another neurotransmitter suggested to have an inhibitory effect towards puberty onset is melatonin. Melatonin (N-acetyl-5-methoxytryptamine) is a hormone predominantly synthetized in the pineal gland of mammals that is best known for its function as a regulator of the circadian rhythm [70]. It can cross biological barriers [71] and exert biological and pharmacological activities through receptor dependent or independent pathways [70, 72, 73]. In humans and monkeys, the levels of melatonin are known to be elevated in early childhood, decreasing later and remaining stable from early puberty to adulthood [74, 75] illustrating that it is a factor to consider when analyzing the puberty of the individual. Observations in hamsters and sheep indicate that melatonin delays puberty onset [76, 77]. Notably, individuals with pineal tumors were shown to have premature puberty onsets [78, 79], whereas the timing of puberty in blind boys (low melatonin) is delayed [80] illustrating that it is necessary a tight control of melatonin to have a normal puberty.

Growth hormone (GH) is a member of a hormone family that comprises prolactins and placental lactogens. The GH peptide is composed of a single-chain of 191 amino acids with 2 disulphide bridges between amino acids 53-165 and 282-189, and four α-helices [81], organized in an up-up-down-down topology. The expression of GH gene is regulated by GH-releasing hormone, glucocorticoids, somatostatin and insulin growth factor-1 (IGF-1). The levels of GH are known to change during life. The increase in estradiol is responsible for the spontaneous secretion of GH. Of note, the levels of this hormone are low in early puberty but increase throughout mid- and late puberty [82 - 84]. The endogenous secretion of GH follows the height increase tendency rate and then decreases [85]. Interestingly, the role of GH in the end stage of somatic maturation during transition loses importance [86]. In studies with GH replacement, it is clear that the action of GH is necessary in the post-pubertal phase in order to achieve adult maturity (for review [86]). However, the when and how GH secretion influence body changes is not clear yet and remains a matter of great debate.

FACTORS THAT CONTROL PUBERTY

The entire complex process of puberty is under the control of multiple genes and other associated regulatory mechanisms. These mechanisms include classical transcription regulation of genes and non-transcriptional regulatory phenomena, such as epigenetics and microRNAs. Some studies suggest that about 50-80% variance in puberty onset could be under genetic influence [87]. Therefore, the timing of puberty appears as a complex genetic trait influenced by variation on multiple genes [23, 88]. The increase in pulsatile release of GnRH is the result of a balance between inhibitory and stimulatory factors. It results from coordinated changes in transynaptic and glial-neuronal communication [89]. Mutations in the gene encoding the GnRH receptor cause hypogonadotropic hypogonadism, and affects the activation of the HPG axis [90]. Mutations on KAL [91] and FGFR1 [92] genes are the number one cause of Kallman syndrome, which is a rare genetic condition characterized by a failure to start or to fully complete puberty. Mutations of KISS1R is identified as a cause of isolated hypogonadotropic hypogonadism, and central precocious puberty [93, 94]. The neurokinin B (NKB) has been described as an important factor on puberty onset and the genes encoding the NKB receptor (TACR3) and NKB (TAC3) have an important role for the activation of the HPG axis in puberty [95, 96]. The MKRN3 was the first gene, with inhibitory effects on GnRH secretion, identified in humans thought the whole-exome sequencing analysis of families with central precocious puberty [97]. In addition, the gene DAX1 encodes transcription factors that play significant roles in the hypothalamus, pituitary, gonad, and adrenal cortex, and mutations in this gene is also reported to be the responsible for hypogonadotropic hypogonadism [98]. Many other mutations are also responsible for an abnormal growth, for example mutations on genes that encode GH or GHR [99], POU1F1, PITX1, PROP1, HESX1 genes [100], COL1A1, FGFR3 genes [101].

The onset of puberty and its genetic effects are influenced by several multifactorial factors, including nutrition, general health, geography, among others. The matter of whether alterations of whole body metabolism connected to energy disposal and metabolic rates could affect the CNS and consequently the onset and progression of puberty has been subject to intense research and discussion. The discovery of the genes encoding leptin, adipocyte satiety factor and its receptor, was responsible for the establishment of a relationship between the amount of fat, fat metabolism, energy balance and the reproductive potential of the individuals [102 - 104]. Indeed, leptin levels are directly proportional to the amount of body fat [105, 106] and the primary site of leptin production is the adipose tissue [106]. However, placenta, brain and stomach may also express low levels of leptin [107 - 109]. This hormone was related to the modulation of GH secretion [110, 111] and thus, suggested to play key roles, that go far beyond food control, in body physiology. In 1995, Tartaglia and co-workers, using an expression-cloning strategy, were able to isolate the leptin receptor (LepR) from the mouse choroid plexus [104]. Later, it was shown that direct or indirect activation of LepR involves multiple signaling pathways. The levels of leptin reflect the energy status of the body, and have an important role in the control of body weight and on the regulation of metabolism, since it acts on the hypothalamus and suppresses appetite [105, 112, 113]. The effect of leptin in the reproductive system is now gathering more interest from the scientific community as it has been shown that it is crucial to determine the reproductive potential of the individuals. The hypothalamic GnRH neurons, even though they do not express LepRb, are the primary responsible for leptin action on the gonadotropic axis, suggesting the contribution of transitional signals [114] such as insulin-like growth factor 1, NPY, proopiomelanocortin, kisspeptin and nitric oxide synthase (for review [32]). This suggestion was supported by the fact that the abolition of leptin signaling in GnRH neurons does not affect reproductive performance. However, the elimination of LepR in all forebrain neurons compromises fertility [115]. In an *in vitro* study, performed using the LβT2 gonadotroph cell line, leptin was shown to increase LH secretion in response to GnRH [116]. The first studies with rodents indicated that leptin administration could induce or delay puberty onset [117, 118]. Other studies in humans and rodents with leptin deficiency indicated that, although leptin is in fact important for puberty onset, this hormone alone is not able to trigger puberty. Therefore, it has been suggested by several authors that leptin can be a metabolic gate of puberty onset [119, 120]. However, this role of leptin in puberty onset is better characterized in females than in males (for review [121, 122]). Nevertheless, it is known that threshold levels of leptin are necessary for the beginning and advance of the puberty in males. Still, leptin alone was reported to be not enough to promote puberty in males [123]. In addition, serum leptin levels display a gradual increase during the pre-pubertal years in boys [124]. Indeed, during puberty in males, leptin levels peak at Tanner stage 2 and decrease to pre-pubertal levels at the genital stage 5 [125], being that this decrease is attributed to the effects of testosterone [126]. Taken together, these studies clearly show that leptin is an important factor for puberty but not the main trigger for its onset. Other hormone linked to the control of food intake is ghrelin, which is usually negatively correlated with the BMI [127, 128]. This is a 28-amino acid orexigenic hormone whose levels increase after food deprivation [129, 130]. In rats, the administration of ghrelin delays male pubertal development, suggesting a relation between malnutrition and a decrease in reproductive development and function [131]. In humans, during puberty, serum levels of ghrelin decline [132]. The consequences of this decrease in the pubertal activation of HPG is not yet clarified. However, it has been suggested that ghrelin may have a main inhibitory role in male puberty onset [133].

In 1963, IGF was reported to hold non-suppressible insulin-like activity [134]. Since then, it was shown that IGF-1 plays an important role in growth, development, and metabolism, being part of a family of secreted single chain polypeptides (for review [135]). The insulin growth factor-I receptor (IGF-IR) is part of a family of transmembrane tyrosine kinases that includes the insulin receptor and the orphan insulin receptor-related receptor and other receptors, that modulate the biological activity of growth factors [136, 137]. The role of both, IGF-1 and IGF-1R, in the central reproductive axis has not been elucidated yet, however, IGF-1 KO mouse were shown to be infertile [138, 139]. It is known that during male puberty the levels of IGF-1 rise, following the pubertal growth spurt and reflecting the increase of GH secretion during this phase [140, 141]. The levels of IGF-1 do increase steeply in individuals during puberty [142], changing progressively with age and ongoing pubertal stage [143]. This reflects the importance of IGF-1 in puberty onset. *in vitro* studies also demonstrated that IGF-1 affects GnRH neuronal function [144, 145]. In fact, IGF-1 stimulates GnRH release from hypothalamic cell line [145] and stimulates GnRH promoter activity [144, 146].

The AMH is 140-kDa dimeric glycoprotein hormone that belongs to the transforming growth factor-β (TGF-β) family which is secreted by Sertoli cells in the prepubertal testis, being that its levels decline at the onset of puberty. It is known that when a defect in testosterone production occurs during the neonatal period or puberty, the levels of AMH are high. When FSH is administered to boys with congenital hypogonadotropic hypogonadism, there is an increase in AMH and inhibin B (a marker of Sertoli cell function) but when FSH is administered with human chorionic gonadotropin (hCG) the levels of AMH decrease with a lower decrease in inhibin B. This complies with the current knowledge on FSH action during childhood since it stimulates AMH and hCG also stimulates testosterone with a higher suppressive effect on AMH than in inhibin B. Thus, it is very important to determine the hormonal profile of boys during childhood and puberty [147] to follow the changes that occur and avoid possible problems.

Men have a major circulating hormone produced by Leydig cells: the insulin-like factor 3 (INSL3). It is a small peptide hormone member of the relaxin–insulin hormone family and is a major secreted product of the mature interstitial Leydig cells. In addition, ISNL3 can readily cross the blood-testis barrier and thus, it can be present in the luminal fluid from seminiferous tubules, *rete* testis and also in the epididymis. It has been shown that the levels of this hormone progressively increase throughout male puberty and remain correlated with the progressive elevation of LH discussed above. This highlights that during puberty, Leydig cell differentiation and function may be under the influence of LH and that determining the levels of INSL3 may be a good marker to identify the occurrence of possible disorders in male puberty [148]. For instance, in boys with Klinefelter syndrome, altered levels of INSL3 are usually described to be associated with abnormal testes. It has been reported that INSL3 levels in Klinefelter boys are similar to those in normal boys during adulthood but those levels reach a plateau at midpuberty in the former while in the later they continue to increase [149].

A BRIEF OVERVIEW ON PUBERTY-ASSOCIATED DISORDERS

The normal pubertal onset is reported to occur at about 9 years of age in boys. When pubertal signs appear before that age, the event is described as a precocious puberty, a condition considered pathological and that requires medical evaluation [150]. Likewise, when boys at 14 years of age do not present signs of puberty it is also considered a pathological condition (often reported as delayed puberty). There are two main types of precocious puberty, the gonadotropin dependent (central) or independent precocious puberty. In the former, the boys present increased levels of LH and FSH, which results in enlarged testicular size, elevated testosterone, advanced bone age and many other clinical signs of puberty. Those boys must be accompanied to rule out severe conditions such as hypothalamic hamartoma, optic gliomas, central nervous system dysfunction, among others. In the latter condition, gonadotropin-independent or peripheral precocious puberty, it should be noted that it may result from testicular tumor, testotoxicosis or some syndromes. It should also be emphasized that boys with delayed puberty usually have a family history associated with that condition but it is highly recommendable to rule out a possible genetic cause related with hypogonatropic hypogonadism or Klinefelter syndrome, among others.

One of the most common problems occurring in male puberty is pubertal gynecomastia which consists of an often benign proliferation of the male breast glandular and fibrous tissue. It can be uni- or bilateral and usually occurs at midpuberty at the Tanner phases 3-4. The causes for this problem are not well understood but it has been suggested that it may result from impaired estrogen/androgen balance. This can occur during a rapid sexual maturation with ongoing steroidogenesis; due to an increased aromatase activity or increased sensitivity to estrogens in breast tissue [151, 152].

Another issue important to take into consideration during puberty is the possible hypogonadism that may occur when the boys experience problems in pubertal development, micropenis, or cryptorchidism. In addition, when testes fail to descend there is a high risk factor for infertility and testicular malignancy [153] and thus, this is a health condition that must be well followed by the clinicians.

CONCLUDING REMARKS

Defining puberty merely as a series of process to achieve sexual maturation is an oversimplification of the topic. Puberty is a very complex process that is accompanied by physical, psychological and biochemical changes coordinated by several factors, including hormones. It follows the life of the individual from the pre-puberty stage until the complete sexual maturation already in the adult life. In this chapter, we described the biochemical events that may impact puberty onset and normal adult fertility, which depends on the successful completion of these changes. Here, we discussed some of the most relevant markers of puberty onset, including growth hormone, IGF-1, leptin and other markers. The mechanisms determining puberty onset are controlled by many factors, such as the genetic background, metabolic and nutritional status. All these factors may impact neuroendocrine control and influence the action of many neurotransmitters which are responsible for the modulation of the secretion of hormones involved in the HPG axis, determinant in the puberty process. The biological or biochemical changes elicited by the puberty are so pronounced that they translate into evident visual physical changes. The evaluation of Tanner stage is still a very valid way to verify the evolution of male puberty. In addition, the calculation of testicular volume is also a reliable marker to assess male pubertal onset. The biochemical signals and pathways that trigger the initiation of puberty remain a matter of intense research and debate between scientists. This is particularly important since maturation of reproductive system has an evolutionary importance and is highly dependent of a complex regulatory network. In the next years, this will remain a hot topic of research, and novel information concerning the mechanisms of the onset of puberty, age of onset, and the physical and hormonal changes that occur during that period are expected.

CONFLICT OF INTEREST

The authors confirm that they have no conflict of interest to declare for this publication.

ACKNOWLEDGEMENTS

This work was supported by the "Fundação para a Ciência e a Tecnologia"–FCT (PTDC/BBB-BQB/1368/2014) and UMIB (PEst-OE/SAU/UI0215/2014); and of FEDER through the POPH and POCI - COMPETE 2020 (POCI-01-01-5-FEDER-007491) funds. Ana D. Martins (SFRH/BD/108726/2015) and João P. Monteiro (within the project PTDC/BBB-BQB/1368/2014) were also financed by FCT.

REFERENCES

[1] Tanner JM, Whitehouse RH, Marshall WA, Carter BS. Prediction of adult height from height, bone age, and occurrence of menarche, at ages 4 to 16 with allowance for midparent height. Arch Dis Child 1975; 50(1): 14-26.
[http://dx.doi.org/10.1136/adc.50.1.14] [PMID: 164838]

[2] Andersson AM, Toppari J, Haavisto AM, *et al.* Longitudinal reproductive hormone profiles in infants: peak of inhibin B levels in infant boys exceeds levels in adult men. J Clin Endocrinol Metab 1998; 83(2): 675-81.
[http://dx.doi.org/10.1210/jcem.83.2.4603] [PMID: 9467591]

[3] Chemes HE. Infancy is not a quiescent period of testicular development. Int J Androl 2001; 24(1): 2-7. [http://dx.doi.org/10.1046/j.1365-2605.2001.00260.x] [PMID: 11168644]

[4] Rey RA, Campo SM, Bedecarrás P, Nagle CA, Chemes HE. Is infancy a quiescent period of testicular development? Histological, morphometric, and functional study of the seminiferous tubules of the cebus monkey from birth to the end of puberty. J Clin Endocrinol Metab 1993; 76(5): 1325-31. [http://dx.doi.org/10.1210/jcem.76.5.8496325] [PMID: 8496325]

[5] Winter JS, Faiman C. Pituitary-gonadal relations in male children and adolescents. Pediatr Res 1972; 6(2): 126-35. [http://dx.doi.org/10.1203/00006450-197202000-00006] [PMID: 5047471]

[6] Burr IM, Sizonenko PC, Kaplan SL, Grumbach MM. Hormonal changes in puberty. I. Correlation of serum luteinizing hormone and follicle stimulating hormone with stages of puberty, testicular size, and bone age in normal boys. Pediatr Res 1970; 4(1): 25-35. [http://dx.doi.org/10.1203/00006450-197001000-00003] [PMID: 5416996]

[7] Sniffen RC. The testis. I. The normal testis. Arch Pathol (Chic) 1950; 50(3): 259-84. [PMID: 15433699]

[8] Martin LJ. Cell interactions and genetic regulation that contribute to testicular Leydig cell development and differentiation. Mol Reprod Dev 2016; 83(6): 470-87. [http://dx.doi.org/10.1002/mrd.22648] [PMID: 27079813]

[9] Wen Q, Cheng CY, Liu YX. Development, function and fate of fetal Leydig cells. Semin Cell Dev Biol 2016; 59: 89-98. [http://dx.doi.org/10.1016/j.semcdb.2016.03.003] [PMID: 26968934]

[10] Paniagua R, Nistal M. Morphological and histometric study of human spermatogonia from birth to the onset of puberty. J Anat 1984; 139(Pt 3): 535-52. [PMID: 6490534]

[11] Gilula NB, Fawcett DW, Aoki A. The Sertoli cell occluding junctions and gap junctions in mature and developing mammalian testis. Dev Biol 1976; 50(1): 142-68. [http://dx.doi.org/10.1016/0012-1606(76)90074-9] [PMID: 1269826]

[12] Almirón I, Chemes H. Spermatogenic onset. II. FSH modulates mitotic activity of germ and Sertoli cells in immature rats. Int J Androl 1988; 11(3): 235-46. [http://dx.doi.org/10.1111/j.1365-2605.1988.tb00998.x] [PMID: 3137178]

[13] Almirón I, Domené H, Chemes HE. The hormonal regulation of premeiotic steps of spermatogenesis in the newborn rat. J Androl 1984; 5(4): 235-42. [http://dx.doi.org/10.1002/j.1939-4640.1984.tb00784.x] [PMID: 6432758]

[14] Abreu AP, Kaiser UB. Pubertal development and regulation. Lancet Diabetes Endocrinol 2016; 4(3): 254-64. [http://dx.doi.org/10.1016/S2213-8587(15)00418-0] [PMID: 26852256]

[15] Pasqualini T, Chemes H, Rivarla MA. Testicular testosterone levels during puberty in cryptorchidism. Clin Endocrinol (Oxf) 1981; 15(6): 545-54. [http://dx.doi.org/10.1111/j.1365-2265.1981.tb00700.x] [PMID: 6120056]

[16] Page ST. Physiologic role and regulation of intratesticular sex steroids. Curr Opin Endocrinol Diabetes Obes 2011; 18(3): 217-23. [http://dx.doi.org/10.1097/MED.0b013e328345d50e] [PMID: 21478750]

[17] Chemes HE, Gottlieb SE, Pasqualini T, Domenichini E, Rivarola MA, Bergadá C. Response to acute hCG stimulation and steroidogenic potential of Leydig cell fibroblastic precursors in humans. J Androl 1985; 6(2): 102-12. [http://dx.doi.org/10.1002/j.1939-4640.1985.tb00824.x] [PMID: 3886616]

[18] Marshall WA, Tanner JM. Variations in the pattern of pubertal changes in boys. Arch Dis Child 1970; 45(239): 13-23.
[http://dx.doi.org/10.1136/adc.45.239.13] [PMID: 5440182]

[19] Shirtcliff EA, Dahl RE, Pollak SD. Pubertal development: correspondence between hormonal and physical development. Child Dev 2009; 80(2): 327-37.
[http://dx.doi.org/10.1111/j.1467-8624.2009.01263.x] [PMID: 19466995]

[20] Foster DL, Jackson LM, Padmanabhan V. Programming of GnRH feedback controls timing puberty and adult reproductive activity. Mol Cell Endocrinol 2006; 254-255: 109-19.
[http://dx.doi.org/10.1016/j.mce.2006.04.004] [PMID: 16723182]

[21] Parent AS, Rasier G, Gerard A, *et al.* Early onset of puberty: tracking genetic and environmental factors. Horm Res 2005; 64 (Suppl. 2): 41-7.
[http://dx.doi.org/10.1159/000087753] [PMID: 16286770]

[22] Phillip M, Lazar L. Precocious puberty: growth and genetics. Horm Res 2005; 64 (Suppl. 2): 56-61.
[http://dx.doi.org/10.1159/000087760] [PMID: 16286772]

[23] Palmert MR, Boepple PA. Variation in the timing of puberty: clinical spectrum and genetic investigation. J Clin Endocrinol Metab 2001; 86(6): 2364-8.
[http://dx.doi.org/10.1210/jcem.86.6.7603] [PMID: 11397824]

[24] Corbier P, Dehennin L, Castanier M, Mebazaa A, Edwards DA, Roffi J. Sex differences in serum luteinizing hormone and testosterone in the human neonate during the first few hours after birth. J Clin Endocrinol Metab 1990; 71(5): 1344-8.
[http://dx.doi.org/10.1210/jcem-71-5-1344] [PMID: 2229291]

[25] Winter JS, Faiman C, Hobson WC, Prasad AV, Reyes FI. Pituitary-gonadal relations in infancy. I. Patterns of serum gonadotropin concentrations from birth to four years of age in man and chimpanzee. J Clin Endocrinol Metab 1975; 40(4): 545-51.
[http://dx.doi.org/10.1210/jcem-40-4-545] [PMID: 1127071]

[26] Plant TM. A study of the role of the postnatal testes in determining the ontogeny of gonadotropin secretion in the male rhesus monkey (Macaca mulatta). Endocrinology 1985; 116(4): 1341-50.
[http://dx.doi.org/10.1210/endo-116-4-1341] [PMID: 3971918]

[27] Terasawa E, Bridson WE, Nass TE, Noonan JJ, Dierschke DJ. Developmental changes in the luteinizing hormone secretory pattern in peripubertal female rhesus monkeys: comparisons between gonadally intact and ovariectomized animals. Endocrinology 1984; 115(6): 2233-40.
[http://dx.doi.org/10.1210/endo-115-6-2233] [PMID: 6499767]

[28] Albertsson-Wikland K, Rosberg S, Lannering B, Dunkel L, Selstam G, Norjavaara E. Twenty-fou--hour profiles of luteinizing hormone, follicle-stimulating hormone, testosterone, and estradiol levels: a semilongitudinal study throughout puberty in healthy boys. J Clin Endocrinol Metab 1997; 82(2): 541-9.
[http://dx.doi.org/10.1210/jcem.82.2.3778] [PMID: 9024251]

[29] Judd HL, Parker DC, Siler TM, Yen SS. The nocturnal rise of plasma testosterone in pubertal boys. J Clin Endocrinol Metab 1974; 38(4): 710-3.
[http://dx.doi.org/10.1210/jcem-38-4-710] [PMID: 4856558]

[30] Mitamura R, Yano K, Suzuki N, Ito Y, Makita Y, Okuno A. Diurnal rhythms of luteinizing hormone, follicle-stimulating hormone, and testosterone secretion before the onset of male puberty. J Clin Endocrinol Metab 1999; 84(1): 29-37.
[http://dx.doi.org/10.1210/jcem.84.1.5404] [PMID: 9920058]

[31] Terasawa E. Hypothalamic control of the onset of puberty. Curr Opin Endocrinol Diabetes 1999; 6: e49.
[http://dx.doi.org/10.1097/00060793-199902000-00008]

[32] Ojeda SR, Lomniczi A, Mastronardi C, *et al.* Minireview: the neuroendocrine regulation of puberty: is the time ripe for a systems biology approach? Endocrinology 2006; 147(3): 1166-74. [http://dx.doi.org/10.1210/en.2005-1136] [PMID: 16373420]

[33] Navarro VM, Tena-Sempere M. Neuroendocrine control by kisspeptins: role in metabolic regulation of fertility. Nat Rev Endocrinol 2011; 8(1): 40-53. [http://dx.doi.org/10.1038/nrendo.2011.147] [PMID: 21912400]

[34] Oakley AE, Clifton DK, Steiner RA. Kisspeptin signaling in the brain. Endocr Rev 2009; 30(6): 713-43. [http://dx.doi.org/10.1210/er.2009-0005] [PMID: 19770291]

[35] Pinilla L, Aguilar E, Dieguez C, Millar RP, Tena-Sempere M. Kisspeptins and reproduction: physiological roles and regulatory mechanisms. Physiol Rev 2012; 92(3): 1235-316. [http://dx.doi.org/10.1152/physrev.00037.2010] [PMID: 22811428]

[36] Ohtaki T, Shintani Y, Honda S, *et al.* Metastasis suppressor gene KiSS-1 encodes peptide ligand of a G-protein-coupled receptor. Nature 2001; 411(6837): 613-7. [http://dx.doi.org/10.1038/35079135] [PMID: 11385580]

[37] Muir AI, Chamberlain L, Elshourbagy NA, *et al.* AXOR12, a novel human G protein-coupled receptor, activated by the peptide KiSS-1. J Biol Chem 2001; 276(31): 28969-75. [http://dx.doi.org/10.1074/jbc.M102743200] [PMID: 11387329]

[38] Kotani M, Detheux M, Vandenbogaerde A, *et al.* The metastasis suppressor gene KiSS-1 encodes kisspeptins, the natural ligands of the orphan G protein-coupled receptor GPR54. J Biol Chem 2001; 276(37): 34631-6. [http://dx.doi.org/10.1074/jbc.M104847200] [PMID: 11457843]

[39] Dhillo WS, Chaudhri OB, Patterson M, *et al.* Kisspeptin-54 stimulates the hypothalamic-pituitary gonadal axis in human males. J Clin Endocrinol Metab 2005; 90(12): 6609-15. [http://dx.doi.org/10.1210/jc.2005-1468] [PMID: 16174713]

[40] Navarro VM, Castellano JM, Fernández-Fernández R, *et al.* Characterization of the potent luteinizing hormone-releasing activity of KiSS-1 peptide, the natural ligand of GPR54. Endocrinology 2005; 146(1): 156-63. [http://dx.doi.org/10.1210/en.2004-0836] [PMID: 15375028]

[41] Goodman RL, Lehman MN, Smith JT, *et al.* Kisspeptin neurons in the arcuate nucleus of the ewe express both dynorphin A and neurokinin B. Endocrinology 2007; 148(12): 5752-60. [http://dx.doi.org/10.1210/en.2007-0961] [PMID: 17823266]

[42] Wakabayashi Y, Nakada T, Murata K, *et al.* Neurokinin B and dynorphin A in kisspeptin neurons of the arcuate nucleus participate in generation of periodic oscillation of neural activity driving pulsatile gonadotropin-releasing hormone secretion in the goat. J Neurosci 2010; 30(8): 3124-32. [http://dx.doi.org/10.1523/JNEUROSCI.5848-09.2010] [PMID: 20181609]

[43] van den Pol AN, Wuarin JP, Dudek FE. Glutamate, the dominant excitatory transmitter in neuroendocrine regulation. Science 1990; 250(4985): 1276-8. [http://dx.doi.org/10.1126/science.1978759] [PMID: 1978759]

[44] Brann DW. Glutamate: a major excitatory transmitter in neuroendocrine regulation. Neuroendocrinology 1995; 61(3): 213-25. [http://dx.doi.org/10.1159/000126843] [PMID: 7898626]

[45] Mahesh VB, Zamorano P, De Sevilla L, Lewis D, Brann DW. Characterization of ionotropic glutamate receptors in rat hypothalamus, pituitary and immortalized gonadotropin-releasing hormone (GnRH) neurons (GT17 cells). Neuroendocrinology 1999; 69(6): 397-407. [http://dx.doi.org/10.1159/000054442] [PMID: 10364691]

[46] Meeker RB, Greenwood RS, Hayward JN. Glutamate receptors in the rat hypothalamus and pituitary. Endocrinology 1994; 134(2): 621-9.
[http://dx.doi.org/10.1210/endo.134.2.7905409] [PMID: 7905409]

[47] Hsu WL, Chung HW, Wu CY, *et al.* Glutamate Stimulates Local Protein Synthesis in the Axons of Rat Cortical Neurons by Activating α-Amino-3-hydroxy-5-methyl-4-isoxazolepropionic Acid (AMPA) Receptors and Metabotropic Glutamate Receptors. J Biol Chem 2015; 290(34): 20748-60.
[http://dx.doi.org/10.1074/jbc.M115.638023] [PMID: 26134564]

[48] Niswender CM, Conn PJ. Metabotropic glutamate receptors: physiology, pharmacology, and disease. Annu Rev Pharmacol Toxicol 2010; 50: 295-322.
[http://dx.doi.org/10.1146/annurev.pharmtox.011008.145533] [PMID: 20055706]

[49] Seeburg PH. The TiPS/TINS lecture: the molecular biology of mammalian glutamate receptor channels. Trends Pharmacol Sci 1993; 14(8): 297-303.
[http://dx.doi.org/10.1016/0165-6147(93)90047-N] [PMID: 7504359]

[50] Brann DW, Mahesh VB. Excitatory amino acids: evidence for a role in the control of reproduction and anterior pituitary hormone secretion. Endocr Rev 1997; 18(5): 678-700.
[http://dx.doi.org/10.1210/edrv.18.5.0311] [PMID: 9331548]

[51] Bourguignon JP, Gerard A, Alvarez Gonzalez ML, Purnelle G, Franchimont P. Endogenous glutamate involvement in pulsatile secretion of gonadotropin-releasing hormone: evidence from effect of glutamine and developmental changes. Endocrinology 1995; 136(3): 911-6.
[http://dx.doi.org/10.1210/endo.136.3.7867599] [PMID: 7867599]

[52] Brito VN, Mendonca BB, Guilhoto LM, Freitas KC, Arnhold IJ, Latronico AC. Allelic variants of the gamma-aminobutyric acid-A receptor alpha1-subunit gene (GABRA1) are not associated with idiopathic gonadotropin-dependent precocious puberty in girls with and without electroencephalographic abnormalities. J Clin Endocrinol Metab 2006; 91(6): 2432-6.
[http://dx.doi.org/10.1210/jc.2005-2657] [PMID: 16569738]

[53] Decavel C, Van den Pol AN. GABA: a dominant neurotransmitter in the hypothalamus. J Comp Neurol 1990; 302(4): 1019-37.
[http://dx.doi.org/10.1002/cne.903020423] [PMID: 2081813]

[54] Rando RR, Bangerter FW, Farb DH. The inactivation of gamma-aminobutyric acid transaminase in dissociated neuronal cultures from spinal cord. J Neurochem 1981; 36(3): 985-90.
[http://dx.doi.org/10.1111/j.1471-4159.1981.tb01690.x] [PMID: 7205286]

[55] Terasawa E, Luchansky LL, Kasuya E, Nyberg CL. An increase in glutamate release follows a decrease in gamma aminobutyric acid and the pubertal increase in luteinizing hormone releasing hormone release in the female rhesus monkeys. J Neuroendocrinol 1999; 11(4): 275-82.
[http://dx.doi.org/10.1046/j.1365-2826.1999.00325.x] [PMID: 10223281]

[56] Mitsushima D, Hei DL, Terasawa E. gamma-Aminobutyric acid is an inhibitory neurotransmitter restricting the release of luteinizing hormone-releasing hormone before the onset of puberty. Proc Natl Acad Sci USA 1994; 91(1): 395-9.
[http://dx.doi.org/10.1073/pnas.91.1.395] [PMID: 8278400]

[57] Mitsushima D, Marzban F, Luchansky LL, *et al.* Role of glutamic acid decarboxylase in the prepubertal inhibition of the luteinizing hormone releasing hormone release in female rhesus monkeys. J Neurosci 1996; 16(8): 2563-73.
[PMID: 8786432]

[58] Kasuya E, Nyberg CL, Mogi K, Terasawa E. A role of gamma-amino butyric acid (GABA) and glutamate in control of puberty in female rhesus monkeys: effect of an antisense oligodeoxynucleotide for GAD67 messenger ribonucleic acid and MK801 on luteinizing hormone-releasing hormone release. Endocrinology 1999; 140: 705-12.
[http://dx.doi.org/10.1210/endo.140.2.6574] [PMID: 9927297]

[59] Weiner RI, Ganong WF. Effect of the depletion of brain catecholamines on puberty and the estrous cycle in the rat. Neuroendocrinology 1971; 8(2): 125-35.
[http://dx.doi.org/10.1159/000122000] [PMID: 5104827]

[60] Flatmark T. Catecholamine biosynthesis and physiological regulation in neuroendocrine cells. Acta Physiol Scand 2000; 168(1): 1-17.
[http://dx.doi.org/10.1046/j.1365-201x.2000.00596.x] [PMID: 10691773]

[61] Cocchi D, Fraschini F, Jalanbo H, Müller EE. Role of brain catecholamines in the postcastration rise in plasma LH of prepuberal rats. Endocrinology 1974; 95(6): 1649-57.
[http://dx.doi.org/10.1210/endo-95-6-1649] [PMID: 4434907]

[62] Kalra SP, Crowley WR. Neuropeptide Y: a novel neuroendocrine peptide in the control of pituitary hormone secretion, and its relation to luteinizing hormone. Front Neuroendocrinol 1992; 13(1): 1-46.
[PMID: 1361458]

[63] Blomqvist AG, Herzog H. Y-receptor subtypeshow many more? Trends Neurosci 1997; 20(7): 294-8.
[http://dx.doi.org/10.1016/S0166-2236(96)01057-0] [PMID: 9223221]

[64] Corder R, Walker CD, Gaillard RG, Aubert ML. Inhibition of sexual maturation in male rats by melatonin: evidence linking the mechanism of action to changes in the regulation of hypothalamic neuropeptide y. J Neuroendocrinol 1992; 4(1): 1-8.
[http://dx.doi.org/10.1111/j.1365-2826.1992.tb00337.x] [PMID: 21554569]

[65] Woodhams PL, Allen YS, McGovern J, *et al.* Immunohistochemical analysis of the early ontogeny of the neuropeptide Y system in rat brain. Neuroscience 1985; 15(1): 173-202.
[http://dx.doi.org/10.1016/0306-4522(85)90131-9] [PMID: 3892361]

[66] El Majdoubi M, Sahu A, Ramaswamy S, Plant TM, Neuropeptide Y. Neuropeptide Y: A hypothalamic brake restraining the onset of puberty in primates. Proc Natl Acad Sci USA 2000; 97(11): 6179-84.
[http://dx.doi.org/10.1073/pnas.090099697] [PMID: 10811877]

[67] Ferin M, Wehrenberg WB, Lam NY, Alston EJ, Vande Wiele RL. Effects and site of action of morphine on gonadotropin secretion in the female rhesus monkey. Endocrinology 1982; 111(5): 1652-6.
[http://dx.doi.org/10.1210/endo-111-5-1652] [PMID: 6813107]

[68] Kesner JS, Kaufman JM, Wilson RC, Kuroda G, Knobil E. The effect of morphine on the electrophysiological activity of the hypothalamic luteinizing hormone-releasing hormone pulse generator in the rhesus monkey. Neuroendocrinology 1986; 43(6): 686-8.
[http://dx.doi.org/10.1159/000124605] [PMID: 3531908]

[69] Ei Terasawa JR. Neuroendocrine Mechanism of Puberty. Handbook of Neuroendocrinolog. 2012; 19: pp. 435-66.
[http://dx.doi.org/10.1016/B978-0-12-375097-6.10019-8]

[70] Rocha CS, Rato L, Martins AD, Alves MG, Oliveira PF. Melatonin and male reproductive health: relevance of darkness and antioxidant properties. Curr Mol Med 2015; 15(4): 299-311.
[http://dx.doi.org/10.2174/1566524015666150505155530] [PMID: 25941822]

[71] Reiter RJ, Tan DX, Qi W, Manchester LC, Karbownik M, Calvo JR. Pharmacology and physiology of melatonin in the reduction of oxidative stress *in vivo.* Biol Signals Recept 2000; 9(3-4): 160-71.
[http://dx.doi.org/10.1159/000014636] [PMID: 10899701]

[72] Macchi MM, Bruce JN. Human pineal physiology and functional significance of melatonin. Front Neuroendocrinol 2004; 25(3-4): 177-95.
[http://dx.doi.org/10.1016/j.yfrne.2004.08.001] [PMID: 15589268]

[73] Ekmekcioglu C. Melatonin receptors in humans: biological role and clinical relevance. Biomed Pharmacother 2006; 60(3): 97-108.
[http://dx.doi.org/10.1016/j.biopha.2006.01.002] [PMID: 16527442]

[74] Waldhauser F, Boepple PA, Schemper M, Mansfield MJ, Crowley WF Jr. Serum melatonin in central precocious puberty is lower than in age-matched prepubertal children. J Clin Endocrinol Metab 1991; 73(4): 793-6.
[http://dx.doi.org/10.1210/jcem-73-4-793] [PMID: 1909703]

[75] Cavallo A, Dolan LM. 6-Hydroxymelatonin sulfate excretion in human puberty. J Pineal Res 1996; 21(4): 225-30.
[http://dx.doi.org/10.1111/j.1600-079X.1996.tb00290.x] [PMID: 8989721]

[76] Tamarkin L, Westrom WK, Hamill AI, Goldman BD. Effect of melatonin on the reproductive systems of male and female Syrian hamsters: a diurnal rhythm in sensitivity to melatonin. Endocrinology 1976; 99(6): 1534-41.
[http://dx.doi.org/10.1210/endo-99-6-1534] [PMID: 1033827]

[77] Bittman EL, Karsch FJ. Nightly duration of pineal melatonin secretion determines the reproductive response to inhibitory day length in the ewe. Biol Reprod 1984; 30(3): 585-93.
[http://dx.doi.org/10.1095/biolreprod30.3.585] [PMID: 6722237]

[78] Rivarola MA, Mendilaharzu H, Warman M, *et al.* Endocrine disorders in 66 suprasellar and pineal tumors of patients with prepubertal and pubertal ages. Horm Res 1992; 37(1-2): 1-6.
[http://dx.doi.org/10.1159/000182272] [PMID: 1398469]

[79] Kuo HC, Sheen JM, Wu KS, Wei HH, Hsiao CC. Precocious puberty due to human chorionic gonadotropin-secreting pineal tumor. Chang Gung Med J 2006; 29(2): 198-202.
[PMID: 16767969]

[80] Bellastella A, Criscuolo T, Sinisi AA, *et al.* Influence of blindness on plasma luteinizing hormone, follicle-stimulating hormone, prolactin, and testosterone levels in prepubertal boys. J Clin Endocrinol Metab 1987; 64(4): 862-4.
[http://dx.doi.org/10.1210/jcem-64-4-862] [PMID: 3102549]

[81] Miller WL, Eberhardt NL. Structure and evolution of the growth hormone gene family. Endocr Rev 1983; 4(2): 97-130.
[http://dx.doi.org/10.1210/edrv-4-2-97] [PMID: 6345149]

[82] Federico G, Baroncelli GI, Vanacore T, Fiore L, Saggese G. Pubertal changes in biochemical markers of growth. Horm Res 2003; 60 (Suppl. 1): 46-51.
[http://dx.doi.org/10.1159/000071225] [PMID: 12955017]

[83] Rose SR, Municchi G, Barnes KM, *et al.* Spontaneous growth hormone secretion increases during puberty in normal girls and boys. J Clin Endocrinol Metab 1991; 73(2): 428-35.
[http://dx.doi.org/10.1210/jcem-73-2-428] [PMID: 1856268]

[84] Mauras N, Rogol AD, Haymond MW, Veldhuis JD. Sex steroids, growth hormone, insulin-like growth factor-1: neuroendocrine and metabolic regulation in puberty. Horm Res 1996; 45(1-2): 74-80.
[http://dx.doi.org/10.1159/000184763] [PMID: 8742123]

[85] Zadik Z, Chalew SA, McCarter RJ Jr, Meistas M, Kowarski AA. The influence of age on the 24-hour integrated concentration of growth hormone in normal individuals. J Clin Endocrinol Metab 1985; 60(3): 513-6.
[http://dx.doi.org/10.1210/jcem-60-3-513] [PMID: 3972964]

[86] Attanasio AF, Shalet SM. Growth hormone and the transition from puberty into adulthood. Endocrinol Metab Clin North Am 2007; 36(1): 187-201.
[http://dx.doi.org/10.1016/j.ecl.2006.11.002] [PMID: 17336740]

[87] Parent AS, Teilmann G, Juul A, Skakkebaek NE, Toppari J, Bourguignon JP. The timing of normal puberty and the age limits of sexual precocity: variations around the world, secular trends, and changes after migration. Endocr Rev 2003; 24(5): 668-93.
[http://dx.doi.org/10.1210/er.2002-0019] [PMID: 14570750]

[88] Lander ES, Schork NJ. Genetic dissection of complex traits. Science 1994; 265(5181): 2037-48. [http://dx.doi.org/10.1126/science.8091226] [PMID: 8091226]

[89] Cooper JD. Progress towards understanding the neurobiology of Batten disease or neuronal ceroid lipofuscinosis. Curr Opin Neurol 2003; 16(2): 121-8. [http://dx.doi.org/10.1097/00019052-200304000-00001] [PMID: 12644737]

[90] de Roux N, Young J, Misrahi M, Schaison G, Milgrom E. Loss of function mutations of the GnRH receptor: a new cause of hypogonadotropic hypogonadism. J Pediatr Endocrinol Metab 1999; 12 (Suppl. 1): 267-75. [PMID: 10698591]

[91] Franco B, Guioli S, Pragliola A, *et al.* A gene deleted in Kallmanns syndrome shares homology with neural cell adhesion and axonal path-finding molecules. Nature 1991; 353(6344): 529-36. [http://dx.doi.org/10.1038/353529a0] [PMID: 1922361]

[92] Dodé C, Levilliers J, Dupont JM, *et al.* Loss-of-function mutations in FGFR1 cause autosomal dominant Kallmann syndrome. Nat Genet 2003; 33(4): 463-5. [http://dx.doi.org/10.1038/ng1122] [PMID: 12627230]

[93] Topaloglu AK, Tello JA, Kotan LD, *et al.* Inactivating KISS1 mutation and hypogonadotropic hypogonadism. N Engl J Med 2012; 366(7): 629-35. [http://dx.doi.org/10.1056/NEJMoa1111184] [PMID: 22335740]

[94] Silveira LG, Noel SD, Silveira-Neto AP, *et al.* Mutations of the KISS1 gene in disorders of puberty. J Clin Endocrinol Metab 2010; 95(5): 2276-80. [http://dx.doi.org/10.1210/jc.2009-2421] [PMID: 20237166]

[95] Topaloglu AK, Reimann F, Guclu M, *et al.* TAC3 and TACR3 mutations in familial hypogonadotropic hypogonadism reveal a key role for Neurokinin B in the central control of reproduction. Nat Genet 2009; 41(3): 354-8. [http://dx.doi.org/10.1038/ng.306] [PMID: 19079066]

[96] Topaloglu AK, Semple RK. Neurokinin B signalling in the human reproductive axis. Mol Cell Endocrinol 2011; 346(1-2): 57-64. [http://dx.doi.org/10.1016/j.mce.2011.07.014] [PMID: 21807065]

[97] Abreu AP, Dauber A, Macedo DB, *et al.* Central precocious puberty caused by mutations in the imprinted gene MKRN3. N Engl J Med 2013; 368(26): 2467-75. [http://dx.doi.org/10.1056/NEJMoa1302160] [PMID: 23738509]

[98] Rojek A, Flader M, Malecka E, Niedziela M. A novel mutation in the NR0B1 (DAX1) gene in a large family with two boys affected by congenital adrenal hypoplasia. Hormones (Athens) 2014; 13(3): 413-9. [http://dx.doi.org/110.14310/horm.2002.1495] [PMID: 25079468]

[99] Godowski PJ, Leung DW, Meacham LR, *et al.* Characterization of the human growth hormone receptor gene and demonstration of a partial gene deletion in two patients with Laron-type dwarfism. Proc Natl Acad Sci USA 1989; 86(20): 8083-7. [http://dx.doi.org/10.1073/pnas.86.20.8083] [PMID: 2813379]

[100] Cohen LE, Radovick S. Molecular basis of combined pituitary hormone deficiencies. Endocr Rev 2002; 23(4): 431-42. [http://dx.doi.org/10.1210/er.2001-0030] [PMID: 12202459]

[101] Superti-Furga A, Bonafé L, Rimoin DL. Molecular-pathogenetic classification of genetic disorders of the skeleton. Am J Med Genet 2001; 106(4): 282-93. [http://dx.doi.org/10.1002/ajmg.10233] [PMID: 11891680]

[102] Spiegelman BM, Flier JS. Adipogenesis and obesity: rounding out the big picture. Cell 1996; 87(3): 377-89. [http://dx.doi.org/10.1016/S0092-8674(00)81359-8] [PMID: 8898192]

[103] Zhang Y, Proenca R, Maffei M, Barone M, Leopold L, Friedman JM. Positional cloning of the mouse obese gene and its human homologue. Nature 1994; 372(6505): 425-32.
[http://dx.doi.org/10.1038/372425a0] [PMID: 7984236]

[104] Tartaglia LA, Dembski M, Weng X, *et al.* Identification and expression cloning of a leptin receptor, OB-R. Cell 1995; 83(7): 1263-71.
[http://dx.doi.org/10.1016/0092-8674(95)90151-5] [PMID: 8548812]

[105] Considine RV, Sinha MK, Heiman ML, *et al.* Serum immunoreactive-leptin concentrations in normal-weight and obese humans. N Engl J Med 1996; 334(5): 292-5.
[http://dx.doi.org/10.1056/NEJM199602013340503] [PMID: 8532024]

[106] Hamnvik OP, Liu X, Petrou M, *et al.* Soluble leptin receptor and leptin are associated with baseline adiposity and metabolic risk factors, and predict adiposity, metabolic syndrome, and glucose levels at 2-year follow-up: the Cyprus Metabolism Prospective Cohort Study. Metabolism 2011; 60(7): 987-93.
[http://dx.doi.org/10.1016/j.metabol.2010.09.009] [PMID: 21056886]

[107] Wilkinson M, Morash B, Ur E. The brain is a source of leptin. Front Horm Res 2000; 26: 106-25.
[http://dx.doi.org/10.1159/000061018] [PMID: 10767944]

[108] Bado A, Levasseur S, Attoub S, *et al.* The stomach is a source of leptin. Nature 1998; 394(6695): 790-3.
[http://dx.doi.org/10.1038/29547] [PMID: 9723619]

[109] Toro AR, Maymó JL, Ibarbalz FM, *et al.* Leptin is an anti-apoptotic effector in placental cells involving p53 downregulation. PLoS One 2014; 9(6): e99187.
[http://dx.doi.org/10.1371/journal.pone.0099187] [PMID: 24922063]

[110] Maqsood AR, Trueman JA, Whatmore AJ, *et al.* The relationship between nocturnal urinary leptin and gonadotrophins as children progress towards puberty. Horm Res 2007; 68(5): 225-30.
[http://dx.doi.org/10.1159/000101335] [PMID: 17389812]

[111] Phillip M, Moran O, Lazar L. Growth without growth hormone. J Pediatr Endocrinol Metab 2002; 15 (Suppl. 5): 1267-72.
[PMID: 12510977]

[112] Myers MG Jr. Leptin receptor signaling and the regulation of mammalian physiology. Recent Prog Horm Res 2004; 59: 287-304.
[http://dx.doi.org/10.1210/rp.59.1.287] [PMID: 14749507]

[113] Halaas JL, Gajiwala KS, Maffei M, *et al.* Weight-reducing effects of the plasma protein encoded by the obese gene. Science 1995; 269(5223): 543-6.
[http://dx.doi.org/10.1126/science.7624777] [PMID: 7624777]

[114] Cunningham MJ, Clifton DK, Steiner RA. Leptins actions on the reproductive axis: perspectives and mechanisms. Biol Reprod 1999; 60(2): 216-22.
[http://dx.doi.org/10.1095/biolreprod60.2.216] [PMID: 9915984]

[115] Quennell JH, Mulligan AC, Tups A, *et al.* Leptin indirectly regulates gonadotropin-releasing hormone neuronal function. Endocrinology 2009; 150(6): 2805-12.
[http://dx.doi.org/10.1210/en.2008-1693] [PMID: 19179437]

[116] Avelino-Cruz JE, Flores A, Cebada J, Mellon PL, Felix R, Monjaraz E. Leptin increases L-type Ca2+ channel expression and GnRH-stimulated LH release in LbetaT2 gonadotropes. Mol Cell Endocrinol 2009; 298(1-2): 57-65.
[http://dx.doi.org/10.1016/j.mce.2008.09.003] [PMID: 18834922]

[117] Ahima RS, Dushay J, Flier SN, Prabakaran D, Flier JS. Leptin accelerates the onset of puberty in normal female mice. J Clin Invest 1997; 99(3): 391-5.
[http://dx.doi.org/10.1172/JCI119172] [PMID: 9022071]

[118] Chehab FF, Mounzih K, Lu R, Lim ME. Early onset of reproductive function in normal female mice treated with leptin. Science 1997; 275(5296): 88-90.
[http://dx.doi.org/10.1126/science.275.5296.88] [PMID: 8974400]

[119] Castellano JM, Roa J, Luque RM, *et al.* KiSS-1/kisspeptins and the metabolic control of reproduction: physiologic roles and putative physiopathological implications. Peptides 2009; 30(1): 139-45.
[http://dx.doi.org/10.1016/j.peptides.2008.06.007] [PMID: 18634841]

[120] Roa J, Tena-Sempere M. Energy balance and puberty onset: emerging role of central mTOR signaling. Trends Endocrinol Metab 2010; 21(9): 519-28.
[http://dx.doi.org/10.1016/j.tem.2010.05.003] [PMID: 20554449]

[121] Elias CF, Purohit D. Leptin signaling and circuits in puberty and fertility. Cell Mol Life Sci 2013; 70(5): 841-62.
[http://dx.doi.org/10.1007/s00018-012-1095-1] [PMID: 22851226]

[122] Tena-Sempere M, Barreiro ML. Leptin in male reproduction: the testis paradigm. Mol Cell Endocrinol 2002; 188(1-2): 9-13.
[http://dx.doi.org/10.1016/S0303-7207(02)00008-4] [PMID: 11911940]

[123] Cheung CC, Thornton JE, Nurani SD, Clifton DK, Steiner RA. A reassessment of leptins role in triggering the onset of puberty in the rat and mouse. Neuroendocrinology 2001; 74(1): 12-21.
[http://dx.doi.org/10.1159/000054666] [PMID: 11435754]

[124] Ahmed ML, Ong KK, Morrell DJ, *et al.* Longitudinal study of leptin concentrations during puberty: sex differences and relationship to changes in body composition. J Clin Endocrinol Metab 1999; 84(3): 899-905.
[http://dx.doi.org/10.1210/jcem.84.3.5559] [PMID: 10084568]

[125] Horlick MB, Rosenbaum M, Nicolson M, *et al.* Effect of puberty on the relationship between circulating leptin and body composition. J Clin Endocrinol Metab 2000; 85(7): 2509-18.
[http://dx.doi.org/10.1210/jcem.85.7.6689] [PMID: 10902802]

[126] Palmert MR, Radovick S, Boepple PA. The impact of reversible gonadal sex steroid suppression on serum leptin concentrations in children with central precocious puberty. J Clin Endocrinol Metab 1998; 83(4): 1091-6.
[http://dx.doi.org/10.1210/jcem.83.4.4700] [PMID: 9543124]

[127] Ybarra J, Bobbioni-Harsch E, Chassot G, *et al.* Persistent correlation of ghrelin plasma levels with body mass index both in stable weight conditions and during gastric-bypass-induced weight loss. Obes Surg 2009; 19(3): 327-31.
[http://dx.doi.org/10.1007/s11695-008-9748-8] [PMID: 18975038]

[128] Shiiya T, Nakazato M, Mizuta M, *et al.* Plasma ghrelin levels in lean and obese humans and the effect of glucose on ghrelin secretion. J Clin Endocrinol Metab 2002; 87(1): 240-4.
[http://dx.doi.org/10.1210/jcem.87.1.8129] [PMID: 11788653]

[129] Shintani M, Ogawa Y, Ebihara K, *et al.* Ghrelin, an endogenous growth hormone secretagogue, is a novel orexigenic peptide that antagonizes leptin action through the activation of hypothalamic neuropeptide Y/Y1 receptor pathway. Diabetes 2001; 50(2): 227-32.
[http://dx.doi.org/10.2337/diabetes.50.2.227] [PMID: 11272130]

[130] Diéguez C, da Boit K, Novelle MG, Martínez de Morentin PB, Nogueiras R, López M. New insights in ghrelin orexigenic effect. Front Horm Res 2010; 38: 196-205.
[http://dx.doi.org/10.1159/000318511] [PMID: 20616512]

[131] Fernandez-Fernandez R, Martini AC, Navarro VM, *et al.* Novel signals for the integration of energy balance and reproduction. Mol Cell Endocrinol 2006; 254-255: 127-32.
[http://dx.doi.org/10.1016/j.mce.2006.04.026] [PMID: 16759792]

[132] Soriano-Guillén L, Barrios V, Chowen JA, *et al.* Ghrelin levels from fetal life through early adulthood: relationship with endocrine and metabolic and anthropometric measures. J Pediatr 2004; 144(1): 30-5. [http://dx.doi.org/10.1016/j.jpeds.2003.08.050] [PMID: 14722515]

[133] Tena-Sempere M. Ghrelin, the gonadal axis and the onset of puberty. Endocr Dev 2013; 25: 69-82. [http://dx.doi.org/10.1159/000346055] [PMID: 23652393]

[134] Froesch ER, Buergi H, Ramseier EB, Bally P, Labhart A. Antibody-Suppressible and Nonsuppressible Insulin-Like Activities in Human Serum and Their Physiologic Significance. An Insulin Assay with Adipose Tissue of Increased Precision and Specificity. J Clin Invest 1963; 42: 1816-34. [http://dx.doi.org/10.1172/JCI104866] [PMID: 14083170]

[135] Gennigens C, Menetrier-Caux C, Droz JP. Insulin-Like Growth Factor (IGF) family and prostate cancer. Crit Rev Oncol Hematol 2006; 58(2): 124-45. [http://dx.doi.org/10.1016/j.critrevonc.2005.10.003] [PMID: 16387509]

[136] Jones JI, Clemmons DR. Insulin-like growth factors and their binding proteins: biological actions. Endocr Rev 1995; 16(1): 3-34. [http://dx.doi.org/10.1210/edrv-16-1-3] [PMID: 7758431]

[137] Adams TE, Epa VC, Garrett TP, Ward CW. Structure and function of the type 1 insulin-like growth factor receptor. Cell Mol Life Sci 2000; 57(7): 1050-93. [http://dx.doi.org/10.1007/PL00000744] [PMID: 10961344]

[138] Baker J, Hardy MP, Zhou J, *et al.* Effects of an Igf1 gene null mutation on mouse reproduction. Mol Endocrinol 1996; 10(7): 903-18. [http://dx.doi.org/10.1210/mend.10.7.8813730] [PMID: 8813730]

[139] Baker J, Liu JP, Robertson EJ, Efstratiadis A. Role of insulin-like growth factors in embryonic and postnatal growth. Cell 1993; 75(1): 73-82. [http://dx.doi.org/10.1016/S0092-8674(05)80085-6] [PMID: 8402902]

[140] Murray PG, Clayton PE. Endocrine Control of Growth. Am J Med Genet C Semin Med Genet 2013. [http://dx.doi.org/10.1002/ajmg.c.31357]

[141] Wolfe A, Divall S, Wu S. The regulation of reproductive neuroendocrine function by insulin and insulin-like growth factor-1 (IGF-1). Front Neuroendocrinol 2014; 35(4): 558-72. [http://dx.doi.org/10.1016/j.yfrne.2014.05.007] [PMID: 24929098]

[142] Cole TJ, Ahmed ML, Preece MA, Hindmarsh P, Dunger DB. The relationship between Insulin-like Growth Factor 1, sex steroids and timing of the pubertal growth spurt. Clin Endocrinol (Oxf) 2015; 82(6): 862-9. [http://dx.doi.org/10.1111/cen.12682] [PMID: 25418044]

[143] Löfqvist C, Andersson E, Gelander L, Rosberg S, Blum WF, Albertsson Wikland K. Reference values for IGF-I throughout childhood and adolescence: a model that accounts simultaneously for the effect of gender, age, and puberty. J Clin Endocrinol Metab 2001; 86(12): 5870-6. [http://dx.doi.org/10.1210/jcem.86.12.8117] [PMID: 11739455]

[144] Zhen S, Zakaria M, Wolfe A, Radovick S. Regulation of gonadotropin-releasing hormone (GnRH) gene expression by insulin-like growth factor I in a cultured GnRH-expressing neuronal cell line. Mol Endocrinol 1997; 11(8): 1145-55. [http://dx.doi.org/10.1210/mend.11.8.9956] [PMID: 9212061]

[145] Anderson RA, Zwain IH, Arroyo A, Mellon PL, Yen SS. The insulin-like growth factor system in the GT17 GnRH neuronal cell line. Neuroendocrinology 1999; 70(5): 353-9. [http://dx.doi.org/10.1159/000054496] [PMID: 10567861]

[146] Longo KM, Sun Y, Gore AC. Insulin-like growth factor-I effects on gonadotropin-releasing hormone biosynthesis in GT17 cells. Endocrinology 1998; 139(3): 1125-32. [http://dx.doi.org/10.1210/endo.139.3.5852] [PMID: 9492046]

[147] Young J, Chanson P, Salenave S, *et al.* Testicular anti-mullerian hormone secretion is stimulated by recombinant human FSH in patients with congenital hypogonadotropic hypogonadism. J Clin Endocrinol Metab 2005; 90(2): 724-8.
[http://dx.doi.org/10.1210/jc.2004-0542] [PMID: 15536161]

[148] Ferlin A, Garolla A, Rigon F, Rasi Caldogno L, Lenzi A, Foresta C. Changes in serum insulin-like factor 3 during normal male puberty. J Clin Endocrinol Metab 2006; 91(9): 3426-31.
[http://dx.doi.org/10.1210/jc.2006-0821] [PMID: 16804040]

[149] Wikström AM, Bay K, Hero M, Andersson AM, Dunkel L. Serum insulin-like factor 3 levels during puberty in healthy boys and boys with Klinefelter syndrome. J Clin Endocrinol Metab 2006; 91(11): 4705-8.
[http://dx.doi.org/10.1210/jc.2006-0669] [PMID: 16926256]

[150] Carel JC, Léger J. Clinical practice. Precocious puberty. N Engl J Med 2008; 358(22): 2366-77.
[http://dx.doi.org/10.1056/NEJMcp0800459] [PMID: 18509122]

[151] Nordt CA, DiVasta AD. Gynecomastia in adolescents. Curr Opin Pediatr 2008; 20(4): 375-82.
[http://dx.doi.org/10.1097/MOP.0b013e328306a07c] [PMID: 18622190]

[152] Derkacz M, Chmiel-Perzyńska I, Nowakowski A. Gynecomastia - a difficult diagnostic problem. Endokrynol Pol 2011; 62(2): 190-202.
[PMID: 21528484]

[153] Thorup J, McLachlan R, Cortes D, *et al.* What is new in cryptorchidism and hypospadiasa critical review on the testicular dysgenesis hypothesis. J Pediatr Surg 2010; 45(10): 2074-86.
[http://dx.doi.org/10.1016/j.jpedsurg.2010.07.030] [PMID: 20920735]

CHAPTER 7

Biochemical Events Occurring in the Epididymis

Tânia R. Dias[1,2,3,*] and **Raquel L. Bernardino**[2]

[1] *Health Sciences Research Center, University of Beira Interior, Rua Marquês d'Ávila e Bolama, 6201-001, Covilhã, Portugal*

[2] *Department of Microscopy, Laboratory of Cell Biology, Institute of Biomedical Sciences Abel Salazar and Unit for Multidisciplinary Research in Biomedicine, University of Porto, Rua de Jorge Viterbo Ferreira, 4050-313, Porto, Portugal*

[3] *LAQV/REQUIMTE — Laboratory of Bromatology and Hydrology, Faculty of Pharmacy, University of Porto, Rua do Campo Alegre, 4150-755, Porto, Portugal*

Abstract: The epididymis is a long convoluted organ of the male reproductive tract. Its functionality has been overlooked for many years, but it is currently accepted that it has a preponderant role in spermatozoa post-testicular maturation. The epididymis presents a high secretory activity. Several proteins can be released in bulk through apical blebs or can be associated with epididymosomes, which fuse with sperm plasma membrane becoming integral proteins. The interaction of epididymal proteins with spermatozoa is a very important factor in the regulation of spermatozoa maturation along their passage through the different epididymal regions. A mature sperm cell recovered from the epididymal caudal region should present the ability to move (activated motility) and to fertilize the oocyte. The atmosphere created within the epididymal lumen is very dynamic, since the epididymal fluid composition is relatively different between the tubule compartments. The blood-epididymal barrier (BEB) created by junctions between principal cells of the epididymal epithelium is not only responsible for the control of epididymal luminal fluid composition, but also acts as a defense mechanism to protect spermatozoa from the immune system, harmful xenobiotics and oxidative stress. While the caput and corpus of epididymis are mainly involved in sperm maturation, the caudal region is the site of mature sperm storage in a quiescent and protected state. In this chapter, we discuss the biochemical events occurring during the transit of spermatozoa through the epididymis. We will focus on the involvement and structural organization of epididymal epithelial cells and secretory proteins on spermatozoa modifications during their maturational process.

Keywords: Androgens, Apical blebs, Blood-epididymal barrier, Coating proteins, Epididymal epithelial cells, Epididymal secreted proteins, Epididymis, Epididymosomes, Fertilizing ability, Integral membrane proteins, Luminal micro-

* **Corresponding author Tânia R. Dias:** Avenida Infante D. Henrique 6200-506 Covilhã, Portugal; Tel: +351 275 329 002; Fax: +351 275 329 099; E-mail: taniairdias@gmail.com

Marco G. Alves and Pedro F. Oliveira (Eds.)

environment, Motility acquisition, Sperm protection, Sperm maturation, Sperm storage.

INTRODUCTION

Spermatozoa development goes far beyond their complex process of production in the seminiferous tubules. Their post-testicular progress involves ultrastructural and macromolecular modifications during their course to reach the site of fertilization in the oviduct [1]. These alterations result from sequential, temporally controlled interactions between male reproductive tract secretions and the transiting male gamete [2]. After being shed from the testes, spermatozoa follow their pathway through the rete testis and efferent ducts, reaching the epididymis. The epididymis is a long convoluted tubule that is structurally organized into three principal regions: the caput (head), the corpus (body) and the distal cauda epididymis (tail) [3]. The epididymal epithelium is constituted by a diverse set of cell types: principal, narrow, apical, clear, basal, halo and surrounding peritubular myoid cells [4, 5]. Each cell type has a particular function and compartmentalization throughout the epididymal duct. Though, all cellular types contribute to the establishment and regulation of the epididymal luminal environment, which is crucial for the attainment of spermatozoa peculiar morphological and functional characteristics [1, 4]. Among the wide range of epididymal functions, we can highlight the following: (1) sperm concentration, to facilitate ejaculation; (2) functional maturation, to acquire motility and fertilizing ability; (3) storage in a quiescent viable state until ejaculation; (4) removal of degenerating sperm and (5) protection of spermatozoa [6].

From the rete testis to the end of the epididymis, spermatozoa are bathed in a continuously and progressively changing medium of fluid proteins and other chemical components [7]. The epididymal fluid composition is highly regulated by a selective structure known as blood-epididymal barrier (BEB). The formation of this barrier is a critical factor for sperm maturation, since it enables the development of the proper epididymal luminal environment for spermatozoa maturational process. Besides, the epididymis has a great proteinaceous secretory activity [8]. In fact, it releases a wide range of proteins that directly influence the composition of the epididymal epithelium (*e.g.* pH, osmolality), but also contributes for sperm protection, since it modulates oxidative stress (OS) [9]. The maturational process of spermatozoa includes many changes in sperm physiological properties, such as the acquisition of forward motility, the ability to recognize and bind to the zona pellucida, and the capacity to fuse with the plasma membrane of an oocyte [10]. During epididymal transit, spermatozoa acquire new proteins, some of which are coating proteins that can be removed by washing with isotonic or hypertonic solutions, while others are assimilated by sperm plasma membrane as integral membrane proteins. These latter are incorporated in spermatozoa membranes by small vesicles called epididymosomes [11]. However, the underlying mechanisms are not yet fully understood.

The mature spermatozoa are finally stored in a quiescent state in the cauda epididymis [12]. Since they can be stored for several days until ejaculation, the characteristic microenvironment of this epididymal section should also be controlled. Particularly, there is a need to protect spermatozoa from OS, since they are highly susceptible to reactive oxygen species (ROS) damage [13]. Moreover, at this stage, it is essential to remove degenerating spermatozoa, since they can damage the viable quiescent cells [14]. This chapter is focused on the major sequential modifications of spermatozoa during their transit through the epididymis, highlighting the role of epididymal secretome and the biochemical modifications occurring from the immotile testicular spermatozoa to the quiescent, but actively motile, spermatozoa at the end of the epididymal duct.

STRUCTURE AND FUNCTION OF THE EPIDIDYMIS

The epididymis is an accessory organ derived from the Wolffian duct, anatomically connected to the testes, which at birth essentially consist of mesenchymal tissue [15]. During prenatal development, cell proliferation in Wolffian duct is dependent on the presence of androgens and mesenchymal factors, whereas postnatal development is influenced by lumicrine factors, such as androgens, growth factors and several enzymes secreted by the testes [16]. The epididymal postnatal development consists of three major stages: an undifferentiated period, a period of differentiation and a last period of expansion or proliferation [15]. In the first period, from birth to early infancy, the proximal regions of epididymis begin to coil, while the cauda coiling still uncomplete. Moreover, this accessory organ undergoes extensive remodeling and duct elongation/convolution until puberty, where it becomes fully differentiated [15, 17]. In the second period, from infancy to puberty, the epididymal epithelium differentiates into specific cells: principal, apical, basal, clear and narrow cells. During puberty, the epithelial cell differentiation is completed, since there is a high rate of cell division and epididymal expansion. In the third period, there is a continued growth of the epididymis and spermatozoa appear in the lumen of the duct [15]. The adult epididymis consists in a several meters-long contorted duct that, if uncoiled, measures about 5.5 meters in humans [3], 1 meter in mice [18], 3 meters in rat [19] and up to 80 meters in horses [20]. Human epididymis is quite different from that of other mammalians. The macroscopic aspect of the human epididymis allows the anatomically division of the duct, which includes the proximal region (caput), corpus and distal cauda (Fig. **7.1**). This segmentation is also based on structural and functional parameters of each region. In most mammals, each region of the epididymis is structured into lobules that are separated by connective tissue septa [1]. Although, histological and ultrastructural segmentation in humans differs among the different phylogenies of mammalians [10]. While the epididymis of mammals, such as mouse and rat, can be divided into initial segment, caput, corpus and cauda, the human epididymis is poorly differentiated, since no initial segment can be distinguished [21]. The human proximal caput is formed by efferent ducts and the presence of poorly defined and incomplete septa, which do not clearly demark epididymal compartments [10]. However, 10, 19 and 7 intraregional segments can be distinguished in the epididymis of the mouse, rat and human, respectively. These segments are separated by connective tissue septa that can establish borders for epididymal gene expression, protein content and epithelial responses to lumicrine factors [4, 22]. Each anatomical region consists of a lumen and polarized epithelium, which are easily identified in adult mammals. Histologically, the human epididymis is a tube of smooth muscle lined by a pseudostratified epithelium. This duct presents characteristics that allow the easy recognition of the anterior and posterior border, since the thickness is different in the proximal and caudal segment. The caudal region is thinnest than the caput, whereas the luminal diameter increases from the caput to the distal regions [2, 23]. Moreover, from proximal to distal segments, the muscular wall increases from a single circular layer to three layers. Epididymal proximal region presents smooth muscle with slow rhythmic contractility, which slightly moves spermatozoa towards the vas deferens. On the other hand, the distal region is richly innervated by the sympathetic nervous system, creating intense contractions of the lower part of the epididymis during ejaculation [3]. The mechanism responsible for driving luminal contents has been attributed to the peristaltic contractions of the smooth muscle cells lining the epididymal tubule [24 - 26]. All the epididymal duct is also surrounded by interstitial components including blood vessels, lymphatic vessels, connective tissue septa, macrophages and lymphocytes [5].

Epididymal Cell Types

The functionality of each epididymal region depends on the segment-specific epithelial cell populations. In fact, the specific regionalization and luminal environment of the different epididymal segments is ensured by the cell types that populate each region.

Among the several types of epithelial cells identified in the epididymis are the principal, the narrow, the apical, the clear, the basal and the halo cells, surrounded by multiple layers of peritubular myoid cells (Fig. **7.1**) [4, 5] Some of these cells are found throughout the duct (*e.g.* principal cells and basal cells), while others are exclusively located in specific segments (*e.g.* narrow cells, apical cells, clear cells and halo cells). Although the localization of the epithelial cell types differs between species (partly due to the inconsistency of the identification methods and definition of the different regions in some species), in general, all the cell types appear to be expressed in mammalian species [27]. The establishment and regulation of a unique luminal environment is crucial for the maturation, concentration, storage and viability of spermatozoa [1, 4]. The epididymis has a high degree of regionalization according to the different functionalities of the distinct cell types. Specifically, principal cells are responsible for protein secretion and absorption, clear and apical cells for endocytosis, clear and narrow cells for the acidification of the luminal fluid, halo cells for the immune defense and phagocytosis, and the basal cells for the production of antioxidants [28, 29]. In this section, we will present a brief description of the major cell types present along the epididymis and their potential functions.

Principal Cells

The main cell type found in the epididymis are the principal cells, constituting approximately 80% of all the epithelium [1]. However, this percentage of principal cells decreases along the epididymal duct from proximal to distal [30]. The height of these columnar cells extends the full thickness of the epithelium, from the basement lamina to the lumen through prominent stereocilia (Fig. **7.1**). Moreover, this columnar structure present in the initial region is converted into low cuboidal cells in the cauda epididymis [31 - 33]. Their structure and function dramatically differ between each segments [30, 34]. The appearance and organization of the secretory apparatus, such as endoplasmic reticulum, secretory granules and Golgi apparatus, and endocytic apparatus (vesicular bodies, endosomes and lysosomes) varies between each epididymal region [27].

Principal cells of epididymal initial region present two types of endoplasmic reticulum. At the base of the cell, and commonly arranged in parallel arrays, appears a typical flattened rough endoplasmic reticulum cisterna. The other type of endoplasmic reticulum appears as irregularly-shaped dilated elements, presents few ribosomes and is referred to as sparsely granulated endoplasmic reticulum [27, 31]. This latter is found in the apical and supranuclear regions of the principal cells, which are interconnected with each other in an opposite way to the apical plasma membrane on one side and Golgi apparatus on the other side [35, 36]. The most remarkable feature of these cells is their highly developed secretory activity. A large number of secreted proteins to epididymal lumen are synthesized by principal cells and are directly involved in the control of luminal protein concentrations [27]. Rough endoplasmic reticulum is associated to protein synthesis, which undergo glycosylation in the Golgi apparatus [37].

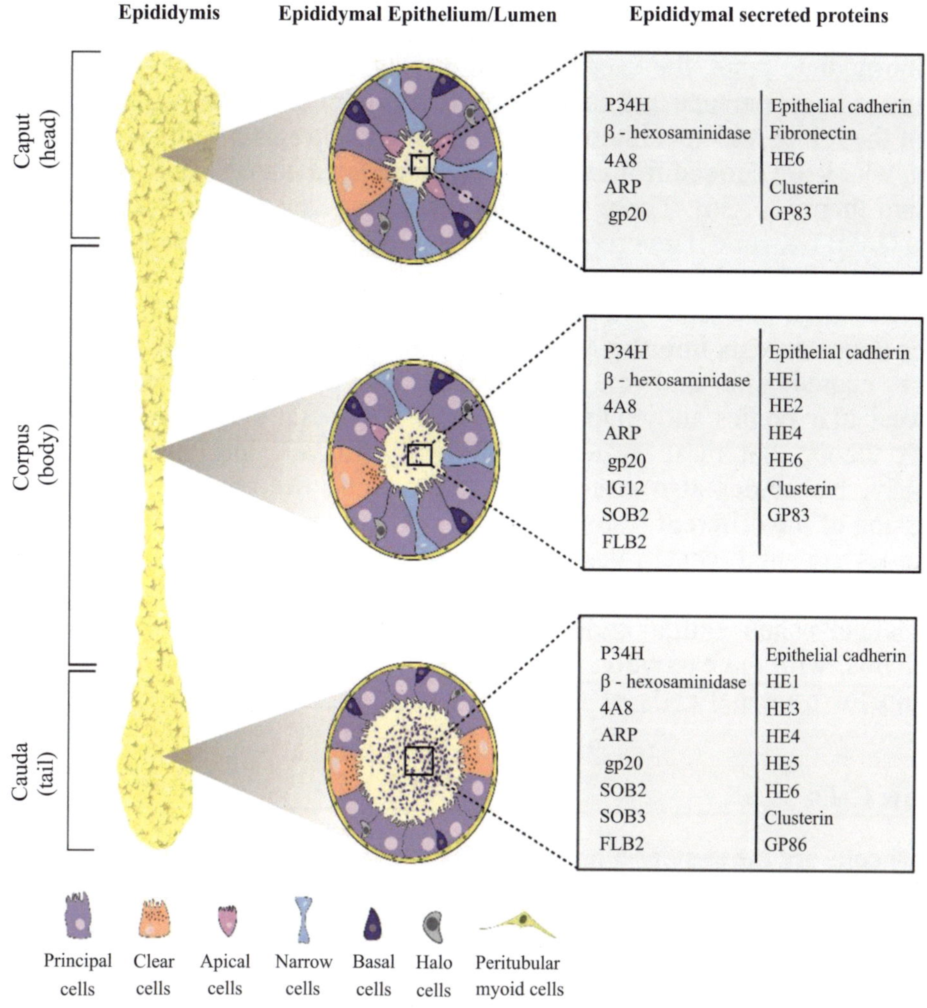

Fig. (7.1). Schematic representation of human epididymal duct. It is constituted by the caput (head), corpus (body) and cauda (tail). The epididymal epithelium comprises a diverse set of cell types: principal, clear, apical, narrow, basal, halo and peritubular myoid cells. There are evident differences in the distribution of epithelial cells along each epididymal segment. Principal cells are the most abundant cells, being largely present in caput region and gradually decreasing until cauda region. Narrow and apical cells are only present in caput and corpus regions, and their expression decreases from the proximal to the distal segment. Clear and basal cells are present in all epididymal regions, though the percentage of basal cells is higher. Besides, clear cells are more active in the cauda epididymis. Halo cells are small cells located on the base of all the epithelium, but do not touch the basement membrane. Peritubular myoid cells are the cells that surround all the other cellular types. The diameter of the epididymal lumen, as well as the number of spermatozoa, increases along the epididymal duct. The epididymis presents a high secretory activity, which is variable from one region to the other. Here are also presented some of the main proteins secreted by the epididymal epithelium in each region. Abbreviations: gp20: sialylglycoprotein; ARP: AEG-Related Protein.

The Golgi apparatus in principal cells also varies between each epididymal region. The initial region contains some elaborated Golgi stacks made up of a cis Golgi network, some flattened saccules and several trans Golgi networks [36]. In the intermediate zone, the saccules of the Golgi stack are strongly tubular and fenestrated in appearance and show fewer trans Golgi networks [30, 38]. Principal cells of the initial region contain vesicular tubular aggregates in their supranuclear region, which are derived from the sparsely granulated endoplasmic reticulum that surround them [35, 36]. These vesicular tubular aggregates transport proteins to the cis Golgi network. The proteins pass the Golgi stacks of saccules, where they are glycosylated, and are segregated into secretory granules formed in the trans Golgi networks. Secretory granules reach and fuse with the apical cell surface to deliver their contents into the lumen [35]. Principal cells present on their apical surface coated pits and on their subsurface lysosomes, coated vesicles, multivesicular bodies and endosomes. There is enough evidence supporting the current theory that these structures gradually convert into one another [34]. Similarly, lysosomes also structurally differ along the epididymis, due to the expression of the different lysosomal enzymes. These enzymes are transported by lysosomes via small coated vesicles derived from the Golgi apparatus. Some of these vesicles may bind to cell surface [27, 39, 40]. In the intermediate zone, principal cells show similar endocytic organelles, as found in other regions of the epididymis, with the exception of endosomes. This suggests a possibly different function for principal cells of this region in relation to their endocytic activity [38].

Narrow Cells

Narrow cells are the slender elongated cells that only appear within the epithelium of the initial region and intermediate zone of the epididymis (Fig. **7.1**) [41, 42]. They constitute 3% of the total epithelial cells in the initial region, increasing to 6% in the intermediate segment [27]. The cytoplasm of these cells tapers between principal cells as it touches the basement membrane, but its apical cytoplasm may bulge slightly into the lumen [43]. They are characterized by several apically located cup-shaped vesicles and mitochondria, presenting a small flattened nucleus found in the upper half of the cell cytoplasm. Narrow cells are involved in endocytosis and in the process of intracellular transport between the epididymal lumen and the epithelial cells [43]. These cells are crucial for the degradation of specific proteins and carbohydrates within their lysosomes and for the protection of spermatozoa against an electrolytic imbalance [15, 42]. Narrow cells are different from the other epididymal cells in their morphological appearance, distribution and expression of different proteins, such as the glutathione S-transferases (GSTs) and lysosomal enzymes [42].

Apical Cells

Apical cells constitute approximately 10% of the initial region epithelium and approximately 1% of the total epithelium of the intermediate segment [41, 42]. They are characterized by the presence of many mitochondria in the apical cytoplasm, by few microvilli at the luminal border and by a spherical nucleus that is located in the upper half of the cell cytoplasm. These cells do not contact with the basement membrane [15]. Clearly, apical cells differ from adjacent narrow and principal cells concerning their protein expression profile. Although little is known about the specific functions of these cells, a possible role has been suggested in relation to the maintenance of sperm quiescence and pH regulation in the lumen, through the production of enzymes of the carbonic anhydrase family [44] (see Chapter 8).

Clear Cells

Clear cells are evenly distributed rough the caput, corpus and the cauda of the epididymis, constituting fewer than 5% of the total epithelial cell population [15, 27]. These cells are known to be responsible for endocytosis, and they were proposed to play an essential role in the removal of factors from the lumen. They are characterized by the lack of microvilli, an apical region with several coated pits, vesicles, endosomes, multivesicular bodies, lysosomes, as well as a basal region presenting the nucleus and a variable amount of lipid droplets [32, 45]. Clear cells are the epididymal cells with the major endocytic activity and they are particularly active in the cauda epididymis [45, 46]. Spermatozoa crossing the epididymis release cytoplasmic droplets that usually are taken up by the clear cells [45]. These cytoplasmic droplets are created at the time of sperm release and contain Golgi saccular components that can be related to alterations of the sperm plasma membrane [47]. These cells are also responsible for the clearance of proteins from the epididymal lumen and participate in the regulation of luminal fluid acidification [45].

Basal Cells

Basal cells are triangular and flat cells located on the basal side of the epithelium [48]. They are present in all epididymal segments, and constitute 15%–20% of the total epithelium [27, 30, 49]. Basal cells do not access the luminal compartment and are in close association with the overlying principal cells, as indicated by the presence of basal cell cytoplasmic extensions between principal cells. Thus, basal cells may regulate principal cells functions [48, 50]. Basal cells possess coated pits on the plasma membrane, suggesting a function associated with receptor-mediated endocytosis of factors from the blood or principal cells. They also assist the regulation of electrolyte and water transportation [48, 51]. Basal cells present an accumulation of secretory vesicles within mid and trans Golgi saccules and distinct secretory granules that appear next to the Golgi apparatus. These secretory granules may be used to regulate cell function or enter the circulation to perform functions yet to be determined [27]. Some reports have suggested that basal cells may have an important role in the epithelial immune system and in the regulation of electrolytes by principal cells, but the exact roles for these cells are not yet clear [15].

Halo Cells

The halo cells, which are present throughout the epididymal epithelium, are characterized by its small dense nucleus surrounded by a very pale cytoplasm [30]. These cells are located in the base of the epithelium and they do not touch the basement membrane [15]. Rough endoplasmic reticulum is not frequently found in these cells, but free ribonucleoprotein particles and occasional polyribosome rosettes are normally dispersed throughout the cytoplasm, as well as large mitochondria and occasional multivesicular bodies [31]. Halo cells appear to be the primary immune cell in the epididymis [52], having been described either as lymphocytes [30] or monocytes [53].

Functions of Mammalian Epididymis

The mammalian epididymis is a complex tubule that comprises several important functions: transport of spermatozoa; development of sperm functional maturation (acquisition of motility and fertilizing ability); maintenance of BEB to establish the specialized luminal environment required for sperm protection; and storage of sperm in a quiescent, but viable, state until ejaculation [6]. The absence or depletion of any of these functions may be a significant factor for male infertility [15]. The major function of the adult epididymis is to provide the optimal conditions to ensure the transport of maturing sperm along the duct, culminating in the development and conservation of fertilization.

Spermatozoa released from the seminiferous tubules are transported through the rete testis and efferent ducts until begin their course along the epididymis. This transport occurs against an increasing hydrostatic pressure gradient from seminiferous tubules to cauda epididymis [12]. The duration of this process is variable and dependent on the species, size of the duct, and number of produced spermatozoa. Usually, the standard transit time of mammals' spermatozoa through the epididymis is between 10 and 12 days [30]. However, in humans the sperm transit is relatively more rapid (2-4 days) [54]. The progression of spermatozoa within the epididymal luminal fluid is a dynamic process controlled by the electrical and contractile activity of the epididymal duct [55, 56]. The rate of luminal fluid is not uniform in all epididymal segments and the progression decreases from proximal to distal regions and vas deferens [25]. In fact, there are frequent contractions of smooth muscle fibers along the caput and corpus regions, whilst cauda epididymis exhibit low-frequency segmental contractions [26, 57]. The smooth muscle contractions that cause movement of sperm along the epididymal duct are influenced by some hormonal and neuronal factors. For instance, epididymal cells express specific receptors for oxytocin, vasopressin and endothelin [58, 59]. It has been described that these neurohypophysial peptides can increase epididymal contractility [60, 61]. Interestingly, the effects of oxytocin may be interplayed with estrogens, since these hormones demonstrated an upregulation of both gene and protein expression of oxytocin receptor in rabbit epididymis [62]. It is also known that testosterone is able to control the contractility of the epididymal duct to ensure a right rate of sperm transport [15]. Moreover, previous studies have suggested that prostaglandins are important regulators of proximal epididymis contractions, thus regulating epididymal motility and sperm transport [63].

The acquisition of sperm motility and fertilizing ability are the maturational events that occur within the epididymis, mostly in caput and corpus segments [15]. The distal cauda is essentially a storage site for functionally mature spermatozoa [1]. Maturation implicates biochemical and morphological alterations in the sperm surface caused by epididymal secretions of proteins, glycoproteins and enzymes that are essential in the process of fertilization [64] (see below). During this maturational process several sperm characteristics change. An evident change in epididymal sperm is the shedding of the cytoplasmic droplet. Sperm in the cauda epididymis still possesses the droplet of residual cytoplasm that remains after the reshaping of the cell during spermiogenesis. In most species, the droplet moves distally along the flagellum during epididymal passage and is shed prior to or during ejaculation [65]. The appearance and topographical configuration of the sperm plasma membrane also changes during its passage through the epididymis, involving a reduction in size to facilitate ejaculation, the alteration of the shape of the apical segment, changes in the appearance of the acrosomal contents [66], and in the density and distribution of membrane constituents [67]. For instance, there is a selective and progressive loss of phospholipids that results in an elevated amount of cholesterol. This alteration is associated with the stabilization of the membrane of the mature sperm for storage in the cauda epididymis [68]. Sperm epididymal maturation also includes the activation of motility. Testicular spermatozoa are immotile, just exhibiting a faint twitch of the flagellum, while spermatozoa released by the cauda of epididymis move progressively and vigorously forward (see Chapter **9**) [15].

The cauda epididymis is where spermatozoa remain stored in appropriated conditions until ejaculation. Spermatozoa can be stored in the cauda epididymis during days or weeks and retain their functions [69, 70]. This feature makes the amount of spermatozoa in the ejaculate more controllable and less dependent on testicular production, which can be normally maintained while spermatozoa are transported to the epididymis [71]. The survival of spermatozoa in the cauda epididymis is species-specific and is also dependent on the temperature of incubation [14]. In scrotal mammals, the combination of a unique luminal milieu and lower temperatures (30–32 ºC) is thought to be major contributor to sperm survival. However, if spermatozoa are removed from the cauda epididymis and incubated at 32 ºC *in vitro*, their fertility and viability are measured in hours rather than days. This caudal region is also responsible for the removal or sequestration of degenerating spermatozoa in order to protect the viable spermatozoa [14]. This is an important function because some attrition of sperm is likely during storage and the release of enzymes from dead sperm could damage the remaining sperm [72]. It is known that epididymal caudal region presents mechanisms to remove or sequestrate these degenerating spermatozoa [14]. Generally, defective sperm is marked for phagocytosis by the protein ubiquitin that is produced by the epididymis [73]. Although the mechanisms of sperm survival in the distal epididymis are still poorly understood, the characteristic sperm chromatin by itself creates a defense mechanism against possible damages during sperm epididymal transit due to its high condensation (see Chapter **9**). This is the process that makes spermatozoa in the distal region quiescent cells, *i.e.*, transcriptionally and translationally silent [9]. It has been suggested that pH control is also essential for storage of quiescent spermatozoa for long periods [74, 75] (see Chapter 8). It involves the control of luminal epididymal fluid composition, which includes a complex mixture of water, inorganic ions, small organic molecules and proteins [76]. The composition of epididymal lumen is crucial not only for maturation, but also for protection and storage of epididymal spermatozoa.

The proper functionality of the spermatozoa also requires a delicate balance in ROS production and recycling. Spermatozoa need to be protected from damage caused by OS and immune system, while their motility needs to be suppressed until it is required to conserve energy and maintain structural integrity [71]. Thus, sperm redox activity is physiologically important in promoting normal sperm function [77]. In fact, small amounts of ROS are required for sperm capacitation, hyperactive motility and acrosome reaction (see Chapter 10) [78]. However, to avoid premature capacitation, epididymal spermatozoa should be protected from ROS during their storage at cauda epididymis. Spermatozoa are particularly susceptible to ROS damages due to the high concentration of polyunsaturated fatty acids (PUFAs) in their plasma membranes [13]. When the uncontrolled production of ROS exceeds the antioxidant capacity of spermatozoa, all cellular components including lipids, proteins, nucleic acids, and sugars are potential targets of OS [79]. Thus, the production of ROS by spermatozoa correlates with lipid peroxidation, DNA oxidation, poor sperm quality and reduced fertility [80, 81]. The epididymis possesses the enzyme glutathione-S-transferase (different expression and activity among epididymal regions), which is part of the machinery used to protect the sperm from OS or to help maintaining quiescence by inhibiting ROS, which could trigger premature capacitation [82]. Another important structure to protect spermatozoa is the BEB, which is created by tight junctions between epididymal epithelial cells. It functions as a selective barrier to protect maturing spermatozoa and control the luminal fluid microenvironment. The BEB creates a defense mechanism that protects spermatozoa from the immune system, harmful xenobiotics and excessive ROS [15, 83]. The isolation of the epididymal lumen from the rest of the body is vital because certain sperm proteins are recognized as foreign objects by the immune system [84]. However, since immune cells are isolated from the epididymal lumen, it is required an alternative method to protect the spermatozoa against harmful microorganisms. With the high incidence of sexually transmitted infections and deleterious effects on fertility in humans, increased interest towards such factors has arisen [85]. It has been described that genes expressed in the epididymis encoding cysteine-rich secreted proteins are not only involved in sperm maturation, but also have antimicrobial properties [86 - 88]. However, further studies will be needed to clarify these findings.

EPIDIDYMAL PROTEINS AND THEIR FUNCTIONS

The fluid secreted by the seminiferous tubules (see Chapter 8), which contains a wide range of proteins, is mainly reabsorbed when reaching the initial region of epididymis. However, it is known that this tubule has also a great secretory activity [10]. Consequently, most proteins found in epididymal fluid are secreted by the epididymal epithelium (Fig. **7.1**) [9]. Many luminal proteins may not play direct roles in sperm maturation, but rather help to create the appropriate environment that is conducive for this process to occur [89]. The formation of this luminal environment is the result of net secretory and absorptive processes of the epithelium, which continually changes along the duct [11]. Thus, epididymal proteins are involved in the regulation of luminal pH, osmolality, regulation of OS and regulation of protein folding/misfolding. There are also mechanisms to remove secreted proteins from the lumen, presumably once their functions have been carried out or if misfolding occurs [90].

Epididymal protein production can occur by two different mechanisms of apocrine secretion. Epididymis can release secretory products in bulk through apical blebs, or integral membrane proteins injected with epididymosomes can fuse with sperm plasma membrane. Apical blebs are balloon-like structures that can be attached to the apical membrane by thin stalks or exist as free vesicles within the epididymal lumen [27]. This type of vesicles contains free ribosomes and cisternae of endoplasmic reticulum, and is mostly found in the initial and distal epididymal regions. When reaching the middle of the epididymal lumen, the apical blebs are believed to disintegrate to release their contents as near as possible of spermatozoa, without necessarily having to bind to the spermatozoa [91]. Concerning epididymosomes, these are electron dense vesicles with about 50-500 nm in diameter [92]. Epididymosomes-associated proteins are not processed through the endoplasmic reticulum and Golgi apparatus, being characterized by unusual glycosylation patterns. These vesicles contain lipid rafts (cholesterol and phospholipid-enriched microdomains), where glycosylphosphatidylinositol (GPI)-anchored and transmembrane proteins are contained, as well as signaling molecules such as protein tyrosine kinases [93]. Epididymosomes originate from the various regions of the epididymis and have corresponding differences in protein composition. These exosomes provide a way of transferring the proteins secreted by the epididymal epithelium to a maturing sperm membrane [92].

There are several types of proteins described in human epididymis, which are classified according to their function. However, there are also many epididymal proteins, which functions remain to be identified. Some epididymal secreted proteins are related to the interaction between the male and female gametes, including the binding of sperm to zona pellucida of the oocyte and sperm-egg fusion [23]. The main proteins involved in the interaction of the spermatozoon with zona pellucida are: P34H (34 kDa) [94], β-hexosaminidase (65 kDa) [95], 4A8 (110 kDa) [96], 1G12 (15-25 kDa) [97] and SOB3 (18-19 kDa) [98]. Capacitated spermatozoa interact with zona pellucida through sperm receptors that recognize glycoconjugates in zona pellucida (see Chapter 10). P34H is a protein of epididymal origin predominantly secreted by the principal cells in the proximal and distal regions of the epididymal corpus [94]. The expression of this protein has been detected in the acrosomal cap of human spermatozoa recovered from the caput, but the expression is higher in the cauda epididymis. The expression of P34H in sperm is lost during the acrosome reaction, suggesting that P34H is an epididymal protein involved in sperm interaction with zona pellucida [99]. β-Hexosaminidase is a glycosidase that hydrolyses the non-reducing terminal N-acetylglucosamine (GlcNAc) residues from β-glycosidic boundaries in several glycoconjugates [95]. It has been described that GlcNAc residues are involved on the interaction of human sperm and zona pellucida. When placing capacitated spermatozoa in contact with bovine serum albumin (mechanism that resembles the contact with zona pellucida), non-reducing terminal GlcNAc triggers the acrosome reaction [100]. However, the mechanisms by which this epididymal enzyme is involved on the sperm-zona pellucida interaction remains to be fully elucidated. The 1G12 protein stands out for its ability to immobilize and agglutinate human spermatozoa [97], whereas SOB3 is involved in secondary binding to the zona pellucida [98].

In relation to the process of sperm-egg fusion, there are numerous proteins involved, such as: AEG-Related Protein (ARP-30 kDa) [101], SOB2 (17.5, 18 and 19 kDa) [102], FLB1 (94-100 kDa) [102], sialylglycoprotein (gp20-20 kDa) [103], epithelial cadherins (120-130 kDa) and fibronectin (30-35 kDa) [104]. ARP belongs to the cysteine-rich secretory protein (CRISP) family members that contains a highly conserved cluster of cysteines near the carboxyl-terminus. ARP is secreted by epithelial cells of epididymis and has been detected on the human sperm head after the acrosome reaction. Human oocytes present in their surface the presence of complementary sites to ARP [101]. Therefore, this suggests a role for ARP in human's sperm-egg fusion. While SOB2 is expressed in spermatozoa of the caput and corpus epididymis [102], FLB1 is detected in some ejaculated spermatozoa [102], and gp20 is founded in principal cells of the epididymis epithelium and in capacitated spermatozoa [103]. Cadherins are a family of cell adhesion molecules known to bind to other cadherins located on adjacent cells [105]. These proteins are dependent on ion calcium and are related with several signal transduction pathways through tyrosine kinases associated with adhesion sites [106]. Epithelial cadherins were identified in human epididymal epithelium and on the surface of both human gametes [107], thus suggesting a possible role in sperm-egg interaction. Fibronectin, human egg plasma membrane and spermatozoa contain an RGD (Arg-Gly-Asp) sequence that is essential to the binding and penetration of human spermatozoa into the oocyte [108 - 110]. Fibronectin has been identified as an epididymal secretory protein and can be a marker of human sperm maturation [111].

Additionally, six major secretory proteins of human epididymal epithelial cells have been identified as HE1-HE6 [23]. HE1 is the major secretory glycoprotein of the human epididymis (25-27 kDa), being detected in high amounts in the corpus epididymal epithelium, as well as in the cauda epididymal fluid [112]. It is estimated that this protein is involved in cholesterol transport, since it contains a N-terminus almost identical to the same amino acid sequence of ram lipid transfer proteins [23]. Therefore, HE1 may represent a decapacitation factor that control the cholesterol content of sperm during maturation, storage and capacitation [113]. HE2 is a small secretory protein (10 kDa), specifically produced by the proximal region of epididymal epithelium [113]. This protein is considered the human sperm antigen due to its localization in the acrosome and equatorial regions of the sperm. In addition, it has been suggested that HE2 might be involved in gamete fusion [114]. Similarly to HE2, HE3 is abundant in proximal region, and is poorly conserved among mammals, therefore its role in sperm maturation is speculative [23]. HE4 is a small acidic secretory protein (10 kDa) with structural similarity to secretory leukocyte proteinase inhibitor of seminal plasma. HE4 has a generalized expression in epididymis and over the entire surface of spermatozoa [113]. Dissociation of HE4 from the spermatozoa during capacitation suggested that HE4 also act as a decapacitating factor [64]. HE5 (23-37 kDa) was found to be abundant in the epithelial cells of the distal epididymis and in spermatozoa. This protein is identical to the CD52 antigen, which is expressed on the cell surface of human lymphocytes [115]. Different from the others HE, which bind loosely to sperm, HE5/CD52 is linked to the sperm membrane in the cauda of epididymis via a GPI anchor. Therefore, HE5 may have a role in protecting spermatozoa from immune system along maturation, storage and fertilization [112]. HE6 is expressed mainly in epithelial cells lining the caput region of human epididymal duct. The amino acid sequence of HE6 has homology with the seven transmembrane-domain (Tm7) receptor superfamily, majority with G-protein coupled cell surface hormone receptors and with low homology to the secretin/VIP family. This protein may be involved in the signal transduction mechanisms, thought the exact mechanisms remain largely unknown [116]. Furthermore, clusterin is an abundant glycoprotein, also secreted by the caput region of the epididymis that is associated with sperm, suggesting a role in sperm maturation [117]. GP83 is located in the corpus and cauda epididymis, specifically in the supranuclear region and cell membrane of principal cells as well in the luminal content and spermatozoa [118]. The epididymis produces and secretes several proteins with a wide range of functions, but mainly associated to spermatozoa maturation. This illustrates the essential role for the proper functionality of this organ to a successful fertilization. However, the epididymal proteome and secretome need to be further investigated in order to understand the involved mechanisms in the processes that occur in the epididymis.

BIOCHEMICAL CONTROL OF SPERM MODIFICATIONS/SPERM MATURATION

During epididymal transit, spermatozoa undergo several morphological and biochemical changes (Box **7.1**). Among the major modifications are included: (1) changes in the composition of plasma membrane glycoproteins and sterols [119]; (2) extensive cross-linking of nuclear protamines by disulfide bonds [120]; (3) an increase in total surface negative charge; (4) relocation of surface antigens; and (5) addition, elimination or modification of surface proteins [92]. These alterations are behind the control of sperm maturational process. In addition, other events also occur in spermatozoa during epididymal transit and are essential for the acquisition of forward motility and fertilizing ability [2]. The attainment of motility is progressive along the epididymis and is the clearest evidence of sperm maturation. In fact, a gradual increase in the percentage of motile spermatozoa recovered from the caput, corpus and cauda regions of the epididymis has been demonstrated [121]. The motile capacity of spermatozoa is mostly regulated by the interaction with the epididymal milieu. However, intrinsic sperm proteins actively contribute to this process (see Chapter **9**). Though, the concept of sperm maturation goes far beyond motility. In fact, it is generally reflected by the acquisition of spermatozoa fertilizing ability, which is only fully attained when reaching the proximal cauda epididymis [122]. Generally, it refers to the ability of the spermatozoon to fuse with a physiologically normal and structurally intact oocyte, either *in vivo* or *in vitro* [123]. Sperm maturation involves several changes in the sperm plasma membrane in response to epididymal secretions and their numerous proteins (as described above) [6]. Interestingly, analytic data of epididymal secretome reported the presence of 408 proteins in the epididymal intraluminal compartment. Among those, 207 were also detected on spermatozoa, which reinforces the interaction between epididymis and spermatozoa [124]. Even though some of these proteins can be of testicular origin or secreted by both the epididymis and the prostate [125], it became clear that spermatozoa acquire new proteins during epididymal transit [23]. This affirmation is supported by the fact that most proteins of testes-released spermatozoa are assimilated until the developing germ cells reach the elongated spermatid stage, since at this moment sperm DNA starts to condensate, ceasing spermatozoa biosynthetic capacity [126]. Therefore, the attainment of proteins by epididymal spermatozoa is mediated by the interaction between the spermatozoa proteins acquired during spermatogenesis and proteins from the epididymal duct [8]. This interaction may occur by different mechanisms: loose binding, that potentially maintains quiescence; tight binding, needed for the interaction with the oocyte in the female tract; post-membrane-insertion modification of membrane proteins (masking/unmasking); or functioning within the epididymal lumen in order to maintain the proper environment [6]. The proteins that spermatozoa assimilate during their transit along the epididymal duct are classically referred to as "coating proteins", since they can be removed by washing with isotonic or hypertonic solutions [123]. Epididymal sperm-coating proteins may exert their effects on maturating-spermatozoa or become functional only in the female tract. Some of the epididymal secretory proteins are known as "decapacitation factors", since they contribute to the stabilization of the sperm plasma membrane, preventing the occurrence of premature capacitation [127]. Contrastingly, other proteins have been related to the ability of spermatozoa to recognize and bind to the zona pellucida and oocyte plasma membrane (see Chapter **10**) [128 - 130]. These proteins are incorporated in sperm plasma membrane, thus acting as integral-like proteins [123]. One of the main examples of this latter category are the GPI-anchored proteins expressed by epididymal cells. These proteins are inserted in sperm plasma membrane as they pass through the epididymis in a mechanism mediated by epididymosomes [14]. However, the mechanisms used by the epididymosomes to transfer their contents into the sperm plasma membrane are not yet fully understood.

Box 7.1 | Summary

- Sperm concentration, i.e., reduction in the volume of sperm nuclei: loss of water, increase in the formation of disulphide bonds, alteration of the shape of the apical segment, changes in the appearance of the acrosomal contents, and changes in the density and distribution of membrane constituents (e.g. phospholipids, cholesterol) for membrane stabilization;
- Increase in total surface negative charge;
- Relocation of surface antigens;
- Addition, elimination or modification of surface proteins: epididymis secretes several proteins that through apical blebs or epididymosomes reach the sperm surface, becoming a coating protein or an integral membrane protein, respectively;
- Spermatozoa acquire the ability to move and to fuse with the oocyte (fertilizing ability).

The unique luminal environment of epididymis is among the main regulators of sperm maturation. All regions of the epididymis provide aeration, nourishment, waste removal and physical/biochemical protection for the sperm [6]. The process of sperm maturation is androgen-dependent. In fact, testosterone is found at much higher concentrations in the intraluminal fluid of the proximal epididymis than the levels found in circulation [131]. After reaching the epididymal fluid, testosterone is rapidly endocytosed by principal cells, which rapidly metabolize it to dihydrotestosterone (most active androgen) by the action of 5α-reductase [132]. Epididymis also contain the P450 aromatase that transforms androgens to estradiol [133]. Thus both the androgens and estrogens are behind the control of epididymal gene expression, which is crucial for sperm maturational process. Moreover, the characteristic atmosphere of epididymis is not only dependent on the secretion and absorption of several proteins and ions by the epithelium, but also on the selective transport of molecules across the BEB [134, 135]. This barrier creates a seal between the epididymal cells that leads to a selective transport of molecules across the epididymal epithelium [136]. The composition of the epididymal luminal fluid is associated with another mechanism for altering sperm integral membrane proteins. It has been demonstrated that some integral membrane proteins were not detectable on sperm from epididymal proximal regions, but were detectable on sperm recovered from the cauda epididymis or ejaculated sperm [6]. Since spermatozoa are transcriptionally and translationally silent, it was proposed an unmasking mechanism on mature sperm proteins related to changes in glycosylation (the attachment of sugar moieties to proteins) [6]. Moreover, the enzymes involved in glycosylation are only minimally active at the relatively basic pH of the epididymal fluid [137]. The optimal pH for many enzymes is modified by the present substrates, thus the luminal composition on each epididymal segment influences the activity of these enzymes and the level of glycosylation. A clear example is the spermatozoal fucosyltransferase activity which is higher in rat sperm harvested from the distal caput and lower in sperm harvested from more distal regions [137].

Several molecules expressed in the adult epididymis may also regulate epididymal functions, and consequently sperm maturation. Some examples include the reproductive homeobox X-linked (Rhox) genes and sonic hedgehog (Shh). Particularly, Rhox5 seems to be involved in sperm motility acquisition, since spermatozoa from mice lacking Rhox5 exhibited reduced fertility in part because of impaired motility [138]. The inhibition of Shh pathway led to a reduced ability of mouse spermatozoa from cauda epididymis to initiate motility [139]. The fox (forkhead box) transcription factors also carry out multiple roles in the epididymis. The Foxa2 is involved in the responsiveness of several gene promoters to steroid hormones [140]. Moreover, the expression of Foxl1 by epididymis is important for normal sperm function. In fact, it has been demonstrated that mice lacking this protein present a high incidence of tail angulation and a decreased ability to migrate through the female tract resulting in decreased fertility [141]. The acidification of the epididymal lumen requires the function of the vacuolar H^+-ATPase proton pump and is necessary for sperm maturation [142, 143]. Since Foxl1 is involved in the regulation of vacuolar H^+-ATPase proton pump, the decreased fertility observed in mice lacking Foxl1 may reflect impaired epididymal sperm maturation as a result of increased luminal pH [141]. Overall, the biochemical control of sperm modifications during maturation is not only dependent on hormones (like androgens), but also on luminal proteins, lipids, signaling molecules and transcription factors.

CONCLUDING REMARKS

The epididymis is the male accessory organ responsible for spermatozoa maturation after being released from the seminiferous tubules. This physiological complex duct is also a site of storage of mature spermatozoa until they are expelled at the moment of ejaculation. During spermatozoa transit through the epididymis, they encounter a constantly-changing and dynamic luminal microenvironment. The proper composition, pH and osmolality of epididymal fluid in each epididymal region is mainly controlled by the BEB, and is essential for the acquisition of sperm motility and fertilizing ability. Although the mechanisms underlying the morphological and biochemical alterations involved in sperm maturation have to be further disclosed, in recent years, there was a substantial increase in the understanding of the functions of several epididymal proteins and their interaction with the proteinaceous spermatozoa coat. These proteins are crucial not only for the progression of spermatozoa from an immotile immature state in epididymal proximal regions, to a fully functional mature state in distal regions, but also for sperm-egg fusion, evidencing the importance of this tubule to male fertilization.

CONFLICT OF INTEREST

The authors confirm that they have no conflict of interest to declare for this publication.

ACKNOWLEDGEMENT

This work was supported by the “Fundação para a Ciência e a Tecnologia”–FCT (PTDC/BBB-BQB/1368/2014), CICS (UID/Multi/00709/2013), UMIB (PEst-OE/SAU/UI0215/2014) and REQUIMTE (UID/QUI/50006/2013); and of FEDER through the POPH and POCI - COMPETE 2020 (POCI-01-0145-FE-ER-007491) funds. Tânia R. Dias (SFRH/BD/109284/2015) and Raquel L. Bernardino (SFRH/BD/103105/2014) were also funded by FCT.

REFERENCES

[1] Cornwall GA. New insights into epididymal biology and function. Hum Reprod Update 2009; 15(2): 213-27.
[http://dx.doi.org/10.1093/humupd/dmn055] [PMID: 19136456]

[2] Toshimori K. Biology of spermatozoa maturation: an overview with an introduction to this issue. Microsc Res Tech 2003; 61(1): 1-6.
[http://dx.doi.org/10.1002/jemt.10311] [PMID: 12672117]

[3] Kent M. Male Reproductive System Human anatomy. McGraw-Hill 2001; pp. 697-724.

[4] Shum WW, Ruan YC, Da Silva N, Breton S. Establishment of cell-cell cross talk in the epididymis: control of luminal acidification. J Androl 2011; 32(6): 576-86.
[http://dx.doi.org/10.2164/jandrol.111.012971] [PMID: 21441423]

[5] Mital P, Hinton BT, Dufour JM. The blood-testis and blood-epididymis barriers are more than just their tight junctions. Biol Reprod 2011; 84(5): 851-8.
[http://dx.doi.org/10.1095/biolreprod.110.087452] [PMID: 21209417]

[6] Marengo SR. Maturing the sperm: unique mechanisms for modifying integral proteins in the sperm plasma membrane. Anim Reprod Sci 2008; 105(1-2): 52-63.
[http://dx.doi.org/10.1016/j.anireprosci.2007.11.018] [PMID: 18255240]

[7] Guyonnet B, Dacheux F, Dacheux JL, Gatti JL. The epididymal transcriptome and proteome provide some insights into new epididymal regulations. J Androl 2011; 32(6): 651-64.
[http://dx.doi.org/10.2164/jandrol.111.013086] [PMID: 21764898]

[8] Dacheux JL, Gatti JL, Dacheux F. Contribution of epididymal secretory proteins for spermatozoa maturation. Microsc Res Tech 2003; 61(1): 7-17.
[http://dx.doi.org/10.1002/jemt.10312] [PMID: 12672118]

[9] Gatti JL, Castella S, Dacheux F, *et al.* Post-testicular sperm environment and fertility. Anim Reprod Sci 2004; 82-83: 321-39.
[http://dx.doi.org/10.1016/j.anireprosci.2004.05.011] [PMID: 15271463]

[10] Sullivan R, Mieusset R. The human epididymis: its function in sperm maturation. Hum Reprod Update 2016; 22(5): 574-87.
[http://dx.doi.org/10.1093/humupd/dmw015] [PMID: 27307387]

[11] Sullivan R, Frenette G, Girouard J. Epididymosomes are involved in the acquisition of new sperm proteins during epididymal transit. Asian J Androl 2007; 9(4): 483-91.
[http://dx.doi.org/10.1111/j.1745-7262.2007.00281.x] [PMID: 17589785]

[12] Foldesy RG, Bedford JM. Biology of the scrotum. I. Temperature and androgen as determinants of the sperm storage capacity of the rat cauda epididymidis. Biol Reprod 1982; 26(4): 673-82.
[http://dx.doi.org/10.1095/biolreprod26.4.673] [PMID: 7082731]

[13] Lenzi A, Gandini L, Picardo M, Tramer F, Sandri G, Panfili E. Lipoperoxidation damage of spermatozoa polyunsaturated fatty acids (PUFA): scavenger mechanisms and possible scavenger therapies. Front Biosci 2000; 5: E1-E15.
[PMID: 10702376]

[14] Jones R. Sperm survival *versus* degradation in the Mammalian epididymis: a hypothesis. Biol Reprod 2004; 71(5): 1405-11.
[http://dx.doi.org/10.1095/biolreprod.104.031252] [PMID: 15215193]

[15] Robaire B, Hinton BT, Orgebin-Crist M-C. The epididymis. Phys Rep 2006; 1071-48.
[http://dx.doi.org/10.1016/B978-012515400-0/50027-0]

[16] Hinton BT, Lan ZJ, Lye RJ, Labus JC. Regulation of epididymal function by testicular factors: the lumicrine hypothesis The testis. Springer 2000; pp. 163-73.

[17] Rodriguez CM, Kirby JL, Hinton BT. The development of the epididymis The Epididymis: From Molecules to Clinical Practice. New york: Kluwer Academic/Plenum Publishers 2002; pp. 251-67.
[http://dx.doi.org/10.1007/978-1-4615-0679-9_14]

[18] Takano H, Abe K, Ito T. [Changes in the mouse epididymis after ligation of the ductuli efferentes or proximal epididymal duct: qualitative and quantitative histological studies (authors transl)]. Kaibogaku Zasshi 1981; 56(2): 79-90. [Changes in the mouse epididymis after ligation of the ductuli efferentes or proximal epididymal duct: qualitative and quantitative histological studies (author's transl)].
[PMID: 7293728]

[19] Turner TT, Gleavy JL, Harris JM. Fluid movement in the lumen of the rat epididymis: effect of vasectomy and subsequent vasovasostomy. J Androl 1990; 11(5): 422-8.
[PMID: 2254175]

[20] Maneely R. Epididymal structure and function: a historical and critical review. Acta Zoologica 1959; 40: 1-21.
[http://dx.doi.org/10.1111/j.1463-6395.1959.tb00389.x]

[21] Turner TT. De Graafs thread: the human epididymis. J Androl 2008; 29(3): 237-50.
[http://dx.doi.org/10.2164/jandrol.107.004119] [PMID: 18222912]

[22] Turner TT, Johnston DS, Finger JN, Jelinsky SA. Differential gene expression among the proximal segments of the rat epididymis is lost after efferent duct ligation. Biol Reprod 2007; 77(1): 165-71.
[http://dx.doi.org/10.1095/biolreprod.106.059493] [PMID: 17377138]

[23] Lasserre A, Barrozo R, Tezón JG, Miranda PV, Vazquez-Levin MH. Human epididymal proteins and sperm function during fertilization: un update. Biol Res 2001; 34(3-4): 165-78. [http://dx.doi.org/10.4067/S0716-97602001000300004] [PMID: 11715855]

[24] Jaakkola UM, Talo A. Effects of oxytocin and vasopressin on electrical and mechanical activity of the rat epididymis *in vitro*. J Reprod Fertil 1981; 63(1): 47-51. [http://dx.doi.org/10.1530/jrf.0.0630047] [PMID: 7277332]

[25] Jaakkola UM, Talo A. Relation of electrical activity to luminal transport in the cauda epididymidis of the rat *in vitro*. J Reprod Fertil 1982; 64(1): 121-6. [http://dx.doi.org/10.1530/jrf.0.0640121] [PMID: 7054487]

[26] Jaakkola UM, Talo A. Movements of the luminal contents in two different regions of the caput epididymidis of the rat *in vitro*. J Physiol 1983; 336: 453-63. [http://dx.doi.org/10.1113/jphysiol.1983.sp014590] [PMID: 6875914]

[27] Hermo L, Robaire B. Epididymal cell types and their functions. Springer 2002. [http://dx.doi.org/10.1007/978-1-4615-0679-9_5]

[28] França LR, Avelar GF, Almeida FF. Spermatogenesis and sperm transit through the epididymis in mammals with emphasis on pigs. Theriogenology 2005; 63(2): 300-18. [http://dx.doi.org/10.1016/j.theriogenology.2004.09.014] [PMID: 15626401]

[29] Robaire B, Syntin P, Jervis K. The coming of age of the epididymis Testis, Epididymis and Technologies in the year 2000. Springer 2000; pp. 229-62. [http://dx.doi.org/10.1007/978-3-662-04050-8_14]

[30] Robaire B, Hermo L. Efferent ducts, epididymis and vas deferens: structure, functions and their regulation The physiology of reproduction. New York: Raven press 1988; pp. 999-1080.

[31] Hoffer AP, Hamilton DW, Fawcett DW. The ultrastructure of the principal cells and intraepithelial leucocytes in the initial segment of the rat epididymis. Anat Rec 1973; 175(2): 169-201. [http://dx.doi.org/10.1002/ar.1091750205] [PMID: 4685557]

[32] Abou-Haïla A, Fain-Maurel MA. Regional differences of the proximal part of mouse epididymis: morphological and histochemical characterization. Anat Rec 1984; 209(2): 197-208. [http://dx.doi.org/10.1002/ar.1092090207] [PMID: 6465530]

[33] Abe K, Takano H, Ito T. Response of epididymal duct to the temporary depletion of spermatozoa induced by testicular irradiation in mice. Anat Rec 1983; 207(1): 17-24. [http://dx.doi.org/10.1002/ar.1092070103] [PMID: 6638530]

[34] Hermo L, Oko R, Morales CR. Secretion and endocytosis in the male reproductive tract: a role in sperm maturation. Int Rev Cytol 1994; 154: 106-89. [http://dx.doi.org/10.1016/S0074-7696(08)62199-3] [PMID: 8083031]

[35] Hermo L, Smith CE. The structure of the Golgi apparatus: a sperms eye view in principal epithelial cells of the rat epididymis. Histochem Cell Biol 1998; 109(5-6): 431-47. [http://dx.doi.org/10.1007/s004180050246] [PMID: 9681626]

[36] Hermo L, Green H, Clermont Y. Golgi apparatus of epithelial principal cells of the epididymal initial segment of the rat: structure, relationship with endoplasmic reticulum, and role in the formation of secretory vesicles. Anat Rec 1991; 229(2): 159-76. [http://dx.doi.org/10.1002/ar.1092290203] [PMID: 1849381]

[37] Flickinger CJ, Howards SS, English HF. Ultrastructural differences in efferent ducts and several regions of the epididymis of the hamster. Am J Anat 1978; 152(4): 557-85. [http://dx.doi.org/10.1002/aja.1001520409] [PMID: 678334]

[38] Hermo L. Structural features and functions of principal cells of the intermediate zone of the epididymis of adult rats. Anat Rec 1995; 242(4): 515-30. [http://dx.doi.org/10.1002/ar.1092420408] [PMID: 7486022]

[39] Friend DS, Farquhar MG. Functions of coated vesicles during protein absorption in the rat vas deferens. J Cell Biol 1967; 35(2): 357-76.
[http://dx.doi.org/10.1083/jcb.35.2.357] [PMID: 6055991]

[40] Hermo L, Adamali HI, Mahuran D, Gravel RA, Trasler JM. β-Hexosaminidase immunolocalization and α- and β-subunit gene expression in the rat testis and epididymis. Mol Reprod Dev 1997; 46(3): 227-42.
[http://dx.doi.org/10.1002/(SICI)1098-2795(199703)46:3<227::AID-MRD1>3.0.CO;2-R] [PMID: 9041125]

[41] Sun EL, Flickinger CJ. Morphological characteristics of cells with apical nuclei in the initial segment of the adult rat epididymis. Anat Rec 1980; 196(3): 285-93.
[http://dx.doi.org/10.1002/ar.1091960304] [PMID: 7406221]

[42] Adamali HI, Hermo L. Apical and narrow cells are distinct cell types differing in their structure, distribution, and functions in the adult rat epididymis. J Androl 1996; 17(3): 208-22.
[PMID: 8792211]

[43] Hermo L, Adamali HI, Andonian S. Immunolocalization of CA II and H+ V-ATPase in epithelial cells of the mouse and rat epididymis. J Androl 2000; 21(3): 376-91.
[PMID: 10819445]

[44] Hermo L, Chong DL, Moffatt P, Sly WS, Waheed A, Smith CE. Region- and cell-specific differences in the distribution of carbonic anhydrases II, III, XII, and XIV in the adult rat epididymis. J Histochem Cytochem 2005; 53(6): 699-713.
[http://dx.doi.org/10.1369/jhc.4A6575.2005] [PMID: 15928319]

[45] Hermo L, Dworkin J, Oko R. Role of epithelial clear cells of the rat epididymis in the disposal of the contents of cytoplasmic droplets detached from spermatozoa. Am J Anat 1988; 183(2): 107-24.
[http://dx.doi.org/10.1002/aja.1001830202] [PMID: 2849296]

[46] Sun EL, Flickinger CJ. Development of cell types and of regional differences in the postnatal rat epididymis. Am J Anat 1979; 154(1): 27-55.
[http://dx.doi.org/10.1002/aja.1001540104] [PMID: 760488]

[47] Oko R, Hermo L, Chan PT, Fazel A, Bergeron JJ. The cytoplasmic droplet of rat epididymal spermatozoa contains saccular elements with Golgi characteristics. J Cell Biol 1993; 123(4): 809-21.
[http://dx.doi.org/10.1083/jcb.123.4.809] [PMID: 8227142]

[48] Veri JP, Hermo L, Robaire B. Immunocytochemical localization of the Yf subunit of glutathione S-transferase P shows regional variation in the staining of epithelial cells of the testis, efferent ducts, and epididymis of the male rat. J Androl 1993; 14(1): 23-44.
[PMID: 8473235]

[49] Marengo SR, Amann RP. Morphological features of principal cells in the ovine epididymis: a quantitative and qualitative study. Biol Reprod 1990; 42(1): 167-79.
[http://dx.doi.org/10.1095/biolreprod42.1.167] [PMID: 2310815]

[50] Seiler P, Cooper TG, Yeung CH, Nieschlag E. Regional variation in macrophage antigen expression by murine epididymal basal cells and their regulation by testicular factors. J Androl 1999; 20(6): 738-46.
[PMID: 10591613]

[51] Hermo L, Papp S. Effects of ligation, orchidectomy, and hypophysectomy on expression of the Yf subunit of GST-P in principal and basal cells of the adult rat epididymis and on basal cell shape and overall arrangement. Anat Rec 1996; 244(1): 59-69.
[http://dx.doi.org/10.1002/(SICI)1097-0185(199601)244:1<59::AID-AR6>3.0.CO;2-A] [PMID: 8838424]

[52] Cheung KH, Leung GP, Leung MC, Shum WW, Zhou WL, Wong PY. Cell-cell interaction underlies formation of fluid in the male reproductive tract of the rat. J Gen Physiol 2005; 125(5): 443-54. [http://dx.doi.org/10.1085/jgp.200409205] [PMID: 15851503]

[53] Hamilton DW. The mammalian epididymis. Reprod Biol 1972; 268-337.

[54] Bedford JM. The status and the state of the human epididymis. Hum Reprod 1994; 9(11): 2187-99. [http://dx.doi.org/10.1093/oxfordjournals.humrep.a138416] [PMID: 7868697]

[55] Talo A, Jaakkola U-M, Markkula-Viitanen M. Spontaneous electrical activity of the rat epididymis *in vitro*. J Reprod Fertil 1979; 57(2): 423-9. [http://dx.doi.org/10.1530/jrf.0.0570423] [PMID: 513032]

[56] Jaakkola U-M. Regional variations in transport of the luminal contents of the rat epididymis *in vivo*. J Reprod Fertil 1983; 68(2): 465-70. [http://dx.doi.org/10.1530/jrf.0.0680465] [PMID: 6864663]

[57] Turner TT. Spermatozoa are exposed to a complex microenvironment as they traverse the epididymis. Ann N Y Acad Sci 1991; 637: 364-83. [http://dx.doi.org/10.1111/j.1749-6632.1991.tb27323.x] [PMID: 1785781]

[58] Whittington K, Assinder SJ, Parkinson T, Lapwood KR, Nicholson HD. Function and localization of oxytocin receptors in the reproductive tissue of rams. Reproduction 2001; 122(2): 317-25. [http://dx.doi.org/10.1530/rep.0.1220317] [PMID: 11467983]

[59] Einspanier A, Ivell R. Oxytocin and oxytocin receptor expression in reproductive tissues of the male marmoset monkey. Biol Reprod 1997; 56(2): 416-22. [http://dx.doi.org/10.1095/biolreprod56.2.416] [PMID: 9116141]

[60] Filippi S, Vannelli GB, Granchi S, *et al.* Identification, localization and functional activity of oxytocin receptors in epididymis. Mol Cell Endocrinol 2002; 193(1-2): 89-100. [http://dx.doi.org/10.1016/S0303-7207(02)00101-6] [PMID: 12161007]

[61] Filippi S, Morelli A, Vignozzi L, *et al.* Oxytocin mediates the estrogen-dependent contractile activity of endothelin-1 in human and rabbit epididymis. Endocrinology 2005; 146(8): 3506-17. [http://dx.doi.org/10.1210/en.2004-1628] [PMID: 15860558]

[62] Filippi S, Luconi M, Granchi S, *et al.* Estrogens, but not androgens, regulate expression and functional activity of oxytocin receptor in rabbit epididymis. Endocrinology 2002; 143(11): 4271-80. [http://dx.doi.org/10.1210/en.2002-220384] [PMID: 12399422]

[63] Hib J, Oscar P. Effects of prostaglandins and indomethacin on rat epididymal responses to norepinephrine and acetylcholine. Arch Androl 1978; 1(1): 43-7. [http://dx.doi.org/10.3109/01485017808988316] [PMID: 742941]

[64] Kirchhoff C, Osterhoff C, Pera I, Schröter S. Function of human epididymal proteins in sperm maturation. Andrologia 1998; 30(4-5): 225-32. [http://dx.doi.org/10.1111/j.1439-0272.1998.tb01164.x] [PMID: 9739419]

[65] Cooper TG. The epididymis, cytoplasmic droplets and male fertility. Asian J Androl 2011; 13(1): 130-8. [http://dx.doi.org/10.1038/aja.2010.97] [PMID: 21076437]

[66] Olson GE, Winfrey VP, Nagdas SK. Structural modification of the hamster sperm acrosome during posttesticular development in the epididymis. Microsc Res Tech 2003; 61(1): 46-55. [http://dx.doi.org/10.1002/jemt.10316] [PMID: 12672122]

[67] López ML, Olea N, Retamal CA. Post-testicular changes in the density and distribution of intramembrane particles of stallion sperm surface domains. Anim Reprod Sci 2007; 100(1-2): 204-10. [http://dx.doi.org/10.1016/j.anireprosci.2006.08.027] [PMID: 17014974]

[68] Jones R. Plasma membrane structure and remodelling during sperm maturation in the epididymis. J Reprod Fertil Suppl 1998; 53: 73-84.
[PMID: 10645268]

[69] Yanagimachi R, Kamiguchi Y, Mikamo K, Suzuki F, Yanagimachi H. Maturation of spermatozoa in the epididymis of the Chinese hamster. Am J Anat 1985; 172(4): 317-30.
[http://dx.doi.org/10.1002/aja.1001720406] [PMID: 3887886]

[70] Orgebin-Crist M, Danzo B, Davies J. Endocrine control of the development and maintenance of sperm fertilizing ability in the epididymis 1975.

[71] Jones RC. To store or mature spermatozoa? The primary role of the epididymis. Int J Androl 1999; 22(2): 57-67.
[http://dx.doi.org/10.1046/j.1365-2605.1999.00151.x] [PMID: 10194636]

[72] Olson GE, Winfrey VP, NagDas SK, Melner MH. Region-specific expression and secretion of the fibrinogen-related protein, fgl2, by epithelial cells of the hamster epididymis and its role in disposal of defective spermatozoa. J Biol Chem 2004; 279(49): 51266-74.
[http://dx.doi.org/10.1074/jbc.M410485200] [PMID: 15377663]

[73] Sutovsky P, Moreno R, Ramalho-Santos J, Dominko T, Thompson WE, Schatten G. A putative, ubiquitin-dependent mechanism for the recognition and elimination of defective spermatozoa in the mammalian epididymis. J Cell Sci 2001; 114(Pt 9): 1665-75.
[PMID: 11309198]

[74] Shum WW, Da Silva N, Brown D, Breton S. Regulation of luminal acidification in the male reproductive tract *via* cell-cell crosstalk. J Exp Biol 2009; 212(Pt 11): 1753-61.
[http://dx.doi.org/10.1242/jeb.027284] [PMID: 19448084]

[75] Carr DW, Usselman MC, Acott TS. Effects of pH, lactate, and viscoelastic drag on sperm motility: a species comparison. Biol Reprod 1985; 33(3): 588-95.
[http://dx.doi.org/10.1095/biolreprod33.3.588] [PMID: 4052526]

[76] Rato L, Socorro S, Cavaco JE, Oliveira PF. Tubular fluid secretion in the seminiferous epithelium: ion transporters and aquaporins in Sertoli cells. J Membr Biol 2010; 236(2): 215-24.
[http://dx.doi.org/10.1007/s00232-010-9294-x] [PMID: 20697886]

[77] Aitken RJ, Jones KT, Robertson SA. Reactive oxygen species and sperm functionin sickness and in health. J Androl 2012; 33(6): 1096-106.
[http://dx.doi.org/10.2164/jandrol.112.016535] [PMID: 22879525]

[78] Agarwal A, Nallella KP, Allamaneni SS, Said TM. Role of antioxidants in treatment of male infertility: an overview of the literature. Reprod Biomed Online 2004; 8(6): 616-27.
[http://dx.doi.org/10.1016/S1472-6483(10)61641-0] [PMID: 15169573]

[79] Agarwal A, Makker K, Sharma R. Clinical relevance of oxidative stress in male factor infertility: an update. Am J Reprod Immunol 2008; 59(1): 2-11.
[http://dx.doi.org/10.1111/j.1600-0897.2007.00559.x] [PMID: 18154591]

[80] Aitken RJ, Koppers AJ. Apoptosis and DNA damage in human spermatozoa. Asian J Androl 2011; 13(1): 36-42.
[http://dx.doi.org/10.1038/aja.2010.68] [PMID: 20802502]

[81] Moustafa MH, Sharma RK, Thornton J, *et al.* Relationship between ROS production, apoptosis and DNA denaturation in spermatozoa from patients examined for infertility. Hum Reprod 2004; 19(1): 129-38.
[http://dx.doi.org/10.1093/humrep/deh024] [PMID: 14688171]

[82] Vernet P, Fulton N, Wallace C, Aitken RJ. Analysis of reactive oxygen species generating systems in rat epididymal spermatozoa. Biol Reprod 2001; 65(4): 1102-13.
[http://dx.doi.org/10.1095/biolreprod65.4.1102] [PMID: 11566731]

[83] Cyr DG, Finnson K, Dufresne J, Gregory M. Cellular interactions and the blood-epididymal barrier The epididymis: from molecules to clinical practice. Springer 2002; pp. 103-18. [http://dx.doi.org/10.1007/978-1-4615-0679-9_6]

[84] Itoh M, Terayama H, Naito M, Ogawa Y, Tainosho S. Tissue microcircumstances for leukocytic infiltration into the testis and epididymis in mice. J Reprod Immunol 2005; 67(1-2): 57-67. [http://dx.doi.org/10.1016/j.jri.2005.06.007] [PMID: 16111766]

[85] Hall SH, Hamil KG, French FS. Host defense proteins of the male reproductive tract. J Androl 2002; 23(5): 585-97. [PMID: 12185087]

[86] Zhao Y, Diao H, Ni Z, Hu S, Yu H, Zhang Y. The epididymis-specific antimicrobial peptide β-defensin 15 is required for sperm motility and male fertility in the rat (Rattus norvegicus). Cell Mol Life Sci 2011; 68(4): 697-708. [http://dx.doi.org/10.1007/s00018-010-0478-4] [PMID: 20694738]

[87] Hall SH, Yenugu S, Radhakrishnan Y, Avellar MC, Petrusz P, French FS. Characterization and functions of beta defensins in the epididymis. Asian J Androl 2007; 9(4): 453-62. [http://dx.doi.org/10.1111/j.1745-7262.2007.00298.x] [PMID: 17589782]

[88] Diao H, Yu HG, Sun F, Zhang YL, Tanphaichitr N. Rat recombinant β-defensin 22 is a heparin-binding protein with antimicrobial activity. Asian J Androl 2011; 13(2): 305-11. [http://dx.doi.org/10.1038/aja.2010.93] [PMID: 21151152]

[89] Cornwall GA, Von Horsten HH, Whelly S. Cystatin-related epididymal spermatogenic aggregates in the epididymis. J Androl 2011; 32(6): 679-85. [http://dx.doi.org/10.2164/jandrol.111.012963] [PMID: 21764901]

[90] Dacheux JL, Dacheux F. Protein secretion in the epididymis The Epididymis: From Molecules to Clinical Practice. New York: Kluwer Academic/Plenum Publishers 2002; pp. 151-68. [http://dx.doi.org/10.1007/978-1-4615-0679-9_9]

[91] Hermo L, Jacks D. Natures ingenuity: bypassing the classical secretory route *via* apocrine secretion. Mol Reprod Dev 2002; 63(3): 394-410. [http://dx.doi.org/10.1002/mrd.90023] [PMID: 12237956]

[92] Sullivan R, Saez F, Girouard J, Frenette G. Role of exosomes in sperm maturation during the transit along the male reproductive tract. Blood Cells Mol Dis 2005; 35(1): 1-10. [http://dx.doi.org/10.1016/j.bcmd.2005.03.005] [PMID: 15893944]

[93] Kawano N, Yoshida K, Miyado K, Yoshida M. Lipid rafts: keys to sperm maturation, fertilization, and early embryogenesis. J lipids 2011; 2011

[94] Légaré C, Gaudreault C, St-Jacques S, Sullivan R. P34H sperm protein is preferentially expressed by the human corpus epididymidis. Endocrinology 1999; 140(7): 3318-27. [PMID: 10385429]

[95] Miranda PV, González-Echeverría F, Blaquier JA, Mahuran DJ, Tezón JG. Evidence for the participation of β-hexosaminidase in human sperm-zona pellucida interaction *in vitro*. Mol Hum Reprod 2000; 6(8): 699-706. [http://dx.doi.org/10.1093/molehr/6.8.699] [PMID: 10908279]

[96] Batova IN, Ivanova MD, Mollova MV, Kyurkchiev SD. Human sperm surface glycoprotein involved in sperm-zona pellucida interaction. Int J Androl 1998; 21(3): 141-53. [http://dx.doi.org/10.1111/j.1365-2605.1998.00104.x] [PMID: 9669198]

[97] Komori S, Kameda K, Sakata K, *et al.* Characterization of fertilization-blocking monoclonal antibody 1G12 with human sperm-immobilizing activity. Clin Exp Immunol 1997; 109(3): 547-54. [http://dx.doi.org/10.1046/j.1365-2249.1997.4801380.x] [PMID: 9328135]

[98] Martin Ruiz C, Duquenne C, Treton D, Lefèvre A, Finaz C. SOB3, a human sperm protein involved in zona pellucida binding: physiological and biochemical analysis, purification. Mol Reprod Dev 1998; 49(3): 286-97.
[http://dx.doi.org/10.1002/(SICI)1098-2795(199803)49:3<286::AID-MRD9>3.0.CO;2-K] [PMID: 9491381]

[99] Boué F, Blais J, Sullivan R. Surface localization of P34H an epididymal protein, during maturation, capacitation, and acrosome reaction of human spermatozoa. Biol Reprod 1996; 54(5): 1009-17.
[http://dx.doi.org/10.1095/biolreprod54.5.1009] [PMID: 8722620]

[100] Brandelli A, Miranda PV, Tezon JG. Participation of glycosylated residues in the human sperm acrosome reaction: possible role of N-acetylglucosaminidase. Biochimica et Biophysica Acta (BBA)-. Molecular Cell Research 1994; 1220: 299-304.

[101] Cohen DJ, Ellerman DA, Busso D, *et al.* Evidence that human epididymal protein ARP plays a role in gamete fusion through complementary sites on the surface of the human egg. Biol Reprod 2001; 65(4): 1000-5.
[http://dx.doi.org/10.1095/biolreprod65.4.1000] [PMID: 11566719]

[102] Lefèvre A, Martin Ruiz C, Chokomian S, Duquenne C, Finaz C. Characterization and isolation of SOB2, a human sperm protein with a potential role in oocyte membrane binding. Mol Hum Reprod 1997; 3(6): 507-16.
[http://dx.doi.org/10.1093/molehr/3.6.507] [PMID: 9239740]

[103] Focarelli R, Giuffrida A, Capparelli S, *et al.* Specific localization in the equatorial region of gp20, a 20 kDa sialylglycoprotein of the capacitated human spermatozoon acquired during epididymal transit which is necessary to penetrate zona-free hamster eggs. Mol Hum Reprod 1998; 4(2): 119-25.
[http://dx.doi.org/10.1093/molehr/4.2.119] [PMID: 9542968]

[104] Andersson AM, Edvardsen K, Skakkebaek NE. Expression and localization of N- and E-cadherin in the human testis and epididymis. Int J Androl 1994; 17(4): 174-80.
[http://dx.doi.org/10.1111/j.1365-2605.1994.tb01239.x] [PMID: 7995652]

[105] Takeichi M. Cadherins: a molecular family important in selective cell-cell adhesion. Annu Rev Biochem 1990; 59: 237-52.
[http://dx.doi.org/10.1146/annurev.bi.59.070190.001321] [PMID: 2197976]

[106] Takeichi M. Morphogenetic roles of classic cadherins. Curr Opin Cell Biol 1995; 7(5): 619-27.
[http://dx.doi.org/10.1016/0955-0674(95)80102-2] [PMID: 8573335]

[107] Rufas O, Fisch B, Ziv S, Shalgi R. Expression of cadherin adhesion molecules on human gametes. Mol Hum Reprod 2000; 6(2): 163-9.
[http://dx.doi.org/10.1093/molehr/6.2.163] [PMID: 10655458]

[108] Bronson RA, Fusi F. Sperm-oolemmal interaction: role of the Arg-Gly-Asp (RGD) adhesion peptide. Fertil Steril 1990; 54(3): 527-9.
[http://dx.doi.org/10.1016/S0015-0282(16)53775-3] [PMID: 2397797]

[109] Fusi FM, Vignali M, Busacca M, Bronson RA. Evidence for the presence of an integrin cell adhesion receptor on the oolemma of unfertilized human oocytes. Mol Reprod Dev 1992; 31(3): 215-22.
[http://dx.doi.org/10.1002/mrd.1080310309] [PMID: 1554507]

[110] Schaller J, Glander HJ, Dethloff J. Evidence of β 1 integrins and fibronectin on spermatogenic cells in human testis. Hum Reprod 1993; 8(11): 1873-8.
[http://dx.doi.org/10.1093/oxfordjournals.humrep.a137952] [PMID: 7507130]

[111] Miranda PV, Tezon JG. Characterization of fibronectin as a marker for human epididymal sperm maturation. Mol Reprod Dev 1992; 33(4): 443-50.
[http://dx.doi.org/10.1002/mrd.1080330411] [PMID: 1472375]

[112] Kirchhoff C, Osterhoff C, Young L. Molecular cloning and characterization of HE1, a major secretory protein of the human epididymis. Biol Reprod 1996; 54(4): 847-56.
[http://dx.doi.org/10.1095/biolreprod54.4.847] [PMID: 8924505]

[113] Kirchhoff C, Pera I, Derr P, Yeung C-H, Cooper T. The molecular biology of the sperm surface The fate of the male germ cell. Springer 1997; pp. 221-32.

[114] Osterhoff C, Kirchhoff C, Krull N, Ivell R. Molecular cloning and characterization of a novel human sperm antigen (HE2) specifically expressed in the proximal epididymis. Biol Reprod 1994; 50(3): 516-25.
[http://dx.doi.org/10.1095/biolreprod50.3.516] [PMID: 8167223]

[115] Kirchhoff C, Krull N, Pera I, Ivell R. A major mRNA of the human epididymal principal cells, HE5, encodes the leucocyte differentiation CDw52 antigen peptide backbone. Mol Reprod Dev 1993; 34(1): 8-15.
[http://dx.doi.org/10.1002/mrd.1080340103] [PMID: 8418821]

[116] Osterhoff C, Ivell R, Kirchhoff C. Cloning of a human epididymis-specific mRNA, HE6, encoding a novel member of the seven transmembrane-domain receptor superfamily. DNA Cell Biol 1997; 16(4): 379-89.
[http://dx.doi.org/10.1089/dna.1997.16.379] [PMID: 9150425]

[117] OBryan MK, Murphy BF, Liu DY, Clarke GN, Baker HW. The use of anticlusterin monoclonal antibodies for the combined assessment of human sperm morphology and acrosome integrity. Hum Reprod 1994; 9(8): 1490-6.
[http://dx.doi.org/10.1093/oxfordjournals.humrep.a138736] [PMID: 7989511]

[118] Sun GH, Lin YC, Guo YW, Chang SY, Liu HW. Purification of GP-83, a glycoprotein secreted by the human epididymis and conjugated to mature spermatozoa. Mol Hum Reprod 2000; 6(5): 429-34.
[http://dx.doi.org/10.1093/molehr/6.5.429] [PMID: 10775646]

[119] Retamal C, Urzúa J, Lorca C, López ML, Alves EW. Changes in the plasma membrane proteins of stallion spermatozoa during maturation in the epididymis. J Submicrosc Cytol Pathol 2000; 32(2): 229-39.
[PMID: 11085212]

[120] Dias GM, Retamal CA, Tobella L, Arnholdt AC, López ML. Nuclear status of immature and mature stallion spermatozoa. Theriogenology 2006; 66(2): 354-65.
[http://dx.doi.org/10.1016/j.theriogenology.2005.10.024] [PMID: 16423383]

[121] Moore HD, Hartman TD, Pryor JP. Development of the oocyte-penetrating capacity of spermatozoa in the human epididymis. Int J Androl 1983; 6(4): 310-8.
[http://dx.doi.org/10.1111/j.1365-2605.1983.tb00545.x] [PMID: 6618687]

[122] Yanagimachi R. Mammalian fertilization The Physiology of Reproduction. New York: Raven Press 1994; pp. 189-317.

[123] Sostaric E, Aalberts M, Gadella BM, Stout TA. The roles of the epididymis and prostasomes in the attainment of fertilizing capacity by stallion sperm. Anim Reprod Sci 2008; 107(3-4): 237-48.
[http://dx.doi.org/10.1016/j.anireprosci.2008.04.011] [PMID: 18550301]

[124] Li J, Liu F, Wang H, *et al.* Systematic mapping and functional analysis of a family of human epididymal secretory sperm-located proteins. Mol Cell Proteomics 2010; 9(11): 2517-28.
[http://dx.doi.org/10.1074/mcp.M110.001719] [PMID: 20736409]

[125] Li J, Liu F, Liu X, *et al.* Mapping of the human testicular proteome and its relationship with that of the epididymis and spermatozoa. Mol Cell Proteomics 2011; 10 M110. 004630
[http://dx.doi.org/10.1074/mcp.M110.004630]

[126] Dominguez K, Arca CD, Ward SW. The relationship between chromatin structure and DNA damage in mammalian spermatozoa Sperm Chromatin. Springer 2011; pp. 61-8.

[127] Clauss A, Lilja H, Lundwall A. A locus on human chromosome 20 contains several genes expressing protease inhibitor domains with homology to whey acidic protein. Biochem J 2002; 368(Pt 1): 233-42. [http://dx.doi.org/10.1042/bj20020869] [PMID: 12206714]

[128] Cohen DJ, Maldera JA, Vasen G, *et al.* Epididymal protein CRISP1 plays different roles during the fertilization process. J Androl 2011; 32(6): 672-8. [http://dx.doi.org/10.2164/jandrol.110.012922] [PMID: 21441424]

[129] Lefebvre J, Boileau G, Manjunath P. Recombinant expression and affinity purification of a novel epididymal human sperm-binding protein, BSPH1. Mol Hum Reprod 2009; 15(2): 105-14. [http://dx.doi.org/10.1093/molehr/gan077] [PMID: 19091820]

[130] Joseph A, Shur BD, Hess RA. Estrogen, efferent ductules, and the epididymis. Biol Reprod 2011; 84(2): 207-17. [http://dx.doi.org/10.1095/biolreprod.110.087353] [PMID: 20926801]

[131] Viger RS, Robaire B. The mRNAs for the Steroid 5a-Reductase Isozymes, Types 1 and 2, Are Differentially. J Androl 1996; 17: 27-34. [PMID: 8833738]

[132] Robaire B, Hamzeh M. Androgen action in the epididymis. J Androl 2011; 32(6): 592-9. [http://dx.doi.org/10.2164/jandrol.111.014266] [PMID: 21764895]

[133] Shayu D, Rao AJ. Expression of functional aromatase in the epididymis: role of androgens and LH in modulation of expression and activity. Mol Cell Endocrinol 2006; 249(1-2): 40-50. [http://dx.doi.org/10.1016/j.mce.2006.01.016] [PMID: 16569475]

[134] Hinton BT, Palladino MA. Epididymal epithelium: its contribution to the formation of a luminal fluid microenvironment. Microsc Res Tech 1995; 30(1): 67-81. [http://dx.doi.org/10.1002/jemt.1070300106] [PMID: 7711321]

[135] Dacheux JL, Belghazi M, Lanson Y, Dacheux F. Human epididymal secretome and proteome. Mol Cell Endocrinol 2006; 250(1-2): 36-42. [http://dx.doi.org/10.1016/j.mce.2005.12.022] [PMID: 16431015]

[136] Dube E, Hermo L, Chan PT, Cyr DG. Alterations in the human blood-epididymis barrier in obstructive azoospermia and the development of novel epididymal cell lines from infertile men. Biol Reprod 2010; 83(4): 584-96. [http://dx.doi.org/10.1095/biolreprod.110.084459] [PMID: 20505168]

[137] Tulsiani DR. Glycan modifying enzymes in luminal fluid of rat epididymis: are they involved in altering sperm surface glycoproteins during maturation? Microsc Res Tech 2003; 61(1): 18-27. [http://dx.doi.org/10.1002/jemt.10313] [PMID: 12672119]

[138] Maclean JA II, Chen MA, Wayne CM, *et al.* Rhox: a new homeobox gene cluster. Cell 2005; 120(3): 369-82. [http://dx.doi.org/10.1016/j.cell.2004.12.022] [PMID: 15707895]

[139] Turner TT, Bang HJ, Attipoe SA, Johnston DS, Tomsig JL. Sonic hedgehog pathway inhibition alters epididymal function as assessed by the development of sperm motility. J Androl 2006; 27(2): 225-32. [http://dx.doi.org/10.2164/jandrol.05114] [PMID: 16278368]

[140] Yu X, Suzuki K, Wang Y, *et al.* The role of forkhead box A2 to restrict androgen-regulated gene expression of lipocalin 5 in the mouse epididymis. Mol Endocrinol 2006; 20(10): 2418-31. [http://dx.doi.org/10.1210/me.2006-0008] [PMID: 16740652]

[141] Blomqvist SR, Vidarsson H, Söder O, Enerbäck S. Epididymal expression of the forkhead transcription factor Foxi1 is required for male fertility. EMBO J 2006; 25(17): 4131-41. [http://dx.doi.org/10.1038/sj.emboj.7601272] [PMID: 16932748]

[142] Pastor-Soler N, Piétrement C, Breton S. Role of acid/base transporters in the male reproductive tract and potential consequences of their malfunction. Physiology (Bethesda) 2005; 20: 417-28. [http://dx.doi.org/10.1152/physiol.00036.2005] [PMID: 16287991]

[143] Yeung CH, Breton S, Setiawan I, Xu Y, Lang F, Cooper TG. Increased luminal pH in the epididymis of infertile c-ros knockout mice and the expression of sodium-hydrogen exchangers and vacuolar proton pump H+-ATPase. Mol Reprod Dev 2004; 68(2): 159-68. [http://dx.doi.org/10.1002/mrd.20067] [PMID: 15095336]

CHAPTER 8

Formation and Biochemistry of Seminal Plasma and Male Accessory Fluids

Raquel L. Bernardino*

Department of Microscopy, Laboratory of Cell Biology, Institute of Biomedical Sciences Abel Salazar and Unit for Multidisciplinary Research in Biomedicine, University of Porto, Rua de Jorge Viterbo Ferreira, 4050-313, Porto, Portugal

Abstract: An appropriate microenvironment in each segment of the male reproductive tract is crucial for the successful maturation and motility of sperm and thereby for male fertility. Spermatozoa are produced in the testes and transported to the epididymis along with the seminiferous tubular fluid. The epididymis contains an epididymal milieu that maintains the optimal conditions necessary for sperm maturation and storage. The composition of the luminal fluid is gradually changed along the epididymal duct due to absorption and secretion processes. The main changes in epididymal fluid and other fluids produced by accessory glands will be reflected in the ionic content, osmolality, pH and spermatocrit. Sperm motility is a good predictor of human male fertility that is controlled by some parameters such as bicarbonate and calcium concentrations, which constantly fluctuate throughout the reproductive ducts. The spermatozoa leaving the epididymis along with the epididymal fluid will join the secretions from the prostate and seminal vesicles, thus forming the seminal plasma. More attention should be paid to male reproductive tract fluids, namely its ionic composition and pH in order to unravel the causes of idiopathic infertility, which represents an elevated percentage of infertile men.

Keywords: Bicarbonate, Calcium, Epididymal fluid, Epididymis, Ions, Ionic transporters, pH, Seminal plasma, Seminal vesicles, Seminiferous tubular fluid, Sperm capacitation and motility, Spermatozoa, Prostate.

INTRODUCTION

The male reproductive system is very complex and highly sophisticated. Spermatozoa are generated in the testes and undergo a maturational process while traveling through the long epididymal tubule, until they reach the cauda epididymis. The sperms are continually exposed to a specialized luminal fluid microenvironment. The composition of the fluid that bathes spermatozoa is

* **Corresponding author Raquel L. Bernardino:** Rua de Jorge Viterbo Ferreira, 4050-313, Porto, Portugal; Tel: +351 938626516; Fax: +351 220 428 000; E-mail: raquellbernardino@gmail.com

Marco G. Alves and Pedro F. Oliveira (Eds.)

unique in all ducts of the male reproductive tract and is rather different from blood plasma and interstitial fluid [1]. The composition of the testicular fluid and epididymal fluid is variable, and major changes from one region to the next may be detected. The processes underlying the formation of seminal fluid are essential for male reproduction, since the biochemical composition of this fluid is critical for sperm function. Seminal fluid contributes to the process of sperm capacitation and fertilization, controlling pH, nourishing spermatozoa and creating a proper environment for immunological protection [2]. The motility of spermatozoa is also severely affected by the composition of seminal plasma and is, in fact, favored by a controlled pH in the seminal fluid [3].

Failure to maintain pH homeostasis along the male reproductive tract may impair the production and maturation of spermatozoa, therefore causing subfertility or infertility [4, 5]. The importance of understanding the functional relevance of the luminal fluids of the male reproductive tract relies in the fact that up to 40% of infertile men present idiopathic infertility, which may be a reflection of disorders in sperm maturation and storage [6]. This chapter will discuss some of the key components of the testicular fluid, epididymal fluid and seminal plasma and briefly explain how these very specific microenvironments are created.

THE EPIDIDYMAL MILIEU

The epididymis is an organ consisting of a highly convoluted duct system supposed to cover a total length of about 20 meters in man. The whole duct is strictly dependent upon testicular products for the maintenance of its structure as well as secretory, reabsorptive, biosynthetic and metabolic activity [7, 8]. The epididymal lumen has usually the most complex fluid found in any exocrine gland. This may be due to the continuous changes in its composition, such as the presence of some substances in unusually high concentrations for unknown reasons, or the presence of others, not found in any other body fluids [9]. The epididymal fluid compostition is largely influenced by the end-product of the exocrine activity of the testes, testicular fluid or testicular plasma. Besides being dependent on the presence of androgens [10], the epididymis also relies on the presence of luminal fluid factors obtained from the testes and the epididymis itself. Some studies described that without testicular luminal fluid factors, many cells within the initial segment of epididymis would undergo apoptosis [11, 12]. Therefore, factors originated from testes are responsible for the preservation of the integrity and survival of cells within epididymis. The testicular fluid that goes to epididymis is mainly composed by the seminiferous tubular fluid (STF). There is a layer of spindle-shaped cells that fills the space among the external and internal lamella of the seminiferous tubules surrounding tissue, to which the tubules owe their contractibility [13]. STF was thought to be a mixture of primary fluid, most likely secreted by Sertoli cells [7]. However, the seminiferous epithelium secretes a fluid that is later modified when enters the rete testis, by alterations in potassium, bicarbonate, sodium, chloride, proteins and steroid concentrations [14]. For instance, STF is characterized by being potassium-rich, and is later altered to a sodium chloride-rich when entering the rete testis [7]. Thereby, the epithelium of rete testis is active in the regulation of the luminal fluid microenvironment, and not as much in controlling the volume of fluid produced in the STF that goes to the epididymis [7]. Nevertheless, the role of the rete testis in the regulation of luminal fluid environment has been overlooked. The testicular fluid undergoes a sequence of changes before it entries the epididymis, and along its passage through the seminiferous tubules, rete testis and, lastly, the efferent ducts. Therefore, the "testicular semen" is a suspension of spermatozoa released by the germinal epithelium into a combination of fluids originated from different compartments of the testes and referred to as testicular fluid [15]. The epididymal lumen has a complex fluid that is controlled by the blood-epididymal barrier (BEB), which maintains a specialized luminal fluid, providing a suitable environment for sperm maturation and survival [16]. Luminal fluid microenvironment is important in the processes of sperm maturation and storage. The epididymal epithelium is composed by very active cells in intermediary metabolism that generate products of energy metabolism and reactive oxygen species [6, 16]. The epididymal lumen is rich in inorganic ions and small organic molecules, which create an environment that is hyperosmotic when compared to serum [17]. Perturbations in the microenvironment that surrounds the spermatozoa, such as alterations in the luminal pH or extreme temperatures, can affect maturation and development [4].

LUMINAL FLUID COMPOSITION: RELEVANCE OF BICARBONATE

The luminal fluid surrounding the spermatozoa displays peculiarities between each region of male reproductive tract. The production process begins inside the testes where spermatozoa are released into the lumen of the seminiferous tubule. Inside the seminiferous tubules the spermatozoa are bathed in STF, which is mainly produced and released by Sertoli cells [18]. The establishment of the ionic composition of the STF implies the net movement of water, K^+ secretion and Cl^-, Na^+ and HCO^-_3 reabsorption, which contribute for luminal acidification [18]. Substantial differences in ionic composition of STF have been reported comparatively to blood plasma, particularly concerning the concentration of K^+, Na^+, Cl^- and HCO^-_3. The reported composition of the STF differs according to the method of collection [19 - 22]. The study of male reproductive tract fluids is very complex, with micropuncture, which has originally been used to study renal physiology, being the most common method. The major problem of micropuncture analysis is the available quantity of sample, since it obtains very low volumes, in the order of nanoliters or picoliters [23]. Therefore, the analysis of these samples is really difficult, hence the few studies focused on the composition of the fluids in human reproductive tract that are available using this technique. Even though, STF collected from rat seminiferous tubules by micropuncture evidenced more K^+ than in fluid collected from rete testis, in a concentration about ten times higher when compared to blood plasma. However, the HCO^-_3 and Na^+ concentrations were lower in rat STF than in blood plasma (Table **8.1**). Ca^{2+} concentration in STF was similar to that of blood plasma, and Mg^{+2} and phosphate levels were higher in STF. With a pH of approximately 7.3, STF is more acid that blood and the osmolality of the fluid available inside the seminiferous tubules is isosmotic in the rat [1, 22 - 24] (Table **8.1**). The electrical potential difference across the seminiferous tubules epithelium is approximately 4.8 mV, lumen negative to the interstitial medium. K^+ and Cl^- enter the tubule against their electrochemical gradient, whereas Na^+ and HCO^-_3 entrance into the lumen is favored by that gradient [24]. The STF flows through the rete testis and the efferent ducts into the epididymis. Rete testis fluid arises within the seminiferous tubules, thus containing some of the same components present in STF. Rete testis fluid contains more Na^+ and Ca^{2+} than STF, however the concentrations of K^+, phosphate and Mg^{+2} are lower [1, 22, 23] (Table **8.1**).

Table 8.1. Electrolyte concentrations, osmolality, pH and spermatocrit in the seminiferous tubular fluid, rete testis fluid, epididymis fluids, vas deferens fluid and plasma of the rat. STF- Seminiferous tubular fluid.

	STF	**Rete Testis Fluid**	**Epididymis Fluids**			***Vas Deferens* Fluid**	**Plasma**
			Caput	**Corpus**	**Cauda**		
Na^+ (mM/L)	110±5 [24]	142±10 [1, 22, 23]	104±3 [23]	94±11 [23]	37±3 [23]	23±4 [24]	139±4 [23]
K^+ (mM/L)	40±1 [22, 23]	12±0.5 [22, 23]	21±2 [23]	37±2 [24]	50±1 [31]	52±2 [24]	4±1 [1]
HCO^-_3 (mM/L)	20±0.4 [1, 24]	21±5 [1, 22]	3±0.3 [24]	----------	7±0.3 [24]	7±0.3 [24]	30±0.1 [24]
Cl^- (mM/L)	143±12 [23]	136±5 [1, 22, 23]	24±2 [23]	39±5 [23]	27±2 [23, 24]	11±2 [24]	122±4 [23]
Phosphate (mM/L)	9±1 [23]	2±0.5 [23]	59±5 [23]	94±3 [23]	84±5 [23]	----------	2±0.1 [23]
Ca^{2+} (mM/L)	0.4±0.03 [1, 23]	0.8±0.1 [1, 23]	0.9±0.1 [23]	0.5±0.1 [23]	0.3±0.1 [23]	----------	0.5±0.1 [23]
Mg^{2+} (mM/L)	1.2±0.2 [1, 23]	0.4±0.1 [1, 23]	2±0.3 [23]	3±0.2 [23]	1±0.1 [23]	----------	0.4±0.02 [23]
Osmolality (mOsm/Kg)	338±7 [22, 24]	328±23 [22]	315±4 [24]	340±8 [24]	329±5 [24]	339±4 [24]	311±3 [22, 24]

(Table 8.1) contd.....

	STF	Rete Testis Fluid	Epididymis Fluids			*Vas Deferens* Fluid	Plasma
			Caput	Corpus	Cauda		
pH	7.3 [24, 30]	----------	6.6 [24, 30]	----------	6.9 [24]	6.9 [24]	7.5 [24]
Spermatocrit	0.2±0.02 [24]	----------	0.4±0.02 [24]	0.6±0.04 [24]	0.5±0.03 [24]	0.7±0.02 [24]	----------

The concentration of ions, small organic solutes and proteins are all dependent on the movement of water in and out of the lumen. Thus, the concentration of ions in the luminal fluid are not only due to direct secretion into the lumen, but also dependent on the volume of water that is reabsorbed. In many species, 70-96% of the fluid leaving the testes is reabsorbed in the efferent ducts. Particularly in rats, 96% of the fluid is reabsorbed [14]. Other studies in rats demonstrated that when the efferent duct connection is compromised for 24 hours there is a rise of about 50% in testicular volume due to accumulated fluid, thus illustrating the efficiency of the efferent ducts and epididymis in the control of the volume of fluid [25]. Additionally, there is another parameter that demonstrates the absorption of water by the efferent ducts and initial segment of epididymis, which is the fractional volume occupied by sperm (spermatocrit). The spermatocrit increases from 0.2±0.02 in seminiferous tubules to 0.4±0.2 in epididymal caput and to 0.5±0.03 in cauda epididymis [24], indicating that about 50% of the fluid leaving the seminiferous tubules is absorbed by the efferent ducts. Moreover, water reabsorption by vas deferens leads to a spermatocrit of 0.7±0.02, 0.2 more than in the epididymal cauda [24] (Table **8.1**). Apparently, most of the reabsorption process occurs before the cauda of the epididymis, because the ion concentrations are not significantly altered when compared to those observed in the vas deferens. Luminal fluid composition can be regulated by hormonal influence, through the modulation of membrane ion transporters expression and functionality in the male reproductive tract. It has been described that estrogen can regulate the expression of ion transporters involved in pH homeodynamics in the fluids of the male reproductive tract. Mice treated with antiestrogens presented a decreased expression of $Na/^{+}H^{+}$ exchanger 3 (NHE3) in efferent ducts, which results in alterations in the exchange of Na^{+} and H^{+} in mediating water transport [26].

Micropuncture studies have showed that the concentration of Na^{+} decreases and K^{+} increases in the epididymal fluid along the epididymis (Table **8.1**). This suggests that both Na^{+} and water are reabsorbed by the epididymal epithelium. Some in vitro and in vivo studies performed in rats indicate that fluid reabsorption is a passive process, secondary to active Na^{+} transport [27 - 29]. The rates of the ionic transport of Na^{+}, Cl^{-}, K^{+} and water have been found to fluctuate with the region of the duct, but it became clear that epididymis absorbs Na^{+}, Cl^{-} and water and secretes K^{+}. Notably, the more distal parts of the rat epididymis absorb Na^{+}

and water and secrete K^+ at a higher rate than more distal parts of the epididymal duct [29]. Therefore, Na^+ is actively reabsorbed by the epididymal epithelium, thereby creating an osmotic gradient for water reabsorption. The ionic transport that occurs along the epididymis is linked to a progressive increase in the potential difference across the epithelial wall. That difference is 5.6±0.1 mV, lumen negative, in the caput of epididymis and increases to 27±0.6mV, lumen negative, in the cauda and vas deferens. The process of Na^+ reabsorption occurs against an electrochemical potential difference. The rising K^+ concentration can be mainly due to the removal of water, but there is also a contribution from epithelial secretion into the lumen [24]. Potassium concentration is quite different between epididymis and vas deferens regarding blood plasma, diverging from electrochemical equilibrium, what should happen through a more complex process than simple equilibration. Moreover, Cl^- is also reabsorbed against an electrochemical gradient, but the rate of Cl^- reabsorption is only a fraction of the Na^+ reabsorption rate in the epididymis [24].

Levine and Kelly [30] described the first measurement of pH made in vivo in the male reproductive tract of rat. They were able to precisely locate the primary site of acidification in the initial segment of epididymis. The authors observed that at the beginning of the initial segment of epididymis, the pH is about 7.20±0.06 while in the end of the initial segment it is 6.79±0.06, so the fluid becomes more acid, reaching 6.6 in the caput [30]. The pH value of the epididymal fluid increases very slightly again at the end of the epididymis (Table **8.1**).

Luminal acidification depends on several processes, such as HCO^-_3 reabsorption and proton secretion, which occurs in different cell types and in different regions of the epididymis. The most important physiological buffer system in mammals, which controls and maintains the pH range is HCO^-_3. HCO^-_3 originated in the testes (20 mM) is partially reabsorbed between the seminiferous tubules and the caput of the epididymis by the HCO^-_3 transporters [32] and by the action of carbonic anhydrases [33]. Bicarbonate reabsorption is essentially performed by the main cells in the initial segment of the epididymis [4]. In the rat epididymis, HCO^-_3 concentration is around 3-7 mM, with a slight increase in the cauda and vas deferens, related to HCO^-_3 reabsorption in the initial segment [4, 34]. The presence of HCO^-_3 in the luminal fluid is essential for spermatogenesis and spermatozoa maturation. The intratubular concentration of HCO^-_3 in the epididymis and epididymal spermatozoa is regulated by HCO^-_3 transporters, namely HCO^-_3 permeable proteins and carbonic anhydrase activity [32]. Bicarbonate has been shown to stimulate mammalian sperm motility and metabolism through activation of adenylate cyclase. Soluble adenylyl cyclase (sAC) is a HCO^-_3 chemosensor for immature and mature spermatozoa. In vivo studies showed that HCO^-_3 modulates the enzymatic activity of sAC by direct interaction with the allosteric site of the enzyme to produce cAMP, under pH independent conditions [35]. Bicarbonate-regulated sAC was initially purified from testes cytosol, which is an alternative source for cAMP. sAC is not only a soluble protein but has well-defined intracellular targets, such as mitochondria, centrioles, mitotic spindles, midbodies and nuclei [36]. Therefore, adenylyl cyclases are in close association to cAMP effectors, and adenylyl cyclases are in turn regulated by HCO^-_3 [36]. High concentrations of HCO^-_3 should be linked with high cAMP production while the reverse also occurs. Modulation of key ion channels, activation of the sAC/cAMP signaling pathway and protein phosphorylation events are essential for maintaining spermatozoa in a quiescent state during their maturation and storage in the epididymis only. During ejaculation and release into the female reproductive tract, the increase in pH and HCO^-_3 concentration induces sperm capacitation [36, 37] (see Chapter **10**).

Bicarbonate Transporters in Epididymis

Acid-base transporters are classified according to their operation into two distinct groups: acid-extruders (Na^+-H^+ exchangers, Na^+-driven HCO^-_3/Cl^- transporters, Na^+/HCO^-_3 cotransporters, and V-ATPases), used to increase intracellular pH when acidosis occurs, and acid-loaders (Na^+-independent HCO^-_3/Cl^- transporters and Na^+/HCO^-_3 co-transporters), used to decrease intracellular pH when alkalosis occurs [38]. The function as acid-loader or as acid-extruder is also dependent on the ionic gradient established through the membranes [39].

Bicarbonate transporters are largely expressed and involved in the regulation of pH, cell migration, determination of cell volume, transepithelial acid/base transport and Cl^- secretion. Like in other physiological systems, in the male reproductive tract, luminal HCO^-_3 combines with a proton to form H_2CO_3, which is then converted into CO_2 and H_2O by catalysis by carbonic anhydrase [33]. Since this reaction may be reversible in epithelial cells, CO_2 may be conversely hydrated under the action of carbonic anhydrase and then dissociated into HCO^-_3 and a proton [32]. The involvement of HCO^-_3 in epididymal proton secretion is suggested by studies showing that the use of an inhibitor (acetazolamide) of carbonic anhydrase causes an increase in the luminal pH in the cauda epididymis [40]. HCO^-_3 is extruded via HCO^-_3 transporters and protons are recycled into the lumen via V-type H^+-ATPase [41, 42] or Na^+-H^+ exchanger [43]. In the male reproductive tract, HCO^-_3 transporters are highly expressed, particularly in the epididymis. The main families of HCO^-_3 transporters are identified in the epididymis: Solute carrier 4 (SLC4) and Solute carrier 26 (SLC26) families [5]. Intracellular and extracellular HCO^-_3 is transported in and out of the cell across the epididymal membrane mostly by the HCO^-_3 exchanger (Anion exchanger - AE), or the Na^+- HCO^-_3 cotransporter. The "housekeeping AE", AE2, is widely distributed in the male reproductive tract [5, 44]. AE2 was identified in the initial segment, intermediate zone and caput epididymis and in relative low abundance in the distal regions, including the cauda epididymis [45, 46]. AE2 plays a key role in intracellular pH regulation, and its operation is stimulated by exposure to alkaline media and inhibited by the presence of acidic media [5]. The presence of AE2 in the basolateral membrane of the epithelial cells in the proximal parts of the epididymis is associated with the low luminal HCO^-_3 concentration attained in this segment. Along with other HCO^-_3 transporters, AE2 might contribute to net HCO^-_3 reabsorption. The expression of this important HCO^-_3 transporter is increased in some pathological cases, as was observed in prediabetic-induced rats [45]. The significant increase of abnormal sperm morphology in prediabetic rats [47] was suggested to be related with the alteration of HCO^-_3 transepithelial epididymal fluxes.

The Na^+-dependent members of the SLC4 family also contribute to the transport of HCO^-_3 in the epididymis. Due to their transport stoichiometry, they are divided into two sub-groups: electrogenic (NBCe) and electroneutral (NBCn). The direction and stoichiometry of the transport depends on the tissues in which they are expressed. In the epididymis, the NBCe1 and NBCn1 uptake the ions (HCO^-_3 and Na^+) into the cytosol [45]. The NDCBE (Na^+-driven Cl^-/HCO^-_3 exchanger) is an intracellular pH regulator that transports extracellular HCO^-_3 and Na^+ in exchange for intracellular Cl^- and H+, playing an essential role in cellular alkalinisation. The expression of NDCBE has also been detected throughout all the male reproductive tract, including in the epididymis, and was found to be altered in some pathological states (e.g. prediabetes) [45]. Bicarbonate-permeable members of the SLC26 family make the second major subfamily of HCO^-_3 transporters, and some of them are also expressed along the male reproductive tract. However, their function is not as well studied when compared with the SLC4 family. In the epididymis, four members of HCO^-_3 transporters of SLC26 family were identified: SLC26A3, SLC26A4, SLC26A6 and SLC26A7 [32, 45]. The SLC26A3 transporter is highly expressed in the testes, but has a low expression in the epididymis. It was only identified in the luminal side of the apical mitochondria-rich cells (AMRC), located in the caput epididymis and only occasionally in the corpus epididymis [48]. The expression of SLC26A4, SLC26A6 and SLC26A7 [49, 50] has also been reported in the epididymis. However, functional studies concerning the role of some of these transporters in the male reproductive tract tissues are still very scare or inexistent.

In addition to the discussed HCO^-_3 transporters, cystic fibrosis transmembrane conductance regulator (CFTR) is also expressed in the epididymis, and contributes to the ionic composition of the luminal fluid. CFTR has an important role in transepithelial salt absorption, as well as in the HCO^-_3 secretion and in the regulation of fluid volume in epithelial cells [32]. The epithelial cells of the head epididymis present more intense expression of CFTR, while the distribution is irregular in the epithelial cells of the body and tail [51]. A study with primary cultures of rat epididymal epithelial cells confirmed the expression of CFTR and revealed its important role in the regulation of Cl^- secretion and epididymal fluid formation [52]. Several studies have demonstrated that the movement of water could be directly linked with the expression and activity of CFTR, through the production of cAMP, which stimulates aqueous pore, or by interaction with aquaporins [53]. Aquaporins play a major role in water transport [54] across the epididymal epithelium and have been identified throughout the epididymis, including in the efferent ducts and vas deferens [55 - 61], but not necessarily in every region or in epithelial cells [58, 62, 63]. Therefore, besides being an ion channel, CFTR also regulates water permeability in some tissues or cells of the male reproductive tract. Hence, the abnormal functioning of CFTR may involve altered water transport and changes in HCO^-_3 transport, resulting in alterations in the composition of the luminal tubular fluid [64]. HCO^-_3 transport can be affected by hormonal deregulation, namely by increased levels of estrogens. Human SCs with higher levels of estrogens exhibited an increase on the expression of the three HCO^-_3 transporters of the SLC4 family, causing an increase in the influx of HCO^-_3 to the intracellular milieu, and contributing not only to a raise in intracellular pH but also to a decrease in Cl^- intracellular concentration [65]. This alterations can be the result of modifications in the composition of the STF. Thereby, HCO^-_3 is not only essential to ionic homeostasis, but it also plays a crucial role in the maintenance of pH along the male reproductive tract while also playing a central role in spermatozoa activation and capacitation.

Water movement across the male reproductive tract is a fundamental process in the production of luminal fluid and in the maintenance in the equilibrium of ionic concentrations within suitable limits. The essential water transporter channels are aquaporins (AQPs), which facilitate permeation of water and uncharged solutes through cellular membranes [54, 66]. In testis, water is secreted into the lumen of seminiferous tubules by Sertoli cells, contributing for the production of a proper environment for spermatogenesis, and providing a means of transport for the spermatozoa from the testis and through the efferent ducts into the epididymal duct [67]. Most of the testicular fluid that reaches the efferent ducts is reabsorbed, and the luminal fluid is also constantly reabsorbed and secreted along the epididymal duct, in order to create an adequate environment for maintaining the fertility and motility of the spermatozoa [68, 69]. AQPs have an important role in the determination of the composition of the luminal fluids that fill the testicular ducts which serve as vehicles to move spermatozoa from the epididymal ducts. Biophysical properties of AQPs allow their division into two categories: orthodox AQPs, permeable to water (AQP0, AQP1, AQP2, AQP4, AQP5, AQP6 and

AQP8), and aquaglyceroporins, AQPs which transport small uncharged solutes, such as urea and glycerol in addition to water (AQP3, AQP7, AQP9, AQP10) [54, 70]. The conducting properties of other two isoforms, AQP11 and AQP12 are unclear. Some isoforms of AQPs are expressed in the mammalian male reproductive tract [64]. Those identified in testis include AQP0 [61], AQP1 [71], AQP2 [72], AQP4 [73], AQP5 [72], AQP7 [74], AQP8 [74], AQP9 [75], AQP10 [72] and AQP11 [76], and contribute for the establishment of an adequate luminal environment within the seminiferous tubules. In efferent ducts, the expression of AQP1 [56], AQP2 [77] and AQP9 [59] was reported, suggesting that these isoforms participate in the absorption of the large amounts of fluid occurring in these ducts. In rete testis (AQP1) [77, 78], epididymis (AQP2 [62], AQP3 [61], AQP5 [72], AQP7 [72], AQP9 [72], AQP10 [72], AQP11 [63]) and accessory glands [66], some isoforms of AQPs were also identified. Notably, expression of the AQPs and water reabsorption seems to be modulated by hormones. In rat epididymis, AQP9 is downregulated by estrogen, but these effects elicited by estrogens may be prevented by testosterone [60]. The reabsorption of water taking place in the efferent ducts is also affected by estrogens. Knockout rats for estrogen receptors presented a decreased reabsorption of fluid in ductules, with dilatations in rete testis and protrusion into the testis. Therefore, in this case, luminal fluid was not removed by the efferent ducts, resulting in fluid accumulation in the rete testis and seminiferous tubules [79].

LUMINAL CALCIUM AND SPERM FUNCTION

Immature sperm formed in the seminiferous tubules of the testes becomes mature and motile in the epididymis. Sperm motility has been shown to be a good predictor of human male fertility *in vivo* and *in vitro* [80], and is controlled by various parameters, such as Ca^{2+} and HCO^-_3 concentrations in the luminal fluid. Both Ca^{2+} and HCO^-_3 concentrations are important features of the luminal epididymal fluid that could be important for sperm capacitation and motility (**Fig. 8.1**). It has been suggested that Ca^{2+}-binding proteins in sperm membrane directly stimulate the contractile apparatus of the sperm flagella [81]. Extracellular Ca^{2+} in the tail portion of the epididymis is required for motility in epididymal sperm, and Ca^{2+} is directly correlated with activated and hyperactivated sperm motility [82]. The Ca^{2+} concentration in the epididymal fluid controls intracellular cAMP levels of spermatozoa through the regulation of sAC. This will lead to protein phosphorylation, which is the key to understand the initial activation of motility during epididymal transit [37]. Besides sAC regulation, other Ca^{2+} pathways independent of cAMP and protein kinase A (PKA) phosphorylation are involved, such as the calmodulin pathway [83].

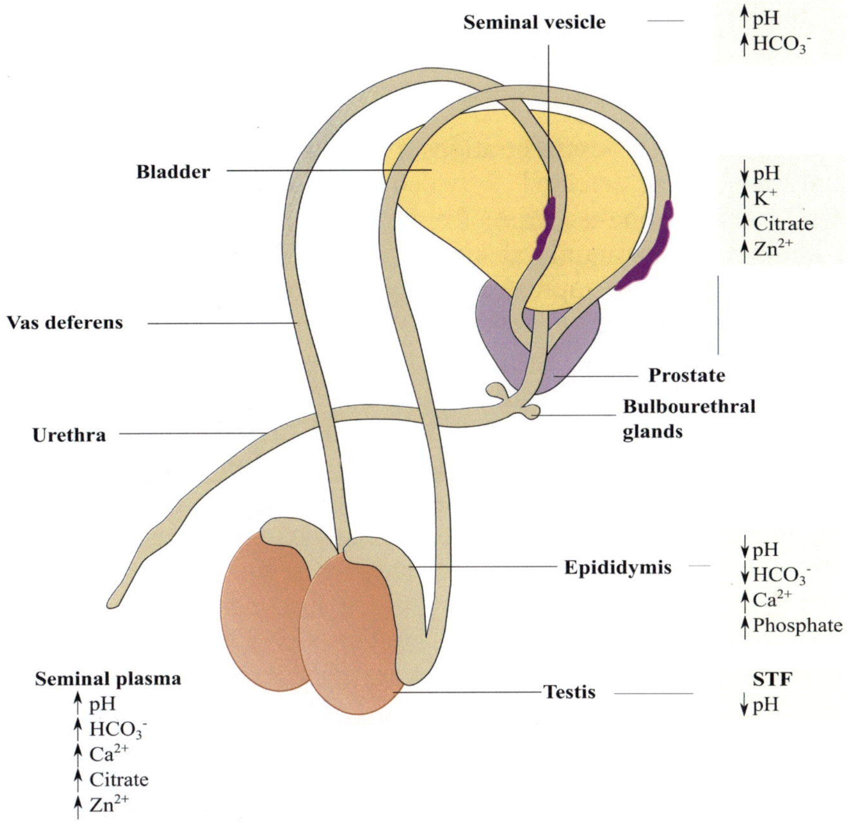

Fig. (8.1). Representative image of the most significant electrolyte composition that constitutes the male reproductive tract fluid, which is strongly correlated with pH establishment. Seminiferous tubular fluid is produced in the testes and presents an acidic pH. In the epididymis, the pH is also acidic due to the low concentration of HCO^-_3, and high concentrations of Ca^{2+} and phosphate. Prostate gland produces a prostatic fluid with elevated concentrations of K^+, citrate and Zn^{2+} with acidic pH. Seminal vesicle is the main contributor of HCO^-_3 for seminal plasma and consequently, the seminal liquid has a more alkaline pH. Seminal plasma is formed by the addition of some fluids, more notably the STF, prostatic and seminal fluid. Some of the ions contributing to an alkaline pH in seminal plasma are HCO^-_3, Ca^{2+}, citrate and Zn^{2+}. Abbreviations: STF, Seminiferous tubular fluid.

Several channels contributing to the control of membrane permeability to Ca^{2+} in the sperm membrane have been identified. Luminal Ca^{2+} is mainly absorbed by the membrane transient receptor potential Ca^{2+} channel (TRP channels), which consist of six transmembrane helices and intracellular N- and C-terminals [84]. Two ubiquitous Ca^{2+} sensor calmodulin (CaM) binding sites have been identified so far in TRP channels [84, 85]. CaM is a constitutive or dissociable Ca^{2+}-sensing subunit for a large variety of ion channels, including TRP family channels. Nevertheless, at the moment, not much is known about the functional role of the

CaM molecules bound to a single functional channel [85]. For numerous TRP channels, binding of CaM to the C-terminal intracellular segment has been described to be essential for Ca^{2+}-dependent inactivation [86, 87], but very few details about the molecular mechanisms involved are yet described [88].

Luminal variations in Ca^{2+} concentrations in the fluid that surrounds sperm during epididymal transit were detected. Between the caput and the cauda epididymis, luminal Ca^{2+} concentration decreases from 0.8 to 0.3 mM in the rat (Table **8.1**) [1, 23]. The luminal Ca^{2+} is mainly absorbed by the TRPV6 channel. At the end of TRPV6 structure there are approximately 30 amino acids that corresponds to the CaM binding sites, and Ca^{2+}-dependent channel inactivation is enabled by CaM binding to this fragment [86]. Recent studies showed that there is a disruption of Ca^{2+} absorption by the epididymal epithelium when the Trpv6 gene is deleted, resulting in increased Ca^{2+} concentrations in the caudal epididymal fluid [89]. When Ca^{2+} concentration is altered in rat epididymal fluid, a partial loss of sperm motility and fertilization capacity is observed [89]. It was reported that cellular Ca^{2+} levels are six times higher in caput spermatozoa than in caudal spermatozoa, and that the rate of uptake in caput spermatozoa seems to be about three times higher than that of caudal spermatozoa [90]. At least some of the effects of Ca^{2+} on sperm motility are believed to be mediated through CaM, since CaM inhibition decreases sperm motility [90, 91]. However, the effects of Ca^{2+} on sAC are not dependent of CaM [83], which suggests that Ca^{2+} affects sperm motility via distinct pathways. Hence, there are at last two different Ca^{2+} activated pathways in sperm: one that is dependent of CaM and another that is not.

Briefly, CaM can regulate some cellular functions and control the intracellular concentrations of Ca^{2+} and cAMP. It has been suggested that in cells with endocrine activity, the mechanisms of Ca^{2+}-CaM are similar to the events that take place between steroid hormones and their receptor proteins in the cytoplasm [92]. Ca^{2+}/CaM is involved in multiple functions in sperm, including motility, capacitation and the acrosome reaction [91, 93]. CaM is located in the principal piece of the flagellum, where the main proteins directly involved in the regulation of motility are found. CaM inhibitors decrease sperm motility, but this inhibition was shown to be largely reversed by stimulation of PKA, although only when substrates for oxidative respiration (lactate and pyruvate) were present in the medium. Additionally, when there is substrate for glycolysis (glucose) in the medium, but there is no lactate and pyruvate, increased intracellular cAMP is not able restore sperm motility. This suggests that CaM is implicated in the regulation of glycolysis [94]. Therefore, the inhibition of CaM indirectly affects glycolysis, and consequently sperm motility.

Ca^{2+} can also be directly linked to flagellar function, through regulation of the atypical sAC, which generates cAMP to activate PKA. sAC is required for sperm motility, and is different from transmembrane adenylyl cyclases, since sAC is the only one that is sensitive to both HCO^-_3 and Ca^{2+} [95]. sAC activity is molecularly distinct from transmembrane AC, since its activity is dependent on the presence of Mn^{+2}, and is insensitive to forskolin (which is known to increase cAMP levels in most cell types) and G protein regulation. Purified sAC exhibited 10-fold lower affinity for ATP regarding transmembrane AC (transmembrane AC Km for ATP-Mn^{+2} is approximately 100 μM, and purified rat testes sAC Km for ATP-Mn^{+2} is approximately 1 mM) [96]. There is a synergistic interaction between HCO^-_3 and Ca^{2+}, where HCO^-_3 increases the Vmax (maximum velocity or rate at which the enzyme catalyzed a reaction) of the enzyme, while Ca^{2+} increases its affinity for ATP-Mn^{+2} as a substrate [96]. sAC activity can be responsive for the elevated Ca^{2+} concentrations established during acrosome reaction and sperm motility, or it may be located close to the Ca^{2+} channel, where it may mediate cAMP regulation of channel opening [97]. PKA, the classic cAMP target, catalyzes the phosphorylation of several flagellar proteins, thus regulating sperm motility. The cAMP-PKA signaling pathway also induces phosphorylation of various proteins required for capacitation response [98].

ELECTROLYTES, PHOSPHATASES AND SEMINAL PLASMA COMPOSITION

Seminal plasma is a fluid that originates from the testes, epididymis, prostate, and seminal vesicles secretions. As already described, a part of STF goes into the epididymis with spermatozoa, thus joining the epididymal fluid. Seminal plasma contains fluids originated by epididymal fluids, which join the fluids released by male accessory glands, prostatic fluid and the one produced by seminal vesicles. Human seminal plasma contains calcium, citrate, zinc and magnesium in higher concentrations than those present in other body fluids [99] (Fig. **8.1**). A comparison between these electrolytes in prostatic and seminal fluid confirms that most of them are originated from the prostate.

Prostate is a glandular structure enclosed by a fibrous capsule, which is structurally divided in three regions: the larger region, the peripheral zone, which comprises 70% of the total volume of the gland, and a central zone and a transition zone, which account for the remaining 30% [100, 101]. The epithelium of prostate is composed of two histologically distinct layers. The secretory luminal layer is constituted by columnar cells that express androgen receptors and produce prostatic secretions, prostate specific antigen (PSA) and keratinocyte growth factor receptor [100]. The other layer that supports the columnar cells consists of epithelial cuboid cells. The basal cells, are essentially responsible for the production of p63, cytokeratin 5 and 14, and keratin, and express some receptors, such as estrogen receptors, insulin-like growth factor receptors, and epidermal growth factor receptors [100, 102]. Neuroendocrine cells are also present in the prostate and are thought to be involved in the growth and secretory activity of this gland [103]. The main function of the prostate is its secretory activity. It essentially secretes PSA, citric acid, prostaglandins and prostatic acid phosphatase, which are essential for sperm motility and fertilization capacity (see Chapter **10**). Prostate secretions are regulated by sex hormones, being dependent on androgens and estrogens, and their respective receptors [104, 105]. For instance, testosterone was shown to stimulate prostate citrate production [106]. The prostatic secretions are important for the control of seminal plasma pH, and are able for neutralizing the acid environment of the other fluids (Table **8.1**) and of the female reproductive tract (see Chapter **10**) [3].

Prostate is the major source of seminal K^+ (66.8 mM from prostate and 27.2 mM from seminal vesicles) [99] (Fig. **8.1**). Less attention has been given to Na^+ and Cl^-, which are also secreted by the prostate gland and seminal vesicles [107]. While the concentrations of Cl^- are identical in prostatic and seminal fluid, Na^+ is slightly lower in the later, what may evidence the fact that both contribute similarly to the two fluids [99]. The pH of the fluids is strongly correlated with the electrolytic composition. The pH in seminal plasma is maintained around 7.5, essentially by the HCO^-_3 produced by accessory reproductive glands [24, 108]. The regulation of HCO^-_3 levels in the seminal plasma is achieved by of cytosolic carbonic anhydrase isozyme activity, secreted by the seminal vesicle, prostate and bulbourethral gland [108]. It has been shown that citrate and zinc levels as well as the pH (6.2 in prostate fluid) (Fig. **8.1**) in prostatic secretions are correlated with secretory enzyme activities, such as acid phosphatases, aminopeptidases and ATPases [109]. Prostatic acid phosphatase (PAP) is the essential phosphatase responsible for the degradation of lysophosphatidic acid (LPA) in human seminal plasma [110]. LPA is a phospholipid that activates specific G protein coupled receptors, inducing multiple cellular responses [111]. The expression of LPA in seminal plasma and sperm is considerable, although its physiological role is not known [110]. Alkaline phosphatase (AP) is another enzyme reported to be present in seminal plasma from numerous species. AP catalyzes the hydrolysis of organic phosphate at basic pH values [112]. The physiological role of these enzymes is speculative in male reproductive tract, but they have been suggested to have an essential action in the active transport of substances across membranes. It is known that there are considerable variations among the AP activities of seminal plasma among different species. Human semen is relatively poor in AP when compared with that of other species, such as in bull semen. There is an inverse relationship between the amounts of AP ejaculated and serum AP activity [113]. Seminal plasma contains prostasomes, which are vesicles secreted by prostate gland that contain cholesterol, sphingomyelin, Ca^{2+} and some other enzymes [114]. It is known that prostasomes fuse to sperm at slightly acidic pH values, and that this phenomenon involves lipid and protein transfers, modifying the properties of sperm membranes [115]. Prostasomes improve sperm motility under conditions of low pH, affecting the sperm competition in the vagina which tends to be acidic [3]. Seminal plasma has a high buffering capacity which is essential for sperm motility and fertilizing ability in environments with different ionic compositions and different pH.

CONCLUDING REMARKS

It is evident that the maintenance of a proper fluid environment for spermatozoa storage and maturation depends on the regulation of absorption/reabsorption and secretion of electrolytes and fluids along the male reproductive tract, with greater emphasis on the processes that occur in the epididymal duct. Significant progress has been made in our understanding of the composition of seminal plasma and fluids secreted by accessory glands, providing new insights that ultimately could lead to improvement of human reproductive health. Given the general concern regarding a putative progressive decline in male fertility, it seems imperative that seminal plasma alterations should become an area of intense future research with proper justified funds.

Box 8.1 | Summary

- Epididymal milieu provides a specialized environment for sperm storage and maturation.
- Luminal fluid microenvironment has a different composition than that of blood plasma.
- Luminal acidification in epididymis depends on HCO_3^- reabsorption and proton secretion.
- The Ca^{2+} and HCO_3^- concentrations in luminal epididymal fluid are important for sperm capacitation and motility.
- Seminal fluid has a high buffering capacity that is essential for sperm motility and fertilizing ability.

CONFLICT OF INTEREST

The authors confirm that they have no conflict of interest to declare for this publication.

ACKNOWLEDGEMENT

This work was supported by the "Fundação para a Ciência e a Tecnologia"–FCT (PTDC/BBB-BQB/1368/2014), UMIB (PEst-OE/SAU/UI0215/2014). Raquel L. Bernardino was also funded by (SFRH/BD/103105/2014).

REFERENCES

[1] S M, DE B. Anatomy, Vasculature, and Innervation of the Male Reproductive Tract. In: The Physiology of Reproduction. In: Knobil E, Neill J, Eds. Int J Biochem. Raven Press 1994; pp. 1063-175.

[2] Poiani A. Complexity of seminal fluid: a review. Behav Ecol Sociobiol 2006; 60: 289-310. [http://dx.doi.org/10.1007/s00265-006-0178-0]

[3] Arienti G, Carlini E, Nicolucci A, Cosmi EV, Santi F, Palmerini CA. The motility of human spermatozoa as influenced by prostasomes at various pH levels. Biol Cell 1999; 91(1): 51-4. [http://dx.doi.org/10.1111/j.1768-322X.1999.tb01083.x] [PMID: 10321022]

[4] Pastor-Soler N, Piétrement C, Breton S. Role of acid/base transporters in the male reproductive tract and potential consequences of their malfunction. Physiology (Bethesda) 2005; 20: 417-28. [http://dx.doi.org/10.1152/physiol.00036.2005] [PMID: 16287991]

[5] Bernardino RL, Jesus TT, Martins AD, *et al.* Molecular basis of bicarbonate membrane transport in the male reproductive tract. Curr Med Chem 2013; 20(32): 4037-49. [http://dx.doi.org/10.2174/15672050113109990200] [PMID: 23931280]

[6] Cornwall GA. New insights into epididymal biology and function. Hum Reprod Update 2009; 15(2): 213-27. [http://dx.doi.org/10.1093/humupd/dmn055] [PMID: 19136456]

[7] Rodríguez CM, Hinton BT. The testicular and epididymal luminal fluid microenvironment Introduction to Mammalian Reproduction. Springer 2003; pp. 61-77. [http://dx.doi.org/10.1007/978-1-4615-0273-9_4]

[8] Arrotéia KF, Pereira LA, Barbieri MF, Justino ML, Garcia PV. The epididymis: embryology, structure, function and its role in fertilization and infertility. In: Pereira LA, Ed. Embryology - Updates and Highlights on Classic Topics. INTECH Open Access Publisher 2012; pp. 41-66. [http://dx.doi.org/10.5772/35847]

[9] Dacheux J-L, Dacheux F. Protein secretion in the epididymis The Epididymis: From molecules to clinical practice. Springer 2002; pp. 151-68. [http://dx.doi.org/10.1007/978-1-4615-0679-9_9]

[10] Verjans HL, de Jong FH, Cooke BA, van der Molen HJ, Eik-Nes KB. Effect of oestradiol benzoate on pituitary and testis function in the normal adult male rat. Acta Endocrinol 1974; 77(4): 636-42. [PMID: 4479701]

[11] Keller R. Shaping the vertebrate body plan by polarized embryonic cell movements. Science 2002; 298(5600): 1950-4. [http://dx.doi.org/10.1126/science.1079478] [PMID: 12471247]

[12] Di Giovanni V, Alday A, Chi L, Mishina Y, Rosenblum ND. Alk3 controls nephron number and androgen production *via* lineage-specific effects in intermediate mesoderm. Development 2011; 138(13): 2717-27.
[http://dx.doi.org/10.1242/dev.059030] [PMID: 21613322]

[13] Farr CH, Ellis LC. In-vitro contractility of rat seminiferous tubules in response to prostaglandins, cyclic GMP, testosterone and 2,4-dibromoacetophenone. J Reprod Fertil 1980; 58(1): 37-42.
[http://dx.doi.org/10.1530/jrf.0.0580037] [PMID: 6244406]

[14] Hinton B, Setchell B. Fluid secretion and movement. Sertoli Cell 1993; 12: 249-67.

[15] Mann T, Lutwak-Mann C. Testis and testicular semen Male Reproductive Function and Semen. Springer 1981; pp. 83-138.
[http://dx.doi.org/10.1007/978-1-4471-1300-3_4]

[16] Elzanaty S, Richthoff J, Malm J, Giwercman A. The impact of epididymal and accessory sex gland function on sperm motility. Hum Reprod 2002; 17(11): 2904-11.
[http://dx.doi.org/10.1093/humrep/17.11.2904] [PMID: 12407047]

[17] Turner T. Necessity's potion: inorganic ions and small organic molecules in the epididymal lumen The Epididymis: From Molecules to Clinical Practice. Springer 2002; pp. 131-50.
[http://dx.doi.org/10.1007/978-1-4615-0679-9_8]

[18] Rato L, Socorro S, Cavaco JE, Oliveira PF. Tubular fluid secretion in the seminiferous epithelium: ion transporters and aquaporins in Sertoli cells. J Membr Biol 2010; 236(2): 215-24.
[http://dx.doi.org/10.1007/s00232-010-9294-x] [PMID: 20697886]

[19] Fisher D. New light shed on fluid formation in the seminiferous tubules of the rat. J Physiol 2002; 542(Pt 2): 445-52.
[http://dx.doi.org/10.1113/jphysiol.2002.018648] [PMID: 12122144]

[20] Henning RD, Young JA. Electrolyte transport in the seminiferous tubules of the rat studied by the stopped-flow microperfusion technique. Experientia 1971; 27(9): 1037-9.
[http://dx.doi.org/10.1007/BF02138866] [PMID: 5116125]

[21] Levine N, Marsh DJ. Micropuncture study of the fluid composition of Sertoli cell-only seminiferous tubules in rats. J Reprod Fertil 1975; 43(3): 547-9.
[http://dx.doi.org/10.1530/jrf.0.0430547] [PMID: 1142341]

[22] Tuck RR, Setchell BP, Waites GM, Young JA. The composition of fluid collected by micropuncture and catheterization from the seminiferous tubules and rete testis of rats. Pflugers Arch 1970; 318(3): 225-43.
[http://dx.doi.org/10.1007/BF00593663] [PMID: 5465176]

[23] Jenkins AD, Lechene CP, Howards SS. Concentrations of seven elements in the intraluminal fluids of the rat seminiferous tubules, rate testis, and epididymis. Biol Reprod 1980; 23(5): 981-7.
[http://dx.doi.org/10.1095/biolreprod23.5.981] [PMID: 7470534]

[24] Levine N, Marsh DJ. Micropuncture studies of the electrochemical aspects of fluid and electrolyte transport in individual seminiferous tubules, the epididymis and the vas deferens in rats. J Physiol 1971; 213(3): 557-70.
[http://dx.doi.org/10.1113/jphysiol.1971.sp009400] [PMID: 5551402]

[25] Tao L, Zupp JL, Setchell BP. Effect of efferent duct ligation on the function of the blood-testis barrier in rats. J Reprod Fertil 2000; 120(1): 13-8.
[PMID: 11006141]

[26] Zhou Q, Clarke L, Nie R, *et al.* Estrogen action and male fertility: roles of the sodium/hydrogen exchanger-3 and fluid reabsorption in reproductive tract function. Proc Natl Acad Sci USA 2001; 98(24): 14132-7.
[http://dx.doi.org/10.1073/pnas.241245898] [PMID: 11698654]

[27] Wong PY, Yeung CH. Inhibition by amiloride of sodium-dependent fluid reabsorption in the rat isolated caudal epididymis. Br J Pharmacol 1976; 58(4): 529-31.
[http://dx.doi.org/10.1111/j.1476-5381.1976.tb08620.x] [PMID: 1000131]

[28] Wong YC, Wong PY, Yeung CH. Ultrastructural correlation of water reabsorption in isolated rat cauda epididymidis. Experientia 1978; 34(4): 485-7.
[http://dx.doi.org/10.1007/BF01935943] [PMID: 639945]

[29] Wong P, Au C, Ngai H. Electrolyte and water transport in rat epididymis; its possible role in sperm maturation. Int J Androl 1978; 1: 608-28.
[http://dx.doi.org/10.1111/j.1365-2605.1978.tb00512.x]

[30] Levine N, Kelly H. Measurement of pH in the rat epididymis *in vivo*. J Reprod Fertil 1978; 52(2): 333-5.
[http://dx.doi.org/10.1530/jrf.0.0520333] [PMID: 24738]

[31] Wong PY, Lee WM. Potassium movement during sodium-induced motility initiation in the rat caudal epididymal spermatozoa. Biol Reprod 1983; 28(1): 206-12.
[http://dx.doi.org/10.1095/biolreprod28.1.206] [PMID: 6299413]

[32] Liu Y, Wang D-K, Chen L-M. The physiology of bicarbonate transporters in mammalian reproduction. Biol Reprod 2012; 86(4): 99.
[http://dx.doi.org/10.1095/biolreprod.111.096826] [PMID: 22262691]

[33] Hermo L, Chong DL, Moffatt P, Sly WS, Waheed A, Smith CE. Region- and cell-specific differences in the distribution of carbonic anhydrases II, III, XII, and XIV in the adult rat epididymis. J Histochem Cytochem 2005; 53(6): 699-713.
[http://dx.doi.org/10.1369/jhc.4A6575.2005] [PMID: 15928319]

[34] Okamura N, Tajima Y, Sugita Y. Decrease in bicarbonate transport activities during epididymal maturation of porcine sperm. Biochem Biophys Res Commun 1988; 157(3): 1280-7.
[http://dx.doi.org/10.1016/S0006-291X(88)81013-1] [PMID: 2849935]

[35] Chen Y, Cann MJ, Litvin TN, *et al.* Soluble adenylyl cyclase as an evolutionarily conserved bicarbonate sensor. Science 2000; 289(5479): 625-8.
[http://dx.doi.org/10.1126/science.289.5479.625] [PMID: 10915626]

[36] Zippin JH, Chen Y, Nahirney P, *et al.* Compartmentalization of bicarbonate-sensitive adenylyl cyclase in distinct signaling microdomains. FASEB J 2003; 17(1): 82-4.
[PMID: 12475901]

[37] Dacheux J-L, Dacheux F. New insights into epididymal function in relation to sperm maturation. Reproduction 2013; 147(2): R27-42.
[http://dx.doi.org/10.1530/REP-13-0420] [PMID: 24218627]

[38] Boron WF. Regulation of intracellular pH. Adv Physiol Educ 2004; 28(1-4): 160-79.
[http://dx.doi.org/10.1152/advan.00045.2004] [PMID: 15545345]

[39] Oliveira PF, Sousa M, Barros A, Moura T, Rebelo da Costa A. Membrane transporters and cytoplasmatic pH regulation on bovine Sertoli cells. J Membr Biol 2009; 227(1): 49-55.
[http://dx.doi.org/10.1007/s00232-008-9139-z] [PMID: 19050954]

[40] Au CL, Wong PY. Luminal acidification by the perfused rat cauda epididymidis. J Physiol 1980; 309: 419-27.
[http://dx.doi.org/10.1113/jphysiol.1980.sp013517] [PMID: 7252873]

[41] Breton S, Smith PJ, Lui B, Brown D. Acidification of the male reproductive tract by a proton pumping (H+)-ATPase. Nat Med 1996; 2(4): 470-2.
[http://dx.doi.org/10.1038/nm0496-470] [PMID: 8597961]

[42] Martins AD, Bernardino RL, Neuhaus-Oliveira A, *et al.* Physiology of Na^{+}/h+ exchangers in the male reproductive tract: relevance for male fertility. Biol Reprod 2014; 91(1): 11. [http://dx.doi.org/10.1095/biolreprod.114.118331] [PMID: 24876406]

[43] Pushkin A, Clark I, Kwon TH, Nielsen S, Kurtz I. Immunolocalization of NBC3 and NHE3 in the rat epididymis: colocalization of NBC3 and the vacuolar H+-ATPase. J Androl 2000; 21(5): 708-20. [PMID: 10975418]

[44] Bernardino RL, Martins AD, Jesus TT, *et al.* Estrogenic regulation of bicarbonate transporters from SLC4 family in rat Sertoli cells. Mol Cell Biochem 2015; 408(1-2): 47-54. [http://dx.doi.org/10.1007/s11010-015-2481-4] [PMID: 26100313]

[45] Bernardino RL, Martins AD, Socorro S, Alves MG, Oliveira PF. Effect of prediabetes on membrane bicarbonate transporters in testis and epididymis. J Membr Biol 2013; 246(12): 877-83. [http://dx.doi.org/10.1007/s00232-013-9601-4] [PMID: 24105628]

[46] Jensen LJ, Stuart-Tilley AK, Peters LL, Lux SE, Alper SL, Breton S. Immunolocalization of AE2 anion exchanger in rat and mouse epididymis. Biol Reprod 1999; 61(4): 973-80. [http://dx.doi.org/10.1095/biolreprod61.4.973] [PMID: 10491632]

[47] Rato L, Alves MG, Dias TR, *et al.* High-energy diets may induce a pre-diabetic state altering testicular glycolytic metabolic profile and male reproductive parameters. Andrology 2013; 1(3): 495-504. [http://dx.doi.org/10.1111/j.2047-2927.2013.00071.x] [PMID: 23495257]

[48] Hihnala S, Kujala M, Toppari J, Kere J, Holmberg C, Höglund P. Expression of SLC26A3, CFTR and NHE3 in the human male reproductive tract: role in male subfertility caused by congenital chloride diarrhoea. Mol Hum Reprod 2006; 12(2): 107-11. [http://dx.doi.org/10.1093/molehr/gal009] [PMID: 16421216]

[49] Kujala M, Hihnala S, Tienari J, *et al.* Expression of ion transport-associated proteins in human efferent and epididymal ducts. Reproduction 2007; 133(4): 775-84. [http://dx.doi.org/10.1530/rep.1.00964] [PMID: 17504921]

[50] Schweinfest CW, Henderson KW, Suster S, Kondoh N, Papas TS. Identification of a colon mucosa gene that is down-regulated in colon adenomas and adenocarcinomas. Proc Natl Acad Sci USA 1993; 90(9): 4166-70. [http://dx.doi.org/10.1073/pnas.90.9.4166] [PMID: 7683425]

[51] Tizzano EF, Silver MM, Chitayat D, Benichou J-C, Buchwald M. Differential cellular expression of cystic fibrosis transmembrane regulator in human reproductive tissues. Clues for the infertility in patients with cystic fibrosis. Am J Pathol 1994; 144(5): 906-14. [PMID: 7513949]

[52] Wong PY. CFTR gene and male fertility. Mol Hum Reprod 1998; 4(2): 107-10. [http://dx.doi.org/10.1093/molehr/4.2.107] [PMID: 9542966]

[53] Schreiber R, Greger R, Nitschke R, Kunzelmann K. Cystic fibrosis transmembrane conductance regulator activates water conductance in Xenopus oocytes. Pflugers Arch 1997; 434(6): 841-7. [http://dx.doi.org/10.1007/s004240050473] [PMID: 9306020]

[54] Bernardino RL, Marinelli RA, Maggio A, *et al.* Hepatocyte and Sertoli Cell Aquaporins, Recent Advances and Research Trends. Int J Mol Sci 2016; 17(7): 1096. [http://dx.doi.org/10.3390/ijms17071096] [PMID: 27409609]

[55] Brown D, Verbavatz JM, Valenti G, Lui B, Sabolić I. Localization of the CHIP28 water channel in reabsorptive segments of the rat male reproductive tract. Eur J Cell Biol 1993; 61(2): 264-73. [PMID: 8223717]

[56] Fisher JS, Turner KJ, Fraser HM, Saunders PT, Brown D, Sharpe RM. Immunoexpression of aquaporin-1 in the efferent ducts of the rat and marmoset monkey during development, its modulation by estrogens, and its possible role in fluid resorption. Endocrinology 1998; 139(9): 3935-45. [PMID: 9724049]

[57] Elkjaer M, Vajda Z, Nejsum LN, *et al.* Immunolocalization of AQP9 in liver, epididymis, testis, spleen, and brain. Biochem Biophys Res Commun 2000; 276(3): 1118-28. [http://dx.doi.org/10.1006/bbrc.2000.3505] [PMID: 11027599]

[58] Pastor-Soler N, Bagnis C, Sabolic I, *et al.* Aquaporin 9 expression along the male reproductive tract. Biol Reprod 2001; 65(2): 384-93. [http://dx.doi.org/10.1095/biolreprod65.2.384] [PMID: 11466204]

[59] Badran HH, Hermo LS. Expression and regulation of aquaporins 1, 8, and 9 in the testis, efferent ducts, and epididymis of adult rats and during postnatal development. J Androl 2002; 23(3): 358-73. [PMID: 12002438]

[60] Pastor-Soler N, Isnard-Bagnis C, Herak-Kramberger C, *et al.* Expression of aquaporin 9 in the adult rat epididymal epithelium is modulated by androgens. Biol Reprod 2002; 66(6): 1716-22. [http://dx.doi.org/10.1095/biolreprod66.6.1716] [PMID: 12021052]

[61] Hermo L, Krzeczunowicz D, Ruz R. Cell specificity of aquaporins 0, 3, and 10 expressed in the testis, efferent ducts, and epididymis of adult rats. J Androl 2004; 25(4): 494-505. [http://dx.doi.org/10.1002/j.1939-4640.2004.tb02820.x] [PMID: 15223838]

[62] Da Silva N, Piétrement C, Brown D, Breton S. Segmental and cellular expression of aquaporins in the male excurrent duct. Biochimica et Biophysica Acta (BBA)-Biomembranes 2006; 1758: 1025-33. [http://dx.doi.org/10.1016/j.bbamem.2006.06.026]

[63] Hermo L, Schellenberg M, Liu LY, *et al.* Membrane domain specificity in the spatial distribution of aquaporins 5, 7, 9, and 11 in efferent ducts and epididymis of rats. J Histochem Cytochem 2008; 56(12): 1121-35. [http://dx.doi.org/10.1369/jhc.2008.951947] [PMID: 18796408]

[64] Alves MG, Sá R, Jesus TT, Sousa M, Oliveira PF. CFTR regulation of Aquaporin-mediated water transport: a target in male fertility. Curr Drug Targets 2015; 16(9): 993-1006. [http://dx.doi.org/10.2174/1573399811666150615144108] [PMID: 26073863]

[65] Bernardino RL, Costa AR, Martins AD, *et al.* Estradiol modulates Na(+) -dependent HCO3 (-) transporters altering intracellular pH and ion transport in human Sertoli cells: A role on male fertility? Biol Cell 2016; 108(7): 179-88. [http://dx.doi.org/10.1111/boc.201500094] [PMID: 26888167]

[66] Huang H-F, He R-H, Sun C-C, Zhang Y, Meng Q-X, Ma Y-Y. Function of aquaporins in female and male reproductive systems. Hum Reprod Update 2006; 12(6): 785-95. [http://dx.doi.org/10.1093/humupd/dml035] [PMID: 16840793]

[67] Setchell BP, Scott TW, Voglmayr JK, Waites GM. Characteristics of testicular spermatozoa and the fluid which transports them into the epididymis. Biol Reprod 1969; 1: 1-, 40-66. [http://dx.doi.org/10.1095/biolreprod1.Supplement_1.40] [PMID: 5406327]

[68] Ilio KY, Hess RA. Structure and function of the ductuli efferentes: a review. Microsc Res Tech 1994; 29(6): 432-67. [http://dx.doi.org/10.1002/jemt.1070290604] [PMID: 7873793]

[69] Wong P, Gong X, Leung G, Cheuk B. Formation of the epididymal fluid microenvironment The epididymis: from molecules to clinical practice. Springer 2002; pp. 119-30. [http://dx.doi.org/10.1007/978-1-4615-0679-9_7]

[70] Preston G, Agre P. Molecular cloning of the red cell integral protein of Mr 28000: a member of an ancient channel family. Proc Natl Acad Sci USA 1991; 88: 11110-4. [http://dx.doi.org/10.1073/pnas.88.24.11110] [PMID: 1722319]

[71] Nicòtina PA, Romeo C, Arena S, *et al.* Immunohistology of aquaporin-1 and stem cell factor-receptor in human undescended testes. Pediatr Surg Int 2004; 20(4): 271-5. [http://dx.doi.org/10.1007/s00383-003-1125-z] [PMID: 15133700]

[72] Klein C, Troedsson MH, Rutllant J. Region-specific expression of aquaporin subtypes in equine testis, epididymis, and ductus deferens. Anat Rec (Hoboken) 2013; 296(7): 1115-26. [http://dx.doi.org/10.1002/ar.22709] [PMID: 23712968]

[73] Jesus TT, Bernardino RL, Martins AD, *et al.* Aquaporin-4 as a molecular partner of cystic fibrosis transmembrane conductance regulator in rat Sertoli cells. Biochem Biophys Res Commun 2014; 446(4): 1017-21. [http://dx.doi.org/10.1016/j.bbrc.2014.03.046] [PMID: 24657265]

[74] Ishibashi K, Kuwahara M, Kageyama Y, Tohsaka A, Marumo F, Sasaki S. Cloning and functional expression of a second new aquaporin abundantly expressed in testis. Biochem Biophys Res Commun 1997; 237(3): 714-8. [http://dx.doi.org/10.1006/bbrc.1997.7219] [PMID: 9299432]

[75] Jesus TT, Bernardino RL, Martins AD, *et al.* Aquaporin-9 is expressed in rat Sertoli cells and interacts with the cystic fibrosis transmembrane conductance regulator. IUBMB Life 2014; 66(9): 639-44. [http://dx.doi.org/10.1002/iub.1312] [PMID: 25270793]

[76] Yeung CH, Callies C, Tüttelmann F, Kliesch S, Cooper TG. Aquaporins in the human testis and spermatozoa - identification, involvement in sperm volume regulation and clinical relevance. Int J Androl 2010; 33(4): 629-41. [PMID: 19840149]

[77] Domeniconi RF, Orsi AM, Justulin LA Jr, Leme Beu CC, Felisbino SL. Immunolocalization of aquaporins 1, 2 and 7 in rete testis, efferent ducts, epididymis and vas deferens of adult dog. Cell Tissue Res 2008; 332(2): 329-35. [http://dx.doi.org/10.1007/s00441-008-0592-x] [PMID: 18340467]

[78] Hermo L, Smith CE. Thirsty business: cell, region, and membrane specificity of aquaporins in the testis, efferent ducts, and epididymis and factors regulating their expression. J Androl 2011; 32(6): 565-75. [http://dx.doi.org/10.2164/jandrol.110.012831] [PMID: 21441426]

[79] Hess R, Gist D, Bunick D, *et al.* Estrogen Receptor (p) Expression in the Excurrent Ducts of the Adult Male Rat Reproductive Tract. J Androl 1997; 18.

[80] Auger J, Serres C, Wolf J, Jouannet P. Sperm motility and fertilization. Contracept Fertil Sex 1992; 1994(22): 314-8.

[81] Babcock DF, Stamerjohn DM, Hutchinson T. Calcium redistribution in individual cells correlated with ionophore action on motility. J Exp Zool 1978; 204(3): 391-9. [http://dx.doi.org/10.1002/jez.1402040310] [PMID: 351135]

[82] Morton BE, Sagadraca R, Fraser C. Sperm motility within the mammalian epididymis: species variation and correlation with free calcium levels in epididymal plasma. Fertil Steril 1978; 29(6): 695-8. [http://dx.doi.org/10.1016/S0015-0282(16)43348-0] [PMID: 658483]

[83] Jaiswal BS, Conti M. Calcium regulation of the soluble adenylyl cyclase expressed in mammalian spermatozoa. Proc Natl Acad Sci USA 2003; 100(19): 10676-81. [http://dx.doi.org/10.1073/pnas.1831008100] [PMID: 12958208]

[84] Zhu MX. Multiple roles of calmodulin and other Ca(2+)-binding proteins in the functional regulation of TRP channels. Pflugers Arch 2005; 451(1): 105-15. [http://dx.doi.org/10.1007/s00424-005-1427-1] [PMID: 15924238]

[85] Saimi Y, Kung C. Calmodulin as an ion channel subunit. Annu Rev Physiol 2002; 64: 289-311. [http://dx.doi.org/10.1146/annurev.physiol.64.100301.111649] [PMID: 11826271]

[86] Niemeyer BA, Bergs C, Wissenbach U, Flockerzi V, Trost C. Competitive regulation of CaT-lik--mediated Ca^{2+} entry by protein kinase C and calmodulin. Proc Natl Acad Sci USA 2001; 98(6): 3600-5.
[http://dx.doi.org/10.1073/pnas.051511398] [PMID: 11248124]

[87] Lambers TT, Weidema AF, Nilius B, Hoenderop JG, Bindels RJ. Regulation of the mouse epithelial Ca2(+) channel TRPV6 by the Ca(2+)-sensor calmodulin. J Biol Chem 2004; 279(28): 28855-61.
[http://dx.doi.org/10.1074/jbc.M313637200] [PMID: 15123711]

[88] Gordon-Shaag A, Zagotta WN, Gordon SE. Mechanism of Ca(2+)-dependent desensitization in TRP channels. Channels (Austin) 2008; 2(2): 125-9.
[http://dx.doi.org/10.4161/chan.2.2.6026] [PMID: 18849652]

[89] Weissgerber P, Kriebs U, Tsvilovskyy V, *et al.* Excision of Trpv6 gene leads to severe defects in epididymal Ca^{2+} absorption and male fertility much like single D541A pore mutation. J Biol Chem 2012; 287(22): 17930-41.
[http://dx.doi.org/10.1074/jbc.M111.328286] [PMID: 22427671]

[90] White DR, Aitken RJ. Relationship between calcium, cyclic AMP, ATP, and intracellular pH and the capacity of hamster spermatozoa to express hyperactivated motility. Gamete Res 1989; 22(2): 163-77.
[http://dx.doi.org/10.1002/mrd.1120220205] [PMID: 2540081]

[91] Si Y, Olds-Clarke P. Evidence for the involvement of calmodulin in mouse sperm capacitation. Biol Reprod 2000; 62(5): 1231-9.
[http://dx.doi.org/10.1095/biolreprod62.5.1231] [PMID: 10775171]

[92] Means AR, Dedman JR. Calmodulinan intracellular calcium receptor. Nature 1980; 285(5760): 73-7.
[http://dx.doi.org/10.1038/285073a0] [PMID: 6990273]

[93] Bendahmane M, Lynch C II, Tulsiani DR. Calmodulin signals capacitation and triggers the agonist-induced acrosome reaction in mouse spermatozoa. Arch Biochem Biophys 2001; 390(1): 1-8.
[http://dx.doi.org/10.1006/abbi.2001.2364] [PMID: 11368508]

[94] Schlingmann K, Michaut MA, McElwee JL, Wolff CA, Travis AJ, Turner RM. Calmodulin and CaMKII in the sperm principal piece: evidence for a motility-related calcium/calmodulin pathway. J Androl 2007; 28(5): 706-16.
[http://dx.doi.org/10.2164/jandrol.106.001669] [PMID: 17460096]

[95] Esposito G, Jaiswal BS, Xie F, *et al.* Mice deficient for soluble adenylyl cyclase are infertile because of a severe sperm-motility defect. Proc Natl Acad Sci USA 2004; 101(9): 2993-8.
[http://dx.doi.org/10.1073/pnas.0400050101] [PMID: 14976244]

[96] Litvin TN, Kamenetsky M, Zarifyan A, Buck J, Levin LR. Kinetic properties of soluble adenylyl cyclase. Synergism between calcium and bicarbonate. J Biol Chem 2003; 278(18): 15922-6.
[http://dx.doi.org/10.1074/jbc.M212475200] [PMID: 12609998]

[97] Darszon A, Labarca P, Nishigaki T, Espinosa F. Ion channels in sperm physiology. Physiol Rev 1999; 79(2): 481-510.
[PMID: 10221988]

[98] Kaupp UB, Weyand I. Cell biology. A universal bicarbonate sensor. Science 2000; 289(5479): 559-60.
[http://dx.doi.org/10.1126/science.289.5479.559] [PMID: 10939966]

[99] Kavanagh JP. Sodium, potassium, calcium, magnesium, zinc, citrate and chloride content of human prostatic and seminal fluid. J Reprod Fertil 1985; 75(1): 35-41.
[http://dx.doi.org/10.1530/jrf.0.0750035] [PMID: 4032375]

[100] Knobil E, Neill JD. Knobil and Neill's physiology of reproduction. Gulf Professional Publishing 2006.

[101] McNeal JE. Normal histology of the prostate. Am J Surg Pathol 1988; 12(8): 619-33.
[http://dx.doi.org/10.1097/00000478-198808000-00003] [PMID: 2456702]

[102] Long RM, Morrissey C, Fitzpatrick JM, Watson RW. Prostate epithelial cell differentiation and its relevance to the understanding of prostate cancer therapies. Clin Sci 2005; 108(1): 1-11. [http://dx.doi.org/10.1042/CS20040241] [PMID: 15384949]

[103] Wang Y, Hayward S, Cao M, Thayer K, Cunha G. Cell differentiation lineage in the prostate. Differentiation 2001; 68(4-5): 270-9. [http://dx.doi.org/10.1046/j.1432-0436.2001.680414.x] [PMID: 11776479]

[104] Pritchard CC, Nelson PS. Gene expression profiling in the developing prostate. Differentiation 2008; 76(6): 624-40. [http://dx.doi.org/10.1111/j.1432-0436.2008.00274.x] [PMID: 18462436]

[105] Lau K-M, LaSpina M, Long J, Ho S-M. Expression of estrogen receptor (ER)-α and ER-β in normal and malignant prostatic epithelial cells: regulation by methylation and involvement in growth regulation. Cancer Res 2000; 60(12): 3175-82. [PMID: 10866308]

[106] Humphrey GF, Mann T. Studies on the metabolism of semen. 5. Citric acid in semen. Biochem J 1949; 44(1): 97-105. [http://dx.doi.org/10.1042/bj0440097] [PMID: 16748486]

[107] Huggins C, Scott WW, Heinen JH. Chemical composition of human semen and of the secretions of the prostate and seminal vesicles. American Journal of Physiology--Legacy Content 1942; 136: 467-73.

[108] Asari M, Sasaki K, Miura K, Ichihara N, Nishita T. Immunohistolocalization of the carbonic anhydrase isoenzymes (CA-I, CA-II, and CA-III) in the reproductive tract of male horses. Am J Vet Res 1996; 57(4): 439-43. [PMID: 8712504]

[109] Kavanagh JP, Darby C. The interrelationships between acid phosphatase, aminopeptidase, diamine oxidase, citric acid, β-glucuronidase, pH and zinc in human prostatic fluid. Int J Androl 1982; 5(5): 503-12. [http://dx.doi.org/10.1111/j.1365-2605.1982.tb00282.x] [PMID: 6816744]

[110] Tanaka M, Kishi Y, Takanezawa Y, Kakehi Y, Aoki J, Arai H. Prostatic acid phosphatase degrades lysophosphatidic acid in seminal plasma. FEBS Lett 2004; 571(1-3): 197-204. [http://dx.doi.org/10.1016/j.febslet.2004.06.083] [PMID: 15280042]

[111] Moolenaar WH, Kranenburg O, Postma FR, Zondag GC. Lysophosphatidic acid: G-protein signalling and cellular responses. Curr Opin Cell Biol 1997; 9(2): 168-73. [http://dx.doi.org/10.1016/S0955-0674(97)80059-2] [PMID: 9069262]

[112] Harris H. The human alkaline phosphatases: what we know and what we dont know. Clin Chim Acta 1990; 186(2): 133-50. [http://dx.doi.org/10.1016/0009-8981(90)90031-M] [PMID: 2178806]

[113] McComb RB, Bowers GN Jr, Posen S. Alkaline phosphatase. New York: Springer Science & Business Media 2013; pp. 1-915.

[114] Kravets FG, Lee J, Singh B, Trocchia A, Pentyala SN, Khan SA. Prostasomes: current concepts. Prostate 2000; 43(3): 169-74. [http://dx.doi.org/10.1002/(SICI)1097-0045(20000515)43:3<169::AID-PROS2>3.0.CO;2-D] [PMID: 10797491]

[115] Carlini E, Palmerini CA, Cosmi EV, Arienti G. Fusion of sperm with prostasomes: effects on membrane fluidity. Arch Biochem Biophys 1997; 343(1): 6-12. [http://dx.doi.org/10.1006/abbi.1997.9999] [PMID: 9210640]

CHAPTER 9

Functional and Biochemical Aspects of Spermatozoa

Tânia R. Dias[1,2,3,*]

[1] *Health Sciences Research Center, University of Beira Interior, Rua Marquês d'Ávila e Bolama, 6201-001, Covilhã, Portugal*

[2] *Department of Microscopy, Laboratory of Cell Biology, Institute of Biomedical Sciences Abel Salazar and Unit for Multidisciplinary Research in Biomedicine, University of Porto, Rua de Jorge Viterbo Ferreira, 4050-313, Porto, Portugal*

[3] *LAQV/REQUIMTE — Laboratory of Bromatology and Hydrology, Faculty of Pharmacy, University of Porto, Rua do Campo Alegre, 4150-755, Porto, Portugal*

Abstract: The spermatozoon is a highly specialized cell that is formed through a complex cellular program of differentiation during spermatogenesis. It has a unique structure and chromatin that reflects its vital function. Morphologically it comprises a head, a midpiece and a tail. The sperm DNA is confined to the nucleus of the head and it has a characteristic protamine-based chromatin that makes it the most condensed eukaryotic DNA. This super compaction of sperm chromatin enhances the protection of DNA from damage since this cell type do not possess robust repair mechanisms. The midpiece is considered the "source of power" of spermatozoa, since it contains many mitochondria, which are responsible for the energy production required for motility. The tail, also known as flagellum, is crucial for spermatozoa movement and transit until they reach the female gamete. The morphological integrity of spermatozoa is of extreme importance for their responsiveness to testicular and epididymal factors involved in maturation. One of the main features that spermatozoa acquire during the maturational process is their motility capacity. This characteristic is not only dependent on the communication of spermatozoa with their surroundings, but also on sperm intrinsic factors, such as adenosine triphosphate (ATP) and specific membrane and secretory proteins. In recent years, sperm epigenome has been a matter of debate among researchers. Its importance is related to its impact on the embryo fate and offspring development. This chapter will discuss the significance of spermatozoa exclusive structure and function for human reproduction and the preservation of generations.

Keywords: Activated motility, Assisted Reproductive Technologies, DNA damage, Epigenetics, Fertilization, Histone, Hyperactivated motility, Protamine, Offspring, Sperm Chromatin, Sperm DNA, Spermatozoa morphology.

* **Corresponding author Tânia R. Dias:** Avenida Infante D. Henrique 6200-506 Covilhã, Portugal; Tel: +351 275 329 002; Fax: +351 275 329 099; E-mail: taniairdias@gmail.com

Marco G. Alves and Pedro F. Oliveira (Eds.)

INTRODUCTION

Spermatozoa are the male gametes shed from the seminiferous tubules after suffering a myriad of changes during the process of spermatogenesis (see Chapter 4). This cell type is essential for human fertilization and reproduction. To accomplish this concrete but fundamental goal, it is necessary that only one spermatozoon delivers its genetic material to the female egg, activates its development, and generates a new individual. The specialized structural features of mammalian spermatozoa reflect their unique functions. While the acrosome contains the essential enzymes to allow the spermatozoon to penetrate the egg and achieve fertilization, the midpiece contains the energy sources and the flagellum the machinery to generate motility [1]. Moreover, the nucleus contains the paternal genome, which is organized in 23 haploid chromosomes with a high degree of condensation. At fertilization, this set of chromosomes combines with the haploid set of the female gamete to form a diploid cell. The chromatin structure of the spermatozoon presents three main features that allow its distinction from the one of somatic cells: (1) the large majority of DNA is packaged by protamines instead of histones; (2) only 5-15% of the histone-bounded DNA is not replaced by protamines; and (3) the DNA is attached to the sperm nuclear matrix at matrix attachment regions (MARs) at medium intervals of roughly 50 kb throughout the genome [2]. Since protamines have about half the size of a typical histone [3], they contribute to the 6-fold condensation of sperm chromatin relative to somatic cells' chromatin. This specific organization presumably increases the protection of DNA during spermatozoa transit from the male to the oocyte prior to fertilization. In addition to the structural integrity of spermatozoa, its maturation and motility acquisition are also crucial factors for a successful natural reproduction. The attainment of motility by spermatozoa, is only possible in proper and controlled environmental conditions during their transit throughout the male and female reproductive tracts (see Chapter **10**). The motile pattern of spermatozoa is vital for the sperm to reach the egg. Firstly, spermatozoa motility is activated during their transit through the epididymis although this capability is only necessary after ejaculation. Then, spermatozoa are hyperactivated in the female tract, so they can achieve their fertilizing ability. In fact, if a spermatozoon lacks motility or presents an altered motile pattern, it will not be able to fertilize the oocyte, unless technological intervention is made.

Nevertheless, sperm chromatin and DNA are always susceptible to damage, which constitutes a risk factor for the development of embryo abnormalities. In fact, exposure to physical agents or chemicals, including therapeutic drugs and environmental toxicants, can affect the integrity of sperm chromatin, inducing structural, genetic and/or epigenetic alterations. Anomalies on sperm chromatin structure such as poor chromatin packaging and/or DNA damage may have an impact on male fertilizing ability. Epigenetics englobes the study of gene expression alterations that occur in the absence of changes in DNA sequence and that are fairly stable across the life of an individual [4]. Histone retention and modification, protamine incorporation into the chromatin, DNA methylation, and spermatozoa RNA transcripts appear to play important roles in the epigenetic state of mature spermatozoa. In fact, the histone-bound chromatin identifies genes that are important for embryonic development. The mechanisms by which such damage is triggered are still largely unresolved and the susceptibility of each individual will depend on their genetic background, lifestyle and exposure to various insults. Depending on the nature of the chemicals, they may directly target the DNA, induce oxidative stress, or modify the epigenetic elements. All these topics will be addressed in the present chapter, highlighting the importance of spermatozoa unique architecture for human reproduction and evolution.

SPERM ULTRASTRUCTURE AND CHROMATIN

Morphology of Human Spermatozoa

Spermatozoa present a unique and complex morphology. In general, they comprise a head, a midpiece and a tail region (Fig. **9.1**), commonly known as flagellum [5]. The spermatozoon is smaller than most cells in the body, but its size does not reflect its fundamental function of generating a new human being. The size, shape of the head, length and relative amount of the different components of the flagellum is species-specific [1]. The head of human seminal spermatozoa is pear-shaped, with a median length of 4.4 μm and width of about 3 μm [6]. The nucleus occupies most of the sperm head area and contains a haploid set of condensed, genetically inactive chromosomes [7]. The apical half of the nucleus is covered by the acrosome (Fig. **9.1**), which represents about 48% of the sperm head surface [6]. This acrosomal cap is a membrane-enclosed cytoplasmic vesicle originating from the Golgi apparatus during sperm formation [8]. It contains several polysaccharides (*e.g.* galactose, mannose, fructose, and hexosamine) [9] and hydrolytic enzymes with a preponderant role in the penetration of the sperm into the egg membranes [5]. The part of the nucleus that is not overlaid by the acrosome cap constitutes the postacrosomal region [10]. The sperm head also contains a small amount of cytoplasm and several cytoskeletal structures, including the dense perinuclear layer that is made of basic proteins (*e.g.* calicin and cylicin) associated with calmodulin and actin filaments [11]. On the base of the sperm head there is a small structure called connecting piece (or neck) that connects the head to the midpiece. The connecting piece harbors the proximal centriole and the empty vault. The proximal centriole is composed of nine microtubule triplets and has a vital role on the orchestration of cell division in the embryo, while the empty vault is originated after the degradation of the distal centriole during spermiogenesis [12]. The connecting piece provides a basal anchor to the axoneme and is covered by several redundant nuclear envelopes [13]. It has also been proposed to be responsible for flagellum beat initiation and alternating directions of bends propagating down the beating flagellum [14].

The midpiece has a cylindrical shape and has about 5-9 μm of length and half the width of the sperm head (Fig. **9.1**) [15]. Its structure consists of numerous mitochondria spirally arranged around the outer dense fibers (ODF) and the central axial filament - axoneme [1]. The mitochondrial sheath is responsible for the production of adenosine triphosphate (ATP), which is the energy supply needed for tail motility during the migration upon the female reproductive tract. The axoneme is essentially a long, specialized cilium formed by a core of microtubules, surrounded by ODF extending from the connecting piece to the principal piece. It has a characteristic "9+2" structure, *i.e.*, two central singlet microtubules encircled by nine outer doublet microtubules (A- and B-tubules). Radial links connect the central microtubule pair to each surrounding microtubule doublet, and nexin bridges connect adjacent doublets [16]. Outer and inner dyneins are observed as projecting "arms" that slide along each outer doublet microtubule. This active sliding has been associated with spermatozoa flagellar movement [17]. A cytoplasmic droplet is frequently found at the midpiece or at the junction of the midpiece with the principal piece in human mature spermatozoa. This tiny droplet-like structure is usually retained after the removal of spermatids cytoplasm by Sertoli cells at the end of spermiogenesis, and is suggested to play a key role in sperm volume adaptation [18]. At the distal part of the mitochondrial sheath of sperm midpiece is a traverse septin-based ring called annulus (Fig. **9.1**) that is the hallmark of the separation between the midpiece and the principal piece [19].

The sperm tail is the only functional flagellum in humans and it can be divided into principal piece and end piece. The principal piece constitutes most of the tail, having an average length of 40-45 μm [15]. It is constituted by the axoneme surrounded by a sheath of supportive fibers composed of two longitudinal columns that run parallel to ODF (Fig. **9.1**). The main function of principal piece is to propel the spermatozoon towards the oocyte, changing both the amplitude and frequency of the whip-like movement of the tail to facilitate sperm hyperactivation and egg penetration.

Finally, the end piece is the narrowest part of the sperm and is about 4-5 μm long [15]. It consists of the axoneme and the ends of ODF and fibrous sheath [7]. Moreover, the whole spermatozoon is enveloped by a plasma membrane that presents a high lipid content, especially of polyunsaturated fatty acids (PUFAs)

[20, 21]. This biochemical constitution confers a fluidity and flexibility to the sperm plasma membrane, which is essential for the fusion with the oocyte membrane at fertilization [21]. Overall, the morphological integrity of spermatozoa is vital for their adequate response to further maturational processes and for the acquisition of fertilizing ability.

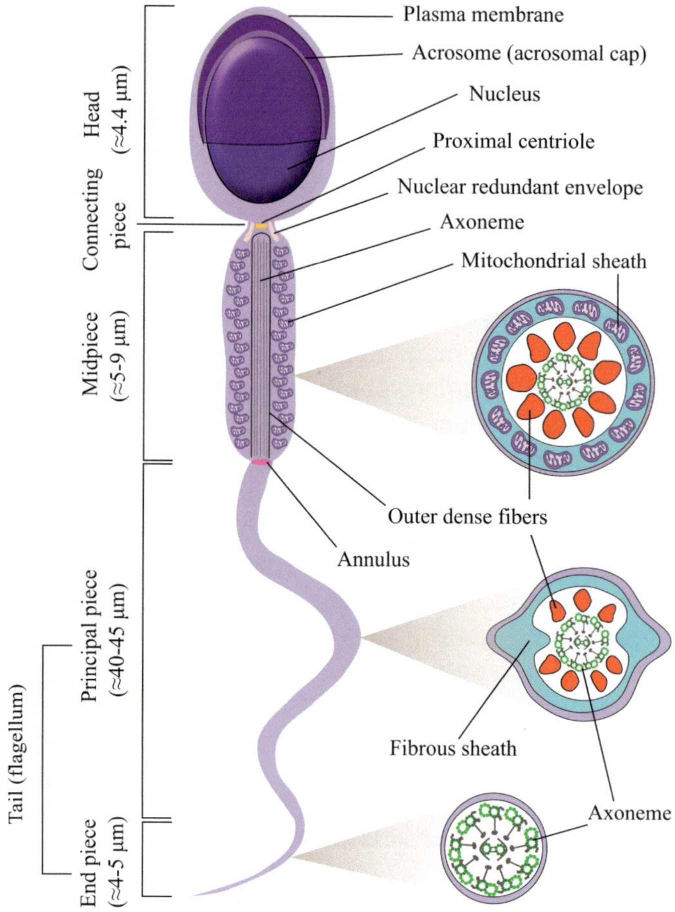

Fig. (9.1). Schematic representation of human spermatozoon structure. It is constituted by the head, connecting piece, midpiece, principal piece and end piece. The head is mainly composed by the nucleus that is enveloped by the acrosome. The connecting piece contains the proximal centriole surrounded by the nuclear redundant envelopes. The midpiece holds the mitochondrial sheath, which is the site of energy production. These several mitochondria are organized around the outer dense fibres and the axoneme. The axoneme extends from the basis of the head (connecting piece) until the end of the sperm flagellum. Separating the midpiece and the beginning of the tail is a ring-like small structure called annulus. The tail comprises the principal piece that is the lengthiest part of the spermatozoon, and the end piece, the narrowest part. Besides the axoneme, the principal piece also contains the outer dense fibres surrounded by a fibrous sheath. The end piece is mainly composed by the axoneme. The spermatozoon is enveloped by a plasma membrane.

Characterization of Sperm Chromatin

The structural arrangement of sperm chromatin is vital to the proper functioning of these cells. The chromatin structure of spermatozoa is organized to resist to conditions that could damage the DNA. At the same time the chromatin must have the property of rapidly making the DNA available to the ooplasm. Sperm DNA is contained in the nucleus of the sperm head, occupying much of the nuclear volume. Though, it is the most tightly condensed eukaryotic DNA, being at least 6-fold more compacted than the DNA in somatic cells [22]. This is mostly due to the different types of DNA packaging. In the case of somatic cell nuclei and mitotic chromosomes, DNA is wrapped around histone octamers forming nucleosomes [23]. The nucleosomes are then further coiled into regular helixes called solenoids [24]. Concerning sperm DNA, it is known that, during spermiogenesis, the vast majority of histones is replaced with transition proteins and then with protamines (Fig. **9.2**) [25]. During this process of remodeling/compaction of sperm chromatin, naturally occurring DNA strand breaks induced by topoisomerase II arise to relieve the torsional stresses that accompany the transition of sperm chromatin from an exclusively nucleosomal to a predominantly protamine-based configuration [26]. Protamines are small and highly basic proteins responsible for the higher degree of sperm chromatin compaction. Human sperm contain two types of protamines, P1 and P2, both present in roughly equal quantities [27]. Alteration in this 1:1 ratio have been correlated with general infertility and poor fertilization ability [28]. These protamines are very rich in positively charged arginine residues (55-79%), which neutralize the strong negative charges of the phosphate groups in the DNA backbone, thus permitting a strong DNA binding [29]. They also contain several cysteines that are responsible for conferring increased stability to sperm chromatin through multiple inter- and intraprotamine disulfide cross-links [29]. During the transit of spermatozoa through the epididymis, a final stage of chromatin organization occurs to originate an even more compacted chromatin. This process involves loss of water, an increase in the formation of disulfide bonds, and an additional reduction in the volume of sperm nuclei. Moreover, throughout this sperm epididymal maturation there is a complete restriction of the facilities for DNA replication and transcription [30]. Typically, this super-compacted sperm DNA occupies a 40-fold lower volume than somatic cells' DNA [31]. Furthermore, the human sperm chromatin contains zinc, more specifically one zinc ion for each protamine molecule [27]. This feature allows the formation of zinc-stabilized structures (zinc fingers) among histidines and cysteines, thus locking the tertiary structure and thereby reducing the number of accessible conformations of the protamine. This increases the conformational stability of these proteins when interacting with DNA [25]. Protamines bounded to sperm DNA form doughnut-loop domains (Fig. **9.2**), known as toroids, that contain roughly 50 kb of DNA [2]. Protamine toroids may be organized to form a linear, side-by-side arrays of chromatin (Fig. **9.2**), resulting in an extremely condensed chromatin, in which most of DNA is hidden within the toroid [32]. Each protamine toroid contains a single DNA loop domain [33]. The toroid exists in a semi-crystalline state and is resistant to nuclease digestion, thus protecting DNA from degradation [34]. However, between each protamine toroid, there is a nuclease sensitive segment of chromatin called the toroid linker (Fig. **9.2**), which is also the site of attachment of DNA to sperm proteinaceous nuclear matrix, commonly known as MARs [35]. The protamine-based configuration of sperm DNA facilitates its protection, transport and safe delivery to the oocyte [36]. Nevertheless, the haploid chromatin of human sperm usually retains 5–15% of histones [37], a higher percentage in comparison to other mammalian species (*e.g.*, bulls, hamsters, and mice) that only retain up to 5% [38]. Therefore, compared to other mammalian species, human sperm chromatin is relatively less compact. Histones are important for the regulation of the degree of DNA compaction and modulation of gene expression, since they can be modified by post-translational modifications (PTMs) that restrict or facilitate the access of transcription factors to the DNA [39]. Several histones have been identified in human sperm, including nuclear proteins histone 2A and 2B (H2A and H2B), histone 3 (H3), histone 4 (H4), and the testis-specific histone (tH2B) [40, 41]. Some studies have demonstrated that the distribution of histones throughout the sperm genome is not random, as they seem to be associated with specific genes [37, 42]. It has been suggested that histones are present in relatively large tracts of DNA, from 10 to 100 kb, and in smaller tracts of DNA interspersed throughout the genome. Moreover, the nuclease sensitivity at MARs suggests that these protamine linker regions are bounded by histones [37, 42].

After fertilization, sperm chromatin decondenses and protamines are completely replaced by histones in the first 2–4 h, so that the paternal chromatin has the same accessible chromatin as all other somatic cells [43]. Sperm nuclear matrix is also disrupted at fertilization, but sperm nuclei contain a unique structure called sperm nuclear annulus to which the entire complement of DNA seems to be anchored [44]. The sperm nuclear matrix acts as a checkpoint for sperm DNA integrity after fertilization, being essential for DNA replication [2]. While protamines are unique to mature spermatozoa, histones and MARs are both found in somatic cells and can be presumed to be residual from the sperm progenitor cells from which spermatozoa are produced [2]. These findings provide evidence for the protective role of protamines during the transit of spermatozoa from testis to the moment of fertilization. The structural organization of both histone-bound chromatin and sperm MARs are probably transmitted to the newly formed paternal pronucleus after fertilization and suggests that both are required for proper embryogenesis. It is possible that the newly fertilized oocytes inherit histone-based chromatin structural organization from the sperm (Fig. **9.2**) [2]. These intricate features of sperm chromatin are essential for sperm function and for the success of fertilization.

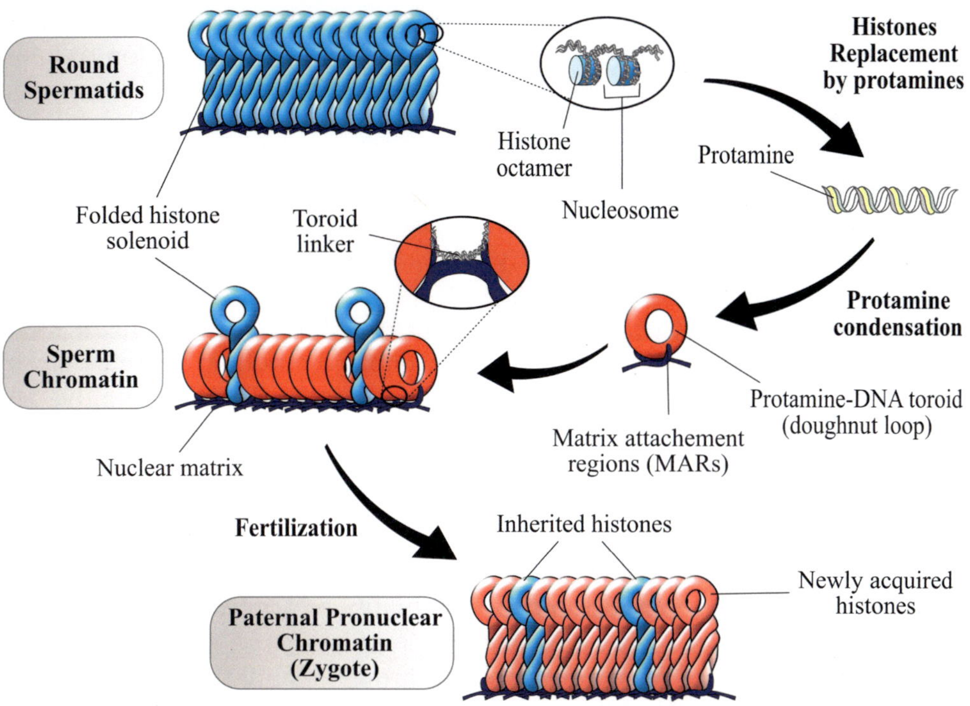

Fig. (9.2). Schematic representation of human sperm chromatin remodelling. The DNA of round spermatids is typically bounded to histone octamers, forming nucleosomes. These structures are folded into regular loops called solenoids. During spermatogenesis, most of this histone-based chromatin is replaced by protamines. However, 5-15% of the histones are retained. Protamines condensation leads to the formation of doughnut loops, known as toroids, to increase DNA protection. Protamine toroids are usually organized side-by-side, linked between each other by a nuclease sensitive segment of chromatin called the toroid linker. This structure also constitutes the site of attachment of DNA to the nuclear matrix - matrix attachment regions (MARs). At fertilization, the sperm chromatin decondenses and protamines are completely replaced by histones. The histones that have not been replaced during spermatogenesis are the inherited ones, whereas those that have been replaced are, at this point, newly acquired histones. It is believed that the retained histones carry the paternal epigenetic marks to the zygote. The MARs are also probably retained in the paternal pronucleus.

NOVEL MODULATORS OF SPERM MOTILITY

The acquisition of motility is one of the most important features of spermatozoa for a successful natural reproduction. Besides their single morphology and chromatin, their uniflagellar movement is essential for their course to encounter the female gamete and fuse with it. Although sperm count and viability are common parameters correlated with fertility, it is necessary only one spermatozoon from a population of hundreds of millions to fertilize the egg. However, a non-motile or abnormally-motile sperm is not able to fertilize unless technological intervention is made [45]. Hence, the assessment of motility is a central part of the evaluation of sperm quality to estimate the fertilizing ability of an individual. The sperm flagellum is a complex structure that contains the essential machinery for sperm movement. In addition, the acquisition of sperm motility is mostly regulated by the communication with the surrounding environment [46].

When spermatozoa are released from the seminiferous epithelium, the flagellum is immotile. During spermatozoa transit through the male reproductive tract, spermatozoa acquire activated motility [47]. This type of motility is mostly characterized by organized movements of the flagellum, as seen in freshly ejaculated sperm [48]. The passage through the epididymis is a key factor for the activation of sperm motility, since the epididymal epithelium secretes several proteins involved in motility acquisition (see Chapter **7**). Surprisingly, it is believed that epididymal spermatozoa are largely immotile (quiescent state) [49]. In the proximal regions of epididymis, spermatozoa are still very immature. Then, once the capacity for motility is acquired by spermatozoa, the composition of the epididymal distal regions keep the sperm flagellar movement almost arrested via the low pH, low concentrations of Na^+ and high concentrations of K^+ [50]. Besides the epididymis, the ionic composition and osmolality of seminal plasma and male accessory fluids are also essential for the regulation of the pH to which spermatozoa are subjected during their transit through the male reproductive tract (see Chapter **8**). On ejaculation, spermatozoa are subjected to changes in the external medium composition, passing through high ionic strength fluids of low osmolality, low K^+ and high Na^+, which contribute for motility activation [51]. The flagellum of an activated sperm generates a symmetrical, lower-amplitude waveform that drives the sperm almost in straight line in relatively non-viscous media, such as seminal plasma [46]. In addition, mammalian sperm display other type of physiological motility, the so-called hyperactivated motility, as seen in most sperm collected from the fertilization site. At some point after the spermatozoon reaches the oviduct, the flagellum is hyperactivated. Subsequently, the pattern of the flagellar beat changes to an asymmetric movement of higher amplitude, resulting in sudden changes in the direction of travel [52, 53]. It has been suggested that hyperactivated motility helps sperm to detach from the oviductal epithelium, move progressively through the oviductal environment to reach the site of fertilization, and penetrate the egg membrane [54].

The communication of spermatozoa with their surroundings is of extreme importance to attain activated and hyperactivated motility, although, these processes are mediated by sperm intrinsic factors, including ATP, specific membrane and secretory proteins [55]. The ATP produced at sperm midpiece constitutes the energy source for sperm motility acquisition. This feature is mediated by the phosphorylation/dephosphorylation and the associated activation and inactivation of the axonemal dynein arms. When dynein become phosphorylated, dynein ATPase enzyme hydrolyzes ATP and convert it into a unidirectional force [56]. Then, each dynein arm interacts with its adjacent microtubular doublet and generate a power stroke that forces the microtubules to slide past one another [57]. Since the axoneme is anchored to the base of the sperm head, this sliding force is translated into a bend in the flagellum. Dephosphorylation of dynein by the calmodulin-dependent protein phosphatase calcineurin reverses this process [46]. This protein phosphorylation and dephosphorylation is tightly regulated by the coordinated and opposed activity of protein kinases and protein phosphatases. While protein kinases transfer a phosphate group from ATP or guanosine triphosphate (GTP) to a given protein, typically at serine, threonine, or tyrosine residues, protein phosphatases catalyze the removal of phosphate groups from specific residues and revert proteins to a non-phosphorylated conformation [58]. Among sperm protein kinases is the protein kinase A (PKA), also known as cAMP-dependent protein kinase, since it is only activated when cAMP is present [59]. Mammalian sperm cAMP synthesis is catalyzed by a unique adenylyl cyclase termed soluble adenylyl cyclase (sAC). At ejaculation, this enzyme is activated by the increased extracellular bicarbonate concentration (9-10-fold increase) [60]. sAC has an affinity for ATP in the millimolar range, rendering the enzyme sensitive to fluctuations in ATP production. cAMP assists sperm protein phosphorylation by PKA, which controls the phosphorylation state of functional proteins in the flagellar axoneme [61]. Mature spermatozoa contain specific A-kinase anchoring proteins (AKAPs), such as AKAP3 and AKAP4, which are associated with the cytoskeletal fibrous sheath of sperm flagella [62]. The PKA binding to AKAP molecules by the interaction with their regulatory subunits regulates sperm motility [63]. In fact, the disruption of this interaction between PKA with AKAPs may lead to the inhibition of sperm motility [64]. Thus, cAMP/PKA signaling evidences a pivotal role in initiation, maintenance and control of sperm motility. Moreover, mitochondrial F1-ATPase is also known to be a target of PKA signaling pathway [65]. Since the activation of this complex leads to an increased production of ATP, the phosphorylation (at serine residues) of F1-ATPase in epididymal spermatozoa is suggested to be relevant for motility [66]. Other protein kinase that correlates with sperm motility is glycogen synthase kinase 3 (GSK3), more specifically α and β isoforms [67, 68]. Phosphorylation of GSK3 leads to the inhibition of its activity, and cAMP-dependent PKA is one of the proteins that negatively regulate GSK3 activity. Serine/tyrosine phosphorylation of GSK3 significantly increases in sperm during their passage through the epididymis [68, 69]. In fact, immotile caput sperm contain 6-fold higher GSK3 activity than sperm at cauda epididymis, which contrastingly are motile-activated [68]. GSK3 activity is correlated with protein phosphatase 1 (PP1) function, which is also a key regulator of sperm motility. The activity of PP1 is controlled by the presence of specific inhibitors, including the inhibitor-2, thus forming a PP1–I2 complex. GSK3 is involved in the dissociation of this complex through the reactivation of PP1. The catalytic activity of this enzyme is known to change during epididymal maturation and a decreased activity has been associated with an increase in sperm motility [70]. In fact, the activity of the testis-specific isoform of PP1 (known as PP1γ2) in immature sperm is two-fold higher than in mature motile caudal spermatozoa. Thus, the inhibition of PP1γ2 activity is involved in both motility initiation and motility stimulation [71]. However, targeted disruption of this phosphatase gene in mice, results in male sterility characterized by sperm tail malformation [72]. Recent studies on mature sperm from mice [73, 74] and humans [75] have revealed that a Src family kinase (SFK) is able to inactivate Serine/Threonine phosphatases, thus being involved in the signaling pathways associated with sperm motility. This tyrosine kinase has been detected in the midpiece of mature mouse sperm, but not in sperm of the caput region, as Src is only incorporated into sperm during their transit from the corpus to the cauda [76]. Src-null mice have demonstrated normal tyrosine phosphorylation, although forward sperm motility has been significantly reduced [76]. Other pathways that have been suggested to be involved in the phosphorylation of proteins associated with mature sperm motility include: phosphatidylinositol 3 kinase-protein kinase B/AKT (PI3K–PKB/AKT) [77, 78], mitogen activate protein kinase (MAPK) [79], Janus kinase/signal transducers and activators of transcription (JAK/STAT) [20], but the intricate mechanisms are not clear.

The influx of Ca^{+2} across spermatozoa membrane is important for triggering several cell functions, including flagellar movement. The intracellular Ca^{+2} in mammalian sperm is controlled by sperm-specific Ca^{+2} channels called cation channels of sperm (CatSper). The CatSper channel complex comprises four homologous α subunits (CatSper 1–4) that are located on the sperm tail and are involved in sperm hyper-activation and fertility by calcium influx [80, 81]. It also includes at least three auxiliary CatSper subunits: β, γ and δ [82]. When reaching the oviduct, progesterone and prostaglandins activate CatSper channels, thus modulating sperm motility hyperactivation [83, 84]. CatSper are members of the voltage-gated ion channel superfamily that includes voltage-gated potassium, sodium, and calcium channels; cyclic nucleotide regulated (CNG) channels; and transient receptor potential (Trp) channels [85]. Both CatSper1 and CatSper2 calcium channels are specifically present in the principal piece of mature sperm flagellum [86, 87]. CatSper1 is required for cAMP-induced calcium influx into sperm [46]. Targeted deletion of the CatSper1 gene results in the ablation of the cAMP-stimulated rise in intracellular sperm calcium, leading to male infertility due to poor sperm motility [86]. It has also been demonstrated that the targeted deletion of the CatSper2 gene results in the absence of hyperactivated sperm motility and hence male infertility [87]. Thus, channel-mediated movement of extracellular calcium into the flagellum is required for both types of motility. Among the calcium permeable channels of spermatozoa, only CatSper1 and CatSper2 are known to be critical for male fertility.

The sperm sodium–hydrogen exchanger (sNHE), also present on the principal piece of the sperm flagellum, is involved in the exchange of cations for protons across the cell membrane [88]. The disruption of the sNHE gene causes complete male-specific infertility as a result of a dramatic effect on spermatozoon motility [89]. sNHE appears to establish a molecular link between spermatozoon pHi and cyclic nucleotide metabolism in the motility signaling system [90]. Although, sNHE signaling pathways are largely unknown, it has been suggested to be important for the stabilization of the functional sAC enzyme [88].

SPERM CHROMATIN INTEGRITY AS A PARAMETER OF SPERM QUALITY

Throughout the years, standard semen parameters have been established to assess whether a male can be considered fertile or infertile. Among those are included: sperm count, viability, motility and morphology [91, 92]. However, these parameters do not evaluate the quality of the sperm nuclear material. Sperm DNA or its chromatin structure are likely susceptible to damage, not only during spermatogenesis, but also through its pathway to encounter the female gamete. Among the several factors that may lead to sperm DNA damages are included: (1) unrepaired DNA breaks during chromatin remodeling and packaging during spermiogenesis; (2) abortive apoptosis, which may lead to the misleading elimination of germ cells from the genetic pool; (3) increased oxidative stress either resulting from internal or external production of reactive oxygen species (ROS); (4) action of endogenous endonucleases and caspases; and (5) exposure to genotoxic agents, either from a certain therapeutic approach or occupational/ environmental reasons [93]. Most likely, these factors are interrelating, and are known to have a negative impact on male fertility rates. Particularly, the excessive generation of ROS has been associated with poor semen quality and sperm DNA fragmentation [94]. The susceptibility of spermatozoon for ROS attack relates to the high content in PUFAs of its plasma membrane, in combination with the lack of antioxidants and DNA repair systems in these cells [21]. Antioxidant defenses such as catalase and superoxide dismutase are present in most somatic cells cytoplasm. Since there is a removal of most spermatozoon cytoplasm during spermatogenesis, these specialized cells lost most of those compounds. Moreover, since they contain a large number of mitochondria, there is an electron leakage that may lead to the generation of high amounts of ROS. Consequently, the antioxidant defensive capacity becomes limited [95].

The increasing rates of subfertility/infertility among young couples has led to a higher demand on the accuracy of sperm parameters analysis. Therefore, the prognostic value of sperm DNA and chromatin integrity tests has been highlighted in the evaluation of fertility problems and reproductive outcomes. Several types of assays have been developed in order to detect chromosomal aberrations [96], DNA fragmentation and compaction [97 - 99], and protamination defects [100]. So far, the test that has demonstrated the most accurate clinical results in terms of fertility outcomes is the sperm chromatin structure assay (SCSA), a flow cytometric test that measures the susceptibility of sperm DNA to acid-induced DNA denaturation in situ [98]. While the DNA of sperm with a normal chromatin structure do not denature, if the DNA is somewhat damaged and contains breaks in the DNA strands it can reach different degrees of denaturation [93]. In this test, spermatozoa are subjected to a mild acid treatment and then are stained with a fluorescent dye called acridine orange [101]. Through a specific SCSA software (SCSA-Soft; SCSA Diagnostics, Inc., Brookings, SD, USA), a scatter plot is created, showing the ratio of green and red sperm [93]. Sperm fluoresces in green when the fluorochrome is intercalated between intact double-stranded DNA and fluoresces in red in single-stranded DNA. The percentage of red sperm reflects the amount of spermatozoa with denatured DNA and is expressed as a DNA fragmentation index (DFI) [101]. Population-based studies have evidenced the excellent prediction power of this assay concerning the achievement of pregnancy [102, 103]. A DFI between 0–20%, reflected a constant chance of spontaneous pregnancy. When DFI was 20%, the chance of obtaining a spontaneous pregnancy was decreased and when the DFI level passed 30–40%, the change was close to zero. Even though, when DFI was <20%, only 13% of all cycles resulted in a pregnancy. These results demonstrate that, in a normal population, not selected because of infertility problems, SCSA is a valuable tool to identify men who are at risk of not giving rise to a pregnancy. It is not possible to get the same information from the traditional sperm parameters [102, 103]. Moreover, other study with the same SCSA test, evidenced the increased risk of being infertile when the DFI was >20% in men with normal standard semen parameters [104].

The evaluation of sperm DNA integrity has also been highlighted in assisted reproductive technologies (ART). In fact, there has been an increasing association between sperm DNA integrity and fertility, success of *in vitro* fertilization (IVF) techniques and pregnancy rates [105]. It has been reported that a DFI value >27% is associated with pregnancy failure in ART [106, 107]. However, recent studies demonstrated that even spermatozoa with high DFI can be used to achieve pregnancy with help of IVF techniques and intracytoplasmic sperm injection (ICSI), but it is still unclear whether the chance of pregnancy is related to the level of DFI [108]. This question needs to be further investigated, but the relevance of DNA fragmentation assays in the evaluation of sperm quality is evidently clear.

SPERM EPIGENOME AND IMPLICATIONS TO OFFSPRING

Epigenetics can be defined as the study of mitotically or meiotically heritable modifications in the function of specific genes, without considering alterations in DNA sequence [109]. Based on previously held beliefs, spermatozoa were thought to be incompetent to drive epigenetic changes in the embryo, since it was believed to occur a total substitution of histones by protamines. Contrastingly to protamines, histones are capable of eliciting gene activation or silencing via tail modifications (*e.g.* methylation or acetylation). Recently, this dogma has changed and it is known that protamination is incomplete and a small percentage of histones is retained, thus probably transmitting certain characteristics of paternal genome to the zygote. It has been shown that histone retention in fertile patients is found at the promoters of genes important in the embryo, including developmental gene promoters, microRNA clusters, and imprinted loci, suggesting that the nucleosome retention is programmatic in nature [37]. Accordingly, an increasing interest has arisen concerning the study of the role of sperm epigenome as a determinant of embryo fate and progeny development [110]. Growing evidence suggests that mature sperm provide appropriate epigenetic marks (Box 9.1) that drive specific genes toward activation and contribute to the pluripotent state of the embryonic cells [111].

Box 9.1 | Summary

- Histone retention and modification:
  - Protamine incorporation into sperm chromatin;
  - Distribution of histones and protamines throughout the genome;
- DNA methylation;
- Spermatozoal RNA transcripts.

DNA Methylation

One of the major epigenetic marks established during spermatogenesis is DNA methylation, which involves the methylation of cytosine residues, mainly (60-

80%) at cytosine-phosphate-guanine (CpG) dinucleotides [112]. Genomic methylation patterns in somatic differentiated cells are generally stable and heritable. Sperm DNA methylation is essential to allele-specific imprinting of certain genes, regulation of gene expression, and inactivation of X chromosome [113]. CpG dinucleotides found in high concentrations near the gene promoter are potent inhibitors of transcription when methylated. While hypermethylation at promoters blocks the access of transcriptional machinery, inhibiting gene expression; hypomethylation facilitates gene activation, since there is an increased accessibility of polymerase to DNA [111]. The process of DNA methylation is catalyzed by enzymes known as DNA methyltransferases (DNMTs) [114]. Recent data concerning the human sperm methylome, classified a 'normal' methylation status of genomic CpGs at 96% [115]. Aberrant methylation of promoters for specific genes was associated with sperm defects and male infertility [116, 117]. The process of DNA methylation is closely related with gametogenesis. After fertilization, there is an active demethylation of sperm DNA that is contrasted with passive demethylation of maternally derived DNA. Subsequently, there is a resetting of the primordial germ cells, resulting in the remodeling of the parental-specific methylation patterns of imprinted genes [117]. Then, de novo monoallelic sex-specific methylation takes place during gametogenesis, so that the offspring imprinted genes are exclusively expressed from either the paternal or the maternal allele [118]. These data suggest that DNA methylation plays an essential role not only in sperm, but also in the embryo.

Histones Retention and Associated Modifications

Histones retention and modification represent other epigenetic chromatin marks, which is critical for transcriptional regulation [119]. Alterations in histone retention can affect sperm function at two levels. Firstly, they could alter protamine content and the tightly regulated P1/P2 ratio, which is indicative of poor semen quality, increased DNA damage and decreased fertility [120, 121]. In fact, sperm concentration, motility, and morphology were found to be significantly reduced in patients with either a low or high P1/P2 ratio, as compared to patients with a normal ratio [122]. An altered P1/P2 ratio has also been correlated with a negative impact on embryo quality and IVF outcome [121]. Moreover, an increased histone to protamine ratio is often present in infertile men when compared to fertile counterparts with a subset of infertile men possessing complete protamine deficiency [28]. Secondly, alterations in histone retention may induce the incorrect distribution of histones and protamines throughout the genome, which may have an impact on normal embryo development [111].

Concerning the PTMs, these occur at lysine and serine residues of histones tail, and can influence targeted gene activation or silencing. The main forms of modifications in sperm include methylation, acetylation, ubiquitination, and phosphorylation, which can act alone or in combination. Histone modifications are dynamic, since they can be easily induced and removed by a wide range of enzymes. Acetylation is the most relevant histone change. It occurs at lysine residues on the amino-terminal tail domains and is regulated by the action of histone acetyl transferase (HAT) and histone deacetylase (HDAC) [123]. Generally, acetylation reduces the affinity of histones for DNA, making genes functionally active, whereas histone deacetylation leads to chromatin condensation, making genes transcriptionally inactive [119]. On the other hand, histone methylation is a key regulator for both activation and inactivation of transcription. Methylation and demethylation are catalyzed by the histone methyltransferase and demethylase [124]. Histone methylation on lysine (K) residues of H3 or H4 can promote gene activation and/or repression. For example, while methylation at lysine 4 of histone H3 (H3-K4) is linked to gene expression, H3K9 and H3K27 di- and tri-methylation is associated with gene silencing [125]. Nevertheless, sperm genome regions that remain bounded to nucleosomes appear to be associated with hypomethylated DNA. This highlights the involvement of transcriptional activation of specific gene families in early cell differentiation and embryogenesis, perhaps in the early embryo [111]. Moreover, altered patterns of sperm DNA and histone methylation have been reported in infertile men, supporting earlier studies into the relationship between DNA methylation and pregnancy outcome in IVF techniques [121].

Spermatozoal RNA Transcripts

The presence of RNA molecules in spermatozoa suggests another type of regulatory mechanism that is implicated in conveying epigenetic information [126]. The types of RNA molecules present in spermatozoa include mRNAs and non-coding RNAs. During spermatogenesis there is an active post-transcriptional protein-coding mRNA regulation, which is especially important at later steps when chromatin compaction induces transcriptional silencing in elongating spermatids [127]. The small non-coding RNAs are not used as a template for protein synthesis, but they function as cellular modulators of gene expression at post-transcriptional or translational level, to control the properties of their target mRNAs. Several small RNAs have been identified in sperm, including Dicer-dependent microRNAs (miRNAs) and endogenous small interfering RNAs (endo-siRNAs), as well as Dicer-independent PIWI-interacting RNAs (piRNAs) [128]. During spermatozoa differentiation, miRNAs mediate the stage-specific control of gene expression by affecting the stability of their target mRNAs or, in some cases, the translation of mRNAs [129]. The post-transcriptional RNA regulation by endo-siRNAs involves the induction of target mRNA degradation or silencing. Although the main targets for the testicular endo-siRNAs are mRNAs (92%), they can also target transcripts of pseudogenes (3%), retrotransposons (1%), and non-coding RNAs (4%) [127]. Concerning piRNAs, their functions are mediated through binding to PIWI proteins, which are predominantly expressed in the germline of a variety of organisms [130]. In mammals, different populations of piRNAs have been identified in spermatogonia, spermatocytes and spermatids. It has been demonstrated that piRNAs are not only involved in male germ line development, but also in retrotransposon repression and epigenetic regulation [131]. Since the retention of spermatozoal RNA transcripts in spermatozoa begins to occur during early stages of spermatogenesis, it came the possibility that these small molecules can carry hereditary information from one generation to the next [119]. It appears that spermatozoal RNA transcripts are capable of inhibiting the protamination process, thus maintaining a histone-bound chromatin structure [126]. RNA transcripts colocalize with nucleosome-bound chromatin near the nuclear envelope in the mature sperm. Although this mechanism is not fully understood, this colocalization seems to provide a possible explanation for the regulation of histone retention. A selective retention in sperm seems to be advantageous for targeted gene activation or silencing in the embryo [111]. Spermatozoal RNAs also seem to possess the capacity to regulate histone modifications and DNA methylation, whereas the chromatin structure and DNA modifications in turn may affect transcription of RNAs [132]. The genetic origins of RNAs identified in sperm are highly correlated with regions of the genome that are hypomethylated and enriched in histone proteins, especially those with H3K4me3 modifications. RNAs present in the mature spermatozoa are delivered to the oocyte, thus triggering essential functions during early embryogenesis [133]. Still, studies should be made to further disclose the biochemical mechanistic behind these processes.

CONCLUDING REMARKS

The spermatozoon has the fundamental function of generating a new individual. This concrete goal is the basis of life and perpetuation of generations. The unique architecture of spermatozoa ultrastructure and chromatin is well-organized and plays a direct role in their functions. There is a preponderant role of all sperm structures in the establishment of the connection between the spermatozoon and the oocyte, at fertilization. The tail motile pattern is crucial for the spermatozoon to travel from the site of its storage in the epididymis, until it reaches the oocyte at the female reproductive tract. The nucleus carries the most important part of spermatozoa, the sperm DNA that will be combined with the genetic material of the oocyte during fertilization. The success of this peculiar process requires not only the physical integrity of spermatozoa, but also the integrity of the paternal genome. Mammalian sperm chromatin has an intricate organization that presumably increases DNA protection, however there are several internal and external factors that can lead to genetic and epigenetic damages. Several tests, mainly SCSA, have demonstrated a high potential in evaluating sperm DNA fragmentation and its association with fertility outcomes. However, more studies should be made to reach clear and clinically useful data for inferring male fertility potential for a semen sample. The combination of several tests is certainly a measure to be considered in the future. Moreover, the findings concerning sperm epigenome challenge the widely-assumed notion that the paternal genome does not provide any epigenetic contribution to the offspring. Despite the advances in the identification of several epigenetic markers, this topic should be further investigated since it constitutes an excellent approach to control the pregnancy outcomes.

CONFLICT OF INTEREST

The authors confirm that they have no conflict of interest to declare for this publication.

ACKNOWLEDGEMENTS

This work was supported by the "Fundação para a Ciência e a Tecnologia" – FCT: CICS (UID/Multi/00709/2013), UMIB (PEst-OE/SAU/UI0215/2014) and REQUIMTE (UID/QUI/50006/2013); and by FEDER through the POPH and POCI - COMPETE 2020 (POCI-01-0145-FEDER-007491) funds. Tânia R. Dias (SFRH/BD/109284/2015) was also funded by FCT.

REFERENCES

[1] Rabbani SI, Devi K, Khanam S. Pioglitazone, a PPAR-gamma ligand inhibited the nicotinamide-streptozotocin induced sperm abnormalities in type-2 diabetic Wistar rats. Pak J Pharm Sci 2010; 23(3): 326-31.
[PMID: 20566448]

[2] Ward WS. Function of sperm chromatin structural elements in fertilization and development. Mol Hum Reprod 2010; 16(1): 30-6.
[http://dx.doi.org/10.1093/molehr/gap080] [PMID: 19748904]

[3] Fuentes-Mascorro G, Serrano H, Rosado A. Sperm chromatin. Arch Androl 2000; 45(3): 215-25.
[http://dx.doi.org/10.1080/01485010050193995] [PMID: 11111870]

[4] Daxinger L, Whitelaw E. Understanding transgenerational epigenetic inheritance *via* the gametes in mammals. Nat Rev Genet 2012; 13(3): 153-62.
[PMID: 22290458]

[5] Vander AJ, Sherman JH, Luciano DS. Human physiology: The mechanism of body function. 8th ed. McGraw Hill 2001; pp. 1-800.

[6] Bellastella G, Cooper TG, Battaglia M, *et al.* Dimensions of human ejaculated spermatozoa in Papanicolaou-stained seminal and swim-up smears obtained from the Integrated Semen Analysis System (ISAS(®)). Asian J Androl 2010; 12(6): 871-9.
[http://dx.doi.org/10.1038/aja.2010.90] [PMID: 20852650]

[7] Saladin KS. The male reproductive system. Anatomy and Physiology: The unit of form and function, McGraw–Hill 2003; 1017-47.

[8] Yao R, Ito C, Natsume Y, *et al.* Lack of acrosome formation in mice lacking a Golgi protein, GOPC. Proc Natl Acad Sci USA 2002; 99(17): 11211-6. [http://dx.doi.org/10.1073/pnas.162027899] [PMID: 12149515]

[9] Boström K, Öckerman PA. Glycosidases in human semen and male genital organs. Scand J Urol Nephrol 1971; 5(2): 117-22. [http://dx.doi.org/10.3109/00365597109133589] [PMID: 5093104]

[10] Knobil E, Neill JD. Knobil and Neill's physiology of reproduction. Gulf Professional Publishing 2006; pp. 1-3230.

[11] Virtanen I, Badley RA, Paasivuo R, Lehto VP. Distinct cytoskeletal domains revealed in sperm cells. J Cell Biol 1984; 99(3): 1083-91. [http://dx.doi.org/10.1083/jcb.99.3.1083] [PMID: 6381503]

[12] Sathananthan AH, Ratnasooriya WD, de Silva PK, Menezes J. Characterization of human gamete centrosomes for assisted reproduction. Ital J Anat Embryol 2001; 106(2) (Suppl. 2): 61-73. [PMID: 11732597]

[13] De Jonge CJ, Barratt C. The sperm cell: production, maturation, fertilization, regeneration. Cambridge University Press 2006; pp. 1-359. [http://dx.doi.org/10.1017/CBO9780511545115]

[14] Vernon GG, Woolley DM. Basal sliding and the mechanics of oscillation in a mammalian sperm flagellum. Biophys J 2004; 87(6): 3934-44. [http://dx.doi.org/10.1529/biophysj.104.042648] [PMID: 15465868]

[15] Saladin KS. Human Anatomy. 7th Ed. McGraw Hill 2007; pp. 1-1242.

[16] Gaffney EA, Gadêlha H, Smith DJ, Blake JR, Kirkman-Brown JC. Mammalian sperm motility: observation and theory. Annu Rev Fluid Mech 2011; 43: 501-28. [http://dx.doi.org/10.1146/annurev-fluid-121108-145442]

[17] Inaba K. Sperm flagella: comparative and phylogenetic perspectives of protein components. Mol Hum Reprod 2011; 17(8): 524-38. [http://dx.doi.org/10.1093/molehr/gar034] [PMID: 21586547]

[18] Xu H, Yuan S-Q, Zheng Z-H, Yan W. The cytoplasmic droplet may be indicative of sperm motility and normal spermiogenesis. Asian J Androl 2013; 15(6): 799-805. [http://dx.doi.org/10.1038/aja.2013.69] [PMID: 23770936]

[19] Lhuillier P, Rode B, Escalier D, *et al.* Absence of annulus in human asthenozoospermia: case report. Hum Reprod 2009; 24(6): 1296-303. [http://dx.doi.org/10.1093/humrep/dep020] [PMID: 19221096]

[20] Flesch FM, Gadella BM. Dynamics of the mammalian sperm plasma membrane in the process of fertilization. Biochim Biophys Acta 2000; 1469(3): 197-235. [http://dx.doi.org/10.1016/S0304-4157(00)00018-6] [PMID: 11063883]

[21] Lenzi A, Gandini L, Picardo M, Tramer F, Sandri G, Panfili E. Lipoperoxidation damage of spermatozoa polyunsaturated fatty acids (PUFA): scavenger mechanisms and possible scavenger therapies. Front Biosci 2000; 5: E1-E15. [PMID: 10702376]

[22] Ward WS, Zalensky AO. The unique, complex organization of the transcriptionally silent sperm chromatin. Crit Rev Eukaryot Gene Expr 1996; 6(2-3): 139-47. [http://dx.doi.org/10.1615/CritRevEukarGeneExpr.v6.i2-3.30] [PMID: 8855386]

[23] Ioannou D, Miller D, Griffin DK, Tempest HG. Impact of sperm DNA chromatin in the clinic. J Assist Reprod Genet 2016; 33(2): 157-66.
[http://dx.doi.org/10.1007/s10815-015-0624-x] [PMID: 26678492]

[24] Finch JT, Klug A. Solenoidal model for superstructure in chromatin. Proc Natl Acad Sci USA 1976; 73(6): 1897-901.
[http://dx.doi.org/10.1073/pnas.73.6.1897] [PMID: 1064861]

[25] Björndahl L, Kvist U. Human sperm chromatin stabilization: a proposed model including zinc bridges. Mol Hum Reprod 2010; 16(1): 23-9.
[http://dx.doi.org/10.1093/molehr/gap099] [PMID: 19933313]

[26] Tarozzi N, Bizzaro D, Flamigni C, Borini A. Clinical relevance of sperm DNA damage in assisted reproduction. Reprod Biomed Online 2007; 14(6): 746-57.
[http://dx.doi.org/10.1016/S1472-6483(10)60678-5] [PMID: 17579991]

[27] Balhorn R. The protamine family of sperm nuclear proteins. Genome Biol 2007; 8(9): 227.
[http://dx.doi.org/10.1186/gb-2007-8-9-227] [PMID: 17903313]

[28] Zhang X, San Gabriel M, Zini A. Sperm nuclear histone to protamine ratio in fertile and infertile men: evidence of heterogeneous subpopulations of spermatozoa in the ejaculate. J Androl 2006; 27(3): 414-20.
[http://dx.doi.org/10.2164/jandrol.05171] [PMID: 16474017]

[29] Agarwal A, Said TM. Role of sperm chromatin abnormalities and DNA damage in male infertility. Hum Reprod Update 2003; 9(4): 331-45.
[http://dx.doi.org/10.1093/humupd/dmg027] [PMID: 12926527]

[30] Jennings C, Powell D. Genome organisation in the murine sperm nucleus. Zygote 1995; 3(2): 123-31.
[http://dx.doi.org/10.1017/S0967199400002495] [PMID: 7582914]

[31] Ward WS. The structure of the sleeping genome: implications of sperm DNA organization for somatic cells. J Cell Biochem 1994; 55(1): 77-82.
[http://dx.doi.org/10.1002/jcb.240550109] [PMID: 8083302]

[32] Miller D, Brinkworth M, Iles D. Paternal DNA packaging in spermatozoa: more than the sum of its parts? DNA, histones, protamines and epigenetics. Reproduction 2010; 139(2): 287-301.
[http://dx.doi.org/10.1530/REP-09-0281] [PMID: 19759174]

[33] Sotolongo B, Huang TT, Isenberger E, Ward WS. An endogenous nuclease in hamster, mouse, and human spermatozoa cleaves DNA into loop-sized fragments. J Androl 2005; 26(2): 272-80.
[http://dx.doi.org/10.1002/j.1939-4640.2005.tb01095.x] [PMID: 15713834]

[34] Ward MA, Ward WS. A model for the function of sperm DNA degradation. Reprod Fertil Dev 2004; 16(5): 547-54.
[http://dx.doi.org/10.1071/RD03072] [PMID: 15355763]

[35] Martins RP, Ostermeier GC, Krawetz SA. Nuclear matrix interactions at the human protamine domain: a working model of potentiation. J Biol Chem 2004; 279(50): 51862-8.
[http://dx.doi.org/10.1074/jbc.M409415200] [PMID: 15452126]

[36] Rousseaux S, Caron C, Govin J, Lestrat C, Faure A-K, Khochbin S. Establishment of male-specific epigenetic information. Gene 2005; 345(2): 139-53.
[http://dx.doi.org/10.1016/j.gene.2004.12.004] [PMID: 15716030]

[37] Hammoud SS, Nix DA, Zhang H, Purwar J, Carrell DT, Cairns BR. Distinctive chromatin in human sperm packages genes for embryo development. Nature 2009; 460(7254): 473-8.
[PMID: 19525931]

[38] Erenpreiss J, Spano M, Erenpreisa J, Bungum M, Giwercman A. Sperm chromatin structure and male fertility: biological and clinical aspects. Asian J Androl 2006; 8(1): 11-29.
[http://dx.doi.org/10.1111/j.1745-7262.2006.00112.x] [PMID: 16372115]

[39] Bowman GD, Poirier MG. Post-translational modifications of histones that influence nucleosome dynamics. Chem Rev 2015; 115(6): 2274-95.
[http://dx.doi.org/10.1021/cr500350x] [PMID: 25424540]

[40] Gatewood JM, Cook GR, Balhorn R, Schmid CW, Bradbury EM. Isolation of four core histones from human sperm chromatin representing a minor subset of somatic histones. J Biol Chem 1990; 265(33): 20662-6.
[PMID: 2243112]

[41] Zalensky AO, Breneman JW, Zalenskaya IA, Brinkley BR, Bradbury EM. Organization of centromeres in the decondensed nuclei of mature human sperm. Chromosoma 1993; 102(8): 509-18.
[http://dx.doi.org/10.1007/BF00368344] [PMID: 8243163]

[42] Arpanahi A, Brinkworth M, Iles D, *et al.* Endonuclease-sensitive regions of human spermatozoal chromatin are highly enriched in promoter and CTCF binding sequences. Genome Res 2009; 19(8): 1338-49.
[http://dx.doi.org/10.1101/gr.094953.109] [PMID: 19584098]

[43] Ajduk A, Yamauchi Y, Ward MA. Sperm chromatin remodeling after intracytoplasmic sperm injection differs from that of *in vitro* fertilization. Biol Reprod 2006; 75(3): 442-51.
[http://dx.doi.org/10.1095/biolreprod.106.053223] [PMID: 16775225]

[44] Barone JG, De Lara J, Cummings KB, Ward WS. DNA organization in human spermatozoa. J Androl 1994; 15(2): 139-44.
[PMID: 8056637]

[45] Zhang ZH, Zhu HB, Li LL, Yu Y, Zhang HG, Liu RZ. Decline of semen quality and increase of leukocytes with cigarette smoking in infertile men. Iran J Reprod Med 2013; 11(7): 589-96.
[PMID: 24639795]

[46] Turner RM. Moving to the beat: a review of mammalian sperm motility regulation. Reprod Fertil Dev 2006; 18(1-2): 25-38.
[http://dx.doi.org/10.1071/RD05120] [PMID: 16478600]

[47] Dacheux J-L, Dacheux F. New insights into epididymal function in relation to sperm maturation. Reproduction 2013; 147(2): R27-42.
[http://dx.doi.org/10.1530/REP-13-0420] [PMID: 24218627]

[48] Cornwall GA. New insights into epididymal biology and function. Hum Reprod Update 2009; 15(2): 213-27.
[http://dx.doi.org/10.1093/humupd/dmn055] [PMID: 19136456]

[49] Verma RJ. Sperm quiescence in cauda epididymis: a mini-review. Asian J Androl 2001; 3(3): 181-3.
[PMID: 11561187]

[50] Carr DW, Usselman MC, Acott TS. Effects of pH, lactate, and viscoelastic drag on sperm motility: a species comparison. Biol Reprod 1985; 33(3): 588-95.
[http://dx.doi.org/10.1095/biolreprod33.3.588] [PMID: 4052526]

[51] Cooper TG. The epididymis, cytoplasmic droplets and male fertility. Asian J Androl 2011; 13(1): 130-8.
[http://dx.doi.org/10.1038/aja.2010.97] [PMID: 21076437]

[52] Suarez SS, Ho HC. Hyperactivated motility in sperm. Reprod Domest Anim 2003; 38(2): 119-24.
[http://dx.doi.org/10.1046/j.1439-0531.2003.00397.x] [PMID: 12654022]

[53] Suarez SS. Control of hyperactivation in sperm. Hum Reprod Update 2008; 14(6): 647-57.
[http://dx.doi.org/10.1093/humupd/dmn029] [PMID: 18653675]

[54] Ho H-C, Suarez SS. Hyperactivation of mammalian spermatozoa: function and regulation. Reproduction 2001; 122(4): 519-26.
[http://dx.doi.org/10.1530/rep.0.1220519] [PMID: 11570958]

[55] Ashrafzadeh A, Karsani SA, Nathan S. Mammalian sperm fertility related proteins. Int J Med Sci 2013; 10(12): 1649-57.
[http://dx.doi.org/10.7150/ijms.6395] [PMID: 24151436]

[56] Tash JS. Protein phosphorylation: the second messenger signal transducer of flagellar motility. Cell Motil Cytoskeleton 1989; 14(3): 332-9.
[http://dx.doi.org/10.1002/cm.970140303] [PMID: 2555066]

[57] Brokaw CJ. Direct measurements of sliding between outer doublet microtubules in swimming sperm flagella. Science 1989; 243(4898): 1593-6.
[http://dx.doi.org/10.1126/science.2928796] [PMID: 2928796]

[58] González-Fernández L, Ortega-Ferrusola C, Macias-Garcia B, Salido GM, Peña FJ, Tapia JA. Identification of protein tyrosine phosphatases and dual-specificity phosphatases in mammalian spermatozoa and their role in sperm motility and protein tyrosine phosphorylation. Biol Reprod 2009; 80(6): 1239-52.
[http://dx.doi.org/10.1095/biolreprod.108.073486] [PMID: 19211810]

[59] Leclerc P, de Lamirande E, Gagnon C. Cyclic adenosine 3,5'monophosphate-dependent regulation of protein tyrosine phosphorylation in relation to human sperm capacitation and motility. Biol Reprod 1996; 55(3): 684-92.
[http://dx.doi.org/10.1095/biolreprod55.3.684] [PMID: 8862788]

[60] Mann T, Lutwak-Mann C. Male reproductive function and semen: themes and trends in physiology, biochemistry and investigative andrology. Springer Science & Business Media 2012; pp. 1-500.

[61] Yoshida M, Kawano N, Yoshida K. Control of sperm motility and fertility: diverse factors and common mechanisms. Cell Mol Life Sci 2008; 65(21): 3446-57.
[http://dx.doi.org/10.1007/s00018-008-8230-z] [PMID: 18622578]

[62] Turner RM, Musse MP, Mandal A, *et al.* Molecular genetic analysis of two human sperm fibrous sheath proteins, AKAP4 and AKAP3, in men with dysplasia of the fibrous sheath. J Androl 2001; 22(2): 302-15.
[PMID: 11229805]

[63] Carr DW, Newell AE. The role of A-kinase anchoring proteins (AKaps) in regulating sperm function. Soc Reprod Fertil Suppl 2007; 63: 135-41.
[PMID: 17566268]

[64] Vijayaraghavan S, Liberty GA, Mohan J, Winfrey VP, Olson GE, Carr DW. Isolation and molecular characterization of AKAP110, a novel, sperm-specific protein kinase A-anchoring protein. Mol Endocrinol 1999; 13(5): 705-17.
[http://dx.doi.org/10.1210/mend.13.5.0278] [PMID: 10319321]

[65] ORourke B, Van Eyk JE, Foster DB. Mitochondrial protein phosphorylation as a regulatory modality: implications for mitochondrial dysfunction in heart failure. Congest Heart Fail 2011; 17(6): 269-82.
[http://dx.doi.org/10.1111/j.1751-7133.2011.00266.x] [PMID: 22103918]

[66] Baker MA, Witherdin R, Hetherington L, Cunningham-Smith K, Aitken RJ. Identification of post-translational modifications that occur during sperm maturation using difference in two-dimensional gel electrophoresis. Proteomics 2005; 5(4): 1003-12.
[http://dx.doi.org/10.1002/pmic.200401100] [PMID: 15712234]

[67] Vijayaraghavan S, Mohan J, Gray H, Khatra B, Carr DW. A role for phosphorylation of glycogen synthase kinase-3α in bovine sperm motility regulation. Biol Reprod 2000; 62(6): 1647-54.
[http://dx.doi.org/10.1095/biolreprod62.6.1647] [PMID: 10819767]

[68] Somanath PR, Jack SL, Vijayaraghavan S. Changes in sperm glycogen synthase kinase-3 serine phosphorylation and activity accompany motility initiation and stimulation. J Androl 2004; 25(4): 605-17.
[http://dx.doi.org/10.1002/j.1939-4640.2004.tb02831.x] [PMID: 15223849]

[69] Vijayaraghavan S, Trautman KD, Goueli SA, Carr DW. A tyrosine-phosphorylated 55-kilodalton motility-associated bovine sperm protein is regulated by cyclic adenosine 3,5-monophosphates and calcium. Biol Reprod 1997; 56(6): 1450-7.
[http://dx.doi.org/10.1095/biolreprod56.6.1450] [PMID: 9166697]

[70] Vijayaraghavan S, Chakrabarti R, Myers K. Regulation of sperm function by protein phosphatase PP1gamma2. Soc Reprod Fertil Suppl 2007; 63: 111-21.
[PMID: 17566266]

[71] Fardilha M, Esteves SL, Korrodi-Gregório L, Pelech S, da Cruz E Silva OA, da Cruz E Silva E. Protein phosphatase 1 complexes modulate sperm motility and present novel targets for male infertility. Mol Hum Reprod 2011; 17(8): 466-77.
[http://dx.doi.org/10.1093/molehr/gar004] [PMID: 21257602]

[72] Chakrabarti R, Kline D, Lu J, Orth J, Pilder S, Vijayaraghavan S. Analysis of Ppp1cc-null mice suggests a role for PP1gamma2 in sperm morphogenesis. Biol Reprod 2007; 76(6): 992-1001.
[http://dx.doi.org/10.1095/biolreprod.106.058610] [PMID: 17301292]

[73] Baker MA, Hetherington L, Aitken RJ. Identification of SRC as a key PKA-stimulated tyrosine kinase involved in the capacitation-associated hyperactivation of murine spermatozoa. J Cell Sci 2006; 119(Pt 15): 3182-92.
[http://dx.doi.org/10.1242/jcs.03055] [PMID: 16835269]

[74] Krapf D, Arcelay E, Wertheimer EV, *et al.* Inhibition of Ser/Thr phosphatases induces capacitation-associated signaling in the presence of Src kinase inhibitors. J Biol Chem 2010; 285(11): 7977-85.
[http://dx.doi.org/10.1074/jbc.M109.085845] [PMID: 20068039]

[75] Battistone MA, Da Ros VG, Salicioni AM, *et al.* Functional human sperm capacitation requires both bicarbonate-dependent PKA activation and down-regulation of Ser/Thr phosphatases by Src family kinases. Mol Hum Reprod 2013; 19(9): 570-80.
[http://dx.doi.org/10.1093/molehr/gat033] [PMID: 23630234]

[76] Krapf D, Ruan YC, Wertheimer EV, *et al.* cSrc is necessary for epididymal development and is incorporated into sperm during epididymal transit. Dev Biol 2012; 369(1): 43-53.
[http://dx.doi.org/10.1016/j.ydbio.2012.06.017] [PMID: 22750823]

[77] Luconi M, Cantini G, Baldi E, Forti G. Role of a-kinase anchoring proteins (AKAPs) in reproduction. Front Biosci (Landmark Ed) 2011; 16: 1315-30.
[http://dx.doi.org/10.2741/3791] [PMID: 21196234]

[78] Sagare-Patil V, Vernekar M, Galvankar M, Modi D. Progesterone utilizes the PI3K-AKT pathway in human spermatozoa to regulate motility and hyperactivation but not acrosome reaction. Mol Cell Endocrinol 2013; 374(1-2): 82-91.
[http://dx.doi.org/10.1016/j.mce.2013.04.005] [PMID: 23623968]

[79] Almog T, Naor Z. The role of Mitogen activated protein kinase (MAPK) in sperm functions. Mol Cell Endocrinol 2010; 314(2): 239-43.
[http://dx.doi.org/10.1016/j.mce.2009.05.009] [PMID: 19467295]

[80] Muratori M, Luconi M, Marchiani S, Forti G, Baldi E. Molecular markers of human sperm functions. Int J Androl 2009; 32(1): 25-45.
[http://dx.doi.org/10.1111/j.1365-2605.2008.00875.x] [PMID: 18298567]

[81] Lobley A, Pierron V, Reynolds L, Allen L, Michalovich D. Identification of human and mouse CatSper3 and CatSper4 genes: characterisation of a common interaction domain and evidence for expression in testis. Reprod Biol Endocrinol 2003; 1: 53.
[http://dx.doi.org/10.1186/1477-7827-1-53] [PMID: 12932298]

[82] Chung J-J, Navarro B, Krapivinsky G, Krapivinsky L, Clapham DE. A novel gene required for male fertility and functional CATSPER channel formation in spermatozoa. Nat Commun 2011; 2: 153.
[http://dx.doi.org/10.1038/ncomms1153] [PMID: 21224844]

[83] Lishko PV, Botchkina IL, Kirichok Y. Progesterone activates the principal Ca2+ channel of human sperm. Nature 2011; 471(7338): 387-91. [http://dx.doi.org/10.1038/nature09767] [PMID: 21412339]

[84] Strünker T, Goodwin N, Brenker C, *et al.* The CatSper channel mediates progesterone-induced Ca2+ influx in human sperm. Nature 2011; 471(7338): 382-6. [http://dx.doi.org/10.1038/nature09769] [PMID: 21412338]

[85] Frank HY, Catterall WA. The VGL-chanome: a protein superfamily specialized for electrical signaling and ionic homeostasis. Sci STKE 2004; 2004: re15.

[86] Ren D, Navarro B, Perez G, *et al.* A sperm ion channel required for sperm motility and male fertility. Nature 2001; 413(6856): 603-9. [http://dx.doi.org/10.1038/35098027] [PMID: 11595941]

[87] Quill TA, Ren D, Clapham DE, Garbers DL. A voltage-gated ion channel expressed specifically in spermatozoa. Proc Natl Acad Sci USA 2001; 98(22): 12527-31. [http://dx.doi.org/10.1073/pnas.221454998] [PMID: 11675491]

[88] Quill TA, Wang D, Garbers DL. Insights into sperm cell motility signaling through sNHE and the CatSpers. Mol Cell Endocrinol 2006; 250(1-2): 84-92. [http://dx.doi.org/10.1016/j.mce.2005.12.031] [PMID: 16413670]

[89] Chen S-R, Chen M, Deng SL, Hao XX, Wang XX, Liu YX. Sodium-hydrogen exchanger NHA1 and NHA2 control sperm motility and male fertility. Cell Death Dis 2016; 7: e2152. [http://dx.doi.org/10.1038/cddis.2016.65] [PMID: 27010853]

[90] Wang D, King SM, Quill TA, Doolittle LK, Garbers DL. A new sperm-specific Na+/H+ exchanger required for sperm motility and fertility. Nat Cell Biol 2003; 5(12): 1117-22. [http://dx.doi.org/10.1038/ncb1072] [PMID: 14634667]

[91] Agarwal A, Deepinder F, Sharma RK, Ranga G, Li J. Effect of cell phone usage on semen analysis in men attending infertility clinic: an observational study. Fertil Steril 2008; 89(1): 124-8. [http://dx.doi.org/10.1016/j.fertnstert.2007.01.166] [PMID: 17482179]

[92] Larsen L, Scheike T, Jensen TK, *et al.* Computer-assisted semen analysis parameters as predictors for fertility of men from the general population. Hum Reprod 2000; 15(7): 1562-7. [http://dx.doi.org/10.1093/humrep/15.7.1562] [PMID: 10875866]

[93] Sakkas D, Alvarez JG. Sperm DNA fragmentation: mechanisms of origin, impact on reproductive outcome, and analysis. Fertil Steril 2010; 93(4): 1027-36. [http://dx.doi.org/10.1016/j.fertnstert.2009.10.046] [PMID: 20080235]

[94] Irvine DS, Twigg JP, Gordon EL, Fulton N, Milne PA, Aitken RJ. DNA integrity in human spermatozoa: relationships with semen quality. J Androl 2000; 21(1): 33-44. [PMID: 10670517]

[95] Koppers AJ, De Iuliis GN, Finnie JM, McLaughlin EA, Aitken RJ. Significance of mitochondrial reactive oxygen species in the generation of oxidative stress in spermatozoa. J Clin Endocrinol Metab 2008; 93(8): 3199-207. [http://dx.doi.org/10.1210/jc.2007-2616] [PMID: 18492763]

[96] Pang MG, Hoegerman SF, Cuticchia AJ, *et al.* Detection of aneuploidy for chromosomes 4, 6, 7, 8, 9, 10, 11, 12, 13, 17, 18, 21, X and Y by fluorescence in-situ hybridization in spermatozoa from nine patients with oligoasthenoteratozoospermia undergoing intracytoplasmic sperm injection. Hum Reprod 1999; 14(5): 1266-73. [http://dx.doi.org/10.1093/humrep/14.5.1266] [PMID: 10325276]

[97] Fernández JL, Muriel L, Rivero MT, Goyanes V, Vazquez R, Alvarez JG. The sperm chromatin dispersion test: a simple method for the determination of sperm DNA fragmentation. J Androl 2003; 24(1): 59-66. [PMID: 12514084]

[98] Bungum M, Bungum L, Giwercman A. Sperm chromatin structure assay (SCSA): a tool in diagnosis and treatment of infertility. Asian J Androl 2011; 13(1): 69-75.
[http://dx.doi.org/10.1038/aja.2010.73] [PMID: 21057512]

[99] Gorczyca W, Gong J, Darzynkiewicz Z. Detection of DNA strand breaks in individual apoptotic cells by the *in situ* terminal deoxynucleotidyl transferase and nick translation assays. Cancer Res 1993; 53(8): 1945-51.
[PMID: 8467513]

[100] Nanassy L, Carrell DT. Analysis of the methylation pattern of six gene promoters in sperm of men with abnormal protamination. Asian J Androl 2011; 13(2): 342-6.
[http://dx.doi.org/10.1038/aja.2010.160] [PMID: 21196940]

[101] Evenson DP, Larson KL, Jost LK. Sperm chromatin structure assay: its clinical use for detecting sperm DNA fragmentation in male infertility and comparisons with other techniques. J Androl 2002; 23(1): 25-43.
[http://dx.doi.org/10.1002/j.1939-4640.2002.tb02599.x] [PMID: 11780920]

[102] Evenson DP, Darzynkiewicz Z, Melamed MR. Relation of mammalian sperm chromatin heterogeneity to fertility. Science 1980; 210(4474): 1131-3.
[http://dx.doi.org/10.1126/science.7444440] [PMID: 7444440]

[103] Spanò M, Bonde JP, Hjøllund HI, Kolstad HA, Cordelli E, Leter G. Sperm chromatin damage impairs human fertility. Fertil Steril 2000; 73(1): 43-50.
[PMID: 10632410]

[104] Giwercman A, Lindstedt L, Larsson M, *et al.* Sperm chromatin structure assay as an independent predictor of fertility *in vivo*: a case-control study. Int J Androl 2010; 33(1): e221-7.
[http://dx.doi.org/10.1111/j.1365-2605.2009.00995.x] [PMID: 19840147]

[105] Zini A, Boman JM, Belzile E, Ciampi A. Sperm DNA damage is associated with an increased risk of pregnancy loss after IVF and ICSI: systematic review and meta-analysis. Hum Reprod 2008; 23(12): 2663-8.
[http://dx.doi.org/10.1093/humrep/den321] [PMID: 18757447]

[106] Larson KL, DeJonge CJ, Barnes AM, Jost LK, Evenson DP. Sperm chromatin structure assay parameters as predictors of failed pregnancy following assisted reproductive techniques. Hum Reprod 2000; 15(8): 1717-22.
[http://dx.doi.org/10.1093/humrep/15.8.1717] [PMID: 10920092]

[107] Larson-Cook KL, Brannian JD, Hansen KA, Kasperson KM, Aamold ET, Evenson DP. Relationship between the outcomes of assisted reproductive techniques and sperm DNA fragmentation as measured by the sperm chromatin structure assay. Fertil Steril 2003; 80(4): 895-902.
[http://dx.doi.org/10.1016/S0015-0282(03)01116-6] [PMID: 14556809]

[108] Oleszczuk K, Giwercman A, Bungum M. Sperm chromatin structure assay in prediction of *in vitro* fertilization outcome. Andrology 2016; 4(2): 290-6.
[http://dx.doi.org/10.1111/andr.12153] [PMID: 26757265]

[109] Bird A. Perceptions of epigenetics. Nature 2007; 447(7143): 396-8.
[http://dx.doi.org/10.1038/nature05913] [PMID: 17522671]

[110] Carrell DT, Hammoud SS. The human sperm epigenome and its potential role in embryonic development. Mol Hum Reprod 2010; 16(1): 37-47.
[http://dx.doi.org/10.1093/molehr/gap090] [PMID: 19906823]

[111] Jenkins TG, Carrell DT. The sperm epigenome and potential implications for the developing embryo. Reproduction 2012; 143(6): 727-34.
[http://dx.doi.org/10.1530/REP-11-0450] [PMID: 22495887]

[112] Portela A, Esteller M. Epigenetic modifications and human disease. Nat Biotechnol 2010; 28(10): 1057-68.
[http://dx.doi.org/10.1038/nbt.1685] [PMID: 20944598]

[113] Bronner C, Chataigneau T, Schini-Kerth VB, Landry Y. The Epigenetic Code Replication Machinery, ECREM: a promising drugable target of the epigenetic cell memory. Curr Med Chem 2007; 14(25): 2629-41.
[http://dx.doi.org/10.2174/092986707782023244] [PMID: 17979715]

[114] Liyanage VR, Jarmasz JS, Murugeshan N, Del Bigio MR, Rastegar M, Davie JR. DNA modifications: function and applications in normal and disease States. Biology (Basel) 2014; 3(4): 670-723.
[http://dx.doi.org/10.3390/biology3040670] [PMID: 25340699]

[115] Molaro A, Hodges E, Fang F, *et al.* Sperm methylation profiles reveal features of epigenetic inheritance and evolution in primates. Cell 2011; 146(6): 1029-41.
[http://dx.doi.org/10.1016/j.cell.2011.08.016] [PMID: 21925323]

[116] Navarro-Costa P, Nogueira P, Carvalho M, *et al.* Incorrect DNA methylation of the DAZL promoter CpG island associates with defective human sperm. Hum Reprod 2010; 25(10): 2647-54.
[http://dx.doi.org/10.1093/humrep/deq200] [PMID: 20685756]

[117] Wu W, Shen O, Qin Y, *et al.* Idiopathic male infertility is strongly associated with aberrant promoter methylation of methylenetetrahydrofolate reductase (MTHFR). PLoS One 2010; 5(11): e13884.
[http://dx.doi.org/10.1371/journal.pone.0013884] [PMID: 21085488]

[118] Reik W, Dean W, Walter J. Epigenetic reprogramming in mammalian development. Science 2001; 293(5532): 1089-93.
[http://dx.doi.org/10.1126/science.1063443] [PMID: 11498579]

[119] Stuppia L, Franzago M, Ballerini P, Gatta V, Antonucci I. Epigenetics and male reproduction: the consequences of paternal lifestyle on fertility, embryo development, and children lifetime health. Clin Epigenetics 2015; 7: 120.
[http://dx.doi.org/10.1186/s13148-015-0155-4] [PMID: 26566402]

[120] Oliva R. Protamines and male infertility. Hum Reprod Update 2006; 12(4): 417-35.
[http://dx.doi.org/10.1093/humupd/dml009] [PMID: 16581810]

[121] Aoki VW, Liu L, Jones KP, *et al.* Sperm protamine 1/protamine 2 ratios are related to *in vitro* fertilization pregnancy rates and predictive of fertilization ability. Fertil Steril 2006; 86(5): 1408-15.
[http://dx.doi.org/10.1016/j.fertnstert.2006.04.024] [PMID: 17011555]

[122] Aoki VW, Liu L, Carrell DT. Identification and evaluation of a novel sperm protamine abnormality in a population of infertile males. Hum Reprod 2005; 20(5): 1298-306.
[http://dx.doi.org/10.1093/humrep/deh798] [PMID: 15705617]

[123] Jenuwein T, Allis CD. Translating the histone code. Science 2001; 293(5532): 1074-80.
[http://dx.doi.org/10.1126/science.1063127] [PMID: 11498575]

[124] Lachner M, Jenuwein T. The many faces of histone lysine methylation. Curr Opin Cell Biol 2002; 14(3): 286-98.
[http://dx.doi.org/10.1016/S0955-0674(02)00335-6] [PMID: 12067650]

[125] Dada R, Kumar M, Jesudasan R, Fernández JL, Gosálvez J, Agarwal A. Epigenetics and its role in male infertility. J Assist Reprod Genet 2012; 29(3): 213-23.
[http://dx.doi.org/10.1007/s10815-012-9715-0] [PMID: 22290605]

[126] Miller D, Ostermeier GC, Krawetz SA. The controversy, potential and roles of spermatozoal RNA. Trends Mol Med 2005; 11(4): 156-63.
[http://dx.doi.org/10.1016/j.molmed.2005.02.006] [PMID: 15823753]

[127] Yadav RP, Kotaja N. Small RNAs in spermatogenesis. Mol Cell Endocrinol 2014; 382(1): 498-508.
[http://dx.doi.org/10.1016/j.mce.2013.04.015] [PMID: 23632103]

[128] Meikar O, Da Ros M, Korhonen H, Kotaja N. Chromatoid body and small RNAs in male germ cells. Reproduction 2011; 142(2): 195-209.
[http://dx.doi.org/10.1530/REP-11-0057] [PMID: 21652638]

[129] Carthew RW, Sontheimer EJ. Origins and Mechanisms of miRNAs and siRNAs. Cell 2009; 136(4): 642-55.
[http://dx.doi.org/10.1016/j.cell.2009.01.035] [PMID: 19239886]

[130] Gan H, Lin X, Zhang Z, *et al.* piRNA profiling during specific stages of mouse spermatogenesis. RNA 2011; 17(7): 1191-203.
[http://dx.doi.org/10.1261/rna.2648411] [PMID: 21602304]

[131] Chuma S, Nakano T. piRNA and spermatogenesis in mice. Philos Trans R Soc Lond B Biol Sci 2013; 368(1609): 20110338.
[http://dx.doi.org/10.1098/rstb.2011.0338] [PMID: 23166399]

[132] Soubry A, Hoyo C, Jirtle RL, Murphy SK. A paternal environmental legacy: evidence for epigenetic inheritance through the male germ line. BioEssays 2014; 36(4): 359-71.
[http://dx.doi.org/10.1002/bies.201300113] [PMID: 24431278]

[133] Sendler E, Johnson GD, Mao S, *et al.* Stability, delivery and functions of human sperm RNAs at fertilization. Nucleic Acids Res 2013; 41(7): 4104-17.
[http://dx.doi.org/10.1093/nar/gkt132] [PMID: 23471003]

CHAPTER 10

Biochemistry Behind the Journey of Spermatozoa Through the Female Reproductive Tract

Luís Rato*

Health Sciences Research Centre, University of Beira Interior, Rua Marquês d'Ávila e Bolama, 6201-001, Covilhã, Portugal

Abstract: Sperm released in the lumen of seminiferous tubules are functionally immature. These cells acquire maturation during their passage through the epididymis. The epididymis exhibits an extraordinary structure showing different segments with distinct luminal composition, which act as a whole for the gradual differentiation of sperm. This organ is permanently targeted by neuronal and hormonal factors, in particular by androgens. The study of the biochemical mechanisms that mediate sperm maturation has been a matter of intense debate. The current advances on the knowledge of sperm physiology was possible due to studies conducted in laboratory and domestic species, whereas in humans these processes remain to be fully explored. This is a subject with high relevance in the field of reproductive biology since defects in these events may end-up in infertility. Maturation of sperm begins in the epididymis, but does not end in this organ, since after ejaculation sperms are still unable to fertilize the oocyte. After being deposited in the reproductive female tract, sperm undergo a number of structural and biochemical changes to become "capacitated". Non-capacitated sperm cannot interact with eggs *In vivo* as their failure to hyperactivate motility precludes ascent to the site of fertilization. Sperm and egg must interact so that gamete fusion and the introduction of paternal information into the egg occurs, and the program of development must be activated. Male gametes are the "vehicle" by which the genetic information is passed from fathers to the offspring. In this context, there is increasing evidence that parental lifestyle and the environment influence phenotypes of the next generation. Sperm epigenome has huge implications for the success of male fertility, fertilization, pregnancy and in the transmission of undesirable information to the next generations. In this chapter we will discuss these topics from a biochemical point of view by exploring the mechanisms that govern the most relevant processes.

Keywords: Acrosome reaction, Capacitation, Epididymis, Fertilization, Glycosylation, Male Reproductive tract, Phosphorylation, Post-translational modifications, Sperm-egg interactions, Sperm Epigenome, Sperm proteins.

* **Corresponding author Luís Rato:** Health Sciences Research Centre, Av. Infante D. Henrique, 6201-506, Covilhã, Portugal; Tel: +351 275 329 002; Fax: +351 275 329 099; E-mail: luis.pedro.rato@gmail.com

Marco G. Alves and Pedro F. Oliveira (Eds.)

INTRODUCTION

During spermiation, sperm are released in the lumen of the seminiferous tubules morphologically mature, however the proteome of spermatozoa with testicular source does not allow for itself that the spermatozoa is functionally competent. In the later stages of spermatogenesis, sperm are devoid of transcriptional, as well as translational activity. To become mature, sperm require two post-testicular maturation steps; the first occurs in the epididymis and is known as epididymal maturation. During their passage through the epididymis, sperm are exposed to a unique environment, since these cells remain "isolated" due to the blood-epididymal barrier. In the epididymal lumen, sperms are bathed in fluid produced by the cells of the epididymal epithelium, which results from an extraordinary absorptive and secretory activity. At this site there is a constant exchange of proteins between protein epididymal epithelium and sperm where the epididymosomes were reported as main "actors" in this process. At the same time, sperms suffer several modifications known as post-translational modifications (PTMs), namely phosphorylation and glycosylation. Acquisition of motility is one of the significant changes mediated by protein phosphorylation, which begins in the epididymal environment. Sperm motility is regulated by the phosphorylation profile in the several parts of the flagellum and axoneme. This process is coordinated by protein kinases and phosphatases.

The second step of sperm maturation occurs within the female tract after ejaculation in an event known as capacitation. Capacitation is essential for fertilization since sperms are prepared to undergo an exocytosis process known as acrosome reaction, as well as changes in the sperm motility known as hyperactivated movement. At the molecular level, capacitation is associated with molecular changes such as loss of cholesterol from sperm plasma membrane, changes in intracellular ion concentrations, namely HCO_3^- and Ca^{2+}, hyperpolarization of sperm plasma membrane, increased activity of protein kinase A (PKA), and protein tyrosine (Tyr) phosphorylation. All these points will be discussed in detail below. These events have been independently studied and the information regarding how they interconnect to regulate sperm motility and to prepare sperm to undergo the acrosome reaction is still poorly explained. Mammalian fertilization comprises sperm migration through the reproductive female tract, where it undergoes biochemical and morphological alterations and sperm-egg interactions in the oviduct as well. Fertilization occurs through a series of coordinated steps, which ends with the fusion of the two gametes to produce a genetically distinct individual. In this regard, there is an increasing awareness that the molecular changes that occur in the genome, called epigenetic alterations, not only influence the success of male fertility but also fertilization and even pregnancy. Furthermore, the most recent evidence demonstrated that the genetic information transmitted through male gametes has enormous implications in the subsequent generations, particularly due to the transmission of undesired information that predispose the offspring to metabolic diseases. In this chapter we will discuss, from the biochemical point of view, all steps that sperm experiment from the moment that enters in the epididymal duct till fusion with oocyte.

SPERM EJACULATION

After being released in the lumen of seminiferous tubules, sperms proceed through the rete testis, efferent ducts and begin their journey towards the epididymis which acts as a site for sperm storage until ejaculation. Ejaculation involves a series of events triggered by central nervous system activation of the sympathetic nervous system that creates an emission containing the semen and the secretions from seminal vesicles, prostate, and bulbourethral glands [1, 2]. This process can be divided into two distinct phases: emission and expulsion. The emission phase involves the distal epididymis, vas deferens, seminal vesicles, prostate gland, prostatic urethra, and the bladder neck. The initial step in emission starts with closure of the bladder neck due to sympathetic innervation of the base of the bladder. After bladder neck closure, secretion of fluid from the prostate (10% of total ejaculate volume) provides zinc ions, citric acid and prostate specific antigen (PSA), which facilitates the liquefaction of semen after ejaculation. Subsequently, seminal vesicles contribute to most of the volume (75–80% of total volume) of the ejaculate presenting a rich concentration in HCO_3^- (alkalinization), prostaglandins, fructose, ascorbic acid, and seminogelin I and II. A minor contribution also includes excretion of fluid from bulbourethral glands. The expulsion phase follows the emission and consists of discharge of the semen from the urethra through the coordinated actions of the bladder neck, urethra, and pelvic striated muscles in a process mediated by somatic nervous system [2].

Beyond the neural control, ejaculation is also target of neurocrine regulation. Indeed, androgens can affect the ejaculation process, thus affecting sexual behavior in men because acts both on central and peripheral nervous system, where many areas of which are connected to ejaculatory reflex [3]. Evidences from animal models demonstrated that testosterone (T) regulates the central serotonin pathway. Treatment with T decreased the serotonin release and its metabolite, 5-hydroxyindoleacetic acid by the hypothalamus, thus suggesting that high levels of T may induce premature ejaculation, which is associated with impaired serotonin pathway [4]. At peripheral level T regulates the activity of nitric oxide (NO), as well the expression and activity of phosphodiesterase-5 (PDE-5), an important system involved in the penile erection and in the contractility of genital male tract during emission phase [5]. The initial part of the ejaculatory reflex is also targeted by estrogens, in particular by 17β-estradiol [6]. The use of animal models of estrogen deprivation (inducing hypogonadotropic hypogonadism and blocking aromatase activity) has showed that 17β-estradiol regulates the epididymal contractile activity. These works also show that endogenous estrogens are key players in the epididymal responsiveness to the contractile agents; oxytocin and endothelin-1 [7, 8]. In addition to this, the epididymal hyporesponsiveness in hypogonadal animals has been normalized by administration with estradiol valerate or with tamoxifen—a selective estrogen receptor modulator but not with testosterone enanthate, illustrating a direct role of estrogens. These data suggest that ejaculation is under hormonal control of sex steroids, nevertheless there are other key players in this process. Animal studies have highlighted the vital role of neurotransmitters in the control of ejaculation, such as dopamine, serotonin or NO. Dopamine plays an excitatory role in ejaculation. This has been supported by the injection of the dopamine agonist apomorphine into the medial preoptic area that increases the frequency of ejaculation [9, 10], while injection of dopamine antagonists decrease the occurrence of ejaculation [11]. Contrastingly, serotonin generally exerts an inhibitory effect in the neuromodulation of ejaculation, though this may vary according to the receptor subtype [12]. Until now there are 15 known serotonin receptors, also termed as 5-hydroxytryptamine (5-HT) receptors. Due to their heterogeneity, 5-HT receptors have been grouped into seven major families (5-HT1–7) based on their function and location. All members of 5-HT1–7 family are G-protein-coupled receptors, with the exception of 5-HT3. All receptors are post-synaptically located, except for 5-HT1A, 5-HT1B, and 5-HT1D receptors, which are presynaptic and involved in negative feedback [13].

It is well-known the role of NO in erection and recent evidence have also enlightened its role in the ejaculatory process, mainly due to ejaculatory disorders such as premature ejaculation. This dysfunction occurs in nearly 30% of adult men being one of the most common forms of male sexual disorders. It can be caused by erectile dysfunction, anxiety and nerve hypersensitivity, but is quite treatable *via* PDE-5 inhibitors (PDE5-I) [14, 15]. PDE5-I is used to block the degradative action of cyclic guanosine monophosphate (cGMP)-specific PDE5-I on cGMP in the smooth muscle cells lining the blood vessels that supply corpus cavernosum in the penis [15]. Peripherally, nitronergic innervation and NO synthase/cGMP and cyclic adenosine monophosphate (cAMP) signaling pathways have been identified in the smooth muscle of the vas deferens, seminal vesicles, prostate, and urethra [16 - 18]. Drugs such as PDE5-I or NO donors that increase intracellular cGMP or cAMP diminish seminal vesicle contraction and inhibit seminal emission [19].

FACTORS THAT REGULATE SPERM CAPACITATION

After ejaculation sperm have not yet completed the maturation and are still not capable to fertilize. The first evidence are dated from 1951 when Chang [20] and Austin [21, 22] observed that freshly ejaculated mammalian sperm were unable to fertilize eggs *in vivo* until they had resided for a period of time within the female reproductive tract. Sperm that have completed this process acquire "capacitation" [22]. Capacitation was initially observed due to its protracted time course, which in certain species (humans included) may take several hours. In contrast, sperm of many invertebrates, and some non-mammalian vertebrates, fertilize eggs quickly following release from the male reproductive tract. This is often interpreted as capacitation being a uniquely mammalian phenomenon and, at least in regard to these events, there are fundamental differences in the control of fertilization between mammalian and non-mammalian organisms. Capacitation encompasses a series of changes in the cellular physiology and biochemistry of sperm. Such alterations take place in surface membrane, through alteration of peripheral membrane protein composition, antigen localization and surface charge; plasma membrane properties, such as membrane potential, lipid composition and transmembrane phospholipids asymmetry, and the lateral diffusion of lipids and proteins; metabolism; apparent intracellular pH as well as in the cytosolic activities of calcium and other ions; altered cyclic nucleotide metabolism; and changes in protein phosphorylation (Fig. **10.1**). All these alterations take place from the head to flagellum. Capacitation occurs within the female reproductive tract and is completed in the oviduct [23] being influenced by female reproductive tract factors, which apparently provide signals that regulate the process even if those signals are not unique to this region.

Several factors have been proposed to be involved in sperm capacitation and different experimental approaches have been used in order to assess the effects of the oviductal secretions on sperm capacitation. However, the molecular mechanisms by which oviductal secretory products induce the capacitation of spermatozoa need to be clarified. It has been reported that sperm incubated in the presence of oviductal fluid or co-cultured with oviduct epithelial cells showed a pattern of hyperactivated motility which was related to the capacitation state [24]. Furthermore, the adequate levels of HCO_3^- and Ca^{2+} in the oviduct are essential for sperm capacitation [25, 26]. The presence of hyaluronan and sulfated glycosaminoglycans, such as heparin, in the fluid of oviduct seems to play a role in the sperm capacitation [27 - 29]. On other hand, albumin and high density lipoproteins, found in the oviductal fluid seem to participate in the cholesterol efflux from sperm membrane, one of the key steps of sperm capacitation [26, 30]. The epithelial cells of the oviduct secretes proteins whose functions have not been clarified, but recent evidences support their role in the regulation in sperm capacitation. The oviductin, an oviduct-specific glycoprotein with 70–130 kDa, has been found in the oviduct of several mammals and it has been indicated that this protein binds to the anterior acrosomal region of the sperm and enhances sperm capacitation [31, 32], though the molecular mechanism has not been elucidated.

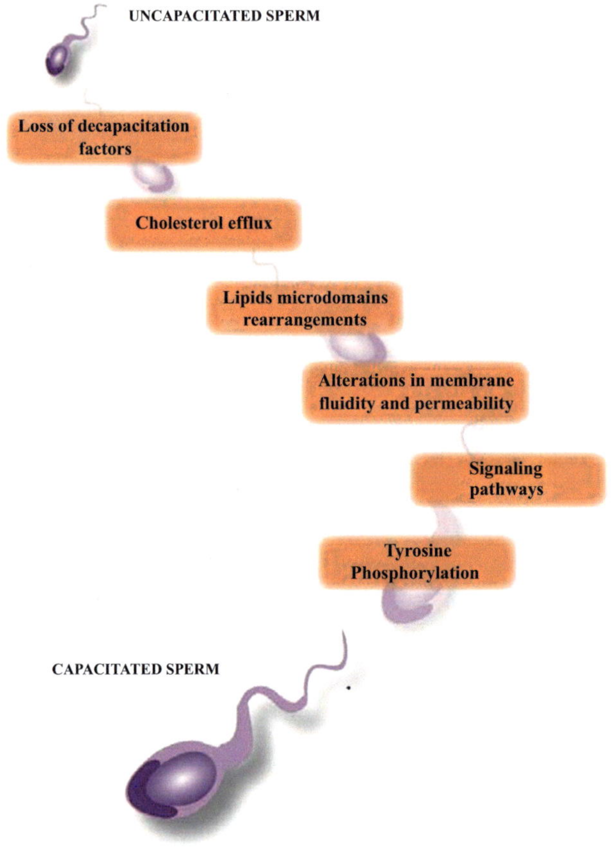

Fig. (10.1). Schematic representation of the proposed process for sperm capacitation. The initial step is the loss of decapacitation factors, which promotes the cholesterol efflux. The loss of cholesterol is associated with decreased cholesterol:phospholipid ratio altering the protein-lipid reorganization and contributes to the lipid reorganization and fluidization of the sperm membrane. The membrane fluidization induced by loss of cholesterol will activate signal transduction pathways, leading to the Tyr phosphorylation of sperm proteins.

The starting point of capacitation reaction is in sperm membrane. The functional changes that this event comprises are: (i) the ability of sperm to bind the oocyte's extracellular matrix, the zona pellucida (ZP) [33] and subsequently acrosome reaction [34]; (ii) hyperactivation, the whiplash flagellar motion required to penetrate the egg [35], and (iii) the capacity to fuse with the oocyte [36]. Capacitation is under control of both extrinsic and intrinsic factors being the major extrinsic signals mediating capacitation sterol acceptors (traditionally albumin) and ion fluxes, namely HCO_3^- and Ca^{2+}. Together, these signaling molecules activate PKA and protein Tyr kinase (PTK) pathways that regulate capacitation [37].

Decapacitation factors are also vital since they protect and stabilize sperm surface membrane in such a way that they do not suffer premature capacitation, otherwise their will not be able to fertilize the oocyte. In fact, the first event that initiates the capacitation reaction is the loss of decapacitation factors. Among the best characterized decapacitation factors are the bovine seminal plasma proteins (BSPs; now known as the Binder of Sperm family), which bind to sperm choline phospholipids, then are stripped from sperm by heparin or components in the genital tract, taking certain membrane lipids (cholesterol and phospholipids) along with them [38]. Other decapacitation factors include cholesterol [39], protease inhibitors (including the Serine (Ser) protease inhibitor Kasal-type-like protein (SPINKL)) [40] and Ser protein inhibitor [41], platelet-activating factor acetylhydrolase [42], phosphatidylethanolamine binding protein 1 [43], NYD-SP27 (an isoform of phospholipase C Zeta 1 localized to the sperm acrosome) [44], HongrES1 (a cauda epididymis-specific protein involved in the capacitation of spermatozoa) [45] and mouse seminal plasma protein (SVS2), which interacts with the monosialotetrahexosylganglioside, also known ganglioside GM1 [46]. A putative mechanism by which sperm undergo capacitation in the oviduct could involve binding of heparin-like molecules present in the oviductal fluid to seminal plasma protein PDC-109, thereby displacing it from the epithelium and releasing the sperm from the reservoir. The PDC-109 is subsequently removed along with membrane cholesterol, triggering the signaling cascade that leads to capacitation.

The complex cascade of molecular events that occur during capacitation may be divided into events that initiate capacitation and events that are a consequence of this process. Molecular events implicated in the initiation of capacitation include lipid rearrangements in sperm plasma membrane, ion fluxes that result in alteration of sperm membrane potential, and increased Tyr phosphorylation of proteins involved in induction of hyperactivation and the acrosome reaction.

Cholesterol Efflux

It is thought that large amounts of cholesterol, incorporated into the sperm during epididymal transit, stabilize the plasma membrane as they pass throughout the female tract [47]. This hypothesis is supported by observations that non-albumin cholesterol acceptors can replace albumin, such as high density lipoproteins [38, 48] and beta-cyclodextrins [49, 50]. It has been proposed that the cholesterol: phosphatidylserine exposure facilitate cell-cell a phospholipid ratio is a major determinant of capacitation, and removal of cholesterol decreases this ratio to destabilize the sperm head plasma membrane, thus increasing its potential for fusion with the outer acrosomal membrane [39]. Cholesterol removal alters the protein-lipid organization of the sperm head plasma membrane [51] and increases its fluidity [52]. Sperm membranes exhibit a high heterogeneity and amongst the several components and/or compartments of the lipid bilayer are lipid rafts. Lipid rafts are dynamic microdomains of the membrane bilayer, enriched in cholesterol, glycosphingolipids, glycosyl-phosphatidylinositol and GPI-anchored proteins. These lipid microdomains are involved in membrane signaling and trafficking platforms [53]. It has been suggested that during capacitation, lipid rafts with enhanced ZP-binding potential cluster to reposition sperm membrane proteins that are involved in gamete recognition, or form signaling complexes leading to downstream reactions during capacitation or acrosomal exocytosis [54]. The loss of cholesterol is associated with decreased cholesterol: phospholipid ratio and a lipid reorganization that contributes to the fluidization of the sperm membrane. The ATP-binding cassette membrane transporter G2 (ABCG2) is one of the sperm proteins that have shown to be phosphorylated in Tyr residues. ABCG2 is present in the plasma membrane overlying the sperm acrosome and is proposed to play a role in the translocation of cholesterol across the plasma membrane in epididymal spermatozoa [55]. The Tyr phosphorylation of ABCG2 has been shown to be necessary for its function within epididymal spermatozoa, while dephosphorylation is believed to result in its inactivation.

The membrane fluidization induced by loss of cholesterol is known to activate signal transduction pathways, leading to the Tyr phosphorylation of sperm proteins [48, 56]. Some of these modifications affect other events such as the ion flux, pump and enzymes activities.

Ion Flux and Sperm Capacitation: The Role of HCO_3^- Transport

The microenvironment within female reproductive tract is rich in HCO_3^- [57], which influences sperm capacitation, while the sperm reservoir secretions are suggested to have low concentration of bicarbonate [57]. HCO_3^- is particularly responsible for inducing capacitation as it rapidly increases the fluidity of sperm membranes [58]. HCO_3^- is able to induce several compositional changes in phospholipid distribution across sperm membrane [59]. Specifically, HCO_3^- activated the outward translocation of sphingomyelin, phosphatidylcholine, phosphatidylserine, and phosphatidylethanolamine, possibly by activating a "scramblase" activity. In addition, it was noted phospholipase activation and membrane fluidization due to bicarbonate. The effect of HCO_3^--induced scramblase activity was reported to vary among different regions of sperm according to the specific lipid population, thus reducing phospholipid asymmetry over the head, but not in the flagellum [59]. Such observations are relevant to capacitation since both, decreased phospholipid asymmetry and phosphatidylserine exposure facilitate cell-cell adhesion, which would enhance sperm-oocyte interaction [60, 61]. These changes are induced by HCO_3^-, *via* cAMP-dependent protein kinase, as cyclic nucleotide PDE-I and phosphatase inhibitors (which prolong PKA-mediated protein phosphorylation) all mimicked the effect of HCO_3^- [62]. It is now accepted that a major regulatory role of HCO_3^- on capacitation is mediated by a non-transmembrane soluble adenylyl cyclase (sAC), which is distinct from classical G protein-regulated, transmembrane adenylyl cyclases. The relevance of sAC has been demonstrated by sAC knockout animals that exhibit normal testicular morphology, epididymis, and sperm, but are infertile due to sperm motility defects [63].

Calcium Influx Modulates Sperm Capacitation

Capacitation is also Ca^{2+} dependent and the initiation and/or regulation of capacitation by Ca^{2+} occurs *via* different targets, some of them being involved with cAMP metabolism. For instance, Ca^{2+} activate both the synthesis of cAMP by sAC [64], as well as degradation by cAMP cyclic nucleotide phosphodiesterase [65] showing the ambiguity of its effects in sperm capacitation. Increased intraflagellar Ca^{2+} occurs during capacitation [66], which is more involved in hyperactivated motility than in capacitation *per se*. Potential transporters involved in Ca^{2+} influx during capacitation include voltage-gated channels, cation channels of spermatozoa generally termed as CatSper, Na^+/Ca^{2+} pumps, Ca^{2+}ATPases, stromal interaction molecule 1 which function as Ca^{2+} sensor and the calcium release-activated calcium channel protein 1. On the other hand, the influx of Ca^{2+} can also be induced by mobilization of $[Ca^{2+}]_i$ through the receptors inositol-1,4,5-trisphosphate, riadone and Ca^{2+} ATPases.

Phosphorylation Events during Capacitation

During capacitation there is an increase in the sperm protein phosphorylation events. Phosphorylation occurring at Ser/Threonine (Thr) or Tyr (by protein kinases) and/or dephosphorylation (by phosphoprotein phosphatases) are pivotal in many cellular processes, including the transduction of extracellular signals, intracellular transport, and cell cycle progression. Sperm essentially do not synthesize proteins, so the dynamic nature of sperm proteome will depend in part on the acquisition of new proteins by PTMs of already manufactured proteins. Indeed, PTMs on existing proteins are essential in the regulation of sperm function, especially during maturation and acquisition of fertilizing potential. Any failure in the control of these complex molecular processes could be detrimental or fatal to a cell because large amounts of defective PTMs and their substrates can lead to male infertility. Studies have showed the potential involvement of altered protein phosphorylation in the asthenozoospermia and reported a direct link between the former and aberrant sperm motility. A deficiency in Tyr phosphorylation of tail proteins, especially those related to hyperactivated motility, was also reported to be associated to asthenozoospermia [67]. Hypophosphorylation of proteins during capacitation in these groups was thought to be caused by decreased membrane fluidity [68].

The capacitation-associated increase in protein Tyr phosphorylation is downstream of cAMP/PKA pathway in mouse sperm [69] and other species [70, 71]. Although the relevance of this PTM for capacitation has not been fully established, the appearance of a cohort of Tyr phosphorylated proteins is accepted as essential for acrosomal sensitivity and fertilization *in vitro* [37, 69] and is thus considered as an endpoint for capacitation. However, this is a matter of some controversy, since others have proposed that Tyr phosphoprotein appearance may not be always an endpoint for capacitation. Studies where capacitation was induced identified many Tyr phosphorylated sperm proteins in the flagellum, highlighting their possible role to initiate and sustain hyperactivation [72 - 74]. In fact, accomplishment of functional competence during capacitation is marked by high levels of Tyr phosphorylation in pre-existing sperm proteins [75], which makes Tyr phosphorylation a hallmark of capacitation. Other important proteins undergoing Tyr phosphorylation during capacitation in human sperm are proteins members of the A-kinase anchor proteins family (AKAPs). The most prominent Tyr phosphorylated proteins appearing in capacitated human sperm are AKAP4 and proAKAP82, which are localized in the cytoskeletal fibrous sheath of the principal piece [76]. These results advocate an interaction between PKA and PTK pathways, while suggesting that protein Tyr phosphorylation may be part of the signaling pathway probably involved in hyperactivation. Similarly Ca^{2+}-binding Tyr phosphorylation regulated-protein (CABYR) undergoes Tyr phosphorylation during capacitation and is localized to the principal piece of the human sperm flagellum in association with the fibrous sheath [77]. The profile of phosphorylated proteins of human sperm revealed that at least 18 proteins are Tyr phosphorylated during capacitation [73]. Valosin-containing protein (VCP), a homologue of the soluble N-ethylmaleimide-sensitive factor activating protein receptor (SNARE)- interacting N-ethylmaleimide sensitive factor (NSF), is phosphorylated in Tyr residues after capacitation being relocalized from the connecting piece to the anterior head [73]. SNARE proteins regulate membrane fusion and exocytosis, so Tyr phosphorylation of VCP could either directly mediate acrosomal responsiveness, or act as a chaperone to carry membrane fusion proteins to the site of plasma-acrosomal membrane fusion [73]. Indeed, Tyr phosphorylated NSF is maintained in an inactive state and protein Tyr phosphatase action reduces the phosphotyrosine content of NSF to promote membrane fusion [78]. On the other hand, the phosphorylation of Tyr residues is triggered by interleukin 6 secreted by cells of endometrium being mediated by Janus kinase 1 (JAK1) signaling pathway [79]. Indeed, extracellular signal-regulated kinase (ERK) modulation of MAPK pathway appears to play a role in generating Tyr phosphorylated sperm proteins during capacitation. ERK signaling seems to be particularly directed to modifications in sperm head. ERK is active in human sperm during capacitation [80] and modulation of ERK cascade with specific inhibitors indicates that it plays a role upstream of protein Tyr phosphorylation [81]. Family members of ERK, in particular ERK1 and ERK2 participate in ERK1/2 phosphorylation and activation which is concomitant with enhanced phosphorylation during capacitation. Moreover, ERK1/2 activation is evident by enhanced phosphorylation during capacitation, and ERK1/2 inhibitors block both protein Tyr phosphorylation and the ability of sperm to acrosome-react. It has been demonstrated that other pathways participate in Tyr phosphorylation-related capacitation (such as BSA, cAMP analogues, and reactive oxygen species) and stimulates the phosphorylation (and presumably the activation) of three MEK-like proteins [82]. MEK is a dual-specificity kinase that phosphorylates Tyr and Thr residues on ERK1/2 mediated mechanisms required for activation. Interestingly, inhibition of both the PKA pathway and non-receptor PTK completely blocked the MEK-like phosphorylation, although protein kinase C and receptor PTK inhibition only prevented the phosphorylation of one of the MEK-like proteins [82].

Serine/Threonine Phosphorylation

The phosphorylation of Ser and Thr during human sperm capacitation is mediated by PKA and PKC [83]. At least 8 proteins with distinct molecular weights, namely 18 kDa, 35 kDa, 43-55 kDa, 94-62 kDa, 110 kDa, and 190 kDa, have been detected as a target for phosphorylation. One of these proteins in the 43-55 kDa region is the FA-1 antigen, which has been shown to be phosphorylated in Tyr residues during capacitation, but also at Ser and Thr residues. PKA appears to regulate the activity of the proteasome that is involved in the modulation of phosphorylation during capacitation. In human sperm, proteasomes have been located (but not exclusively) in plasma membrane overlying the sperm acrosome, allowing for degradation of proteins prior to or during sperm capacitation [84]. Proteasomes have also been detected in sperm tail-connecting piece and also in the midpiece. Their relevance in the regulation of phosphorylation of those residues [85] has been demonstrated and proteasomes seem to be active during the capacitation process since their inhibition results in incomplete capacitation. Also, proteasomal activity may contribute to the release of capacitated spermatozoa from the oviductal sperm reservoir *in vivo*.

SPERM PROTEINS AND BIOCHEMICAL EVENTS IN SPERM-EGG INTERACTIONS

Oocyte is surrounded by ZP which is composed by glycosaminoglycans and the four glycoproteins ZP1, ZP2, ZP3 and ZP4. All proteins of ZP are synthesized by oocytes and post-translationally modified by glycosylation at Ser/Thr (O-linked) and at asparagine (N-linked) residues. Closest to ZP, a layer composed by follicular cells constitutes the zona radiata and is followed by another layer of follicular cells separated by an extracellular matrix, the . Altogether these form a complex called the oocyte cumulus complex. After ovulation, follicular cells secrete chemotactic agents to promote the motility of sperm towards the oocyte in the oviduct. Sperm orient motility in gradients of factors in a conditioned medium by the female reproductive tract. At least one of the active factors in follicular and oviduct fluids appears to be progesterone [86, 87], but floral odorants and bourgeonal-like molecules are also present [87, 88].

At the oviduct, sperm will interact with oocyte, primarily reaching the outer surface of the ZP, with the primary connection to the ZP occurring through the glycosylated ZP3 region (primary receptor for acrosome-intact sperm), which has species-specific glycosylated residues that recognize and bind to a species-specific receptor, fixing sperm to ZP. Then ZP3 and ZP4 bind to specific receptors present in sperm membrane and induce acrosome reaction (Fig. **10.2**). The sperm of many animal species, including all mammals, contain a single large secretory vesicle, or acrosome, in the apical region of the anterior head overlying the nucleus. It consists of an acidic vesicle, containing a variety of proteins such as hyaluronidase, sp56 other proteolytic proteins, bioactive peptides and other proteins with unknown functions.

Only acrosome-intact sperm bind to the ZP tenaciously and undergo the acrosome reaction [89 - 91], illustrating that ZP actively induces acrosome reaction, leading to the release of all contents of the acrosomal vesicle. Thereafter, a new cell surface domain in the apical region of the sperm is formed. This process is imperative and must be completed, otherwise sperm will be unable to penetrate the ZP. Evidence indicated that mannose glycan and N-acetylglucosamine residues are involved in the induction of sperm acrosome reaction [92 - 94]. Furthermore, it was reported that PKA, PKC and G proteins mediate the activation of signaling pathways of the acrosomal exocytosis. The suggested order of signal transduction is (1) Gi protein activation of PKA pathway by regulation of adenylyl cyclase and elevation of cAMP, which, in turn, (2) activates phospholipase C; resulting in (3) hydrolysis of phosphatidylinositol bisphosphate and (4) activation of the PKC pathway (by diacylglycerol and inositol triphosphate) and a separate pathway involving Tyr kinase [95]. Molecules like adhesin and sperm protein sp56 intervene to stabilize the adhesion of spermatozoa to ZP. The posterior third of the vesicular acrosomic contains pro-acrosin enzyme, which is converted in its proteolytic form acrosin by ZP2. Acrosin acts as a secondary receptor for acrosome-reacted sperm. Together with the hyaluronidase, these proteins digest ZP allowing the penetration of sperm to the perivitelline space and the surface of the oocyte. When sperm contacts the cytoplasmic membrane of the oocyte, it is positioned horizontally and immobilize (Fig. **10.3**). The fusion of the two gametes is a critical component of sexual reproduction in which two terminally differentiated cells carrying the genomes of two different individuals originate the zygote that will produce a new genetically distinct individual. After being fertilized, the eggs themselves mount blocks to polyspermy to prevent fertilization by other sperm. Blocks to polyspermy occur primarily at the egg plasma membrane and at the egg coat or ZP. The egg coat block involves the exocytosis of cortical granules (CGs) from the cortex of the egg and causes the conversion of the ZP to a form that cannot support sperm binding [96]. It should also be noted that the mammalian membrane block is established in approximately the same time frame as the ZP block. *In vivo* studies have used fertilized eggs to provide evidence of how mammalian eggs prevent polyspermy. After fertilization, sperm release Ca^{2+} into the egg cytoplasm which triggers transient increases, or oscillations, in intracellular Ca^{2+} levels in the fertilized egg [97]. Fluctuations in the Ca^{2+} levels give rise to a set of events known collectively as egg activation, which includes CG exocytosis, giving rise to the ZP block to polyspermy.

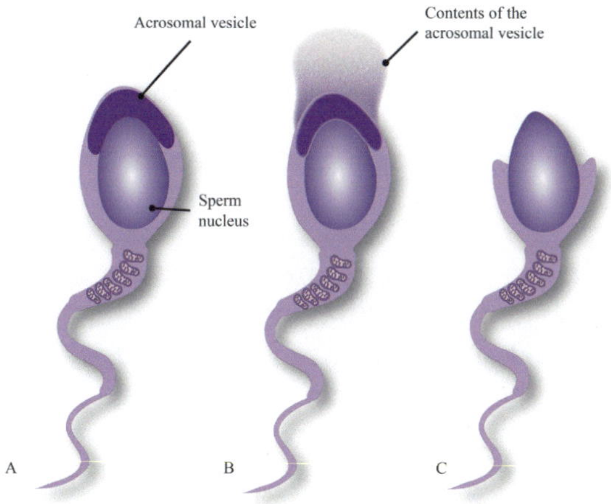

Fig. (10.2). Schematic representation of acrosome reaction. **(A)** During early stages of the acrosome reaction the plasma and acrosomal membranes fuse at several points allowing the release of contents **(B)**. After releasing all acrosomal vesicle contents, a new cell surface domain in the apical membrane of the head of spermatozoa is formed **(C)**. Acrosomal reaction must be completed so spermatozoa can penetrate the zona pellucida and fuse with the oocyte.

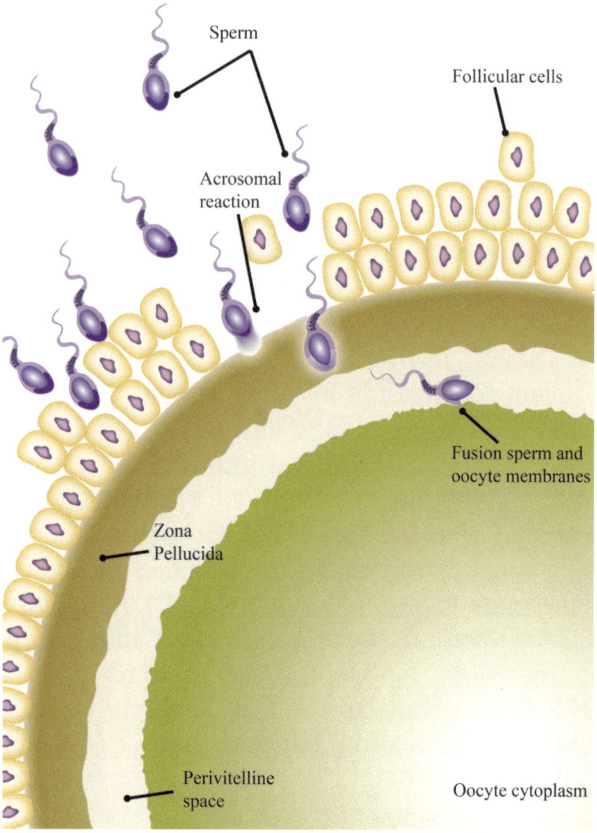

Fig. (10.3). Schematic representation of spermatozoa-egg interactions. The egg is surrounded by extracellular layers: cumulus layer and zona pellucida. The spermatozoa penetrates through these two layers to gain access to perivitelline space. This penetration of the spermatozoa is accomplished by a surface-bound hyaluronidase and by the release of acrosomal enzymes by spermatozoa. The binding of spermatozoa is mediated by several adhesion molecules on both, spermatozoa and egg.

Eggs can be "artificially" fertilized by injecting a spermatozoa into the egg cytoplasm, a process called intracytoplasmic sperm injection (ICSI). However, it has been observed that ICSI-fertilized mouse eggs are unable to prevent polyspermy, since incorporated as many sperm as do unfertilized eggs. The Ca^{2+} signaling may be linked with this, because the Ca^{2+} fluctuations generated by ICSI differ from those generated by natural fertilization [98, 99].

Before considering some of the proteins that mediate the interactions between sperm and oocyte, there are some concepts that must be understood to avoid possible misleading. Until now, we have used the term sperm-egg interactions, which comprises a series of sequential complex events. Sperm-egg interactions consist in the interaction of the sperm membrane with the egg membrane and include sperm-egg adhesion and membrane fusion. These processes are distinct, since sperm-egg fusion refers to the membrane fusion event resulting in cytoplasmic continuity between the two gametes. Sperm-egg binding (or sperm-egg adhesion) refers to the cell-cell interaction that precedes membrane fusion and that is defined experimentally a status that maintained after a specific series of washes.

Gamete plasma membrane interactions occur following sperm penetration of the cumulus layer and the ZP, so that sperm gain access to the perivitelline space between the egg plasma membrane and the ZP. Mammalian sperm-egg membrane interactions occur in a spatially restricted manner. Several proteins are involved in this process and glycolytic enzymes seem to have particular relevance, though their role in these events remains to be clarified. According to what has been recently observed, it is possible that glycolytic enzymes act as potential sites of recognition and/or binding for ZP glycoproteins located in sperm head. It has been showed that aldolase A (ALDOA) directly interacts with ZP glycoprotein (ZP4). Sperm receptors for ZP act as lectin-like proteins that recognize sugar chains on ZP. It was proposed that glycolytic enzymes which have oligosaccharides as substrates in the flagellum, bind to the sugar moieties substrates of the ZP glycoproteins without exerting their catalytic activity when located on the sperm head. Multimolecular complexes involving glycolytic enzymes have already been described [100]. In spermatozoa, three testis-specific isozymes, (spermatogenic cell-specific type 1 hexokinase, muscle-type phosphofructokinase and glutathione S-transferase mu 5 (GSTM5)) form a molecular complex associated with the mouse fibrous sheath [101]. The mu class of glutathione S-transferases (GSTM) has been identified as a ligand for human ZP4 and ZP3, confirming a receptor activity of this GSTM [102]. GSTM was found at the surface of the human sperm head in a region overlying the acrosome of intact sperm and was not maintained after acrosome reaction. Nixon and collaborators [103] proposed the concept of multi-recognition molecules, which are assembled in a functional complex located in lipid rafts of the sperm membrane. They propose that these molecules would interact with the carbohydrate segment of ZP glycoproteins. Thus, it is possible that GSTM-ZP4/ZP3 interaction occurs in the first steps of gamete recognition. Those evidence are consistent with the hypothesis that GSTM is a sperm-specific molecule for ZP3/ZP4 recognition during initial binding. This sperm-specific role of glutathione S-transferases adds the detoxification function of GSTM. By eliminating reactive oxygen species *via* glutathione, it prevents lipid membrane peroxidation, an irreversible and highly damaging process to sperm membrane integrity. Moreover, it seems that the voltage-dependent anion channel 2 (VDAC2) is also involved in the interaction with ZP, namely with ZP2 and ZP3 glycoproteins, since VDAC2 was found on the acrosomic region, in addition to its localization on the flagellum [104, 105].

Others have focused their research on the molecular foundations of fertilization and have identified proteins involved in sperm-egg interactions, such as ADAM1, ADAM2 and izumo spermatozoa-egg fusion protein 1 (IZUMO1) [106]. The relevance of IZUMO1 in fertilization has been demonstrated by using knockout animal models. Although these animals exhibit normal mating behavior and ejaculation, as well as normal sperm motility and migration into the oviduct, they are infertile [107]. The complete sterility of IZUMO1 null animals has been attributed to a defect in sperm–egg fusion, although the sperm is able to bind. In fact, this is corroborated by *in vitro* fertilization (IVF) assays with IZUMO1-deficient sperm. It was observed that sperm penetrate ZP and then accumulate in the perivitelline space, suggesting a defective interaction with the egg plasma membrane, since eggs fertilized by intracytoplasmic sperm injection with IZUMO1-deficient sperm develop into normal embryos. Other testicular sperm surface proteins (such as ADAM3) appear to be strongly associated with sperm fertility. The sterility of ADAM3 knockout mice is mainly linked to a lack of sperm migration from the uterus to the oviduct. Sperm from these animals present poor binding affinity to the ZP and egg plasma membrane under *in vitro* conditions, but are fertile after oviduct artificial insemination or IVF with cumulus-intact and ZP-intact eggs. Interestingly, the same phenotype of ADAM3 knockout animals was also obtained after gene knockout for at least ten different sperm genes Ace, Clgn, Adam2, Adam1a, Calr3, Tpst2, Pdilt, Pmis2, Prss37, and Tex101. The loss of ADAM3 from the mature sperm surface was also observed after Rnase10 deletion, which encodes for a protein secreted only in the initial segment of the epididymis and without any sperm membrane affinities [108]. These evidence indicate that the stability, integrity, and location of ADAM3 at the sperm surface are linked to the presence and/or activities of several other proteins. In testis, several chaperone proteins (*e.g.* calmegin, calsperin, and the testis-specific protein disulfide isomerase homolog), different ADAM3-associated proteins (ADAM1b, ADAM2 and ADAM6), and other proteins (such as Tyrosylprotein sulfotransferase 2 and angiotensin-converting enzyme, to further detail see review [109]) are essential for the location of ADAM3 on sperm surface. Proteomic approaches have also identified other proteins as candidates to sperm-egg interactions, such as sperm equatorial segment protein 1 [110, 111], transmembrane protein 190 [112], and three sperm acrosome-associated proteins: sperm acrosomal membrane-associated 32; sperm lysosomal-like protein 1 and sperm acrosomal membrane-associated 14 [113, 114]. The mechanisms involved in sperm–egg interactions in mammals (including humans) are still unclear. The previous evidences clearly demonstrate that interactions between male and female gametes are more complex and not based in a simple ligand–receptor system. The identification of sperm proteins and the exact role of the epididymis in the molecular mechanisms involved in gamete interactions is still a challenge.

EPIGENETIC PATTERNING IN FERTILIZATION

At fertilization, male and female gametes fuse to originate zygote, the first cell of the developing embryo. At this moment the parental genomes exhibit different stages of the cell cycle, different epigenetic profiles and chromatin composition [115]. The paternal genome is single copy (1C) tightly packaged by protamines, whereas the maternal genome (2C) is wrapped around the nucleosomes. The genome of the two gametes remains physically separate in the zygote, where they undergo different chromatin remodeling, under the influence of maternally inherited factors. After fertilization, protamines of paternal genome are replaced by maternally inherited histones [116, 117]. After histone incorporation, acetylation phenomena become detectable [117], most likely because of newly synthesized histones that carry the evolutionary conserved acetylation of lysine 5 and lysine 12 on histone H4 [118]. Afterwards, methylation of histones also occurs, and the onset of mono-, di- and trimethylation exhibits a timing that is specific for each progressive modification [119]. In the early stages of zygote, the conformational changes occurring in chromatin (hyperacetylation and hypomethylation) allow accessibility to the paternal genome. The replacement by acetylated histones is also closely followed by genome-wide demethylation, which is completed before the beginning of DNA replication in the paternal pronucleus [120]. It has been proposed that DNA demethylation proceeds by direct removal of the methyl group from the cytosine base [121], or by replacement of 5-methylcytosine (5meC) by cytosine through a base-excision mechanism [121]. However, demethylation reactions may also occur through indirect mechanisms. These events involve DNA repair, where DNA glycosylases (such as thymine DNA glycosylase (TDG) and methyl-binding domain protein 4 (MBD4)) repair T/G mismatches that may result from initial deamination of 5meC [122]. MBD4 is part of the family of nuclear proteins related by the presence in each of a methyl-CpG-binding domain. TDG and MBD4, however, have been shown to have weak activity on 5meC:G base pairs, leading to base excision repair, where cytosine replaces 5meC [123]. The MBD2 has been proposed as the enzyme responsible for the removal of methyl group [121]. Still, not all sequences in the paternal genome undergo demethylation. In fact, some of them seem to be "protected", such as imprinted genes H19 [124] and Ras Grf1 [125].

Contrarily to what happens with paternal genome, in the maternal genome the modifications of histones acquired during oocyte growth (namely methylated lysines 9 and 27 of histone H3) [126] are maintained, in both the zygote and subsequent cellular divisions [126]. During the subsequent cleavage divisions, passive demethylation may occur, since DNA methyltransferase 1 (Dnmt1) is excluded from the nucleus [127]. Indeed, Dnmt1 protein inherited from the oocyte (Dnmt1o) is seemingly excluded from the nucleus during the first three cleavage divisions [128] thus accounting for the loss of precisely 50% methylation and enlightening the role of Dnmt1o in the maintenance of imprinted methylation during the fourth cell cycle.

Altogether these molecular events create an asymmetry between the male and female epigenomes (as evidenced by H3K9me3 abundance), up to the 4-cell stage [126, 129], whereas other chromatin marks such as H4K20me3 [130], H3K64me3 [131] and H3K4me3 [132] are equalized by the two-cell stage. This asymmetry is also reflected in DNA methylation, which is globally lost in the paternal pronucleus of the zygote, whilst maternal genome retains it (Fig. **10.4**). A possible explanation may rely in the different epigenetic profiles of both gametes. However, as the majority of these mechanisms remain poorly understood it is hard to infer about its biological significance. It has been hypothesized that modifications in the chromatin established in the gametes may be part of a transgenerational program that is required for a proper embryonic development [133]. Noteworthy, the time of activation of embryonic gene expression parallels epigenetic reprogramming, with the male genome being more permissive to transcription from the late zygote stage [134], whereas transcription increases in both genomes thereafter at the 2-cell and 4-cell stages (reviewed in [135]). Recent reports have shown that loss of early zygotic demethylation in the male genome has a deleterious effect in development due to impaired activation of several genes related with pluripotency [136].

In the zygote, Dppa3 (also called Stella) is a protein that is essential for development during preimplantation protecting the methylation of maternal genome from ten-eleven translocation 3 element (Tet3) oxidation [133]. Dppa3 is extremely important and zygotes lacking this protein lose asymmetry of DNA methylation, exhibiting a global loss of 5-meC and acquire 5-hydroximet-hylcytosine in both paternal and maternal pronuclei (Fig. **10.4**) [137]. In both cases, embryonic lethality occurs, thus highlighting the importance of Dppa3 and the potential importance of epigenetic asymmetry during early preimplantation development.

Maintenance of DNA methylation is thought to be essential for proper development by preventing the activation of retrotransposons, maintenance of imprints and stability of chromosomes. It has been shown that in mature sperm, some imprinted regions are enriched for H3K9me2 (for example, H19 and Rasgrf1), relative to other paternal imprints that are independently maintained of

Dppa3 (as for example, Dlk1- Gtl2) [138], thus opening a novel perspective that the protection of DNA methylation at some imprints may rely on the inheritance of histone modifications from the gametes to the next generation. Indeed, the retaining of histones at specific locations in sperm genome [128] and the fact that can be inherited in the zygote [139] may support the previous hypothesis.

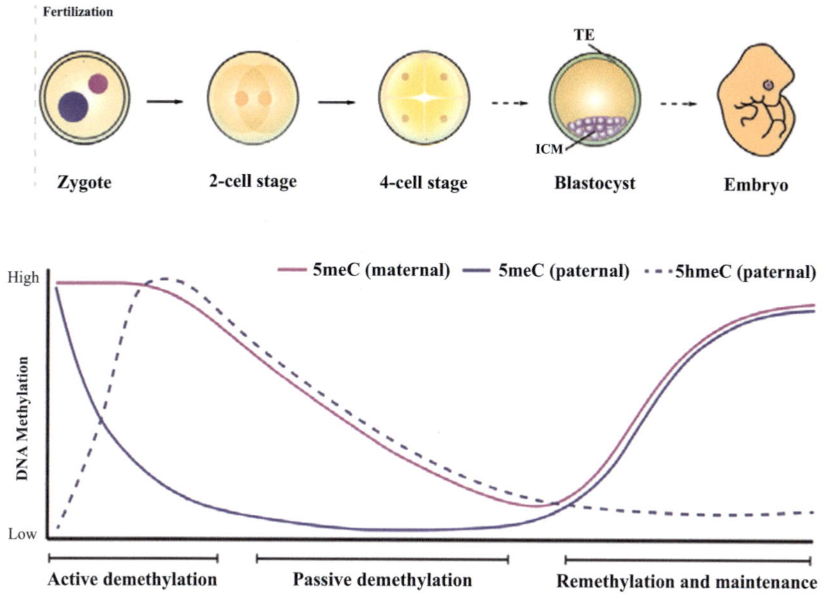

Fig. (10.4). Schematic representation of DNA methylation and imprinting maintenance in preimplantation embryos. Maternal and paternal genomes have distinct characteristics that impose an epigenetic asymmetry in the zygote. The maternal genome (pink pronucleus; pink solid line) undergoes passive DNA demethylation throughout several rounds of DNA replication, while paternal genome (purple pronucleus; purple solid line) undergoes active demethylation before DNA replication in the zygote. The bulk of 5mC in the paternal genome is hydroxylated in the late zygote. Only a few regions were shown to completely revert to unmodified cytosine before the first cleavage division. The bulk of paternal 5hmC is passively diluted, paralleling demethylation of the maternal genome (purple dashed line). Abbreviations: 5hmeC: 5-hydroxymethylcytosine; 5meC: 5-methylcytosine; ICM: inner cell mass; TE: trophectoderm.

Recent studies have revealed chromatin features in sperm that may contribute to totipotency, developmental decisions and imprinting patterns [140, 141]. It has been reported a positive correlation between the extent to which H3K27me3-modified nucleosomes are present around the transcriptional start site of genes in spermatozoa and gene repression in early embryos. It has been proposed that histone methylation in paternal chromatin inheritance as a function of the number of modified nucleosomes that are retained across regulatory regions of loci in sperm [140]. Furthermore, it has been predicted that, in embryos, sperm-inherited modified nucleosomes remain retained in the paternal genome during its remodeling by maternally provided histones in the course of pronucleus formation

[141]. found histones enriched at imprinted gene clusters, and a notable correlation between H3K4me3 and paternally expressed noncoding RNAs and genes.

Another important topic of the epigenetic reprogramming after fertilization is the second wave of global remodeling that occurs during the development of germ cells in the embryo. Primordial germ cells (PGCs) originate from the epiblast cells of the post-implantation embryo, which are cells that have already been primed to a somatic fate [142]. The epigenetic reprogram that occurs during this period must ensure that germ line–specific genes are primed and that an epigenetic landscape that is compatible with restoring totipotency to the next generation is established. This remodeling is a coordinated process with several steps and requires the timely expression of key transcriptional factors as well as appropriate epigenetic modifiers. The earliest global chromatin change occurs during 7.5–10.5 days of embryonic development where PGCs migrate and undergo a reciprocal loss of H3K9me2 and increase in H3K27me3 [143]. The switch between these two repressive chromatin marks has led to the suggestion that germ cells may need to use a more flexible silencing mechanisms at this stage. This idea stems from the description that H3K27me3 mediated by polycomb proteins in ESCs allows the promoters of many developmental regulator genes to be transcriptionally silent [143]. Polycomb group proteins are epigenetic regulators of transcription that have key roles in stem-cell identity, differentiation and disease. Mechanistically, they function within multiprotein complexes, called polycomb repressive complexes (PRCs), which modify histones (and other proteins) and silence target genes. Recently it was reported that the timely down-regulation of H3K27me3 during PGC development is required both for maintaining the expression of pluripotency genes, namely (Oct4, Nanog, Sall4 and SSEA1) and for the derivation of embryonic germ cells *in vitro* [136]. Global demethylation of PCGs occurs between 11.5 and 12.5 days of mouse development and leads to the erasure of methylation in imprinted genes and single copy genes [144] and reactivation of X chromosome [145]. Nevertheless, not all epigenetic marks are erased in imprinted genes in PGCs. For instance, the paternal H19 and the maternal Snrpn alleles are demethylated during PGC development but later during spermatogenesis and oogenesis they need to be methylated again. This de novo methylation of formerly methylated genes seems to occur at an earlier stage than de novo methylation of originally unmethylated genes [146], indicating that other epigenetic marks are not completely erased during PGC development and provide signals for de novo methylation.

A recent time-course analysis of both germline and somatic genes has shown a gradual loss of DNA methylation from 8.5 days of embryonic development, followed by a rapid erasure between 11.5 and 12.5 days [147]. On the basis of these observations, it has been proposed that replication-dependent demethylation occurs during early PGC development, whereas an active mechanism operates at a later stage. Extensive and rapid DNA demethylation has been detected when PGCs enter the gonads (between 11.5 and 12.5 days of embryonic development) at which time most of the cells are in G2 phase [147]. It is thought that this second phase of reprogramming depends on an active process independent of DNA replication. Complete demethylation is achieved after 13.5 days of embryonic development in genes or intergenic regions, including imprinted domains and repeat elements that were previously protected from erasure in the zygote [148]. However, transposable elements belonging to intracisternal A-particle and long-terminal-repeat-containing elements of species-specific endogenous retrovirus 1 family elements and some loci that are located close to these elements or within sub-telomeric regions seem to be exceptions in this case [148]. These mechanisms are extremely relevant since it is thought that are involved in the prevention and transmission of acquired traits to the next generations. While sex-specific imprinted DNA methylation needs to be reestablished, epimutations that may be accumulated throughout parent's life require erasure (at least some of them, due to its detrimental effects in the next generations). This is one of the "hottest" topics that have been debated in the field of developmental biology. Specifically how these germ-cell marks may act post-fertilization to enact long-term changes in offspring behavior or physiology is a matter of debate. The first lineage allocation event in mammalian embryogenesis occurs at the morula stage and results in the formation of the inner cell mass (ICM) and trophectoderm (TE) lineages in the blastocyst. It is possible that molecular changes in sperm induced by paternal environmental experience somehow affect cell fate allocation between ICM and TE by altering cell-cycle dynamics for the first cleavage divisions or, alternatively, TE cell function, with resulting effects on placental development then resulting in metabolic changes in the offspring. Indeed, it has been observed that paternal diet and exercise are linked to pre-implantation growth dynamics [149], possibly providing a link between paternal diet and the findings of common maternal effect phenotypes in the offspring. Such a link would also help explain how epigenetic marks in sperm (see Chapter **9**), namely cytosine methylation or small noncoding RNAs (sncRNAs), which theoretically should be erased, might exert long-term effects, despite operating during a limited time window. However, it has been reported that some of these sncRNAs may be acquired during epididymal transit [150]. Those works strongly suggested that sncRNAs trafficking between epithelium and sperm might be exerted in within epididymal environment, rather than in seminiferous tubules and that this process is mediated by epididymosomes. Studies examining the paternal exposure to environmental factors have proposed that epigenetic marks carried by male gametes transmit the paternal legacy of metabolic traits [151, 152]. However, these nongenetic mechanisms of transgenerational inheritance need to be fully investigated. Recently it has been debated how the interaction between endocrine system and the environmental cues has shaped sperm epigenome and how this may help us to explain the etiology of inherited endocrine disorders. This is where epigenetics meets endocrinology. The primary target of signal transduction is chromatin [153] whereby extracellular signals, including those by hormones and/or chemicals that mimic hormones, are transduced to genomic events *via* specific histone modifications [154]. The adverse effects of the environmental factors promote disturbances in the health state of the next generations through epigenetic modifications passed by male gametes (discussed in detail in chapter 13). The exposure environmental compounds is huge and although these compounds disrupt the endocrine system, it is the long-term response of molecular processes such as epigenetics that will promote downstream developmental events and adult-onset disease. It will be imperative elucidate the role of epigenetics in endocrine disruptor actions and in the etiology of disease, which certainly will provide new insights into diagnostics and therapeutics strategies for environmental exposures, risk assessment and adult-onset disease.

CONCLUDING REMARKS

In this chapter we presented and discussed some biochemical aspects of the various events occurring in sperms throughout their journey once they are deposited in female reproductive tract, with special emphasis on the mechanisms that mediate the fuse with the oocyte to originate a zygote. Sperm are highly differentiated cells with a great interest for research. In fact, in the last decade several breakthroughs on the structural and functional features of spermatozoa have been achieved, mostly due to combination of both modern molecular technologies and classical methods of light and electron microscopy. However and despite all these advances, some of the alterations which take place at sperm surface and/or in sperm cytoplasm still need to be fully clarified. It is expected that in next few years the advent of the high-throughput analysis (next generation sequencing and proteomics) may shed light on the molecular foundations of sperm physiology, functioning and capacitation. In addition, sperm maturation remains as one of the most important steps in the journey, since it defines the functionality of these cells. Many issues are still to be solved, for instance, the molecular basis of the delivery of surface components to specific domains; the fully dissection of the signaling pathways involved in the initiation of motility, capacitation, hyperactivation and acrosome reaction; how these upstream events affect the capacitation and consequently the ability to fuse with the oocyte.

In fact, the role of the spermatozoon is to deliver the male genome into the egg so that it can combine with the oocyte genome to initiate the development of the new individual. It has been speculated that the external insults (*e.g.* environmental contaminants, physical inactivity, eating disorders) associated with current lifestyle of the developed societies may change the epigenetic profile of sperm. These external insults are able to "modify" the genetic information carried by sperm. Some of these alterations are resistant to the normal reprogramming waves occurring during embryo development and therefore heritable. How these epigenetic modifications affect fertilization or the development of the embryo are emerging questions. In addition, there is increasing evidence that some epigenetic modifications acquired throughout parental life are inherited by male germ line thus influencing the phenotypes of the next generations. This will be one of the hottest topics in the field of male reproductive field for years to come.

Box 10.1 | Summary

- Loss of decapacitation factors, HCO_3^- and Ca^{2+} flux regulates the capacitation of spermatozoa.
- The capacitation of spermatozoa is dependent on Tyr, Ser and Thr phosphorylation.
- Only capacitated spermatozoa are able to fertilize oocyte.
- IZUMO and ADAMs proteins are key proteins in the fertilization event.
- Epigenetic profile of spermatozoa influence embryo development.
- Epimutations acquired throughout parent's life are not erased and passed to next generations.

CONFLICT OF INTEREST

The authors confirm that they have no conflict of interest to declare for this publication.

ACKNOWLEDGEMENTS

This work was supported by the "Fundação para a Ciência e a Tecnologia"–FCT (PTDC/BBB-BQB/1368/2014), CICS (UID/Multi/00709/2013), and of FEDER through the POPH and POCI - COMPETE 2020 (POCI-01-0145-FEDER-007491) and National Funds by FCT - Foundation for Science and Technology (Project UID/Multi /00709). Luís Rato is funded by Santander-Totta/University of Beira Interior (BIPD/ICI-CICS-BST-UBI).

REFERENCES

[1] Yeates WK. Ejaculation and its disorders. Arch Ital Urol Nefrol Androl 1990; 62(1): 137-48. [PMID: 2163111]

[2] Marberger H. The Mechanisms of Ejaculation. In: Coutinho EH, Fuchs F, Eds. Physiology and Genetics of Reproduction New York. Springer, US 1974; pp. 99-110. [http://dx.doi.org/10.1007/978-1-4684-2892-6_7]

[3] Corona G, Jannini EA, Mannucci E, *et al.* Different testosterone levels are associated with ejaculatory dysfunction. J Sex Med 2008; 5(8): 1991-8. [http://dx.doi.org/10.1111/j.1743-6109.2008.00803.x] [PMID: 18399946]

[4] Keleta YB, Lumia AR, Anderson GM, McGinnis MY. Behavioral effects of pubertal anabolic androgenic steroid exposure in male rats with low serotonin. Brain Res 2007; 1132(1): 129-38. [http://dx.doi.org/10.1016/j.brainres.2006.10.097] [PMID: 17194457]

[5] Mancina R, Filippi S, Marini M, *et al.* Expression and functional activity of phosphodiesterase type 5 in human and rabbit vas deferens. Mol Hum Reprod 2005; 11(2): 107-15. [http://dx.doi.org/10.1093/molehr/gah143] [PMID: 15640438]

[6] Vignozzi L, Filippi S, Morelli A, *et al.* Regulation of epididymal contractility during semen emission, the first part of the ejaculatory process: a role for estrogen. J Sex Med 2008; 5(9): 2010-6. [http://dx.doi.org/10.1111/j.1743-6109.2008.00914.x] [PMID: 18783525]

[7] Filippi S, Luconi M, Granchi S, *et al.* Estrogens, but not androgens, regulate expression and functional activity of oxytocin receptor in rabbit epididymis. Endocrinology 2002; 143(11): 4271-80. [http://dx.doi.org/10.1210/en.2002-220384] [PMID: 12399422]

[8] Filippi S, Morelli A, Vignozzi L, *et al.* Oxytocin mediates the estrogen-dependent contractile activity of endothelin-1 in human and rabbit epididymis. Endocrinology 2005; 146(8): 3506-17. [http://dx.doi.org/10.1210/en.2004-1628] [PMID: 15860558]

[9] Hull EM, Bitran D, Pehek EA, Warner RK, Band LC, Holmes GM. Dopaminergic control of male sex behavior in rats: effects of an intracerebrally-infused agonist. Brain Res 1986; 370(1): 73-81. [http://dx.doi.org/10.1016/0006-8993(86)91106-6] [PMID: 3011196]

[10] Scaletta LL, Hull EM. Systemic or intracranial apomorphine increases copulation in long-term castrated male rats. Pharmacol Biochem Behav 1990; 37(3): 471-5. [http://dx.doi.org/10.1016/0091-3057(90)90015-A] [PMID: 2087489]

[11] Pehek EA, Warner RK, Bazzett TJ, *et al.* Microinjection of cis-flupenthixol, a dopamine antagonist, into the medial preoptic area impairs sexual behavior of male rats. Brain Res 1988; 443(1-2): 70-6. [http://dx.doi.org/10.1016/0006-8993(88)91599-5] [PMID: 3359281]

[12] Kim SW, Paick JS. Peripheral effects of serotonin on the contractile responses of rat seminal vesicles and vasa deferentia. J Androl 2004; 25(6): 893-9. [http://dx.doi.org/10.1002/j.1939-4640.2004.tb03159.x] [PMID: 15477361]

[13] Azmitia E, Gannon P. The ultrastructural localization of serotonin immunoreactivity in myelinated and unmyelinated axons within the medial forebrain bundle of rat and monkey. J Neurosci 1983; 3(10): 2083-90. [PMID: 6604793]

[14] McMahon CG, McMahon CN, Leow LJ, Winestock CG. Efficacy of type-5 phosphodiesterase inhibitors in the drug treatment of premature ejaculation: a systematic review. BJU Int 2006; 98(2): 259-72. [http://dx.doi.org/10.1111/j.1464-410X.2006.06290.x] [PMID: 16879663]

[15] Wang WF, Minhas S, Ralph DJ. Phosphodiesterase 5 inhibitors in the treatment of premature ejaculation. Int J Androl 2006; 29(5): 503-9. [http://dx.doi.org/10.1111/j.1365-2605.2006.00689.x] [PMID: 16573707]

[16] Hedlund P, Ekström P, Larsson B, Alm P, Andersson KE. Heme oxygenase and NO-synthase in the human prostaterelation to adrenergic, cholinergic and peptide-containing nerves. J Auton Nerv Syst 1997; 63(3): 115-26.
[http://dx.doi.org/10.1016/S0165-1838(96)00139-7] [PMID: 9138243]

[17] Uckert S, Bazrafshan S, Scheller F, Mayer ME, Jonas U, Stief CG. Functional responses of isolated human seminal vesicle tissue to selective phosphodiesterase inhibitors. Urology 2007; 70(1): 185-9.
[http://dx.doi.org/10.1016/j.urology.2007.02.049] [PMID: 17656245]

[18] Kaminski HJ, Andrade FH. Nitric oxide: biologic effects on muscle and role in muscle diseases. Neuromuscul Disord 2001; 11(6-7): 517-24.
[http://dx.doi.org/10.1016/S0960-8966(01)00215-2] [PMID: 11525879]

[19] Hull EM, Lumley LA, Matuszewich L, Dominguez J, Moses J, Lorrain DS. The roles of nitric oxide in sexual function of male rats. Neuropharmacology 1994; 33(11): 1499-504.
[http://dx.doi.org/10.1016/0028-3908(94)90054-X] [PMID: 7532834]

[20] Chang MC. Fertilizing capacity of spermatozoa deposited into the fallopian tubes. Nature 1951; 168(4277): 697-8.
[http://dx.doi.org/10.1038/168697b0] [PMID: 14882325]

[21] Austin CR. Observations on the penetration of the sperm in the mammalian egg. Aust J Sci Res, B 1951; 4(4): 581-96.
[http://dx.doi.org/10.1071/BI9510581] [PMID: 14895481]

[22] Austin CR. The capacitation of the mammalian sperm. Nature 1952; 170(4321): 326.
[http://dx.doi.org/10.1038/170326a0] [PMID: 12993150]

[23] Bedford JM. The status and the state of the human epididymis. Hum Reprod 1994; 9(11): 2187-99.
[http://dx.doi.org/10.1093/oxfordjournals.humrep.a138416] [PMID: 7868697]

[24] Suarez SS. Control of hyperactivation in sperm. Hum Reprod Update 2008; 14(6): 647-57.
[http://dx.doi.org/10.1093/humupd/dmn029] [PMID: 18653675]

[25] Rodriguez-Martinez H. Role of the oviduct in sperm capacitation. Theriogenology 2007; 68 (Suppl. 1): S138-46.
[http://dx.doi.org/10.1016/j.theriogenology.2007.03.018] [PMID: 17452049]

[26] Leese HJ, Hugentobler SA, Gray SM, *et al.* Female reproductive tract fluids: composition, mechanism of formation and potential role in the developmental origins of health and disease. Reprod Fertil Dev 2008; 20(1): 1-8.
[http://dx.doi.org/10.1071/RD07153] [PMID: 18154692]

[27] Kawakami E, Arai T, Oishi I, Hori T, Tsutsui T. Induction of dog sperm capacitation by glycosaminoglycans and glycosaminoglycan amounts of oviductal and uterine fluids in bitches. J Vet Med Sci 2000; 62(1): 65-8.
[http://dx.doi.org/10.1292/jvms.62.65] [PMID: 10676892]

[28] Tienthai P, Johannisson A, Rodriguez-Martinez H. Sperm capacitation in the porcine oviduct. Anim Reprod Sci 2004; 80(1-2): 131-46.
[http://dx.doi.org/10.1016/S0378-4320(03)00134-9] [PMID: 15036522]

[29] Tienthai P, Kjellén L, Pertoft H, Suzuki K, Rodriguez-Martinez H. Localization and quantitation of hyaluronan and sulfated glycosaminoglycans in the tissues and intraluminal fluid of the pig oviduct. Reprod Fertil Dev 2000; 12(3-4): 173-82.
[http://dx.doi.org/10.1071/RD00034] [PMID: 11302427]

[30] Travis AJ, Kopf GS. The role of cholesterol efflux in regulating the fertilization potential of mammalian spermatozoa. J Clin Invest 2002; 110(6): 731-6.
[http://dx.doi.org/10.1172/JCI0216392] [PMID: 12235100]

[31] Saccary L, She YM, Oko R, Kan FW. Hamster oviductin regulates tyrosine phosphorylation of sperm proteins during *in vitro* capacitation. Biol Reprod 2013; 89(2): 38. [http://dx.doi.org/10.1095/biolreprod.113.109314] [PMID: 23843230]

[32] Kimura H, Matsuda J, Ogura A, Asano T, Naiki M. Affinity binding of hamster oviductin to spermatozoa and its influence on *in vitro* fertilization. Mol Reprod Dev 1994; 39(3): 322-7. [http://dx.doi.org/10.1002/mrd.1080390309] [PMID: 7888170]

[33] Topper EK, Killian GJ, Way A, Engel B, Woelders H. Influence of capacitation and fluids from the male and female genital tract on the zona binding ability of bull spermatozoa. J Reprod Fertil 1999; 115(1): 175-83. [http://dx.doi.org/10.1530/jrf.0.1150175] [PMID: 10341736]

[34] Florman HM, Arnoult C, Kazam IG, Li C, OToole CM. A perspective on the control of mammalian fertilization by egg-activated ion channels in sperm: a tale of two channels. Biol Reprod 1998; 59(1): 12-6. [http://dx.doi.org/10.1095/biolreprod59.1.12] [PMID: 9674987]

[35] Ho H-C, Suarez SS. Hyperactivation of mammalian spermatozoa: function and regulation. Reproduction 2001; 122(4): 519-26. [http://dx.doi.org/10.1530/rep.0.1220519] [PMID: 11570958]

[36] Evans JP. Getting sperm and egg together: things conserved and things diverged. Biol Reprod 2000; 63(2): 355-60. [http://dx.doi.org/10.1095/biolreprod63.2.355b] [PMID: 10906037]

[37] Visconti PE, Bailey JL, Moore GD, Pan D, Olds-Clarke P, Kopf GS. Capacitation of mouse spermatozoa. I. Correlation between the capacitation state and protein tyrosine phosphorylation. Development 1995; 121(4): 1129-37. [PMID: 7743926]

[38] Thérien I, Moreau R, Manjunath P. Major proteins of bovine seminal plasma and high-density lipoprotein induce cholesterol efflux from epididymal sperm. Biol Reprod 1998; 59(4): 768-76. [http://dx.doi.org/10.1095/biolreprod59.4.768] [PMID: 9746724]

[39] Davis BK. Timing of fertilization in mammals: sperm cholesterol/phospholipid ratio as a determinant of the capacitation interval. Proc Natl Acad Sci USA 1981; 78(12): 7560-4. [http://dx.doi.org/10.1073/pnas.78.12.7560] [PMID: 6950397]

[40] Lin M-H, Lee RK, Hwu Y-M, *et al.* SPINKL, a Kazal-type serine protease inhibitor-like protein purified from mouse seminal vesicle fluid, is able to inhibit sperm capacitation. Reproduction 2008; 136(5): 559-71. [http://dx.doi.org/10.1530/REP-07-0375] [PMID: 18715980]

[41] Lu C-H, Lee RK, Hwu Y-M, *et al.* SERPINE2, a serine protease inhibitor extensively expressed in adult male mouse reproductive tissues, may serve as a murine sperm decapacitation factor. Biol Reprod 2011; 84(3): 514-25. [http://dx.doi.org/10.1095/biolreprod.110.085100] [PMID: 21084713]

[42] Zhu J, Massey JB, Mitchell-Leef D, Elsner CW, Kort HI, Roudebush WE. Platelet-activating factor acetylhydrolase activity affects sperm motility and serves as a decapacitation factor. Fertil Steril 2006; 85(2): 391-4. [http://dx.doi.org/10.1016/j.fertnstert.2005.07.1303] [PMID: 16595216]

[43] Nixon B, MacIntyre DA, Mitchell LA, Gibbs GM, OBryan M, Aitken RJ. The identification of mouse sperm-surface-associated proteins and characterization of their ability to act as decapacitation factors. Biol Reprod 2006; 74(2): 275-87. [http://dx.doi.org/10.1095/biolreprod.105.044644] [PMID: 16221991]

[44] Bi Y, Xu W-M, Wong HY, *et al.* NYD-SP27, a novel intrinsic decapacitation factor in sperm. Asian J Androl 2009; 11(2): 229-39.
[http://dx.doi.org/10.1038/aja.2009.6] [PMID: 19252507]

[45] Ni Y, Zhou Y, Chen WY, *et al.* HongrES1, a cauda epididymis-specific protein, is involved in capacitation of guinea pig sperm. Mol Reprod Dev 2009; 76(10): 984-93.
[http://dx.doi.org/10.1002/mrd.21063] [PMID: 19565644]

[46] Kawano N, Yoshida K, Iwamoto T, Yoshida M. Ganglioside GM1 mediates decapacitation effects of SVS2 on murine spermatozoa. Biol Reprod 2008; 79(6): 1153-9.
[http://dx.doi.org/10.1095/biolreprod.108.069054] [PMID: 18753612]

[47] Florman HM, Ducibella T. Fertilization in mammals. In: Neill JD, Ed. Physiology of Reproduction. San Diego: Elsevier 2006; pp. 55-112.
[http://dx.doi.org/10.1016/B978-012515400-0/50007-5]

[48] Visconti PE, Galantino-Homer H, Ning X, *et al.* Cholesterol efflux-mediated signal transduction in mammalian sperm. β-cyclodextrins initiate transmembrane signaling leading to an increase in protein tyrosine phosphorylation and capacitation. J Biol Chem 1999; 274(5): 3235-42.
[http://dx.doi.org/10.1074/jbc.274.5.3235] [PMID: 9915865]

[49] Choi Y-H, Toyoda Y. Cyclodextrin removes cholesterol from mouse sperm and induces capacitation in a protein-free medium. Biol Reprod 1998; 59(6): 1328-33.
[http://dx.doi.org/10.1095/biolreprod59.6.1328] [PMID: 9828175]

[50] Nagao Y, Ohta Y, Murakami H, Kato Y. The effects of methyl-β-cyclodextrin on *in vitro* fertilization and the subsequent development of bovine oocytes. Zygote 2010; 18(4): 323-30.
[http://dx.doi.org/10.1017/S0967199409990396] [PMID: 20331909]

[51] Langlais J, Kan FW, Granger L, Raymond L, Bleau G, Roberts KD. Identification of sterol acceptors that stimulate cholesterol efflux from human spermatozoa during *in vitro* capacitation. Gamete Res 1988; 20(2): 185-201.
[http://dx.doi.org/10.1002/mrd.1120200209] [PMID: 3235036]

[52] Smith TT, McKinnon-Thompson CA, Wolf DE. Changes in lipid diffusibility in the hamster sperm head plasma membrane during capacitation *In vivo* and *in vitro*. Mol Reprod Dev 1998; 50(1): 86-92.
[http://dx.doi.org/10.1002/(SICI)1098-2795(199805)50:1<86::AID-MRD11>3.0.CO;2-W] [PMID: 9547514]

[53] Lingwood D, Simons K. Lipid rafts as a membrane-organizing principle. Science 2010; 327(5961): 46-50.
[http://dx.doi.org/10.1126/science.1174621] [PMID: 20044567]

[54] van Gestel RA, Brewis IA, Ashton PR, Helms JB, Brouwers JF, Gadella BM. Capacitation-dependent concentration of lipid rafts in the apical ridge head area of porcine sperm cells. Mol Hum Reprod 2005; 11(8): 583-90.
[http://dx.doi.org/10.1093/molehr/gah200] [PMID: 16051681]

[55] Caballero J, Frenette G, DAmours O, Dufour M, Oko R, Sullivan R. ATP-binding cassette transporter G2 activity in the bovine spermatozoa is modulated along the epididymal duct and at ejaculation. Biol Reprod 2012; 86(6): 181.
[http://dx.doi.org/10.1095/biolreprod.111.097477] [PMID: 22441796]

[56] Shadan S, James PS, Howes EA, Jones R. Cholesterol efflux alters lipid raft stability and distribution during capacitation of boar spermatozoa. Biol Reprod 2004; 71(1): 253-65.
[http://dx.doi.org/10.1095/biolreprod.103.026435] [PMID: 15028630]

[57] Rodríguez-Martínez H, Saravia F, Wallgren M, *et al.* Boar spermatozoa in the oviduct. Theriogenology 2005; 63(2): 514-35.
[http://dx.doi.org/10.1016/j.theriogenology.2004.09.028] [PMID: 15626414]

[58] Harrison RA, Mairet B, Miller NG. Flow cytometric studies of bicarbonate-mediated Ca^{2+} influx in boar sperm populations. Mol Reprod Dev 1993; 35(2): 197-208. [http://dx.doi.org/10.1002/mrd.1080350214] [PMID: 8391278]

[59] Gadella BM, Van Gestel RA. Bicarbonate and its role in mammalian sperm function. Anim Reprod Sci 2004; 82-83: 307-19. [http://dx.doi.org/10.1016/j.anireprosci.2004.04.030] [PMID: 15271462]

[60] Closse C, Dachary-Prigent J, Boisseau MR. Phosphatidylserine-related adhesion of human erythrocytes to vascular endothelium. Br J Haematol 1999; 107(2): 300-2. [http://dx.doi.org/10.1046/j.1365-2141.1999.01718.x] [PMID: 10583215]

[61] Schlegel RA, Prendergast TW, Williamson P. Membrane phospholipid asymmetry as a factor in erythrocyte-endothelial cell interactions. J Cell Physiol 1985; 123(2): 215-8. [http://dx.doi.org/10.1002/jcp.1041230210] [PMID: 3980587]

[62] Harrison RA. Rapid PKA-catalysed phosphorylation of boar sperm proteins induced by the capacitating agent bicarbonate. Mol Reprod Dev 2004; 67(3): 337-52. [http://dx.doi.org/10.1002/mrd.20028] [PMID: 14735495]

[63] Esposito G, Jaiswal BS, Xie F, *et al.* Mice deficient for soluble adenylyl cyclase are infertile because of a severe sperm-motility defect. Proc Natl Acad Sci USA 2004; 101(9): 2993-8. [http://dx.doi.org/10.1073/pnas.0400050101] [PMID: 14976244]

[64] Gross MK, Toscano DG, Toscano WA Jr. Calmodulin-mediated adenylate cyclase from mammalian sperm. J Biol Chem 1987; 262(18): 8672-6. [PMID: 3597392]

[65] Wasco WM, Orr GA. Function of calmodulin in mammalian sperm: presence of a calmodulin-dependent cyclic nucleotide phosphodiesterase associated with demembranated rat caudal epididymal sperm. Biochem Biophys Res Commun 1984; 118(2): 636-42. [http://dx.doi.org/10.1016/0006-291X(84)91350-0] [PMID: 6322756]

[66] Suarez SS, Varosi SM, Dai X. Intracellular calcium increases with hyperactivation in intact, moving hamster sperm and oscillates with the flagellar beat cycle. Proc Natl Acad Sci USA 1993; 90(10): 4660-4. [http://dx.doi.org/10.1073/pnas.90.10.4660] [PMID: 8506314]

[67] Yunes R, Doncel GF, Acosta AA. Incidence of sperm-tail tyrosine phosphorylation and hyperactivated motility in normozoospermic and asthenozoospermic human sperm samples. Biocell 2003; 27(1): 29-36. [PMID: 12847912]

[68] Buffone MG, Calamera JC, Verstraeten SV, Doncel GF. Capacitation-associated protein tyrosine phosphorylation and membrane fluidity changes are impaired in the spermatozoa of asthenozoospermic patients. Reproduction 2005; 129(6): 697-705. [http://dx.doi.org/10.1530/rep.1.00584] [PMID: 15923385]

[69] Visconti PE, Moore GD, Bailey JL, *et al.* Capacitation of mouse spermatozoa. II. Protein tyrosine phosphorylation and capacitation are regulated by a cAMP-dependent pathway. Development 1995; 121(4): 1139-50. [PMID: 7538069]

[70] Leclerc P, de Lamirande E, Gagnon C. Interaction between Ca^{2+}, cyclic 3,5 adenosine monophosphate, the superoxide anion, and tyrosine phosphorylation pathways in the regulation of human sperm capacitation. J Androl 1998; 19(4): 434-43. [PMID: 9733146]

[71] Osheroff JE, Visconti PE, Valenzuela JP, Travis AJ, Alvarez J, Kopf GS. Regulation of human sperm capacitation by a cholesterol efflux-stimulated signal transduction pathway leading to protein kinase A-mediated up-regulation of protein tyrosine phosphorylation. Mol Hum Reprod 1999; 5(11): 1017-26.
[http://dx.doi.org/10.1093/molehr/5.11.1017] [PMID: 10541563]

[72] Baker MA, Smith ND, Hetherington L, *et al.* Label-free quantitation of phosphopeptide changes during rat sperm capacitation. J Proteome Res 2010; 9(2): 718-29.
[http://dx.doi.org/10.1021/pr900513d] [PMID: 19947656]

[73] Ficarro S, Chertihin O, Westbrook VA, *et al.* Phosphoproteome analysis of capacitated human sperm. Evidence of tyrosine phosphorylation of a kinase-anchoring protein 3 and valosin-containing protein/p97 during capacitation. J Biol Chem 2003; 278(13): 11579-89.
[http://dx.doi.org/10.1074/jbc.M202325200] [PMID: 12509440]

[74] Nixon B, Bielanowicz A, Anderson AL, *et al.* Elucidation of the signaling pathways that underpin capacitation-associated surface phosphotyrosine expression in mouse spermatozoa. J Cell Physiol 2010; 224(1): 71-83.
[http://dx.doi.org/10.1002/jcp.22090] [PMID: 20232304]

[75] Mitchell LA, Nixon B, Baker MA, Aitken RJ. Investigation of the role of SRC in capacitation-associated tyrosine phosphorylation of human spermatozoa. Mol Hum Reprod 2008; 14(4): 235-43.
[http://dx.doi.org/10.1093/molehr/gan007] [PMID: 18245108]

[76] Carrera A, Moos J, Ning XP, *et al.* Regulation of protein tyrosine phosphorylation in human sperm by a calcium/calmodulin-dependent mechanism: identification of A kinase anchor proteins as major substrates for tyrosine phosphorylation. Dev Biol 1996; 180(1): 284-96.
[http://dx.doi.org/10.1006/dbio.1996.0301] [PMID: 8948591]

[77] Naaby-Hansen S, Mandal A, Wolkowicz MJ, *et al.* CABYR, a novel calcium-binding tyrosine phosphorylation-regulated fibrous sheath protein involved in capacitation. Dev Biol 2002; 242(2): 236-54.
[http://dx.doi.org/10.1006/dbio.2001.0527] [PMID: 11820818]

[78] Huynh H, Bottini N, Williams S, *et al.* Control of vesicle fusion by a tyrosine phosphatase. Nat Cell Biol 2004; 6(9): 831-9.
[http://dx.doi.org/10.1038/ncb1164] [PMID: 15322554]

[79] Laflamme J, Akoum A, Leclerc P. Induction of human sperm capacitation and protein tyrosine phosphorylation by endometrial cells and interleukin-6. Mol Hum Reprod 2005; 11(2): 141-50.
[http://dx.doi.org/10.1093/molehr/gah142] [PMID: 15665187]

[80] Luconi M, Barni T, Vannelli GB, *et al.* Extracellular signal-regulated kinases modulate capacitation of human spermatozoa. Biol Reprod 1998; 58(6): 1476-89.
[http://dx.doi.org/10.1095/biolreprod58.6.1476] [PMID: 9623609]

[81] de Lamirande E, Gagnon C. The extracellular signal-regulated kinase (ERK) pathway is involved in human sperm function and modulated by the superoxide anion. Mol Hum Reprod 2002; 8(2): 124-35.
[http://dx.doi.org/10.1093/molehr/8.2.124] [PMID: 11818515]

[82] OFlaherty C, de Lamirande E, Gagnon C. Reactive oxygen species and protein kinases modulate the level of phospho-MEK-like proteins during human sperm capacitation. Biol Reprod 2005; 73(1): 94-105.
[http://dx.doi.org/10.1095/biolreprod.104.038794] [PMID: 15772258]

[83] Naz RK. Involvement of protein serine and threonine phosphorylation in human sperm capacitation. Biol Reprod 1999; 60(6): 1402-9.
[http://dx.doi.org/10.1095/biolreprod60.6.1402] [PMID: 10330099]

[84] Morales P, Pizarro E, Kong M, Jara M. Extracellular localization of proteasomes in human sperm. Mol Reprod Dev 2004; 68(1): 115-24.
[http://dx.doi.org/10.1002/mrd.20052] [PMID: 15039955]

[85] Kong M, Diaz ES, Morales P. Participation of the human sperm proteasome in the capacitation process and its regulation by protein kinase A and tyrosine kinase. Biol Reprod 2009; 80(5): 1026-35.
[http://dx.doi.org/10.1095/biolreprod.108.073924] [PMID: 19144957]

[86] Villanueva-Díaz C, Arias-Martínez J, Bermejo-Martínez L, Vadillo-Ortega F. Progesterone induces human sperm chemotaxis. Fertil Steril 1995; 64(6): 1183-8.
[http://dx.doi.org/10.1016/S0015-0282(16)57982-5] [PMID: 7589674]

[87] Sun F, Bahat A, Gakamsky A, *et al.* Human sperm chemotaxis: both the oocyte and its surrounding cumulus cells secrete sperm chemoattractants. Hum Reprod 2005; 20(3): 761-7.
[http://dx.doi.org/10.1093/humrep/deh657] [PMID: 15591080]

[88] Kaupp UB, Kashikar ND, Weyand I. Mechanisms of sperm chemotaxis. Annu Rev Physiol 2008; 70: 93-117.
[http://dx.doi.org/10.1146/annurev.physiol.70.113006.100654] [PMID: 17988206]

[89] Saling PM, Sowinski J, Storey BT. An ultrastructural study of epididymal mouse spermatozoa binding to zonae pellucidae *in vitro*: sequential relationship to the acrosome reaction. J Exp Zool 1979; 209(2): 229-38.
[http://dx.doi.org/10.1002/jez.1402090205] [PMID: 512592]

[90] Florman HM, Storey BT. Mouse gamete interactions: the zona pellucida is the site of the acrosome reaction leading to fertilization *in vitro*. Dev Biol 1982; 91(1): 121-30.
[http://dx.doi.org/10.1016/0012-1606(82)90015-X] [PMID: 7201425]

[91] Saling PM, Storey BT. Mouse gamete interactions during fertilization *in vitro*. Chlortetracycline as a fluorescent probe for the mouse sperm acrosome reaction. J Cell Biol 1979; 83(3): 544-55.
[http://dx.doi.org/10.1083/jcb.83.3.544] [PMID: 574869]

[92] Benoff S, Hurley IR, Mandel FS, Cooper GW, Hershlag A. Induction of the human sperm acrosome reaction with mannose-containing neoglycoprotein ligands. Mol Hum Reprod 1997; 3(10): 827-37.
[http://dx.doi.org/10.1093/molehr/3.10.827] [PMID: 9395260]

[93] Drisdel RC, Mack SR, Anderson RA, Zaneveld LJ. Purification and partial characterization of acrosome reaction inhibiting glycoprotein from human seminal plasma. Biol Reprod 1995; 53(1): 201-8.
[http://dx.doi.org/10.1095/biolreprod53.1.201] [PMID: 7669849]

[94] Miranda PV, Gonzalez-Echeverría F, Marín-Briggiler CI, Brandelli A, Blaquier JA, Tezón JG. Glycosidic residues involved in human sperm-zona pellucida binding *in vitro*. Mol Hum Reprod 1997; 3(5): 399-404.
[http://dx.doi.org/10.1093/molehr/3.5.399] [PMID: 9239724]

[95] Breitbart H, Spungin B. The biochemistry of the acrosome reaction. Mol Hum Reprod 1997; 3(3): 195-202.
[http://dx.doi.org/10.1093/molehr/3.3.195] [PMID: 9237245]

[96] Abbott AL, Ducibella T. Calcium and the control of mammalian cortical granule exocytosis. Front Biosci 2001; 6: D792-806.
[http://dx.doi.org/10.2741/Abbott] [PMID: 11438440]

[97] Kurokawa M, Sato K, Fissore RA. Mammalian fertilization: from sperm factor to phospholipase Czeta. Biol Cell 2004; 96(1): 37-45.
[http://dx.doi.org/10.1016/j.biolcel.2003.11.003] [PMID: 15093126]

[98] Lawrence Y, Whitaker M, Swann K. Sperm-egg fusion is the prelude to the initial Ca^{2+} increase at fertilization in the mouse. Development 1997; 124(1): 233-41.
[PMID: 9006083]

[99] Deguchi R, Shirakawa H, Oda S, Mohri T, Miyazaki S. Spatiotemporal analysis of Ca(2+) waves in relation to the sperm entry site and animal-vegetal axis during Ca(2+) oscillations in fertilized mouse eggs. Dev Biol 2000; 218(2): 299-313. [http://dx.doi.org/10.1006/dbio.1999.9573] [PMID: 10656771]

[100] Campanella ME, Chu H, Low PS. Assembly and regulation of a glycolytic enzyme complex on the human erythrocyte membrane. Proc Natl Acad Sci USA 2005; 102(7): 2402-7. [http://dx.doi.org/10.1073/pnas.0409741102] [PMID: 15701694]

[101] Nakamura N, Mori C, Eddy EM. Molecular complex of three testis-specific isozymes associated with the mouse sperm fibrous sheath: hexokinase 1, phosphofructokinase M, and glutathione S-transferase mu class 5. Biol Reprod 2010; 82(3): 504-15. [http://dx.doi.org/10.1095/biolreprod.109.080580] [PMID: 19889946]

[102] Gopalakrishnan B, Aravinda S, Pawshe CH, *et al.* Studies on glutathione S-transferases important for sperm function: evidence of catalytic activity-independent functions. Biochem J 1998; 329(Pt 2): 231-41. [http://dx.doi.org/10.1042/bj3290231] [PMID: 9425104]

[103] Nixon B, Bielanowicz A, McLaughlin EA, Tanphaichitr N, Ensslin MA, Aitken RJ. Composition and significance of detergent resistant membranes in mouse spermatozoa. J Cell Physiol 2009; 218(1): 122-34. [http://dx.doi.org/10.1002/jcp.21575] [PMID: 18726997]

[104] Hinsch KD, Asmarinah , Hinsch E, Konrad L. VDAC2 (porin-2) expression pattern and localization in the bovine testis. Biochim Biophys Acta 2001; 1518(3): 329-33. [http://dx.doi.org/10.1016/S0167-4781(01)00199-3] [PMID: 11311949]

[105] Triphan X, Menzel VA, Petrunkina AM, *et al.* Localisation and function of voltage-dependent anion channels (VDAC) in bovine spermatozoa. Pflugers Arch 2008; 455(4): 677-86. [http://dx.doi.org/10.1007/s00424-007-0316-1] [PMID: 17647012]

[106] Primakoff P, Hyatt H, Tredick-Kline J. Identification and purification of a sperm surface protein with a potential role in sperm-egg membrane fusion. J Cell Biol 1987; 104(1): 141-9. [http://dx.doi.org/10.1083/jcb.104.1.141] [PMID: 3793758]

[107] Inoue N, Ikawa M, Isotani A, Okabe M. The immunoglobulin superfamily protein Izumo is required for sperm to fuse with eggs. Nature 2005; 434(7030): 234-8. [http://dx.doi.org/10.1038/nature03362] [PMID: 15759005]

[108] Krutskikh A, Poliandri A, Cabrera-Sharp V, Dacheux JL, Poutanen M, Huhtaniemi I. Epididymal protein Rnase10 is required for post-testicular sperm maturation and male fertility. FASEB J 2012; 26(10): 4198-209. [http://dx.doi.org/10.1096/fj.12-205211] [PMID: 22750516]

[109] Cho C. Testicular and epididymal ADAMs: expression and function during fertilization. Nat Rev Urol 2012; 9(10): 550-60. [http://dx.doi.org/10.1038/nrurol.2012.167] [PMID: 22926424]

[110] Wolkowicz MJ, Digilio L, Klotz K, Shetty J, Flickinger CJ, Herr JC. Equatorial segment protein (ESP) is a human alloantigen involved in sperm-egg binding and fusion. J Androl 2008; 29(3): 272-82. [http://dx.doi.org/10.2164/jandrol.106.000604] [PMID: 17978344]

[111] Wolkowicz MJ, Shetty J, Westbrook A, *et al.* Equatorial segment protein defines a discrete acrosomal subcompartment persisting throughout acrosomal biogenesis. Biol Reprod 2003; 69(3): 735-45. [http://dx.doi.org/10.1095/biolreprod.103.016675] [PMID: 12773409]

[112] Nishimura H, Gupta S, Myles DG, Primakoff P. Characterization of mouse sperm TMEM190, a small transmembrane protein with the trefoil domain: evidence for co-localization with IZUMO1 and complex formation with other sperm proteins. Reproduction 2011; 141(4): 437-51. [http://dx.doi.org/10.1530/REP-10-0391] [PMID: 21273369]

[113] Mandal A, Klotz KL, Shetty J, *et al.* SLLP1, a unique, intra-acrosomal, non-bacteriolytic, c lysozyme-like protein of human spermatozoa. Biol Reprod 2003; 68(5): 1525-37.
[http://dx.doi.org/10.1095/biolreprod.102.010108] [PMID: 12606493]

[114] Shetty J, Wolkowicz MJ, Digilio LC, *et al.* SAMP14, a novel, acrosomal membrane-associated, glycosylphosphatidylinositol-anchored member of the Ly-6/urokinase-type plasminogen activator receptor superfamily with a role in sperm-egg interaction. J Biol Chem 2003; 278(33): 30506-15.
[http://dx.doi.org/10.1074/jbc.M301713200] [PMID: 12788941]

[115] Morgan HD, Santos F, Green K, Dean W, Reik W. Epigenetic reprogramming in mammals. Hum Mol Genet 2005; 14(Spec No 1): R47-58.
[http://dx.doi.org/10.1093/hmg/ddi114] [PMID: 15809273]

[116] Braun RE. Packaging paternal chromosomes with protamine. Nat Genet 2001; 28(1): 10-2.
[http://dx.doi.org/10.1038/ng0501-10] [PMID: 11326265]

[117] Adenot PG, Mercier Y, Renard JP, Thompson EM. Differential H4 acetylation of paternal and maternal chromatin precedes DNA replication and differential transcriptional activity in pronuclei of 1-cell mouse embryos. Development 1997; 124(22): 4615-25.
[PMID: 9409678]

[118] Sobel RE, Cook RG, Perry CA, Annunziato AT, Allis CD. Conservation of deposition-related acetylation sites in newly synthesized histones H3 and H4. Proc Natl Acad Sci USA 1995; 92(4): 1237-41.
[http://dx.doi.org/10.1073/pnas.92.4.1237] [PMID: 7862667]

[119] Santos F, Peters AH, Otte AP, Reik W, Dean W. Dynamic chromatin modifications characterise the first cell cycle in mouse embryos. Dev Biol 2005; 280(1): 225-36.
[http://dx.doi.org/10.1016/j.ydbio.2005.01.025] [PMID: 15766761]

[120] Oswald J, Engemann S, Lane N, *et al.* Active demethylation of the paternal genome in the mouse zygote. Curr Biol 2000; 10(8): 475-8.
[http://dx.doi.org/10.1016/S0960-9822(00)00448-6] [PMID: 10801417]

[121] Bhattacharya SK, Ramchandani S, Cervoni N, Szyf M. A mammalian protein with specific demethylase activity for mCpG DNA. Nature 1999; 397(6720): 579-83.
[http://dx.doi.org/10.1038/17533] [PMID: 10050851]

[122] Hendrich B, Hardeland U, Ng H-H, Jiricny J, Bird A. The thymine glycosylase MBD4 can bind to the product of deamination at methylated CpG sites. Nature 1999; 401(6750): 301-4.
[http://dx.doi.org/10.1038/45843] [PMID: 10499592]

[123] Ho L, Crabtree GR. Chromatin remodelling during development. Nature 2010; 463(7280): 474-84.
[http://dx.doi.org/10.1038/nature08911] [PMID: 20110991]

[124] Olek A, Walter J. The pre-implantation ontogeny of the H19 methylation imprint. Nat Genet 1997; 17(3): 275-6.
[http://dx.doi.org/10.1038/ng1197-275] [PMID: 9354788]

[125] Shibata H, Yoda Y, Kato R, *et al.* A methylation imprint mark in the mouse imprinted gene Grf1/Cdc25Mm locus shares a common feature with the U2afbp-rs gene: an association with a short tandem repeat and a hypermethylated region. Genomics 1998; 49(1): 30-7.
[http://dx.doi.org/10.1006/geno.1998.5218] [PMID: 9570946]

[126] Erhardt S, Su IH, Schneider R, *et al.* Consequences of the depletion of zygotic and embryonic enhancer of zeste 2 during preimplantation mouse development. Development 2003; 130(18): 4235-48.
[http://dx.doi.org/10.1242/dev.00625] [PMID: 12900441]

[127] Howell CY, Bestor TH, Ding F, *et al.* Genomic imprinting disrupted by a maternal effect mutation in the Dnmt1 gene. Cell 2001; 104(6): 829-38.
[http://dx.doi.org/10.1016/S0092-8674(01)00280-X] [PMID: 11290321]

[128] Pittoggi C, Renzi L, Zaccagnini G, *et al.* A fraction of mouse sperm chromatin is organized in nucleosomal hypersensitive domains enriched in retroposon DNA. J Cell Sci 1999; 112(Pt 20): 3537-48.
[PMID: 10504302]

[129] Liu H, Kim JM, Aoki F. Regulation of histone H3 lysine 9 methylation in oocytes and early pre-implantation embryos. Development 2004; 131(10): 2269-80.
[http://dx.doi.org/10.1242/dev.01116] [PMID: 15102709]

[130] Kourmouli N, Jeppesen P, Mahadevhaiah S, *et al.* Heterochromatin and tri-methylated lysine 20 of histone H4 in animals. J Cell Sci 2004; 117(Pt 12): 2491-501.
[http://dx.doi.org/10.1242/jcs.01238] [PMID: 15128874]

[131] Daujat S, Weiss T, Mohn F, *et al.* H3K64 trimethylation marks heterochromatin and is dynamically remodeled during developmental reprogramming. Nat Struct Mol Biol 2009; 16(7): 777-81.
[http://dx.doi.org/10.1038/nsmb.1629] [PMID: 19561610]

[132] Lepikhov K, Walter J. Differential dynamics of histone H3 methylation at positions K4 and K9 in the mouse zygote. BMC Dev Biol 2004; 4: 12.
[http://dx.doi.org/10.1186/1471-213X-4-12] [PMID: 15383155]

[133] Gu TP, Guo F, Yang H, *et al.* The role of Tet3 DNA dioxygenase in epigenetic reprogramming by oocytes. Nature 2011; 477(7366): 606-10.
[http://dx.doi.org/10.1038/nature10443] [PMID: 21892189]

[134] Aoki F, Worrad DM, Schultz RM. Regulation of transcriptional activity during the first and second cell cycles in the preimplantation mouse embryo. Dev Biol 1997; 181(2): 296-307.
[http://dx.doi.org/10.1006/dbio.1996.8466] [PMID: 9013938]

[135] Latham KE, Schultz RM. Embryonic genome activation. Front Biosci 2001; 6: D748-59.
[http://dx.doi.org/10.2741/A639] [PMID: 11401780]

[136] Mansour AA, Gafni O, Weinberger L, *et al.* The H3K27 demethylase Utx regulates somatic and germ cell epigenetic reprogramming. Nature 2012; 488(7411): 409-13.
[http://dx.doi.org/10.1038/nature11272] [PMID: 22801502]

[137] Nakamura T, Arai Y, Umehara H, *et al.* PGC7/Stella protects against DNA demethylation in early embryogenesis. Nat Cell Biol 2007; 9(1): 64-71.
[http://dx.doi.org/10.1038/ncb1519] [PMID: 17143267]

[138] Nakamura T, Liu Y-J, Nakashima H, *et al.* PGC7 binds histone H3K9me2 to protect against conversion of 5mC to 5hmC in early embryos. Nature 2012; 486(7403): 415-9.
[http://dx.doi.org/10.1038/nature11093] [PMID: 22722204]

[139] van der Heijden GW, Ramos L, Baart EB, *et al.* Sperm-derived histones contribute to zygotic chromatin in humans. BMC Dev Biol 2008; 8: 34.
[http://dx.doi.org/10.1186/1471-213X-8-34] [PMID: 18377649]

[140] Brykczynska U, Hisano M, Erkek S, *et al.* Repressive and active histone methylation mark distinct promoters in human and mouse spermatozoa. Nat Struct Mol Biol 2010; 17(6): 679-87.
[http://dx.doi.org/10.1038/nsmb.1821] [PMID: 20473313]

[141] Hammoud SS, Nix DA, Zhang H, Purwar J, Carrell DT, Cairns BR. Distinctive chromatin in human sperm packages genes for embryo development. Nature 2009; 460(7254): 473-8.
[http://dx.doi.org/10.1038/nature08162] [PMID: 19525931]

[142] Ohinata Y, Ohta H, Shigeta M, Yamanaka K, Wakayama T, Saitou M. A signaling principle for the specification of the germ cell lineage in mice. Cell 2009; 137(3): 571-84.
[http://dx.doi.org/10.1016/j.cell.2009.03.014] [PMID: 19410550]

[143] Bernstein BE, Mikkelsen TS, Xie X, *et al.* A bivalent chromatin structure marks key developmental genes in embryonic stem cells. Cell 2006; 125(2): 315-26. [http://dx.doi.org/10.1016/j.cell.2006.02.041] [PMID: 16630819]

[144] Lee J, Inoue K, Ono R, *et al.* Erasing genomic imprinting memory in mouse clone embryos produced from day 11.5 primordial germ cells. Development 2002; 129(8): 1807-17. [PMID: 11934847]

[145] Chuva de Sousa Lopes SM, Hayashi K, Shovlin TC, Mifsud W, Surani MA, McLaren A. X chromosome activity in mouse XX primordial germ cells. PLoS Genet 2008; 4(2): e30. [http://dx.doi.org/10.1371/journal.pgen.0040030] [PMID: 18266475]

[146] Lucifero D, Mann MR, Bartolomei MS, Trasler JM. Gene-specific timing and epigenetic memory in oocyte imprinting. Hum Mol Genet 2004; 13(8): 839-49. [http://dx.doi.org/10.1093/hmg/ddh104] [PMID: 14998934]

[147] Hajkova P, Ancelin K, Waldmann T, *et al.* Chromatin dynamics during epigenetic reprogramming in the mouse germ line. Nature 2008; 452(7189): 877-81. [http://dx.doi.org/10.1038/nature06714] [PMID: 18354397]

[148] Guibert S, Forné T, Weber M. Global profiling of DNA methylation erasure in mouse primordial germ cells. Genome Res 2012; 22(4): 633-41. [http://dx.doi.org/10.1101/gr.130997.111] [PMID: 22357612]

[149] McPherson NO, Bakos HW, Owens JA, Setchell BP, Lane M. Improving metabolic health in obese male mice *via* diet and exercise restores embryo development and fetal growth. PLoS One 2013; 8(8): e71459. [http://dx.doi.org/10.1371/journal.pone.0071459] [PMID: 23977045]

[150] Sharma U, Conine CC, Shea JM, *et al.* Biogenesis and function of tRNA fragments during sperm maturation and fertilization in mammals. Science 2016; 351(6271): 391-6. [http://dx.doi.org/10.1126/science.aad6780] [PMID: 26721685]

[151] Chen Q, Yan M, Cao Z, *et al.* Sperm tsRNAs contribute to intergenerational inheritance of an acquired metabolic disorder. Science 2016; 351(6271): 397-400. [http://dx.doi.org/10.1126/science.aad7977] [PMID: 26721680]

[152] Rodgers AB, Morgan CP, Leu NA, Bale TL. Transgenerational epigenetic programming *via* sperm microRNA recapitulates effects of paternal stress. Proc Natl Acad Sci USA 2015; 112(44): 13699-704. [http://dx.doi.org/10.1073/pnas.1508347112] [PMID: 26483456]

[153] Cheung P, Allis CD, Sassone-Corsi P. Signaling to chromatin through histone modifications. Cell 2000; 103(2): 263-71. [http://dx.doi.org/10.1016/S0092-8674(00)00118-5] [PMID: 11057899]

[154] Sun LY, DErcole AJ. Insulin-like growth factor-I stimulates histone H3 and H4 acetylation in the brain *In vivo*. Endocrinology 2006; 147(11): 5480-90. [http://dx.doi.org/10.1210/en.2006-0586] [PMID: 16935839]

CHAPTER 11

Testicular Cancer, Erectile Dysfunction and Male Reproductive Health

Luís Rato*

Health Sciences Research Centre, University of Beira Interior, Rua Marquês d'Ávila e Bolama, 6201-001, Covilhã, Portugal

Abstract: In recent years, there has been growing awareness that male reproductive performance has declined. Numerous studies have focused on various aspects of adverse trends in male reproductive health. There is a wealth of data that congenital disorders, such as hypospadias, undescended testis, testicular atrophy and testicular cancer have increased among young males. Testicular cancer, in particular germ cells tumors, are the most common malignancy among young males accounting more than 10 cases per 100000 men per year in Europe. Both genetic predisposition and environmental contaminants probably contribute for its etiology. Testicular germ cell tumors arise from malignant transformation of testicular germ cells in a multistep process where several aberrant modifications occur in genes involved in proliferation/survival and differentiation. Individuals with testicular germ cell tumors present a high survival rate but during treatments they are exposed to radio- and/or chemotherapy that may induce permanent damages in male fertility. In this context, it is essential to decipher the molecular mechanisms underlying testicular-related cancers. However, other pathologies have also contributed to the decline of male reproductive health, and particularly affect male sexual behavior. Inadequate penile erection, commonly termed as erectile dysfunction (ED) mostly occurs in men older than 40 years. It is quite common in developed countries and compelling evidences have linked the development of ED to diabetes mellitus, hypertension, hyperlipidemia, metabolic syndrome and depression. In fact, it has been shown that certain environmental and factors related to daily life, such as smoking, obesity, and limited or an absence of physical exercise may also be key predictors of ED. Physicians have looked with particular concern to these issues, but also for the sexually transmitted diseases (STDs). Some STDs are resolved without treatment, but others have chronic lifelong infections. In this chapter those topics will be discussed from a biochemical point of view and the pathways that regulate the most relevant processes.

Keywords: *Carcinoma in situ*, Erectile dysfunction, Libido, Phosphodiesterase inhibitors, Testicular cancer, Testicular germ cell tumors, Sexual behavior, Sexual desire, Sexually transmitted diseases.

* **Corresponding author Luís Rato:** Health Sciences Research Centre (CICS-UBI), Av. Infante D. Henrique, 6201-506, Covilhã, Portugal; Tel: +351 275 329 002; Fax:+351 275 329 099; E-mail: luis.pedro.rato@gmail.com

Marco G. Alves and Pedro F. Oliveira (Eds.)

INTRODUCTION

For many years, reproductive health of males has been overlooked. This has occurred because reproductive problems such as infertility have been suggested to have only origin in females. For instance, for many years, women's reproductive capacity has been a target for contraceptive development, which illustrates how the health systems define "priorities" around women's and not men's health needs. However, in the last two-three decades a decline in male reproductive health has been observed, mostly due to the decline in spermatozoa quality. The prevalence of infertility in couples in reproductive age is extremely high and in many developed countries affects one in seven couples, with the "male factor" accounting for the 50% of the cases. Male reproductive health is extremely vulnerable to adverse effects that arise from lifestyle factors. Though there is not yet a direct association, compelling evidence suggested that all these external insults have contributed to several male reproductive disorders that have a common fetal origin, triggered by testicular maldevelopment [1]. This has been termed by "testicular dysgenesis syndrome" (TDS) [1]. Amongst the several reproductive anomalies that may arise from TDS, testicular cancer is one of the most relevant problems since it mostly affects young males. In fact, testicular cancer is the most common malignancy among young men. Most of these cases are treated with radio- and/or chemotherapy, which lead to severe effects for male fertility (most of them permanent). It is therefore imperative to unravel the molecular mechanisms by which testicular-related cancers establish and progress.

On the other hand, the current lifestyle, based on sedentarism and work stress has led to psychological and emotional distress that have also compromised male reproductive health by disturbing male reproductive behavior. All these factors can affect the endocrine system and the molecular pathways that govern it, therefore affecting male sexual behavior (namely libido and erectile function). Physicians have looked with particular concern to these issues but also for the problems caused by pathogens that can be acquired and transmitted through sexual activity. Sexually transmitted diseases (STDs) have accounted to the most common infection diseases. The alarming number of individuals getting STDs has reached pandemic proportions [2]. Most of STDs may be asymptomatic and therefore people may be unaware that have it or are at high risk to be infected. Some of the STDs are resolved without treatment, but others are chronic lifelong infections. In this chapter, those topics will be discussed from a biochemical point of view, with particular focus on the pathways that regulate these processes.

MOLECULAR MECHANISMS INVOLVED IN TESTICULAR CANCER

Testicular cancer is rare accounting to only 1–1.5% of male cancers. It mostly affects young males during their third or fourth decade of life [3, 4]. The World Health Organization (WHO) has classified testicular tumors in three main categories: testicular germ cell tumors (TGCTs) accounting for the most common form of testicular cancer; cord stromal tumors, and miscellaneous germ cell/sex cord stromal tumors [2]. Since TGCTs account for 90-95% of all testicular neoplasia and are a heterogeneous group of neoplasms with diverse histopathology and clinical behavior, we will focus in this type of cancer. TGCTs may occur throughout men's life and are divided into three main types: type I which consists of benign mature teratomas or malignant yolk sac tumors which occur in children usually before four years of age and always become apparent before puberty [5 - 7]; in the type II, TGCTs can be sub-divided into two main types: classic seminoma and nonseminomas, both derived from a common precursor cells, called carcinoma in situ (CIS) or intratubular germ-cell neoplasia. CIS cells are large atypical germ cells that are found between the thickened basement membrane and the Sertoli cell layer within the seminiferous tubules; the third type of TGCTs are known as spermatocytic seminomas and usually occur in men older than 50 years. These benign tumors exhibit slow growth and share some genetic markers with type B spermatogonia [5, 6, 8]. Contrastingly, there has been a marked increase in the incidence of type II germ cell tumors in developed countries in the last 50 years [5, 6, 8]. Type II TGCTs mainly affects men in their reproductive age (20s to 40s years of age). These tumors are associated with a pre-invasive lesion or undifferentiated intratubular germ cell neoplasia. Interestingly the incidence of TGCTs shows geographic and ethnic differences, with Caucasian people being mostly affected in developed countries [8 - 12]. Even within this group, it has been observed marked differences between populations, as evidenced by two North European countries, Denmark and Finland. The rapid increase in the incidence of TGCTs cannot be only explained by genetic predisposition, indicating the possible involvement of environmental or lifestyle factors in its etiology. This is supported by the fact that increased incidence of TGCTs has occurred at the same time with the tendency of other reproductive disorders associated with TDS, such as impaired testicular descent, genital malformations, and male subfertility [13, 14]. Based on these facts, it has been proposed that TGCTs may arise from congenital disorders. For instance, it has been generally accepted that cryptorchidism is one of the best known risk factors for testicular cancer [15], but other components of TDS, such as hypospadias, also arise as good candidates. Interestingly, all these risk factors are directly linked to prenatal or perinatal period of development. TGCTs development is a multistep process that, in its principle, follows the general multiple-hit hypothesis of malignant transformation where accumulation of several aberrations affecting groups of genes involved in proliferation/survival and differentiation/cell repair, at subsequent stages of life, are required for the initiation of tumor. It is likely that tumorigenesis occurs in utero's life during embryonic development, giving rise to the precursor lesion. This is followed by a period of latency until after puberty when, under the influence of sex hormones and alongside the normal spermatogenesis. Morphologically, CIS cells resemble gonocytes, and in post-pubertal testis occupy the place of spermatogonia. There is an intense debate concerning the initiation of malignant transformation of germ cells into tumors cells and according to the most recent hypothesis TGCTs initiate during intra-uterine development, where they are arrested undifferentiated early germ cells, most probably gonocytes [16].

This process is highly sensitive to hormonal fluctuations. Somatic cells secrete hormones and paracrine factors and with other stromal cells they create an adequate "environment" for normal differentiation of germ cells. It is supposed that even subtle imbalances in this microenvironment during development of gonads may disrupt normal differentiation of germ cells leading to prolonged expression of embryonic genes and genes related to the undifferentiated state together with mitosis-meiosis switch errors, premature start and/or abnormal course of meiosis, thus facilitating their neoplastic transformation. A major hallmark of TGCTs is the excess of genetic material at the short arm of chromosome 12, usually in the form of an isochromosome i(12p). The i(12p) results from a structural abnormality upon loss of one arm and duplication of the other, or in other words, one arm of the chromosome mirrors of each other. This genetic abnormality occurs in all primary sites and histologic types [17, 18]. Approximately 80% of TGCT cases exhibit i(12p) and the remainder have excess 12p genetic material in derivative chromosomes [19], however this has been a matter of controversy [20, 21]. This region contains a number of genes associated with pluripotency and proliferation, such as *Nanog, Stellar, Dppa-5, Gdf3, K-Ras, Ccnd2,* and many of these genes are highly expressed in CIS and TGCTs [22 - 30].

Several signaling pathways have been involved in the pathogenesis of TGCT, yet the mechanistic pathways that lead to neoplastic transformation of germ cells remain to be fully clarified. Mutations of p53 tumor suppressor gene are the most common gene alterations in solid tumors and are usually associated with aggressive tumor growth, chemotherapy resistance and poor outcome. p53 is extremely important and acts as a "master guardian". When p53 receives information about metabolic disturbances or genetic damages within a cell it may arrest the advance of the cell through its growth and division cycle to facilitate the repair of damages. If the damages of genome are too severe to be repaired, p53 elicits signals that activate programmed cell death. In TGCTs, mutations in p53 are rare (up to 1–5%) and mainly occur in seminomas [31 - 34]. TGCTs cells often overexpress wild-type p53 protein where the protein was found to be inactive, but its functions could be restored in response to DNA damage [31, 35]. p53 signaling and DNA damage responses seem to function in a different way in TGCTs compared to other cells and tumors, probably reflecting their embryonic and germ cell character. A possible explanation may be due to the increased expression of *Mdm2* gene, due to the amplification of 12p where this gene is located. *Mdm2* encodes for Mdm2 protein that acts on p53 by binding it protein and immediately blocking its function. Mdm2 succeeds in shutting-down p53 driven transcription by preventing the interaction between p53 and p300/Creb-binding protein, which activates transcription via acetylation of histones. Afterwards, Mdm2 directs the attachment of ubiquitin machinery to p53, stimulating the export of p53 from nucleus to the cytoplasm. Thus, subsequent polyubiquitylation leads to its rapid degradation by proteasomes. However, this process can be inhibited by nutlin-3. Nutlin-3 is a small molecular inhibitor of Mdm2/p53 interaction, which leads to the non-genotoxic p53 stabilization, activation of cell cycle arrest and apoptotic pathway [36, 37].

The first alteration that occurs at an early stage of malignant transformation, in cells, sometimes referred to as pre-CIS cells, is an aberrant overexpression of stem cell factor (SCF). SCF also known as steel factor or KIT ligand is a growth factor existing as membrane-bound and soluble form. SCF is a dimeric molecule that exerts its effects by binding to and activating the receptor tyrosine kinase (RTK) c-kit. The activation of c-kit leads to its autophosphorylation and initiation of signal cascade. Its presence may distinguish the pre-malignant germ cells from normal or delayed-mature germ cells [38]. This is an important signaling pathway that may be involved in the development of TGCTs. This RTK pathway plays a key role in the development and progression of many types of cancer. This signaling pathway is extremely complex and in TGCTs have been reported that alterations may occur in multiple parts of this pathway. On one hand, Ras/extracellular signal-regulated kinase (ERK) signal transduction pathway [39] plays an important role in cell differentiation and survival. RTK interacts with GDP/GTP exchange factor Sos and can activate the receptor-linked tyrosine kinases Ras. Sos and the adapter protein Grb2 form a complex through Src homology2 (SH2), and then raise to membrane to act on Ras. Activated Ras will activate the serine/threonine kinase Raf-1, which can then activate the dual specificity kinases mitogen-activated protein kinase 1 (MAPK1) and 2 (MAPK2). The phosphorylation of these two proteins may lead to the re-activation of extracellular signal-regulated kinase 1 (ERK1) and 2 (ERK2), which dimerize and move to the nucleus to regulate gene activities. On the other hand, after c-kit receptor activation, phosphatidylinositol 3-kinase (PI3K) dimerizes through SH2 and then it is recruited to membrane. SH2, which contains an adapter protein, connects esterase subunits to c-kit receptor. As PI3K produces a series of biological signals on the membrane, signal transduction molecules downstream of

PI3K are activated regulating cell survival and angiogenesis [40]. Importantly, functional loss of phosphatase and tensin homolog protein (PTEN) may also be involved [41, 42]. Loss, mutation or inactivation of PTEN, a negative regulator of PI3K and AKT, have been associated with blocked germ cell differentiation, malignant transformation, and the transition from CIS to invasive TGCTs [43, 44]. Increased inactivation of PTEN and up-regulation of AKT may occur upon SCF or estrogen stimulation [45].

SCF/c-kit signaling pathway regulates the survival, proliferation and migration of PGCs, but it is also strongly implicated in TGCTs. Mutations in c-kit are the most common in TGCTs and, together with SCF overexpression, are likely to originate a transient autocrine or paracrine regulation, stimulating malignant proliferation and cell survival, particularly at the early stages of tumorigenesis. This signaling may be further exacerbated by SCF secreted from Sertoli cells, where SCF expression is responsive to hormonal stimulation, particularly to estrogens [45]. Several proteins participate in the SCF/c-kit pathway. For instance, growth factor receptor-bound protein 7 (GRB7) is a protein encoded by Grb7 gene. GRB7 is overexpressed in CIS and TGCT, but is not present in normal testis [46]. A striking increase of GRB7 expression levels were observed in primary tumor samples and in cell lines [47], which are consistent with previous works showing increased expression levels of both GRB7 transcripts and protein in TGCTs [48, 49]. GRB7 is an adapter molecule that interacts with c-kit, epidermal growth factor and Ras through its SH2 domain. GRB7 may have an important role in the regulation of the downstream signaling of these molecules, but also others, such as focal adhesion kinase, platelet-derived growth factor receptor, insulin receptor, fibroblast growth factor receptor and Tek/Tie2 receptor tyrosine kinase [50]. Furthermore, GRB7 is also known to play a role in cell migration through its association with Ephrin type-B receptor 1 and is proposed to modulate the pattern of Ras signaling [50]. Amplification, activating mutations or overexpression of Ras have been detected in invasive TGCTs in up to 10% of cases but not in CIS [34, 42, 46, 47, 49, 51 - 53]. Ras activation can result in signaling through the MAPK/ERK pathway. Similarly, high levels of activated ERK and members of the signal transducer and activator of transcription (STAT) have been described in TGCTs, which are downstream molecules of the SCF/c-kit pathway [41, 42]. In the final steps, activation of SCF/c-kit pathway leads to the activation of transcription factors and up-regulated transcription of several genes, such as, cyclin D1, which promotes proliferation and migration and vascular endothelium growth factor, inducing angiogenesis [54]. Compelling evidence has shown that other genes associated with increased risk of TGCTs interfere with SCF/c-kit pathway. The expression of Spry4 is induced by this pathway and inhibits the MAPK signaling, while Bcl2 antagonist/killer (also termed Bak1), which promotes apoptosis by suppression of Bcl2 and other anti-apoptotic proteins, is down-regulated by SCF/c-kit signaling [55]. The transcription factor AP-2 Gamma (TFAP2C) and its regulator PR domain zinc finger protein 1 (BLIMP1), which are important inhibitors of germ cell differentiation, can also interact with the regulatory effect of SCF/c-kit and were found to be overexpressed in CIS [56]. Recent evidence have also identified Nanos3, Dmrtl and Dnmt3b as potential transcription Factor AP-2 Gamma (TFAP2C) target genes with relevance to development of germ cell tumors.

The steroid pathway is also a common target for unexpected adverse effects of a number of commonly used environmental contaminants, which act as endocrine disruptors. Their possible involvement in the pathogenesis of TDS and testicular cancer has been debated [57]. The fact that the two principal identified etiologic factors predisposing to TGCTs are androgen/estrogen imbalance and genetic background, it suggests a role for genes involved in androgen/estrogen metabolism in TGCT development. So far, genetic polymorphisms in estrogen receptors α and β and the enzymes cytochrome P450 family 1 subfamily B member 1 (CYP1B1) and 17beta-hydroxysteroid dehydrogenase have been related to testicular tumor susceptibility [58 - 61]. Interestingly, certain maternal polymorphisms in CYP1B1 were also associated with increased risk of TGCTs in male offspring [62]. In addition, mutations in androgen receptor (AR) were found in individuals with TGCTs [63].

Several other set of genes involved gonads formation may also be potentially involved in TGCT pathogenesis. The testis-specific protein Y-encoded (TSPY) is the putative gene for the gonadoblastoma locus on the Y chromosome that predisposes dysgenic gonads in XY sex-reversed patients and intersex individuals to gonadoblastoma development. TSPY is overexpressed in pre-invasive lesions and in gonadoblastoma. TSPY is overexpressed in tumor cells in various types of germ cell tumors, including gonadoblastoma, TGCTs and male intracranial germ cell tumors, and has been considered as a key marker that is important in the pathogenesis of these types of human tumors [64 - 66]. The encoded protein TSPY interacts with cyclin B1 by competitively binding at their SET/NAP domains. TSPY colocalizes with cyclin B1 during the cell cycle, particularly on the mitotic spindles at metaphase. TSPY enhances the cyclin B1–CDK1 phosphorylation activity. The stimulatory effect of TSPY has acquired a specialized function in germ cell renewal and differentiation [67]. Additionally, genes responsible for cell division and telomere length regulation may be potentially involved in TGCT tumorigenesis. Telomere regeneration can be accomplished through the actions of the telomerase enzyme, which specifically functions to elongate telomeric DNA. A striking finding is that telomerase activity is clearly detectable in 85 to 90% of human tumor cell samples, while being present at very low levels in the lysates of most types of normal human cells.

Longer telomeres and increased activity of telomerase have been described in TGCTs, where the telomerase activity is related with the degree of tumor differentiation [68]. While this subject needs to be fully disclosed, few studies have reported that telomeric regulation may be via telomerase reverse transcriptase and activating transcription factor 7 interacting protein [69].

BIOCHEMICAL CONTROL OF LIBIDO AND ERECTILE DYSFUNCTION

Libido is an urge that impels individuals to seek out, initiate and/or respond to sexual stimulation. This process is not a subjective sensation. Just like hunger, thirst, heat and cold, libido is built upon a network lying in brain, hypothalamus and limbic system. The control of this process is tightly regulated by several hormones and neurochemicals being most of them important neurotransmitters and/or neuromodulators. Sex steroids are thought to stimulate male sexual behavior largely by acting on AR and estrogen receptors (ERs), expressed in the medial preoptic area (MPOA) [70]. In fact, neurons of MPOA are responsive to sex steroids, after responding to either testosterone (T) or 17β-estradiol in the perfusion medium [71]. Steroid hormone receptors in the MPOA and its afferent connections allow hormones to bias sensory processing to favor sexually relevant stimuli. One step in the translation of long-term steroid effects into rapid behavioral events is probably a change in the release or effectiveness of neurochemical factors. Steroid hormones activate mechanisms of sexual excitation by directing the synthesis of enzymes and receptors for several interactive neurochemical factors that signal male sexual behavior [72, 73]. Among them, dopamine (DA) has been considered one of the most important, however norepinephrine (NE), melanocortin and oxytocin (OT are also known to stimulate male "sex drive" [74, 75]. DA-mediated enhancement of sexual behavior was firstly observed upon administration of L-dopa (3,4-dihydroxy--phenylalanine), a precursor of DA, to men suffering from Parkinson's disease resulting in increased libido and sexual potency [76 - 78]. DA allows hormonally primed output pathways to have easier access to sexually relevant stimuli. Sensory input from a receptive female elicits the release of DA in each of the nigrostriatal, mesolimbic, and in-certohypothalamic systems, which coordinately work to control male sexual behavior. DA exerts its effects through DA receptors expressed in MPOA. There are two families of DA receptors: D1-family, which comprises D1 and D5 receptors coupled with G protein Gsα which activates adenylyl cyclase increasing the intracellular concentration of the cyclic adenosine monophosphate (cAMP) and D2-family, the receptors D2, D3 and D4 are coupled to the G protein Giα (which directly inhibits the activity of adenylyl cyclase and consequently the formation of cAMP). It has been observed that stimulation of

MPOA by high levels of DA during a precopulatory period increased sexual motivation, probably via D1 receptor [79].

MPOA is essential for male sexual behavior [80], since coordinates the genital reflexes necessary for erection and ejaculation [81]. The MPOA receives indirect sensory input from virtually every sensory modality and sends reciprocal connections back to those sources [70]. MPOA can influence sexual motivation and copulation and its relevance to the sexual behavior has been demonstrated by decreased sexual motivation after administration of DA antagonists into the MPOA [82].

The neurotransmitter NE also "shapes" male libido, though its effects may be dose-dependent [83]. Norepinephrine binds to two types of receptors, classically termed "α" and "β" and differentiated according to whether the receptor stimulates (β) or inhibits (α) the action of the second messenger adenylate cyclase. The α receptors are classified into α1 and α2 subtypes, which are found either post-synaptically or pre-synaptically, respectively. Thus, actions of norepinephrine at α1 receptors result in a postsynaptic effect, whereas actions at presynaptic α2 receptors serve as a short-loop inhibitory feedback mechanism that reduces norepinephrine release.

The neuropeptide OT has been termed as a "love hormone" [84, 85]. OT cell bodies are found in the paraventricular and supraoptic nuclei of the hypothalamus. Infusion of oxytocin into the paraventricular nuclei of the hypothalamus stimulated sexual behavior, but the underlying mechanisms are not entirely clear. It has been proposed that oxytocinergic neurons projecting from paraventricular hypothalamic nuclei stimulates dopaminergic neurons in the mesolimbic system, thus stimulating sexual behavior [86].

Apart from the neuroexcitatory effects, other hormones and neurochemical factors exhibit opposite effects to those aforementioned. Progesterone is secreted by adrenal glands and inhibits sexual behavior [87], but it is not clear whether progesterone's effects are mediated via classic receptor or by ligand-independent mechanisms. Furthermore, the activation of opioid signaling pathways is also associated with inhibition of ongoing sexual behavior. Opioid peptides derive from pro-opiomelanocortin (β-endorphin, adrenocorticotrophic hormone and α-melanocyte stimulating hormone), but also from proenkephalins (Met5- and Leu5-enkephalin) and prodynorphin (dynorphin-A, dynorphin-B). These peptides differentially bind to the three classes of opioid receptors, μ, δ, and κ [88]. Several reports have shown that long-term injection of opioids lead to decreased libido [89 - 91], but none of those works added mechanistic insights regarding the effects of opioids in sexual behavior. Recently, it has been reported that administration of μ opioid receptor agonists in the MPOA inhibits sexual behavior in male rats [92 - 94].

Serotonin (5-hydroxytryptamine, or 5-HT) has also been generally associated with decreased libido. This neurotransmitter is synthesized from tryptophan (by the rate-limiting enzyme, tryptophan hydroxylase) producing 5-hydroxytryptophan, which is converted to 5-HT (by aromatic amino acid decarboxylase). It has been suggested that 5-HT acts via anterior lateral hypothalamus and may inhibit sexual motivation by decreasing DA release in the ipsilateral nucleus accumbens, which is a major terminal field of the mesolimbic system [95].

Most of these neurochemical factors are key players in the biochemical pathways underlying sexual arousal and/or sexual desire. One of the first effects of sexual arousal is penile erection. The degree of erection is proportional to the degree of stimulation. Erection is induced by parasympathetic impulses that pass from the sacral portion of the spinal cord through the pelvic nerves to the penis. The parasympathetic nerves use neurochemical factors, (*e.g.* nitric oxide (NO) and/or vasoactive intestinal peptide (VIP), acetylcholine) that elicit relaxation of arteries and arterioles, as well as relaxes the trabecular meshwork of smooth muscles cells (SMCs) of the corpora cavernosum and corpus spongiosum in the penile tissue (Fig. **11.1**). This allows the blood inflow into the large cavernous sinusoids, thus increasing the pressure within sinusoids causing a ballooning of the erectile tissue [81]. All hormones, neurotransmitters, or neuromodulators eliciting the contractile or relaxation responses exert their effects on the cavernosal SMCs through several signaling cascades that can be divided into three major categories: 1) ionic mechanisms; 2) intracellular calcium ($[Ca^{2+}]_i$) mobilization and 3) Ca^{2+} sensitization. Among the ion channels present in SMCs, K^+ channels are of great relevance. At least four distinct K^+ channel subtypes have been identified in SMCs: 1) large-conductance Ca^{2+}-sensitive K^+ channels; 2) metabolically regulated K^+ channels; 3) voltage-regulated K^+ channels and 4) A-type K^+ current. The function of these channels is related to the hyperpolarizing currents that they mediate via the outward flux of K^+ down an electrochemical gradient. This flux together with Ca^{2+} mobilization contributes to the relaxation of arterial and SMCs. During the erectile response, a drop in $[Ca^{2+}]_i$ is important for the relaxation of arteries and SMCs. NO diffuses to SMCs to activate guanylyl cyclase. This enzyme is responsible for the conversion of guanosine triphosphate into the second messenger cyclic guanosine monophosphate (cGMP). Increased levels of cGMP, activates protein kinase G and to a lesser extent protein kinase A (PKA), which further lead to a decrease in $[Ca^{2+}]_i$, (by sequestration of Ca^{2+} in the endoplasmic reticulum, inhibition of cell membrane Ca^{2+} influx channels), and opening K^+ channels with resultant myocyte hyperpolarization and consequently SMCs relaxation [81]. Importantly, all this process ceases when the enzyme phosphodiesterase 5 (PDE-5), present in SMCs, hydrolyses cGMP. In fact, this step is of great interest for therapeutic intervention, since the administration of PDE-5 inhibitors (PDE5-I) is the first line of treatment in men presenting erectile dysfunction (ED) [96 - 100]. It is noteworthy that Ca^{2+} mobilization is extremely important for the maintenance of penile erection. Ca^{2+} mobilization is related with either contraction or relaxation of SMCs and these processes are always preceded by an increase or decrease of $[Ca^{2+}]_i$.

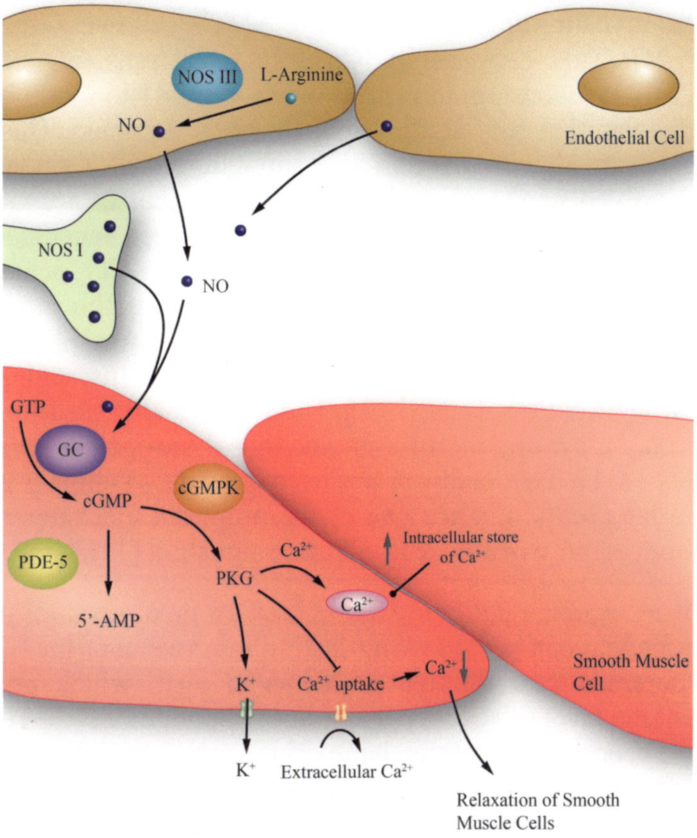

Fig. (11.1). Schematic representation of penile erection by NO. NO is the main mediator of penile SMCs relaxation. After sexual stimulation, NO is produced by nitric oxide synthase I (NOS I) in non-adrenergic non cholinergic nerves or by NOS III present in epithelial cells. NO activates guanylyl cyclase (GC) in smooth muscle cells producing cGMP from GTP. cGMP activates protein kinase G (PKG), which lead to the sequestration of Ca^{2+} into vesicles, open K^+ channels leading to hyperpolarization and consequently closes Ca^{2+} membrane channels. These events decrease Ca^{2+} in SMCs leading to relaxation. These mechanisms cease when phosphodiesterase type 5 hydrolyses cGMP enhancing SMCs contraction and penile flaccidity. Abbreviations: 5'-AMP: adenosine 5'-monophosphate; cGMP: cyclic guanosine monophosphate; GC: guanylyl cyclase; GTP: guanosine triphosphate; NO: nitric oxide; NOS I: nitric oxide synthase; NOS III: nitric oxide synthase III; PKG: protein kinase; Solid arrows: stimulation; Blunted arrows: inhibition.

Sympathetic adrenergic signaling and the activity of substances derived from vascular endothelium, such as endothelins and prostaglandin F2 are involved in these processes [101, 102]. But contrarily to NO, these substances cause penile flaccidity. They activate G-protein coupled receptors that initiate a cascade leading to the increased production of inositol-1,4,5-triphosphate and diacylglycerol. In turn, these substances increase $[Ca^{2+}]_i$ by releasing intracellular stores or opening cell membrane channels to allow Ca^{2+}influx [103]. The elevated $[Ca^{2+}]_i$ binds to calmodulin changing its conformation to expose sites that bind and activate myosin light-chain kinase [103]. The activated myosin light-chain kinase phosphorylates myosin light chains of the SMCs, allowing them to initiate contraction [104]. This increase in $[Ca^{2+}]_i$ is only transient, since following contraction $[Ca^{2+}]_i$ levels return to resting levels within 1 to 2 min in SMCs [105, 106], despite the fact that contractile responses are maintained. This suggests that other mechanisms are also involved in the contraction of SMCs. One of the major mechanisms involved in the contractions of SMCs that is not associated with changes in membrane potential is the regulation of Ca^{2+} sensitization. The Ras homolog gene (Rho)-kinase pathway is a key player in Ca^{2+} sensitization [107, 108]. G-proteins expressed in penile SMCs activate the Rho family member A (RhoA), which activates Rho-kinase. Rho-kinase in-turn phosphorylates the regulatory subunit, preventing dephosphorylation of myofilaments that allow the maintenance of contractility [109, 110]. The Ca^{2+}-sensitizing RhoA/Rho kinase pathway may play a synergistic role in cavernosal vasoconstriction to maintain penile flaccidity [111]. This pathway has been considered another possible target for therapeutic intervention, since one of the proposed mechanisms responsible for ED is the high activity of RhoA/Rho kinase signaling [112].

Despite all advances made until now, there is still a great need for more effective therapeutic drugs that can provide long-lasting improvement for ED. This is one of the most common reproductive problems in men, which presents serious consequences at the level of sexual performance and relationship. These men have difficult to get/keep erection thus hampering a successful intercourse [113]. According to the International Consultation Committee for Sexual Medicine on Definitions/Epidemiology/Risk Factors for Sexual Dysfunction, the prevalence of ED is ranging between 1–10% in men younger than 40 years and increases to 2% to 9% in men from between the ages of 40 and 49 years. After 60 years of age 20–40% of men are affected by ED and in men older than 70 years the prevalence of ED ranges from 50% to 100% [114 - 117]. It is predicted that by 2025 the worldwide prevalence of ED may reach 322 million men [118, 119] but this number may be “masked” by other factors, such as metabolic diseases. ED has been associated to other diseases, namely diabetes mellitus (DM) and obesity. Indeed, type 2 DM (T2DM) is the second most common risk factor for ED, which occurs in 50–75% of diabetics [120]. ED is three times more frequent in diabetics than non-diabetics. Nonetheless, factors associated with lifestyle of industrialized societies, such as physical inactivity, exposure to environmental contaminants, smoke tobacco or alcohol overconsumption are also key factors contributing to the incidence of ED.

BASIC ASPECTS OF SEXUAL TRANSMITTED DISEASES

STDs are infectious diseases spread predominantly through sexual contact, including vaginal, anal and oral sex. Global estimations indicate more than 1 million STDs are acquired every day [2]. The effective programs that have been ensured by health authorities resulted in a substantial decline in new infections [2]. This may be explained by adequate commitment, investment, focus, scale, and quality of implementation of prevention and treatment interventions [121]. Furthermore, most STDs are asymptomatic which increases the risk of transmission among individuals. STDs have a profound impact on sexual and reproductive health worldwide.

An important role in the development of male reproductive disorders is played by chronic infectious and inflammatory diseases in different compartments of the male genital tract, such as urethritis, prostatitis, epididymitis, which can adversely affects sperm function. STDs disrupt male reproduction, but the lack of consensus in literature has made this topic a subject of some controversy. According to the available literature, it seems there be an association between STDs and male infertility, however due to the heterogeneity among studies it is hard to establish it.

To date more than 30 different bacteria, viruses and parasites are transmitted through unprotected sexual intercourse. Eight of these pathogens have been responsible to the greatest incidence of STDs. Of these 8 infections, 4 are currently curable (gonorrhea, syphilis, chlamydia and trichomoniasis), whilst other 4 are incurable viral infections (human immunodeficiency virus (HIV), herpes simplex virus (HSV or herpes), hepatitis B and human papilloma virus). According to the most recent estimations of the WHO, each year there are 357 million new infections with 1 of the 4 curable STDs: gonorrhea (78 million), syphilis (5.6 million), chlamydia (131 million) and trichomoniasis (143 million) [2]. Next, we will briefly discuss the basic aspects of the molecular mechanisms underlying the invasion of some of the most common pathogens in males and how some STDs may affect male reproduction specially in the quality of sperm parameters.

Molecular Mechanisms of HIV Infection

HIV is perhaps one of the most paradigmatic viruses, due to the number of infected individuals since its discovery in the early 1980s. HIV spreads through certain body fluids and attacks the body's immune system, specifically CD4 cells. HIV comprises a viral envelope (Env) containing a capsid with two copies of single-stranded RNA and all molecular machinery needed for reverse transcription. After sexual intercourse, HIV present in the genital fluids enters into the body through genital mucosa. Studies in Rhesus monkeys and humans have shown that the most frequent infection is through genital mucosa, where virus adsorbs to dendritic cells or macrophages of the urethral mucosa [122]. Sexual transmission of HIV depends on the size of the inoculum of virus, the phenotype of the viral isolate, and the susceptibility of the host. Detection of HIV in genital secretions increases in patients with later stages of disease. The mechanisms of urethral HIV transmission are unknown. For HIV to infect and replicate inside their hosts, the viral surface protein Env must first bind to receptor CD4 of the host cells and subsequently to the co-receptors, CCR5 or CXCR4 [122 - 128], which provide stable adsorption. Env is composed by gp120 and gp41subunits and gp120 contains a highly conserved inner domain and a more variable outer domain, whereas gp41 presents an ectodomain followed by a transmembrane domain and C-terminal cytoplasmic tail. Trimeric gp120 on the surface of the virus binds CD4 on the surface of the target cell, inducing a conformational change causing gp41 to become exposed, where it can assist in fusion with the host cell [129]. The hydrophobic, N-terminal gp41 fusion peptide is exposed and likely projected toward the target cell membrane into which it inserts, tethering the viral and host membranes and destabilizing the host lipid bilayer [130]. Assembled as a trimer on the viral membrane, this protein projects three peptides fusion domains that attaches to the lipid bilayer of the target cell. The fusion domains then form hairpin-like structures that draw the virus and cell membranes together to promote fusion, leading to the release of the viral core into the host cell [129]. Once inside, the viral capsid is uncoated releasing viral genome. The viral RNA is then reverse transcribed through reverse transcriptase into double-strand DNA that is transported into the nucleus of the host cell where it integrates host genome. The integrated provirus is then transcribed and translated by host machinery to generate a polyprotein that is autocatalytically cleaved and processed to form new virus that bud from the host cell, enabling additional rounds of replication [131].

Studies from humans have demonstrated an association between HIV and declined male fertility since HIV-infected men exhibited a significant decline in sperm parameters when compared to fertile individuals [132, 133]. Interestingly, there was no significant differences concerning the proportion of sperm with normal morphology and the number of leukocytes in semen between groups. In HIV-infected males the low CD4+ cell counts were associated with reduced sperm motility and normal sperm morphology. These findings were similar to those observed in a subsequent study that correlate several sperm parameters, such as sperm viability, motility and penetration rates with the CD4+ cell number. Patients with high CD4+ counts (350/mm^3) exhibited improved sperm parameters, when compared to those whose CD4+ counts were lower than 350/mm3 [134]. Interestingly, it was also evidenced that antiretroviral treatment may be beneficial for male reproductive health, particularly for fertilization process, since sperm penetration rate was higher in men receiving antiviral therapy, when compared with men that were not treated [134].

Herpes Simplex Virus Infection

Herpes simplex virus, commonly known as herpes, can be divided in two types: herpes simplex virus type 1 (HSV-1) and herpes simplex virus type 2 (HSV-2). HSV-1 is mainly transmitted by oral to oral contact to cause infection in or around the mouth (oral herpes), but can also be transmitted to the genital area through oral-genital contact. HSV-2 is almost exclusively transmitted through sexual contact, causing infection in the genital or anal area (genital herpes). Genital herpes caused by HSV-2 is a global issue, and is estimated that 417 million people worldwide are living with the infection [2]. Curiously, the number of women infected with HSV-2 is higher than men, because the transmission of HSV is more efficient from men to women than from women to men. Contrarily to HIV, the basic structure of HSV consists of double-stranded DNA packaged into an icosahedral capsid [135]. Surrounding the capsid is a layer of mRNAs and proteins known as the tegument, which in turn is covered by a lipid bilayer envelope containing various glycoproteins and proteins. The HSV family can be divided into α, β and γ subgroups [135].

Initial infection occurs in epithelial cells, generally within the skin and the mucosa of the oral and/or genitalia tract [136]. Then, HSV reaches and infects free nerve endings of sensory neurons and colonizes ganglia of the peripheral nervous system. After initial infection, the virus does not manifest and remains latent in neurons. During this period, hosts are still capable to infect other individuals. There are five viral glycoproteins that are involved in the entry process: gB, gC, gD, gH and gL, though gC is not essential for entry. The binding to cells is made by gC and/or gB with heparan sulfate proteoglycans (HSPG). Furthermore, filopodia extensions originating from cellular membrane also facilitate the initial attachment to HSPG-rich sites. Once attached to cellular membrane, virus begins the penetration [136]. In this process, fusion of the virion envelope with the plasma membrane or with the membrane of intracellular vesicle is required. In either case, gB, gC, gH and gL are required to interact with cellular receptors. These receptors include nectin-1 and -2, herpesvirus entry mediator (HVEM) and 3-O sulfated heparan sulfate. Nectin-1 is a member of the immunoglobulin superfamily, and one of four Ca^{2+}-independent immunoglobulin-like cell-cell adhesion molecules that have been described [137]. Nectin-1 is an important entry receptor for HSV [136, 138] acting as a gD receptor. The HVEM is a member of the tumor necrosis factor receptor superfamily that is involved in the inflammatory regulation through interaction with the natural ligands lymphotoxin alpha and the lymphotoxin homolog LIGHT [139]. This receptor is expressed in a variety of cell types, including lymphocytes and other leukocytes, epithelial cells and fibroblasts. Whereas, HVEM and nectin-1 are excellent entry receptors for both HSV-1 and HSV-2, nectin-2 is more active for HSV-2 than for HSV-1 and 3-O-sulfated heparan sulfate is probably more active for HSV-1 than for HSV-2. Fusion of viral envelope with a cellular membrane results in content mixing and eventual release of the viral nucleocapsid and tegument proteins into the cytoplasm of the target cells. Thereafter, HSV nucleocapsids dissociate from tegument proteins and bind a microtubule-dependent, minus end- directed motor, dynein [140]. While most of the tegument proteins are required for activation and modulation of viral gene expression and "shut-down" the protein synthesis of host cells, some may participate in dynein-propelled transport of the nucleocapsids along microtubules toward the nuclear membrane for uncoating and the release of viral DNA into the nucleus. The transcription and replication of viral DNA occurs within the host nucleus. Human pathogens have been recognized to play a considerable role on male infertility. A high prevalence of HSV-1 DNA has been detected in the semen of asymptomatic infertile patients, possibly illustrating an association with altered male reproductive performance. Although HSV-1 infection was not associated with motility and morphology defects of the sperms, it was related with decreased sperm count in the semen fluid [141]. Other studies seem to support that HSV may be associated with male infertility, since the presence of HSV DNA in human sperm, even in low percentage, was significantly associated with reduced sperm motility and sperm count [142]. It has been suggested that HSV impact spermatogenesis, since it was correlated the presence of the pathogen's thymidine kinase in the testis with defects in spermatogenesis and even with sperm structural abnormalities [143]. Those observations were in line with the increased thymidine kinase activity and the loss of germ cells in the testes [144]. However, it must be taken into account that DNA of herpes viruses is frequently detected in the semen of asymptomatic fertile men, as well in infertile male patients [145], so it will be need more studies to clarify how HSV impacts male fertility.

Gonorrhea Infection of the Urogenital Tract

Neisseria gonorrhea (*N. gonorrhoeae*) belongs to the family Neisseriaceae that includes five genera, Neisseria, Kingella, Eikenella, Simonsiella and Alysiella. The genus Neisseria contains two human pathogenic species, *N. gonorrhoeae* and

N. meningitides and approximately 30 apathogenic commensal species that can be found in mouth, upper respiratory tract and rarely in urogenital tract. *N. gonorrhoeae* is primarily transmitted by direct human-to-human contact between the mucosal membranes of the urogenital tract, anal or oropharynx, during sexual intercourse. Gonorrhea infection is initiated as a pyogenic infection of the urethra. It presents an incubation period that varies from 1 to 14 days. *N. gonorrhoeae* is a gram-negative diplococcus which causes gonorrhea. This pathogen is exclusive to humans and primarily affects epithelial cells of the urogenital tract. Studies revealed that the gonococcus can enter human cells, and it has been shown that the organism is intracellular during human infection [146]. The outer membrane structure of *N. gonorrhoeae* is composed by pilus [147, 148], opacity-associated (Opa) outer membrane proteins [149, 150], porin protein (PorB) and lipooligosaccharide (LOS) [151 - 153]. After entering into urogenital tract of the host, it adheres to the mucosal cells initially by means of pili. Pili play a critical role in forming an initial attachment with host cells [154 - 157]. Through their ability to exhibit twitching motility, pili may also provide one mechanism by which nonmotile gonococci are able to colonize and to ascend mucosal surfaces [158, 159]. The outer membranes proteins, namely Opa, LOS, PorB, OmpA and iC3b also facilitate the adhesion and subsequent internalization and transcytosis. Following adherence, bacteria is enfolded by pseudopods and pinocytosed by the host cells. Invasion is mediated by PorB. After adherence, PorB protein is translocated from the bacterial cell membrane to the plasma membrane of the target cell. Afterwards, the organisms are exocytosed into the sub-mucosal region where they elicit a severe neutrophilic response and form microabscesses which are exuded as purulent material into the lumen of urogenital tract. Sialylated gonococci are eventually released from the urethral epithelium, where they can then be transmitted to other partner.

Studies have demonstrated a possible association between *N. gonorrhoeae* and male infertility. The fertility status of 45 men who developed gonococcal urethritis and then epididymo-orchitis were studied prospectively. Before infection, 14 men had proved their fertility through their children. However, two years after infection, only 21% of these fathers and 40% of all subjects showed normal sperm parameters [160], thus suggesting that *N. gonorrhoeae* may be implicated in male infertility. In fact, the urethritis and all chronic infections induced by *N. gonorrhoeae* can cause complications in the epididymis [161]. So, epididymitis can affect the sperm concentration leading to oligospermia and azoospermia in cases of bilateral epididymitis or vas deferens occlusion [162]. A recent case-control study demonstrated that the prevalence of *N. gonorrhoeae* was higher in infertile men when compared with fertile men [163]. Nevertheless the mechanisms involved in the pathophysiology are not completely understood, so further studies will be needed.

Molecular Basis of Syphilis Infection

Syphilis is a chronic infectious disease caused by the *spirochaete Treponema pallidum* (*T. pallidum*). *T. pallidum* is a member of the order Spirochaetales, family *Spirochaetaceae*, and genus *Treponema*, which includes four human pathogens and at least six human nonpathogens [164]. *T. pallidum* is a helically shaped micro-aerophilic bacterium, 6–20μm in length and 0.10–0.18μm in diameter. It consists of a central protoplasmic cylinder bounded by a cytoplasmic membrane, an overlying layer of peptidoglycans and an outer membrane. The outer membrane of *T. pallidum* does not contains lipopolysaccharide and has relatively few surface-exposed transmembrane proteins [165]. Two to three flagella originated from each end of the organism confer motility. *T. pallidum* is a highly motile organism that propels itself by rotating around its longitudinal axis. Unlike most bacterial flagellar filaments, which are comprised of a single protein, the shaft of the *T. pallidum* flagella is made up of several major filament proteins [166, 167]. Three proteins, FlaB1, FlaB2, and FlaB3, constitute the flagellar core [168, 169], which is covered with a sheath composed by subunits of the FlaA proteins [170].

Syphilis is usually acquired by direct sexual contact, with active primary or secondary lesions. Studies have shown that 16 to 30% of individuals who had sexual contact with a syphilis-infected individual in the preceding 30 days become infected [171, 172]. Syphilis is a multistage disease with diverse and wide-ranging manifestations. Infection is initiated when *T. pallidum* penetrates dermal microabrasions or intact mucosal membranes and the initial site of infection is infiltrated with mononuclear cells, forming the primary lesion or chancre. The chancre usually becomes indurated and progress to ulceration, but is not purulent. A few hours after inoculation, and during the evolution of the primary stage, *T. pallidum* disseminates widely and organisms are deposited in a variety of tissues. Manifestations of secondary syphilis usually occur within 3 months of initial infection and are characterized by skin lesions. The most common manifestation is a disseminated mucocutaneous rash. Additionally, pale and discrete macular lesions also appear initially on the trunk and proximal extremities. For the first year after infection, patients are considered to have early latent syphilis. Late latent syphilis is defined as asymptomatic infection of longer than one year or unknown duration and is divided into two stages, based upon an approximation of the time of infection. Late manifestations of syphilis (tertiary syphilis) appear approximately 20 to 40 years after first infection and are divided into three different forms: gummatous syphilis, cardiovascular syphilis and neurological complications [173].

T. pallidum is able to invade and survive in a wide variety of tissues and organs. *T. pallidum* enters into bloodstream within minutes after first inoculation [174], and organisms applied to mucosa are found in deeper tissues within hours. The first step in *T. pallidum* invasion is the attachment of organisms to host cells. *T. pallidum* has been shown to attach to a wide variety of cell types including epithelial, fibroblast like, and endothelial cells of rabbits and humans [175 - 178]. Organisms are also able to adhere to isolated capillary [179], kidney [180], and to other tissues [181]. Microscopic examination of *T. pallidum* associated with cell cultures [175, 182] suggest that the attachment is mediated by adhesins located at the tips of the organisms. However, treponemes have also been observed to be attached to host cells along their length. It is possible that other components of extracellular matrix (ECM), such as laminin, collagen I, and hyaluronic acid, are involved in binding to *T. pallidum* [180, 183]. In the same way, *T. pallidum* adhesins that bind to different ECM components may contribute to the ability of the organism to penetrate different tissues and widely disseminate during infection [173]. At our of the best knowledge there are no studies reporting the effects of *T. pallidum* on male reproductive health, but bearing in mind that severe syphilis infections can likely cause local lesions in organs it is plausible that damages in the testicular tissue and/or in the male reproductive tract may impact testicular function and the quality of sperm thus hampering male fertility.

Chlamydia Trachomatis

Chlamydia trachomatis (*C. trachomatis*) is a small gram-negative bacterium and presently is the most common bacterial sexually transmitted infection in the world [184]. It can infect both men and women and no produces symptoms. *C. trachomatis* is an obligate parasite with a lifecycle comprising two distinct phases: 1) the first consists of small elementary bodies (EB) which are the infectious form of *C. trachomatis*. EB attach to cells and enter and 2) then change into its metabolically active form, called reticulate bodies (RB). RB are responsible for the replication of the organism. The entry process into the host cells is through endocytosis and it is believed that EB surface structures such as major outer membrane proteins and the cysteine rich protein OmcB facilitate this process [185]. EB are internalized within a cell membrane lined vesicle in the cytoplasm of the host cell. These vesicles undergo maturation process to become early endosomes and then late endosomes. The endosomes will not fuse with lysosomes, instead of that they intersect vesicles destined for exocytosis, whilst EB undergo morphological changes to RB. These are multiplied by binary fission and produce RNA, DNA and protein. Afterwards, RB are reorganized into EB form to be delivered from the host as new infectious particle of *C. trachomatis*.

Infected males can suffer from asymptomatic infection of the urethra, epididymis, and prostate, thus indicating a possible negative impact on male fertility. Several studies have reported a reduction in the percentage of progressively motile spermatozoa [186 - 189], which can possibly be attributed to the significant loss mitochondrial potential that *C. trachomatis* induce in sperm mitochondria [190]. Furthermore, it has been demonstrated that *C. trachomatis* declines sperm viability and increase in abnormal morphology [186, 191]. Bezold and collaborators [192] also found an association between the presence of *C. trachomatis* DNA and the reduced sperm concentration in semen. However, others have showed no changes in sperm parameters [187, 193]. There is an obvious inconsistency among studies that can be explained due to a number of reasons, mostly based on methodological aspects [194].

CONCLUDING REMARKS

There is a growing concern about male reproductive health quality. In recent years we have witnessed an increase in the incidence of male reproductive disorders, generally termed testicular dysgenesis syndrome. Testicular cancer, in particular germ cell cancer, is one that mostly affects young individuals. The major concern regarding TGCTs are the side effects that result from the treatment that usually causes irreversible damage in spermatogenesis. TGCTs arise from malignant transformation of PGCs, but the characterization of the underlying molecular mechanisms is far from be fully established. It is expected that the new tools of molecular medicine enable not only the full knowledge of the mechanisms leading to neoplastic transformation of germ cells; but also facilitate the identification of new molecular targets for the management of TGCTs.

On the other hand, erectile dysfunction is one of the most common problems affecting the reproductive performance of males. The biochemical changes induced by factors associated to lifestyle may be the leading cause for this problem, as ED is associated with metabolic diseases. The latest statistical projections suggest that the number of individuals suffering with T2DM and obesity will continue to grow, though these diseases are already considered pandemic. In this sense it is expected that the number of individuals who develop ED will also increase. Thus, it is imperative to search new strategies to treat ED. PDE5-I is in the first line for the management of ED, however there is still a need for more effective therapeutic drugs in order to provide a long-lasting improvement for ED.

Effective strategies to improve male reproductive health will reduce health costs and also the transmission of undesired diseases/infections. The number of STDs is still increasing even in developed countries. Prevention is the most effective way to reduce the risk to be infected with STDs. However, changing behaviors is complex, so we need to focus and carefully define the implementation of prevention and treatment interventions.

Box 11.1 | Summary

- The incidence of TGCTs is increasing among young men.
- TGCTs arise from malignant transformation of PGCs.
- SCF/c-kit signalling pathway is involved in the development of TGCTs.
- Genes responsible for cell division and telomere length regulation may be potentially involved in TGCT tumorigenesis.
- ED is one of the most common problems affecting reproductive performance.
- Ca^{2+} mobilization is related with either contraction or relaxation of SMCs.
- The PDE5-I is the first line in the management of ED.

CONFLICT OF INTEREST

The authors confirm that they have no conflict of interest to declare for this publication.

ACKNOWLEDGEMENTS

This work was supported by the "Fundação para a Ciência e a Tecnologia"–FCT (PTDC/BBB-BQB/1368/2014), CICS (UID/Multi/00709/2013), and of FEDER through the POPH and POCI - COMPETE 2020 (POCI-01-0145-FEER-007491) and National Funds by FCT - Foundation for Science and Technology (Project UID/Multi /00709). Luís Rato is funded by Santander Totta/University of Beira Interior (BIPD/ICI-CICS-BST-UBI).

REFERENCES

[1] Skakkebaek NE, Rajpert-De Meyts E, Main KM. Testicular dysgenesis syndrome: an increasingly common developmental disorder with environmental aspects. Hum Reprod 2001; 16(5): 972-8. [http://dx.doi.org/10.1093/humrep/16.5.972] [PMID: 11331648]

[2] Organization WH. Sexually transmitted infections (STIs). Fact sheet Nº 110. 2015. [Available from: http://www.who.int/mediacentre/factsheets/fs110/en/]

[3] Siegel RL, Miller KD, Jemal A. Cancer statistics, 2016. CA Cancer J Clin 2016; 66(1): 7-30. [http://dx.doi.org/10.3322/caac.21332] [PMID: 26742998]

[4] La Vecchia C, Bosetti C, Lucchini F, *et al.* Cancer mortality in Europe, 20002004, and an overview of trends since 1975. Ann Oncol 2010; 21(6): 1323-60. [http://dx.doi.org/10.1093/annonc/mdp530] [PMID: 19948741]

[5] Bahrami A, Ro JY, Ayala AG. An overview of testicular germ cell tumors. Arch Pathol Lab Med 2007; 131(8): 1267-80. [PMID: 17683189]

[6] Kristensen DM, Sonne SB, Ottesen AM, *et al.* Origin of pluripotent germ cell tumours: the role of microenvironment during embryonic development. Mol Cell Endocrinol 2008; 288(1-2): 111-8. [http://dx.doi.org/10.1016/j.mce.2008.02.018] [PMID: 18420341]

[7] Looijenga LH, Oosterhuis JW. Pathogenesis of testicular germ cell tumours. Rev Reprod 1999; 4(2): 90-100. [http://dx.doi.org/10.1530/ror.0.0040090] [PMID: 10357096]

[8] Huyghe E, Plante P, Thonneau PF. Testicular cancer variations in time and space in Europe. Eur Urol 2007; 51(3): 621-8. [http://dx.doi.org/10.1016/j.eururo.2006.08.024] [PMID: 16963178]

[9] Bray F, Ferlay J, Devesa SS, McGlynn KA, Møller H. Interpreting the international trends in testicular seminoma and nonseminoma incidence. Nat Clin Pract Urol 2006; 3(10): 532-43. [http://dx.doi.org/10.1038/ncpuro0606] [PMID: 17031378]

[10] McKiernan JM, Goluboff ET, Liberson GL, Golden R, Fisch H. Rising risk of testicular cancer by birth cohort in the United States from 1973 to 1995. J Urol 1999; 162(2): 361-3. [http://dx.doi.org/10.1016/S0022-5347(05)68560-6] [PMID: 10411039]

[11] Purdue MP, Devesa SS, Sigurdson AJ, McGlynn KA. International patterns and trends in testis cancer incidence. Int J Cancer 2005; 115(5): 822-7. [http://dx.doi.org/10.1002/ijc.20931] [PMID: 15704170]

[12] Richiardi L, Bellocco R, Adami H-O, *et al.* Testicular cancer incidence in eight northern European countries: secular and recent trends. Cancer Epidemiol Biomarkers Prev 2004; 13(12): 2157-66. [PMID: 15598775]

[13] Møller H, Prener A, Skakkebaek NE. Testicular cancer, cryptorchidism, inguinal hernia, testicular atrophy, and genital malformations: case-control studies in Denmark. Cancer Causes Control 1996; 7(2): 264-74. [http://dx.doi.org/10.1007/BF00051302] [PMID: 8740739]

[14] Toppari J, Larsen JC, Christiansen P, *et al.* Male reproductive health and environmental xenoestrogens. Environ Health Perspect 1996; 104 (Suppl. 4): 741-803. [http://dx.doi.org/10.1289/ehp.96104s4741] [PMID: 8880001]

[15] Dieckmann K-P, Pichlmeier U. Clinical epidemiology of testicular germ cell tumors. World J Urol 2004; 22(1): 2-14. [http://dx.doi.org/10.1007/s00345-004-0398-8] [PMID: 15034740]

[16] Rajpert-De Meyts E. Developmental model for the pathogenesis of testicular carcinoma in situ: genetic and environmental aspects. Hum Reprod Update 2006; 12(3): 303-23. [http://dx.doi.org/10.1093/humupd/dmk006] [PMID: 16540528]

[17] Bartkova J, Bakkenist CJ, Rajpert-De Meyts E, *et al.* ATM activation in normal human tissues and testicular cancer. Cell Cycle 2005; 4(6): 838-45. [http://dx.doi.org/10.4161/cc.4.6.1742] [PMID: 15846060]

[18] Bartkova J, Lukas C, Sørensen CS, *et al.* Deregulation of the RB pathway in human testicular germ cell tumours. J Pathol 2003; 200(2): 149-56. [http://dx.doi.org/10.1002/path.1353] [PMID: 12754735]

[19] Houldsworth J, Korkola JE, Bosl GJ, Chaganti RS. Biology and genetics of adult male germ cell tumors. J Clin Oncol 2006; 24(35): 5512-8.
[http://dx.doi.org/10.1200/JCO.2006.08.4285] [PMID: 17158536]

[20] Oosterhuis JW, Looijenga LH. Current views on the pathogenesis of testicular germ cell tumours and perspectives for future research: highlights of the 5th Copenhagen Workshop on Carcinoma in situ and Cancer of the Testis. APMIS 2003; 111(1): 280-9.
[http://dx.doi.org/10.1034/j.1600-0463.2003.1110131.x] [PMID: 12752274]

[21] Słowikowska-Hilczer J, Romer TE, Kula K. Neoplastic potential of germ cells in relation to disturbances of gonadal organogenesis and changes in karyotype. J Androl 2003; 24(2): 270-8.
[http://dx.doi.org/10.1002/j.1939-4640.2003.tb02672.x] [PMID: 12634315]

[22] Almstrup K, Hoei-Hansen CE, Wirkner U, *et al.* Embryonic stem cell-like features of testicular carcinoma in situ revealed by genome-wide gene expression profiling. Cancer Res 2004; 64(14): 4736-43.
[http://dx.doi.org/10.1158/0008-5472.CAN-04-0679] [PMID: 15256440]

[23] Clark AT, Rodriguez RT, Bodnar MS, *et al.* Human STELLAR, NANOG, and GDF3 genes are expressed in pluripotent cells and map to chromosome 12p13, a hotspot for teratocarcinoma. Stem Cells 2004; 22(2): 169-79.
[http://dx.doi.org/10.1634/stemcells.22-2-169] [PMID: 14990856]

[24] Hart AH, Hartley L, Parker K, *et al.* The pluripotency homeobox gene NANOG is expressed in human germ cell tumors. Cancer 2005; 104(10): 2092-8.
[http://dx.doi.org/10.1002/cncr.21435] [PMID: 16206293]

[25] Hoei-Hansen CE, Almstrup K, Nielsen JE, *et al.* Stem cell pluripotency factor NANOG is expressed in human fetal gonocytes, testicular carcinoma in situ and germ cell tumours. Histopathology 2005; 47(1): 48-56.
[http://dx.doi.org/10.1111/j.1365-2559.2005.02182.x] [PMID: 15982323]

[26] Houldsworth J, Reuter V, Bosl GJ, Chaganti RS. Aberrant expression of cyclin D2 is an early event in human male germ cell tumorigenesis. Cell Growth Differ 1997; 8(3): 293-9.
[PMID: 9056671]

[27] Korkola JE, Houldsworth J, Chadalavada RS, *et al.* Down-regulation of stem cell genes, including those in a 200-kb gene cluster at 12p13.31, is associated with *in vivo* differentiation of human male germ cell tumors. Cancer Res 2006; 66(2): 820-7.
[http://dx.doi.org/10.1158/0008-5472.CAN-05-2445] [PMID: 16424014]

[28] Roelofs H, Mostert MC, Pompe K, *et al.* Restricted 12p amplification and RAS mutation in human germ cell tumors of the adult testis. Am J Pathol 2000; 157(4): 1155-66.
[http://dx.doi.org/10.1016/S0002-9440(10)64631-7] [PMID: 11021820]

[29] Skotheim RI, Lind GE, Monni O, *et al.* Differentiation of human embryonal carcinomas in vitro and *in vivo* reveals expression profiles relevant to normal development. Cancer Res 2005; 65(13): 5588-98.
[http://dx.doi.org/10.1158/0008-5472.CAN-05-0153] [PMID: 15994931]

[30] Sperger JM, Chen X, Draper JS, *et al.* Gene expression patterns in human embryonic stem cells and human pluripotent germ cell tumors. Proc Natl Acad Sci USA 2003; 100(23): 13350-5.
[http://dx.doi.org/10.1073/pnas.2235735100] [PMID: 14595015]

[31] Guillou L, Estreicher A, Chaubert P, *et al.* Germ cell tumors of the testis overexpress wild-type p53. Am J Pathol 1996; 149(4): 1221-8.
[PMID: 8863671]

[32] Kersemaekers A-M, Mayer F, Molier M, *et al.* Role of P53 and MDM2 in treatment response of human germ cell tumors. J Clin Oncol 2002; 20(6): 1551-61.
[http://dx.doi.org/10.1200/JCO.2002.20.6.1551] [PMID: 11896104]

[33] Lutzker SG. P53 tumour suppressor gene and germ cell neoplasia. APMIS 1998; 106(1): 85-9. [http://dx.doi.org/10.1111/j.1699-0463.1998.tb01323.x] [PMID: 9524566]

[34] Sheikine Y, Genega E, Melamed J, Lee P, Reuter VE, Ye H. Molecular genetics of testicular germ cell tumors. Am J Cancer Res 2012; 2(2): 153-67. [PMID: 22432056]

[35] Lutzker SG, Levine AJ. A functionally inactive p53 protein in teratocarcinoma cells is activated by either DNA damage or cellular differentiation. Nat Med 1996; 2(7): 804-10. [http://dx.doi.org/10.1038/nm0796-804] [PMID: 8673928]

[36] Koster R, Timmer-Bosscha H, Bischoff R, Gietema JA, de Jong S. Disruption of the MDM2-p53 interaction strongly potentiates p53-dependent apoptosis in cisplatin-resistant human testicular carcinoma cells *via* the Fas/FasL pathway. Cell Death Dis 2011; 2: e148. [http://dx.doi.org/10.1038/cddis.2011.33] [PMID: 21509038]

[37] Li B, Cheng Q, Li Z, Chen J. p53 inactivation by MDM2 and MDMX negative feedback loops in testicular germ cell tumors. Cell Cycle 2010; 9(7): 1411-20. [http://dx.doi.org/10.4161/cc.9.7.11255] [PMID: 20372076]

[38] Stoop H, Honecker F, van de Geijn GJ, *et al.* Stem cell factor as a novel diagnostic marker for early malignant germ cells. J Pathol 2008; 216(1): 43-54. [http://dx.doi.org/10.1002/path.2378] [PMID: 18566970]

[39] Yasuda T, Kurosaki T. Regulation of lymphocyte fate by Ras/ERK signals. Cell Cycle 2008; 7(23): 3634-40. [http://dx.doi.org/10.4161/cc.7.23.7103] [PMID: 19029810]

[40] Sansal I, Sellers WR. The biology and clinical relevance of the PTEN tumor suppressor pathway. J Clin Oncol 2004; 22(14): 2954-63. [http://dx.doi.org/10.1200/JCO.2004.02.141] [PMID: 15254063]

[41] Kemmer K, Corless CL, Fletcher JA, *et al.* KIT mutations are common in testicular seminomas. Am J Pathol 2004; 164(1): 305-13. [http://dx.doi.org/10.1016/S0002-9440(10)63120-3] [PMID: 14695343]

[42] Sommerer F, Hengge UR, Markwarth A, *et al.* Mutations of BRAF and RAS are rare events in germ cell tumours. Int J Cancer 2005; 113(2): 329-35. [http://dx.doi.org/10.1002/ijc.20567] [PMID: 15386408]

[43] Di Vizio D, Cito L, Boccia A, *et al.* Loss of the tumor suppressor gene PTEN marks the transition from intratubular germ cell neoplasias (ITGCN) to invasive germ cell tumors. Oncogene 2005; 24(11): 1882-94. [http://dx.doi.org/10.1038/sj.onc.1208368] [PMID: 15674339]

[44] Kimura T, Suzuki A, Fujita Y, *et al.* Conditional loss of PTEN leads to testicular teratoma and enhances embryonic germ cell production. Development 2003; 130(8): 1691-700. [http://dx.doi.org/10.1242/dev.00392] [PMID: 12620992]

[45] Moe-Behrens GH, Klinger FG, Eskild W, Grotmol T, Haugen TB, De Felici M. Akt/PTEN signaling mediates estrogen-dependent proliferation of primordial germ cells in vitro. Mol Endocrinol 2003; 17(12): 2630-8. [http://dx.doi.org/10.1210/me.2003-0006] [PMID: 14525951]

[46] Goddard NC, McIntyre A, Summersgill B, Gilbert D, Kitazawa S, Shipley J. KIT and RAS signalling pathways in testicular germ cell tumours: new data and a review of the literature. Int J Androl 2007; 30(4): 337-48. [http://dx.doi.org/10.1111/j.1365-2605.2007.00769.x] [PMID: 17573850]

[47] McIntyre A, Summersgill B, Grygalewicz B, *et al.* Amplification and overexpression of the KIT gene is associated with progression in the seminoma subtype of testicular germ cell tumors of adolescents and adults. Cancer Res 2005; 65(18): 8085-9.
[http://dx.doi.org/10.1158/0008-5472.CAN-05-0471] [PMID: 16166280]

[48] Skotheim RI, Abeler VM, Nesland JM, *et al.* Candidate genes for testicular cancer evaluated by in situ protein expression analyses on tissue microarrays. Neoplasia 2003; 5(5): 397-404.
[http://dx.doi.org/10.1016/S1476-5586(03)80042-8] [PMID: 14670177]

[49] Skotheim RI, Monni O, Mousses S, *et al.* New insights into testicular germ cell tumorigenesis from gene expression profiling. Cancer Res 2002; 62(8): 2359-64.
[PMID: 11956097]

[50] Han DC, Shen T-L, Guan J-L. The Grb7 family proteins: structure, interactions with other signaling molecules and potential cellular functions. Oncogene 2001; 20(44): 6315-21.
[http://dx.doi.org/10.1038/sj.onc.1204775] [PMID: 11607834]

[51] Biermann K, Heukamp LC, Steger K, *et al.* Genome-wide expression profiling reveals new insights into pathogenesis and progression of testicular germ cell tumors. Cancer Genomics Proteomics 2007; 4(5): 359-67.
[PMID: 17993720]

[52] Honecker F, Wermann H, Mayer F, *et al.* Microsatellite instability, mismatch repair deficiency, and BRAF mutation in treatment-resistant germ cell tumors. J Clin Oncol 2009; 27(13): 2129-36.
[http://dx.doi.org/10.1200/JCO.2008.18.8623] [PMID: 19289622]

[53] Rodriguez S, Jafer O, Goker H, *et al.* Expression profile of genes from 12p in testicular germ cell tumors of adolescents and adults associated with i(12p) and amplification at 12p11.2-p12.1. Oncogene 2003; 22(12): 1880-91.
[http://dx.doi.org/10.1038/sj.onc.1206302] [PMID: 12660824]

[54] McIntyre A, Gilbert D, Goddard N, Looijenga L, Shipley J. Genes, chromosomes and the development of testicular germ cell tumors of adolescents and adults. Genes Chromosomes Cancer 2008; 47(7): 547-57.
[http://dx.doi.org/10.1002/gcc.20562] [PMID: 18381640]

[55] Gilbert D, Rapley E, Shipley J. Testicular germ cell tumours: predisposition genes and the male germ cell niche. Nat Rev Cancer 2011; 11(4): 278-88.
[http://dx.doi.org/10.1038/nrc3021] [PMID: 21412254]

[56] Schäfer S, Anschlag J, Nettersheim D, Haas N, Pawig L, Schorle H. The role of BLIMP1 and its putative downstream target TFAP2C in germ cell development and germ cell tumours. Int J Androl 2011; 34(4 Pt 2): e152-8.
[http://dx.doi.org/10.1111/j.1365-2605.2011.01167.x] [PMID: 21564135]

[57] Mayer F, Gillis AJ, Dinjens W, Oosterhuis JW, Bokemeyer C, Looijenga LH. Microsatellite instability of germ cell tumors is associated with resistance to systemic treatment. Cancer Res 2002; 62(10): 2758-60.
[PMID: 12019150]

[58] Ferlin A, Ganz F, Pengo M, Selice R, Frigo AC, Foresta C. Association of testicular germ cell tumor with polymorphisms in estrogen receptor and steroid metabolism genes. Endocr Relat Cancer 2010; 17(1): 17-25.
[http://dx.doi.org/10.1677/ERC-09-0176] [PMID: 19776291]

[59] Figueroa JD, Sakoda LC, Graubard BI, *et al.* Genetic variation in hormone metabolizing genes and risk of testicular germ cell tumors. Cancer Causes Control 2008; 19(9): 917-29.
[http://dx.doi.org/10.1007/s10552-008-9153-6] [PMID: 18415690]

[60] Kristiansen W, Aschim EL, Andersen JM, Witczak O, Fosså SD, Haugen TB. Variations in testosterone pathway genes and susceptibility to testicular cancer in Norwegian men. Int J Androl 2012; 35(6): 819-27.
[http://dx.doi.org/10.1111/j.1365-2605.2012.01297.x] [PMID: 22882535]

[61] Kristiansen W, Haugen TB, Witczak O, Andersen JM, Fosså SD, Aschim EL. CYP1A1, CYP3A5 and CYP3A7 polymorphisms and testicular cancer susceptibility. Int J Androl 2011; 34(1): 77-83.
[http://dx.doi.org/10.1111/j.1365-2605.2010.01057.x] [PMID: 20345875]

[62] Starr JR, Chen C, Doody DR, *et al.* Risk of testicular germ cell cancer in relation to variation in maternal and offspring cytochrome p450 genes involved in catechol estrogen metabolism. Cancer Epidemiol Biomarkers Prev 2005; 14(9): 2183-90.
[http://dx.doi.org/10.1158/1055-9965.EPI-04-0749] [PMID: 16172230]

[63] Garolla A, Ferlin A, Vinanzi C, *et al.* Molecular analysis of the androgen receptor gene in testicular cancer. Endocr Relat Cancer 2005; 12(3): 645-55.
[http://dx.doi.org/10.1677/erc.1.00954] [PMID: 16172197]

[64] Hoei-Hansen CE, Sehested A, Juhler M, *et al.* New evidence for the origin of intracranial germ cell tumours from primordial germ cells: expression of pluripotency and cell differentiation markers. J Pathol 2006; 209(1): 25-33.
[http://dx.doi.org/10.1002/path.1948] [PMID: 16456896]

[65] Kersemaekers A-M, Honecker F, Stoop H, *et al.* Identification of germ cells at risk for neoplastic transformation in gonadoblastoma: an immunohistochemical study for OCT3/4 and TSPY. Hum Pathol 2005; 36(5): 512-21.
[http://dx.doi.org/10.1016/j.humpath.2005.02.016] [PMID: 15948118]

[66] Oram SW, Liu XX, Lee T-L, Chan W-Y, Lau Y-F. TSPY potentiates cell proliferation and tumorigenesis by promoting cell cycle progression in HeLa and NIH3T3 cells. BMC Cancer 2006; 6: 154.
[http://dx.doi.org/10.1186/1471-2407-6-154] [PMID: 16762081]

[67] Li Y, Lau YF. TSPY and its X-encoded homologue interact with cyclin B but exert contrasting functions on cyclin-dependent kinase 1 activities. Oncogene 2008; 27(47): 6141-50.
[http://dx.doi.org/10.1038/onc.2008.206] [PMID: 18591933]

[68] Albanell J, Bosl GJ, Reuter VE, *et al.* Telomerase activity in germ cell cancers and mature teratomas. J Natl Cancer Inst 1999; 91(15): 1321-6.
[http://dx.doi.org/10.1093/jnci/91.15.1321] [PMID: 10433622]

[69] Turnbull C, Rapley EA, Seal S, *et al.* Variants near DMRT1, TERT and ATF7IP are associated with testicular germ cell cancer. Nat Genet 2010; 42(7): 604-7.
[http://dx.doi.org/10.1038/ng.607] [PMID: 20543847]

[70] Simerly RB, Swanson LW. The organization of neural inputs to the medial preoptic nucleus of the rat. J Comp Neurol 1986; 246(3): 312-42.
[http://dx.doi.org/10.1002/cne.902460304] [PMID: 3517086]

[71] Silva NL, Boulant JA. Effects of testosterone, estradiol, and temperature on neurons in preoptic tissue slices. Am J Physiol 1986; 250(4 Pt 2): R625-32.
[PMID: 3963231]

[72] Kow LM, Pfaff DW. Transmitter and peptide actions on hypothalamic neurons in vitro: implications for lordosis. Brain Res Bull 1988; 20(6): 857-61.
[http://dx.doi.org/10.1016/0361-9230(88)90102-5] [PMID: 2900673]

[73] Pfaff D. Drive: Neurobiological and Molecular Mechanisms of Sexual Motivation. Cambridge: Bradford Book (MIT Press) 2005; p. 78.

[74] Bitran D, Hull EM. Pharmacological analysis of male rat sexual behavior. Neurosci Biobehav Rev 1987; 11(4): 365-89.
[http://dx.doi.org/10.1016/S0149-7634(87)80008-8] [PMID: 2830564]

[75] Melis MR, Argiolas A. Dopamine and sexual behavior. Neurosci Biobehav Rev 1995; 19(1): 19-38.
[http://dx.doi.org/10.1016/0149-7634(94)00020-2] [PMID: 7770195]

[76] Bowers MB Jr, Van Woert M, Davis L, Davis L. Sexual behavior during L-dopa treatment for Parkinsonism. Am J Psychiatry 1971; 127(12): 1691-3.
[http://dx.doi.org/10.1176/ajp.127.12.1691] [PMID: 5565858]

[77] Jenkins RB, Groh RH. Mental symptoms in Parkinsonian patients treated with L-dopa. Lancet 1970; 2(7665): 177-9.
[http://dx.doi.org/10.1016/S0140-6736(70)92535-3] [PMID: 4193568]

[78] Mones RJ, Elizan TS, Siegel GJ. Evaluation of L-dopa therapy in Parkinsons disease. N Y State J Med 1970; 70(18): 2309-18.
[PMID: 5272106]

[79] Hull EM, Eaton RC, Markowski VP, Moses J, Lumley LA, Loucks JA. Opposite influence of medial preoptic D1 and D2 receptors on genital reflexes: implications for copulation. Life Sci 1992; 51(22): 1705-13.
[http://dx.doi.org/10.1016/0024-3205(92)90299-5] [PMID: 1359367]

[80] Meisel RL, Sachs BD. The physiology of male sexual behavior. Physiol Rep 1994; 2: 3-105.

[81] Hull EM, Wood RI, McKenna KE. Neurobiology of male sexual behavior. In: Neill's KA, Ed. Physiology of Reproduction. San Diego: Elsevier 2006; pp. 1729-824.
[http://dx.doi.org/10.1016/B978-012515400-0/50038-5]

[82] Warner RK, Thompson JT, Markowski VP, *et al.* Microinjection of the dopamine antagonist cis-flupenthixol into the MPOA impairs copulation, penile reflexes and sexual motivation in male rats. Brain Res 1991; 540(1-2): 177-82.
[http://dx.doi.org/10.1016/0006-8993(91)90505-P] [PMID: 2054609]

[83] Green JD, Clemente CD, De Groot J. Rhinencephalic lesions and behavior in cats: an analysis of the Kluver-Bucy syndrome with particular reference to normal and abnormal sexual behavior. J Comp Neurol 1957; 108(3): 505-45.
[http://dx.doi.org/10.1002/cne.901080308] [PMID: 13525460]

[84] Carter CS, Williams JR, Witt DM, Insel TR. Oxytocin and social bonding. Ann N Y Acad Sci 1992; 652: 204-11.
[http://dx.doi.org/10.1111/j.1749-6632.1992.tb34356.x] [PMID: 1626829]

[85] Young LJ, Wang Z. The neurobiology of pair bonding. Nat Neurosci 2004; 7(10): 1048-54.
[http://dx.doi.org/10.1038/nn1327] [PMID: 15452576]

[86] Kita I, Yoshida Y, Nishino S. An activation of parvocellular oxytocinergic neurons in the paraventricular nucleus in oxytocin-induced yawning and penile erection. Neurosci Res 2006; 54(4): 269-75.
[http://dx.doi.org/10.1016/j.neures.2005.12.005] [PMID: 16427151]

[87] Zumpe D, Clancy AN, Michael RP. Effects of progesterone on the sexual behavior of castrated, testosterone-treated male cynomolgus monkeys (Macaca fascicularis). Physiol Behav 1997; 62(1): 61-7.
[http://dx.doi.org/10.1016/S0031-9384(97)00135-2] [PMID: 9226343]

[88] Zaki PA, Bilsky EJ, Vanderah TW, Lai J, Evans CJ, Porreca F. Opioid receptor types and subtypes: the delta receptor as a model. Annu Rev Pharmacol Toxicol 1996; 36: 379-401.
[http://dx.doi.org/10.1146/annurev.pa.36.040196.002115] [PMID: 8725395]

[89] Abs R, Verhelst J, Maeyaert J, *et al.* Endocrine consequences of long-term intrathecal administration of opioids. J Clin Endocrinol Metab 2000; 85(6): 2215-22.
[http://dx.doi.org/10.1210/jcem.85.6.6615] [PMID: 10852454]

[90] Hallinan R, Byrne A, Agho K, McMahon C, Tynan P, Attia J. Erectile dysfunction in men receiving methadone and buprenorphine maintenance treatment. J Sex Med 2008; 5(3): 684-92.
[http://dx.doi.org/10.1111/j.1743-6109.2007.00702.x] [PMID: 18093096]

[91] Beckman JK, Coniglio JG. The metabolism of polyunsaturated fatty acids in rat Sertoli and germinal cells. Lipids 1980; 15(6): 389-94.
[http://dx.doi.org/10.1007/BF02534061] [PMID: 7401936]

[92] Band LC, Hull EM. Morphine and dynorphin(113) microinjected into the medial preoptic area and nucleus accumbens: effects on sexual behavior in male rats. Brain Res 1990; 524(1): 77-84.
[http://dx.doi.org/10.1016/0006-8993(90)90494-V] [PMID: 1976031]

[93] Hughes AM, Everitt BJ, Herbert J. Selective effects of β-endorphin infused into the hypothalamus, preoptic area and bed nucleus of the stria terminalis on the sexual and ingestive behaviour of male rats. Neuroscience 1987; 23(3): 1063-73.
[http://dx.doi.org/10.1016/0306-4522(87)90181-3] [PMID: 2830562]

[94] Matuszewich L, Ormsby JL, Moses J, Lorrain DS, Hull EM. Effects of morphiceptin in the medial preoptic area on male sexual behavior. Psychopharmacology (Berl) 1995; 122(4): 330-5.
[http://dx.doi.org/10.1007/BF02246262] [PMID: 8657829]

[95] Hull EM, Lorrain DS, Du J, *et al.* Hormone-neurotransmitter interactions in the control of sexual behavior. Behav Brain Res 1999; 105(1): 105-16.
[http://dx.doi.org/10.1016/S0166-4328(99)00086-8] [PMID: 10553694]

[96] Andersson K-E. Mechanisms of penile erection and basis for pharmacological treatment of erectile dysfunction. Pharmacol Rev 2011; 63(4): 811-59.
[http://dx.doi.org/10.1124/pr.111.004515] [PMID: 21880989]

[97] Brant WO, Bella AJ, Lue TF. Treatment options for erectile dysfunction. Endocrinol Metab Clin North Am 2007; 36(2): 465-79.
[http://dx.doi.org/10.1016/j.ecl.2007.02.001] [PMID: 17543730]

[98] Carson CC III. Phosphodiesterase type 5 inhibitors: state of the therapeutic class. Urol Clin North Am 2007; 34(4): 507-515, vi.
[http://dx.doi.org/10.1016/j.ucl.2007.08.013] [PMID: 17983891]

[99] Konstantinos G, Petros P. Phosphodiesterase-5 inhibitors: future perspectives. Curr Pharm Des 2009; 15(30): 3540-51.
[http://dx.doi.org/10.2174/138161209789206953] [PMID: 19860699]

[100] Setter SM, Iltz JL, Fincham JE, Campbell RK, Baker DE. Phosphodiesterase 5 inhibitors for erectile dysfunction. Ann Pharmacother 2005; 39(7-8): 1286-95.
[http://dx.doi.org/10.1345/aph.1E487] [PMID: 15941818]

[101] Andersson KE. Neurophysiology/pharmacology of erection. Int J Impot Res 2001; 13 (Suppl. 3): S8-S17.
[http://dx.doi.org/10.1038/sj.ijir.3900718] [PMID: 11477487]

[102] Saenz de Tejada I, Kim N, Lagan I, Krane RJ, Goldstein I. Regulation of adrenergic activity in penile corpus cavernosum. J Urol 1989; 142(4): 1117-21.
[PMID: 2795742]

[103] Dean RC, Lue TF. Physiology of penile erection and pathophysiology of erectile dysfunction. Urol Clin North Am 2005; 32(4): 379-395, v.
[http://dx.doi.org/10.1016/j.ucl.2005.08.007] [PMID: 16291031]

[104] Berridge MJ. Inositol trisphosphate and calcium signalling mechanisms. Biochim Biophys Acta Mol Cell Res 2009; 1793: 933-40.

[105] Christ GJ, Moreno AP, Melman A, Spray DC. Gap junction-mediated intercellular diffusion of Ca^{2+} in cultured human corporal smooth muscle cells. Am J Physiol 1992; 263(2 Pt 1): C373-83. [PMID: 1325115]

[106] Zhao W, Christ GJ. Endothelin-1 as a putative modulator of erectile dysfunction. II. Calcium mobilization in cultured human corporal smooth muscle cells. J Urol 1995; 154(4): 1571-9. [http://dx.doi.org/10.1016/S0022-5347(01)66931-3] [PMID: 7658593]

[107] Cellek S, Rees RW, Kalsi J. A Rho-kinase inhibitor, soluble guanylate cyclase activator and nitric oxide-releasing PDE5 inhibitor: novel approaches to erectile dysfunction. Expert Opin Investig Drugs 2002; 11(11): 1563-73. [http://dx.doi.org/10.1517/13543784.11.11.1563] [PMID: 12437503]

[108] Walsh MP. The Ayerst Award Lecture 1990. Calcium-dependent mechanisms of regulation of smooth muscle contraction. Biochem Cell Biol 1991; 69(12): 771-800. [http://dx.doi.org/10.1139/o91-119] [PMID: 1818584]

[109] Rees RW, Ziessen T, Ralph DJ, Kell P, Moncada S, Cellek S. Human and rabbit cavernosal smooth muscle cells express Rho-kinase. Int J Impot Res 2002; 14(1): 1-7. [http://dx.doi.org/10.1038/sj.ijir.3900814] [PMID: 11896471]

[110] Somlyo AP, Somlyo AV. Signal transduction by G-proteins, rho-kinase and protein phosphatase to smooth muscle and non-muscle myosin II. J Physiol 2000; 522(Pt 2): 177-85. [http://dx.doi.org/10.1111/j.1469-7793.2000.t01-2-00177.x] [PMID: 10639096]

[111] Jin L, Burnett AL. RhoA/Rho-kinase in erectile tissue: mechanisms of disease and therapeutic insights. Clin Sci 2006; 110(2): 153-65. [http://dx.doi.org/10.1042/CS20050255] [PMID: 16411892]

[112] Vignozzi L, Morelli A, Filippi S, *et al.* Testosterone regulates RhoA/Rho-kinase signaling in two distinct animal models of chemical diabetes. J Sex Med 2007; 4(3): 620-30. [http://dx.doi.org/10.1111/j.1743-6109.2007.00440.x] [PMID: 17498101]

[113] Impotence N. Consensus Conference, 1992. JAMA 1993; 270: 83-90. [PMID: 8510302]

[114] Braun M, Wassmer G, Klotz T, Reifenrath B, Mathers M, Engelmann U. Epidemiology of erectile dysfunction: results of the Cologne Male Survey. Int J Impot Res 2000; 12(6): 305-11. [http://dx.doi.org/10.1038/sj.ijir.3900622] [PMID: 11416833]

[115] Laumann EO, Paik A, Rosen RC. The epidemiology of erectile dysfunction: results from the National Health and Social Life Survey. Int J Impot Res 1999; 11 (Suppl. 1): S60-4. [http://dx.doi.org/10.1038/sj.ijir.3900487] [PMID: 10554933]

[116] Pinnock CB, Stapleton AM, Marshall VR. Erectile dysfunction in the community: a prevalence study. Med J Aust 1999; 171(7): 353-7. [PMID: 10590723]

[117] Nicolosi A, Moreira ED Jr, Shirai M, Bin Mohd Tambi MI, Glasser DB. Epidemiology of erectile dysfunction in four countries: cross-national study of the prevalence and correlates of erectile dysfunction. Urology 2003; 61(1): 201-6. [http://dx.doi.org/10.1016/S0090-4295(02)02102-7] [PMID: 12559296]

[118] Ayta IA, McKinlay JB, Krane RJ. The likely worldwide increase in erectile dysfunction between 1995 and 2025 and some possible policy consequences. BJU Int 1999; 84(1): 50-6. [http://dx.doi.org/10.1046/j.1464-410x.1999.00142.x] [PMID: 10444124]

[119] Bacon CG, Mittleman MA, Kawachi I, Giovannucci E, Glasser DB, Rimm EB. Sexual function in men older than 50 years of age: results from the health professionals follow-up study. Ann Intern Med 2003; 139(3): 161-8.
[http://dx.doi.org/10.7326/0003-4819-139-3-200308050-00005] [PMID: 12899583]

[120] Lewis RW, Fugl-Meyer KS, Corona G, *et al.* Definitions/epidemiology/risk factors for sexual dysfunction. J Sex Med 2010; 7(4 Pt 2): 1598-607.
[http://dx.doi.org/10.1111/j.1743-6109.2010.01778.x] [PMID: 20388160]

[121] Workowski KA, Bolan GA. Sexually transmitted diseases treatment guidelines (2015): Centers for Disease Control and Prevention. 2016. [Available from: http://www.cdc.gov/mmwr/preview/mmwrhtml/rr6403a1.htm]

[122] Ganor Y, Zhou Z, Bodo J, *et al.* The adult penile urethra is a novel entry site for HIV-1 that preferentially targets resident urethral macrophages. Mucosal Immunol 2013; 6(4): 776-86.
[http://dx.doi.org/10.1038/mi.2012.116] [PMID: 23187317]

[123] Alkhatib G, Combadiere C, Broder CC, *et al.* CC CKR5: a RANTES, MIP-1alpha, MIP-1beta receptor as a fusion cofactor for macrophage-tropic HIV-1. Science 1996; 272(5270): 1955-8.
[http://dx.doi.org/10.1126/science.272.5270.1955] [PMID: 8658171]

[124] Choe H, Farzan M, Sun Y, *et al.* The β-chemokine receptors CCR3 and CCR5 facilitate infection by primary HIV-1 isolates. Cell 1996; 85(7): 1135-48.
[http://dx.doi.org/10.1016/S0092-8674(00)81313-6] [PMID: 8674119]

[125] Dalgleish AG, Beverley PC, Clapham PR, Crawford DH, Greaves MF, Weiss RA. The CD4 (T4) antigen is an essential component of the receptor for the AIDS retrovirus. Nature 1984; 312(5996): 763-7.
[http://dx.doi.org/10.1038/312763a0] [PMID: 6096719]

[126] Dragic T, Litwin V, Allaway GP, *et al.* HIV-1 entry into CD4+ cells is mediated by the chemokine receptor CC-CKR-5. Nature 1996; 381(6584): 667-73.
[http://dx.doi.org/10.1038/381667a0] [PMID: 8649512]

[127] Feng HL, Hershlag A, Han YB, Zheng LJ. Localizations of intracellular calcium and Ca^{2+}-ATPase in hamster spermatogenic cells and spermatozoa. Microsc Res Tech 2006; 69(8): 618-23.
[http://dx.doi.org/10.1002/jemt.20329] [PMID: 16741976]

[128] Oberlin E, Amara A, Bachelerie F, *et al.* The CXC chemokine SDF-1 is the ligand for LESTR/fusin and prevents infection by T-cell-line-adapted HIV-1. Nature 1996; 382(6594): 833-5.
[http://dx.doi.org/10.1038/382833a0] [PMID: 8752281]

[129] Chan DC, Kim PS. HIV entry and its inhibition. Cell 1998; 93(5): 681-4.
[http://dx.doi.org/10.1016/S0092-8674(00)81430-0] [PMID: 9630213]

[130] Tamm LK, Han X. Viral fusion peptides: a tool set to disrupt and connect biological membranes. Biosci Rep 2000; 20(6): 501-18.
[http://dx.doi.org/10.1023/A:1010406920417] [PMID: 11426691]

[131] Freed EO. HIV-1 replication. Somat Cell Mol Genet 2001; 26(1-6): 13-33.
[http://dx.doi.org/10.1023/A:1021070512287] [PMID: 12465460]

[132] Muller CH, Coombs RW, Krieger JN. Effects of clinical stage and immunological status on semen analysis results in human immunodeficiency virus type 1-seropositive men. Andrologia 1998; 30 (Suppl. 1): 15-22.
[http://dx.doi.org/10.1111/j.1439-0272.1998.tb02821.x] [PMID: 9629438]

[133] Nicopoullos JD, Almeida PA, Ramsay JW, Gilling-Smith C. The effect of human immunodeficiency virus on sperm parameters and the outcome of intrauterine insemination following sperm washing. Hum Reprod 2004; 19(10): 2289-97.
[http://dx.doi.org/10.1093/humrep/deh426] [PMID: 15242991]

[134] Wang D, Li L, Xie Q, *et al.* Factors affecting sperm fertilizing capacity in men infected with HIV. J Med Virol 2014; 86(9): 1467-72.
[http://dx.doi.org/10.1002/jmv.23991] [PMID: 24898681]

[135] Shukla D, Spear PG. Herpesviruses and heparan sulfate: an intimate relationship in aid of viral entry. J Clin Invest 2001; 108(4): 503-10.
[http://dx.doi.org/10.1172/JCI200113799] [PMID: 11518721]

[136] Akhtar J, Shukla D. Viral entry mechanisms: cellular and viral mediators of herpes simplex virus entry. FEBS J 2009; 276(24): 7228-36.
[http://dx.doi.org/10.1111/j.1742-4658.2009.07402.x] [PMID: 19878306]

[137] Stiles KM, Milne RS, Cohen GH, Eisenberg RJ, Krummenacher C. The herpes simplex virus receptor nectin-1 is down-regulated after trans-interaction with glycoprotein D. Virology 2008; 373(1): 98-111.
[http://dx.doi.org/10.1016/j.virol.2007.11.012] [PMID: 18076965]

[138] Spear PG. Herpes simplex virus: receptors and ligands for cell entry. Cell Microbiol 2004; 6(5): 401-10.
[http://dx.doi.org/10.1111/j.1462-5822.2004.00389.x] [PMID: 15056211]

[139] Kovacs SK, Tiwari V, Prandovszky E, *et al.* Expression of herpes virus entry mediator (HVEM) in the cornea and trigeminal ganglia of normal and HSV-1 infected mice. Curr Eye Res 2009; 34(10): 896-904.
[http://dx.doi.org/10.3109/02713680903184250] [PMID: 19895317]

[140] Sodeik B, Ebersold MW, Helenius A. Microtubule-mediated transport of incoming herpes simplex virus 1 capsids to the nucleus. J Cell Biol 1997; 136(5): 1007-21.
[http://dx.doi.org/10.1083/jcb.136.5.1007] [PMID: 9060466]

[141] Salehi-vaziri M, Monavari S, Khalili M, *et al.* Detection of HSV-1 DNA in the Semen of Infertile Men and Evaluation of its Correlation with Semen Parameters in Iran. Iranian J Virol 2010; 4: 1-6.

[142] Kapranos N, Petrakou E, Anastasiadou C, Kotronias D. Detection of herpes simplex virus, cytomegalovirus, and Epstein-Barr virus in the semen of men attending an infertility clinic. Fertil Steril 2003; 79 (Suppl. 3): 1566-70.
[http://dx.doi.org/10.1016/S0015-0282(03)00370-4] [PMID: 12801561]

[143] Braun RE, Lo D, Pinkert CA, *et al.* Infertility in male transgenic mice: disruption of sperm development by HSV-tk expression in postmeiotic germ cells. Biol Reprod 1990; 43(4): 684-93.
[http://dx.doi.org/10.1095/biolreprod43.4.684] [PMID: 1963095]

[144] Cai LY, Kato T, Nakayama M, *et al.* HSV type 1 thymidine kinase protein accumulation in round spermatids induces male infertility by spermatogenesis disruption and apoptotic loss of germ cells. Reprod Toxicol 2009; 27(1): 14-21.
[http://dx.doi.org/10.1016/j.reprotox.2008.11.052] [PMID: 19063959]

[145] Neofytou E, Sourvinos G, Asmarianaki M, Spandidos DA, Makrigiannakis A. Prevalence of human herpes virus types 17 in the semen of men attending an infertility clinic and correlation with semen parameters. Fertil Steril 2009; 91(6): 2487-94.
[http://dx.doi.org/10.1016/j.fertnstert.2008.03.074] [PMID: 18565516]

[146] Apicella MA, Ketterer M, Lee FK, Zhou D, Rice PA, Blake MS. The pathogenesis of gonococcal urethritis in men: confocal and immunoelectron microscopic analysis of urethral exudates from men infected with Neisseria gonorrhoeae. J Infect Dis 1996; 173(3): 636-46.
[http://dx.doi.org/10.1093/infdis/173.3.636] [PMID: 8627027]

[147] Dehio C, Gray-Owen SD, Meyer TF. Host cell invasion by pathogenic Neisseriae Bacterial Invasion into Eukaryotic Cells. Springer 2000; pp. 61-96.
[http://dx.doi.org/10.1007/978-1-4757-4580-1_4]

[148] Forest KT, Tainer JA. Type-4 pilus-structure: outside to inside and top to bottoma minireview. Gene 1997; 192(1): 165-9.
[http://dx.doi.org/10.1016/S0378-1119(97)00008-5] [PMID: 9224887]

[149] Lemon S, Sparling P. Pathogenesis of sexually transmitted viral and bacterial infections Sexually transmitted diseases. 3rd ed. New York, NY: McGraw-Hill 1999; pp. 433-49.

[150] Sparling PF. Biology of Neisseria gonorrhoeae Sexually Transmitted Diseases. 3rd ed. New York: McGraw-Hill 1999; pp. 433-50.

[151] Danaher RJ, Levin JC, Arking D, Burch CL, Sandlin R, Stein DC. Genetic basis of Neisseria gonorrhoeae lipooligosaccharide antigenic variation. J Bacteriol 1995; 177(24): 7275-9.
[http://dx.doi.org/10.1128/jb.177.24.7275-7279.1995] [PMID: 8522539]

[152] Schneider H, Hammack CA, Apicella MA, Griffiss JM. Instability of expression of lipooligosaccharides and their epitopes in Neisseria gonorrhoeae. Infect Immun 1988; 56(4): 942-6.
[PMID: 3126149]

[153] Yang Q-L, Gotschlich EC. Variation of gonococcal lipooligosaccharide structure is due to alterations in poly-G tracts in lgt genes encoding glycosyl transferases. J Exp Med 1996; 183(1): 323-7.
[http://dx.doi.org/10.1084/jem.183.1.323] [PMID: 8551240]

[154] Brooks G. Structures and characteristics of the gonococcal cell envelope. London, United Kingdom: Gonococcal infection Butler and Tanner, Ltd 1985; pp. 9-12.

[155] Cohen MS, Cannon JG, Jerse AE, Charniga LM, Isbey SF, Whicker LG. Human experimentation with Neisseria gonorrhoeae: rationale, methods, and implications for the biology of infection and vaccine development. J Infect Dis 1994; 169(3): 532-7.
[http://dx.doi.org/10.1093/infdis/169.3.532] [PMID: 8158024]

[156] Kellogg DS Jr, Cohen IR, Norins LC, Schroeter AL, Reising G. Neisseria gonorrhoeae. II. Colonial variation and pathogenicity during 35 months in vitro. J Bacteriol 1968; 96(3): 596-605.
[PMID: 4979098]

[157] McGee ZA, Johnson AP, Taylor-Robinson D. Pathogenic mechanisms of Neisseria gonorrhoeae: observations on damage to human fallopian tubes in organ culture by gonococci of colony type 1 or type 4. J Infect Dis 1981; 143(3): 413-22.
[http://dx.doi.org/10.1093/infdis/143.3.413] [PMID: 6785363]

[158] Henrichsen J. Twitching motility. Annu Rev Microbiol 1983; 37: 81-93.
[http://dx.doi.org/10.1146/annurev.mi.37.100183.000501] [PMID: 6139059]

[159] Wall D, Kaiser D. Type IV pili and cell motility. Mol Microbiol 1999; 32: 01-10.
[http://dx.doi.org/10.1046/j.1365-2958.1999.01339.x]

[160] Osegbe DN. Testicular function after unilateral bacterial epididymo-orchitis. Eur Urol 1991; 19(3): 204-8.
[PMID: 1855525]

[161] Lee YS, Lee KS. Chlamydia and male lower urinary tract diseases. Korean J Urol 2013; 54(2): 73-7.
[http://dx.doi.org/10.4111/kju.2013.54.2.73] [PMID: 23550267]

[162] Ndowa F, Lusti-Narasimhan M. The threat of untreatable gonorrhoea: implications and consequences for reproductive and sexual morbidity. Reprod Health Matters 2012; 20(40): 76-82.
[http://dx.doi.org/10.1016/S0968-8080(12)40653-X] [PMID: 23245412]

[163] Abusarah EA, Awwad ZM, Charvalos E, Shehabi AA. Molecular detection of potential sexually transmitted pathogens in semen and urine specimens of infertile and fertile males. Diagn Microbiol Infect Dis 2013; 77(4): 283-6.
[http://dx.doi.org/10.1016/j.diagmicrobio.2013.05.018] [PMID: 24079950]

[164] Norris S, Larsen S. Treponema and other host-associated spirochetes Manual of clinical microbiology. 6th ed. Washington, DC: American Society for Microbiology 1995; pp. 636-51.

[165] Peeling RW, Hook EW III. The pathogenesis of syphilis: the Great Mimicker, revisited. J Pathol 2006; 208(2): 224-32.
[http://dx.doi.org/10.1002/path.1903] [PMID: 16362988]

[166] Cockayne A, Bailey MJ, Penn CW. Analysis of sheath and core structures of the axial filament of *Treponemapallidum*. J Gen Microbiol 1987; 133(6): 1397-407.
[PMID: 3312473]

[167] Penn CW, Bailey MJ, Cockayne A. The axial filament antigen of *Treponemapallidum*. Immunology 1985; 54(4): 635-41.
[PMID: 3884491]

[168] Champion CI, Miller JN, Lovett MA, Blanco DR. Cloning, sequencing, and expression of two class B endoflagellar genes of *Treponemapallidum* subsp. *pallidum* encoding the 34.5- and 31.0-kilodalton proteins. Infect Immun 1990; 58(6): 1697-704.
[PMID: 2187805]

[169] Pallesen L, Hindersson P. Cloning and sequencing of a *Treponemapallidum* gene encoding a 31.3-kilodalton endoflagellar subunit (FlaB2). Infect Immun 1989; 57(7): 2166-72.
[PMID: 2659537]

[170] Isaacs RD, Hanke JH, Guzman-Verduzco LM, *et al.* Molecular cloning and DNA sequence analysis of the 37-kilodalton endoflagellar sheath protein gene of *Treponemapallidum*. Infect Immun 1989; 57(11): 3403-11.
[PMID: 2680972]

[171] Moore MB Jr, Price EV, Knox JM, Elgin LW. Epidemiologic treatment of contacts to infectious syphilis. Public Health Rep 1963; 78: 966-70.
[http://dx.doi.org/10.2307/4591989] [PMID: 14084872]

[172] Schroeter AL, Turner RH, Lucas JB, Brown WJ. Therapy for incubating syphilis. Effectiveness of gonorrhea treatment. JAMA 1971; 218(5): 711-3.
[http://dx.doi.org/10.1001/jama.1971.03190180033006] [PMID: 5171497]

[173] Lafond RE, Lukehart SA. Biological basis for syphilis. Clin Microbiol Rev 2006; 19(1): 29-49.
[http://dx.doi.org/10.1128/CMR.19.1.29-49.2006] [PMID: 16418521]

[174] Cumberland MC, Turner TB. The rate of multiplication of *Treponemapallidum* in normal and immune rabbits. Am J Syph Gonorrhea Vener Dis 1949; 33(3): 201-12.
[PMID: 18121293]

[175] Fitzgerald TJ, Johnson RC, Miller JN, Sykes JA. Characterization of the attachment of *Treponemapallidum* (Nichols strain) to cultured mammalian cells and the potential relationship of attachment to pathogenicity. Infect Immun 1977; 18(2): 467-78.
[PMID: 336548]

[176] Hayes NS, Muse KE, Collier AM, Baseman JB. Parasitism by virulent *Treponemapallidum* of host cell surfaces. Infect Immun 1977; 17(1): 174-86.
[PMID: 328394]

[177] Lee JH, Choi HJ, Jung J, Lee MG, Lee JB, Lee KH. Receptors for *Treponemapallidum* attachment to the surface and matrix proteins of cultured human dermal microvascular endothelial cells. Yonsei Med J 2003; 44(3): 371-8.
[http://dx.doi.org/10.3349/ymj.2003.44.3.371] [PMID: 12833573]

[178] Thomas DD, Navab M, Haake DA, Fogelman AM, Miller JN, Lovett MA. *Treponemapallidum* invades intercellular junctions of endothelial cell monolayers. Proc Natl Acad Sci USA 1988; 85(10): 3608-12.
[http://dx.doi.org/10.1073/pnas.85.10.3608] [PMID: 3285346]

[179] Quist EE, Repesh LA, Zeleznikar R, Fitzgerald TJ. Interaction of *Treponemapallidum* with isolated rabbit capillary tissues. Br J Vener Dis 1983; 59(1): 11-20.
[PMID: 6337679]

[180] Fitzgerald TJ, Repesh LA, Blanco DR, Miller JN. Attachment of *Treponemapallidum* to fibronectin, laminin, collagen IV, and collagen I, and blockage of attachment by immune rabbit IgG. Br J Vener Dis 1984; 60(6): 357-63.
[PMID: 6394096]

[181] Riviere GR, Thomas DD, Cobb CM. In vitro model of *Treponemapallidum* invasiveness. Infect Immun 1989; 57(8): 2267-71.
[PMID: 2526098]

[182] Fitzgerald TJ, Cleveland P, Johnson RC, Miller JN, Sykes JA. Scanning electron microscopy of *Treponemapallidum* (Nichols strain) attached to cultured mammalian cells. J Bacteriol 1977; 130(3): 1333-44.
[PMID: 324985]

[183] Cameron CE. Identification of a *Treponemapallidum* laminin-binding protein. Infect Immun 2003; 71(5): 2525-33.
[http://dx.doi.org/10.1128/IAI.71.5.2525-2533.2003] [PMID: 12704124]

[184] Stamm WE. Chlamydia trachomatis infections: progress and problems. J Infect Dis 1999; 179 (Suppl. 2): S380-3.
[http://dx.doi.org/10.1086/513844] [PMID: 10081511]

[185] Su H, Raymond L, Rockey DD, Fischer E, Hackstadt T, Caldwell HD. A recombinant Chlamydia trachomatis major outer membrane protein binds to heparan sulfate receptors on epithelial cells. Proc Natl Acad Sci USA 1996; 93(20): 11143-8.
[http://dx.doi.org/10.1073/pnas.93.20.11143] [PMID: 8855323]

[186] Brookings C, Goldmeier D, Sadeghi-Nejad H. Sexually transmitted infections and sexual function in relation to male fertility. Korean J Urol 2013; 54(3): 149-56.
[http://dx.doi.org/10.4111/kju.2013.54.3.149] [PMID: 23526114]

[187] Kokab A, Akhondi MM, Sadeghi MR, *et al.* Raised inflammatory markers in semen from men with asymptomatic chlamydial infection. J Androl 2010; 31(2): 114-20.
[http://dx.doi.org/10.2164/jandrol.109.008300] [PMID: 19779210]

[188] Gallegos G, Ramos B, Santiso R, Goyanes V, Gosálvez J, Fernández JL. Sperm DNA fragmentation in infertile men with genitourinary infection by Chlamydia trachomatis and Mycoplasma. Fertil Steril 2008; 90(2): 328-34.
[http://dx.doi.org/10.1016/j.fertnstert.2007.06.035] [PMID: 17953955]

[189] Gdoura R, Keskes-Ammar L, Bouzid F, Eb F, Hammami A, Orfila J. Chlamydia trachomatis and male infertility in Tunisia. Eur J Contracept Reprod Health Care 2001; 6(2): 102-7.
[http://dx.doi.org/10.1080/ejc.6.2.102.107] [PMID: 11518447]

[190] Sellami H, Znazen A, Sellami A, *et al.* Molecular detection of Chlamydia trachomatis and other sexually transmitted bacteria in semen of male partners of infertile couples in Tunisia: the effect on semen parameters and spermatozoa apoptosis markers. PLoS One 2014; 9(7): e98903.
[http://dx.doi.org/10.1371/journal.pone.0098903] [PMID: 25019616]

[191] Cengiz T, Aydoğanli L, Baykam M, *et al.* Chlamydial infections and male infertility. Int Urol Nephrol 1997; 29(6): 687-93.
[http://dx.doi.org/10.1007/BF02552187] [PMID: 9477368]

[192] Bezold G, Politch JA, Kiviat NB, Kuypers JM, Wolff H, Anderson DJ. Prevalence of sexually transmissible pathogens in semen from asymptomatic male infertility patients with and without leukocytospermia. Fertil Steril 2007; 87(5): 1087-97.
[http://dx.doi.org/10.1016/j.fertnstert.2006.08.109] [PMID: 17433312]

[193] Vigil P, Morales P, Tapia A, Riquelme R, Salgado AM. Chlamydia trachomatis infection in male partners of infertile couples: incidence and sperm function. Andrologia 2002; 34(3): 155-61. [http://dx.doi.org/10.1046/j.1439-0272.2002.00472.x] [PMID: 12059810]

[194] Eley A, Pacey AA, Galdiero M, Galdiero M, Galdiero F. Can Chlamydia trachomatis directly damage your sperm? Lancet Infect Dis 2005; 5(1): 53-7. [http://dx.doi.org/10.1016/S1473-3099(04)01254-X] [PMID: 15620561]

CHAPTER 12

Metabolic Disorders and Male Reproductive Health

Maria J. Meneses[1,2,*]

[1] *ProRegeM PhD Programme, CEDOC – Chronic Diseases Research Center and NOVA Medical School, New University of Lisbon, 1150-082 Lisboa, Portugal*

[2] *Department of Microscopy, Laboratory of Cell Biology, Institute of Biomedical Sciences Abel Salazar (ICBAS) and Unit for Multidisciplinary Research in Biomedicine (UMIB), University of Porto, 4050-313 Porto, Portugal*

Abstract: Metabolic disorders represent a major public health burden nowadays. From these metabolic disorders, obesity and diabetes *mellitus* (DM) may be considered the most significant ones. Obesity is characterized by an excess of body fat, where body mass index (BMI) is used for its classification. When an individual has a BMI between 25 and 30 kg/m^2 is considered overweight, while a BMI over 30 kg/m^2 classifies an individual as obese. This excessive fat is very harmful and may even reduce life expectancy. On the other hand, DM encompasses a cluster of disorders characterized by chronic hyperglycemia that are a result of defects in insulin action, insulin secretion, or both. The exponential increase of these metabolic disorders is, in part, due to erroneous dietary habits that lead to an inadequate intake of essential nutrients. Moreover, while the prevalence of metabolic diseases increases, the fertility trends decrease, illustrating an association that may, or may not, be direct. In fact, there is an increasing number of children, adolescent and men in reproductive age suffering from metabolic disorders. It is well known that the occurrence of a normal spermatogenesis is dependent on the metabolic cooperation established between testicular cells, particularly concerning glucose metabolism and insulin signaling. Therefore, it is crucial to unveil these mechanisms in individuals with metabolic disorders, how they are affected by the disease and how they change the fertility of males. In recent years, several studies have provided new information concerning alterations induced by metabolic disorders in male reproductive health. In addition, it was highlighted that testicular cells possess several mechanisms that react to hormonal fluctuations to counteract hyper- and hypoglycemic events. In this chapter, we will discuss the effects of DM and obesity in the regulation of testicular insulin signaling and glucose metabolism as well as the importance of an adequate diet and how these events are implicated in the reproductive health of males.

[*] **Corresponding author Maria J. Meneses:** CEDOC - Chronic Diseases Research Center, Rua Câmara Pestana, nº 6, 6A, 1150-082 Lisboa, Portugal; Tel: +351 218803101; Fax:+351 218851920; E-mail: mariajoaocmo@gmail.com

Marco G. Alves and Pedro F. Oliveira (Eds.)

Keywords: Antioxidants, Diabetes *mellitus*, Fertility, Glucose, Insulin, Micronutrients, Nutrition, Obesity, Oxidative Stress, Sperm, Vitamins.

INTRODUCTION

In the last years, the world is fronting an emergency in public health, due to the radical increase of metabolic disorders [1], as obesity or diabetes *mellitus* (DM) [2]. Obesity is a metabolic disorder characterized by an excessive body fat accumulation and is measured in part through the body mass index (BMI) [3]. When an individual has a BMI above 25 kg/m^2 but lower than 30 kg/m^2, the individual is considered overweight. However, when BMI surpasses 30 kg/m^2 the individual is considered obese [3]. Obesity may lead to several co-morbidities, being DM one of those [4]. DM is part of a group of metabolic disorders characterized by chronic hyperglycemia. The latter may be due to defects in insulin action, insulin secretion or even both [5]. In this group of diseases, the most representative ones are type 1 DM and type 2 DM. The first one, also known as insulin dependent DM, is an autoimmune disease where T lymphocytes react against insulin-producing pancreatic beta cells [6]. However, the vast majority of diabetic individuals have type 2 DM [5]. It embraces individuals who have insulin resistance and increasing levels of insulin deficiency. Nevertheless, unlike type 1 DM, the key triggering factor of type 2 DM appears to be wrong dietary habits rather than genetic reasons, though the latter can also play a critical role in the appearance of the disease [7]. The deleterious effects of these metabolic disorders is denoted by a widespread list of comorbidities and social problems. Concurrent with a drastic increase in the prevalence of metabolic disorders, we have also been witnessing to a dramatic decline in fertility rates. In fact, research dedicated to fertility trends has been encouraged by reports showing that semen quality has been declining in European populations from a few decades ago until now [8, 9]. Furthermore, these two trends appear to be interrelated for several reasons. One of the possible explanations is the enlarged frequency of men on reproductive age suffering from metabolic disorders [10]. As discussed in the previous chapters, the metabolism of testicular cells is crucial for a normal spermatogenesis. Besides, glucose, insulin and lipids have a key role in the control of the metabolic cooperation established between Sertoli and developing germ cells [11, 12]. Thus, the dysregulation promoted by either obesity or DM in the testicular metabolic cooperation might be a key factor to the decrease in fertility rates observed in countries with high incidence of metabolic diseases. Nowadays, there is evidence from several studies performed either *in vitro* or *in vivo*, that the presence of metabolic disorders or some of their main features have a profound impact on the reproductive potential of males [11, 12]. Moreover, in the last years, several studies have been performed to unveil the mechanisms by which metabolic diseases alter the reproductive potential of males. Therefore, in this we will discuss the possible mechanisms involved in the connection between metabolic disorders, sperm quality and thus (in)fertility. We will also discuss in what way dietary components can act as regulators of testicular metabolism and thus, be useful to counteract the undesirable effects of metabolic disorders.

OXIDATIVE STRESS AND ITS EFFECTS ON MALE REPRODUCTION

Reactive oxygen species (ROS) are byproducts of oxygen metabolism and energy production [13]. This broad term includes both oxygen radicals and certain non-radical oxidizing agents that can be easily converted into radicals, namely superoxide anion radical ($O_{2-}\cdot$), singlet oxygen ($^1O_2$), hydrogen peroxide (H_2O_2), and the highly reactive hydroxyl radical ($\cdot OH$). Free radicals are defined as any species that contain one or more unpaired electrons [14]. ROS are normally produced in cells, playing important roles in cell signaling [15] and being capable of damaging cellular components, namely lipids, proteins and even DNA [16] (Fig. **12.1**). Concerning male reproductive potential, ROS play a crucial role in sperm function as second messengers, namely in capacitation, acrosome reaction [17], and sperm-oocyte fusion when they are produced in small quantities [18]. However, when the antioxidant capacity of the cells is insufficient to neutralize ROS, either by an increase of ROS or by a decrease in antioxidant defenses, oxidative stress (OS) occurs [19] (Fig. **12.1**). OS may then impair sperm cells through damages in plasma membrane and DNA integrity affecting sperm motility and viability, sperm-oocyte fusion, development of embryo and even maintenance of pregnancy [20]. One of the main reasons for spermatozoa being so susceptible to OS is the high percentage of polyunsaturated fatty acids (PUFA) that they contain [21]. The attack to the latter by free radicals leads to the formation of lipid radicals. These combine with oxygen, the universal electron receptor, generating a lipid peroxyl radical [22]. Then, lipid radicals are formed because lipid peroxyl radical extracts hydrogen atoms from adjacent lipids in order to stabilize as a hydroperoxide [23]. In consequence of lipid peroxidation, lipid aldehydes (such as 4-hydroxynonenal) are formed and bind to mitochondrial proteins, stimulating the generation of even more free radicals [22]. This further enhances lipid peroxidation in a vicious cycle that leads spermatozoa to apoptosis. However, and due to the structure of spermatozoa, the nucleases activated in the midpiece, either in the cytoplasm or in mitochondria, cannot enter the nuclear compartment. H_2O_2 is the only product of apoptosis that can pass from the midpiece to the sperm head and consequently damage the DNA. Thus, this is the main reason why the great percentage of DNA damage in spermatozoa has oxidative origin [24].

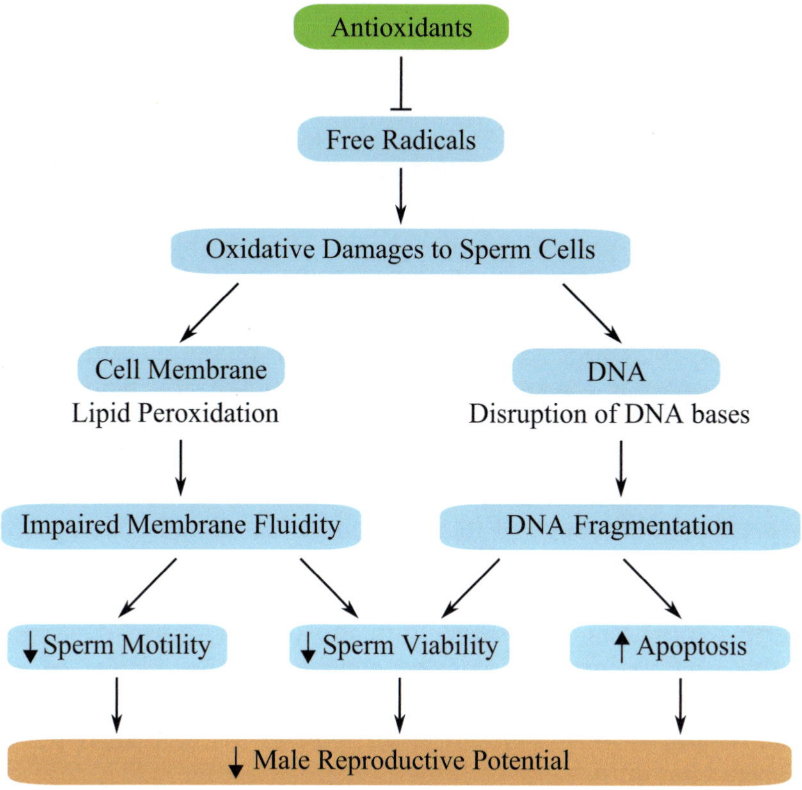

Fig. (12.1). Proposed mechanisms of action for antioxidants in idiopathic male infertility. Antioxidants diminish the amount of free radical that when present in high levels cause oxidative damages to sperm cells. These damages may be exerted through an increase in membrane lipid peroxidation and disruption of DNA bases which consequently lead to impaired membrane fluidity and DNA fragmentation, respectively. All these impairments cause a decrease in male reproductive potential through decreases in either sperm motility, sperm viability and/or apoptosis of developing germ cells. ↓- decrease; ↑- increase.

NUTRITION AND MALE FERTILITY

The impact of nutrition on fertility is widely known for several years. Yet, the knowledge of the relationship between male fertility and nutrition is more recent [25]. In fact, several studies have shown that sperm quality could be improved through supplementation of some specific micronutrients and vitamins [26 - 31]. On the contrary, some elements present in the diet may negatively affect sperm quality and thus male fertility potential. We will briefly discuss the effects of several components of the diet in detail throughout this subchapter.

Vitamin A

Vitamin A is a fat-soluble organic compound found essentially in three main forms: retinal, retinol, and retinoic acid [32]. Dietary vitamin A (retinol) is present in eggs, meat products and many fruits and vegetables, namely carrots, sweet potatoes and pumpkin [33]. Retinol is transported in the serum and converted to retinoic acid in the target tissues [34]. This vitamin is mainly involved in the formation and function of mucous membranes and has a preponderant role in fertility, both male and female [35]. In fact, retinol is delivered to spermatogonia coupled to the retinol-binding protein and is internalized via the stimulation by retinoic acid gene 6 cell membrane receptor (STRA6) [36]. Then, retinol is oxidized to retinal by retinol dehydrogenase 10 and then to retinoic acid by retinaldehyde dehydrogenase 1a1. However, retinoic acid can also directly enter to spermatogonia from Sertoli cells or from the serum. Retinoic acid may then interact with its receptors [37]. The activated receptor will stimulate the transcription of several genes, namely Stra8, known for being essential for meiosis [38]. In fact, vitamin A deficiency in male rats led to a Sertoli cell only situation and to the impairment of the blood/testis barrier due to a decrease in the integrity of Sertoli cell tight junctions [39]. Due to the effects that vitamin A deficiency promotes, blockage of its metabolism has already been proposed as a target in order to develop a male contraceptive [40, 41]. Furthermore, studies show that serum concentrations of retinol are significantly higher in men with normal sperm parameters, compared with those with sperm dysfunction [42]. However, the vast majority of studies concerning the effects of vitamin A supplementation in male fertility are mixed studies, namely with selenium, zinc and vitamins C and E [43]. Thus, it is difficult to distinguish if the beneficial effects are from vitamin A alone or from a synergistic effect [43].

Vitamin B

Vitamin B9, also known as folate, is a water soluble vitamin B that can be found in enriched cereals, potatoes and green vegetables [44]. It is important for DNA synthesis as it is intrinsically involved in purine and pyrimidine production [45]. When folic acid is consumed, it has to be converted by serine hydroxymethyl-transferase to 5,10-methylene tetrahydrofolate. Then, it can be converted into thymidine by thymidylate-synthase or into 10-formyl tetrahydrofolate by C---tetrahydrofolate synthase to follow purine synthesis [45]. Although this micronutrient is so important, it is known that folate-equivalent (folate and folic acid) intake of about 75% of men on reproductive age is below the recommended range [44]. In fact, subfertile men demonstrated a 74% increase in total normal sperm count after supplementation with 5 mg of folic acid (and 66 mg zinc). However, in this double-blind, placebo-controlled interventional study it was also observed a 4% increase in abnormal spermatozoa [46]. On the contrary, men with high folate intake had lower frequencies of several types of aneuploid sperm, namely dissomies X and sex nullisomy [47]. Moreover, in folate-dependent homocysteine remethylation, other vitamin from vitamin B family, cobalamin, is a cofactor for methionine synthase [48]. The deficiency of this vitamin, also known as vitamin B12, leads to folate deficiency, as folate becomes imprisoned in the form of methyltetrahydrofolate [49], thus leading to the defects described above.

Vitamin C

Vitamin C, also known as ascorbic acid, is an essential water-soluble vitamin linked to the synthesis of collagen and proteoglycans and is an important antioxidant [50]. It can be found in several fruits and vegetables, namely citrus and cauliflower [44]. Interestingly, and comparing with blood serum, the concentration of vitamin C in the seminal plasma is about 10 times higher [51]. This is of great importance, as this vitamin helps to prevent sperm damage due to ROS [52]. Indeed, vitamin C scavenges aqueous ROS by rapid electron transfer and thus inhibits lipid peroxidation [53]. Moreover, vitamin C reduces the level of oxidized vitamin E, making these to act synergistically towards the decrease of lipid peroxidation. When vitamin E reacts with a lipid peroxyl radical, a tocopheroxyl radical is formed, and ascorbate can regenerate vitamin E [54]. Men with asthenozoospermia were found to have lower levels of vitamin C and increased levels of ROS on seminal plasma [55]. Besides its antioxidant key role, vitamin C has several other proposed actions in the male reproductive tract. Indeed, this vitamin influences testosterone synthesis [56 - 58]. In line with these observations, a study showed significantly higher levels of vitamin C in the seminal plasma of fertile men, when comparing to infertile individuals. Moreover, they have found a positive correlation between vitamin C levels on seminal fluid and normal sperm morphology [59]. A 60-day study where 30 infertile but healthy men received placebo, 200 mg or 1000 mg vitamin C daily, both treated groups with the vitamin showed significant improvements in sperm parameters. In fact, only a week after the beginning of the study, the group receiving the higher dose of vitamin C showed an increase of 140% in sperm count while the group receiving 200 mg showed an increase of 112%. Additionally, both groups showed a reduction in the number of agglutinated sperm. At the end of the study, every patient receiving vitamin C had impregnated their partner, while no pregnancies occurred in the placebo group [60]. Besides, there are also studies indicating synergistic effects in both sperm motility and concentration when vitamin C is combined with zinc, beta-carotene and vitamin E [61, 62].

Vitamin D

Vitamin D, widely known for its role in the maintenance of calcium and phosphate homeostasis, is a versatile signaling molecule [63]. The vast majority of vitamin D is generated in epidermis with sun exposure, while the other part is obtained through diet. The latter, may be divided in ergocalciferol (vitamin D_2)

that is obtained from plants or cholecalciferol (vitamin D_3) that is obtained from animals [64]. Cholecalciferol, 25-hydroxyvitamin D and 1α,25-dihydroxyvitamin D_3, which are circulating forms of vitamin D, are capable to diffuse across plasma membranes. On the contrary, the ones which are bound to proteins need to be transported into the cell by megalin or cubilin [65], which were already identified in the testis. Moreover, the cell expresses enzymes that are capable of metabolizing vitamin D [66] and, consequently, capable of activating/inactivating it [67]. 1α,25-dihydroxyvitamin D_3, the hormonally active metabolite of vitamin D, exerts its effects through the vitamin D receptor (VDR) [66]. VDR mediates actions in the membrane but also in the cytoplasm, either through modulation of second messengers or ion channels [68]. It is also capable of regulating transcription, since it heterodimerizes with retinoid x receptor and binds to a vitamin D response element in the promoter region of target genes [69]. All of these intervenient were not only identified in the male reproductive tract but also suggested to be crucial for a normal spermatogenesis [70]. In fact, VDR knockout mice were shown to have reproductive dysfunction, both male and female. The male mice had decreased sperm motility and sperm count, as well as histological abnormalities. Furthermore, aromatase gene expression and aromatase activity were decreased. However, testosterone levels remained normal [71]. In addition, it was verified that the gene expression regulation by vitamin D metabolites is modified according to androgen levels [72]. Besides, vitamin peripheral gonadal actions were proven to be important, as the increase in luteinizing hormone (LH) and follicle-stimulating hormone (FSH) levels indicate hypergonadotropic hypogonadism [71]. These data may suggest an interconnection between androgen and vitamin D deficiency. However, VDR effects in mice are not completely translated to human, as VDR is not equally expressed between these species. In fact, while in humans VDR is mainly present in germ cells and fetal or immature Sertoli cells [66], in mice VDR is expressed in germ cells and immature and mature adult Sertoli cells [73]. In what concerns to human reproduction, it was shown that normospermic and subfertile men have a clearly distinct expression profiles of both VDR and enzymes related to vitamin D metabolism [64]. This profile is so distinct that the use of the distinct localization of CYP24A1 (a vitamin D-inactivating enzyme that is transcriptionally regulated by vitamin D) at sperm annulus has already been hypothesized as a sperm quality marker [74]. Besides annulus, there is a distinct proposed mechanism for vitamin D action on spermatozoa. In this, 1α,25-dihydroxyvitamin D_3 activates VDR in the neck region that causes phospholipase C activation and inositol trisphosphate production. This leads to the opening of inositol trisphosphate receptor gated calcium channels in the nuclear envelope and increases intracellular Ca^{2+} concentration [75]. The initial release of Ca^{2+} from redundant nuclear envelope may be supported by store-operated calcium entry. As discussed in the previous chapters, the increase in intracellular Ca^{2+} concentration leads to induction of sperm motility in both capacitated [76] and uncapacitated sperm [77], improves sperm–egg binding *in vitro* and triggers the acrosome reaction [78], which is a prerequisite to fertilize the oocyte. Moreover, in a study investigating human sperm cells at the molecular level, 1α,25-dihydroxyvitamin D_3 had a significant effect on protein phosphorylation, cholesterol efflux, and increased sperm survival [79]. Although the mechanisms by which vitamin D influences male reproductive potential need to be fully elucidated, it seems that vitamin D plays an important role in the maturation of sperm by influencing capacitation and thus by modulating male fertility potential.

Vitamin E

Vitamin E, a fat soluble organic chemical compound, is part of the tocopherol family. It may be found in fruits, vegetables, cereals, grains, vegetable oils, eggs and meat [44]. It is a potent antioxidant that helps to prevent lipid peroxidation and inhibits free radical induced damage to cell membranes [80, 81]. Vitamin E is a potent scavenger of peroxyl radicals, helping to maintain the integrity of long-chain PUFA in cell membrane and thus being the main inhibitor of the free radical-mediated chain reaction of lipid peroxidation [82]. Consequently, and concerning male reproductive function, it is expected that vitamin E protects sperm cell membrane components from oxidative damage [83]. In fact, it was described that vitamin E has the ability to reduce seminal ROS levels in infertile males [62, 84]. Moreover, men with oligozoospermia and asthenozoospermia were found to have decreased levels of α-tocopherol when compared to men with normal sperm parameters [42]. Prospective studies have also showed an improvement of several sperm parameters and even higher pregnancy rates after supplementation with 300-600 mg of vitamin E per day. Despite the advantages that vitamin E has for male reproductive function, around 50% of men in reproductive age do not consume the recommended dose of this organic compound [35]. A retrospective study showed a direct correlation between vitamin E intake and increase in sperm count and a 5% increase in total progressive motility ($p<0.5$) [85]. Moreover, vitamin E supplementation also leads to decreased lipid peroxidation, increased sperm motility, and improved pregnancy rates [86]. The decreased lipid peroxidation is due to a decreased sperm production of malonic dialdehyde (MDA) that is the end product of lipid peroxidation [86]. Furthermore, MDA is an indirect indicator of lipid peroxidation in the cell and it was found that its concentration in the semen is twice high in men with asthenozoospermia when compared with men with normozoospermia. However, supplementation with vitamin E needs to be carefully monitored, as the exaggerated intake may lead to cardiovascular complications [87].

Selenium

Selenium is a crucial trace element, also important for normal testicular development, spermatogenesis, and sperm motility and function [88, 89]. It can be obtained through plants because it is directly absorbed from the soil [44]. Selenium deficiency leads to decreased sperm motility, decreased spermatozoa midpiece stability and increased abnormal sperm morphology [90]. Moreover, it was also described that the lack of selenium may lead to atrophy of the seminiferous epithelium and to reduction of testis volume [27]. On the contrary, selenium supplementation was demonstrated to improve sperm motility, sperm count and morphology, either used alone or with other nutraceutics [31]. In fact, selenium was also found to increase sperm motility by almost 13% in a 3-month placebo-controlled study [91]. These effects may be due to a link between sperm quality, selenium and selenium proteins. Selenium is a constituent of selenoproteins, structural components of mature spermatozoa and some of the major players in protecting against oxidative damage [92]. Therefore, selenium and selenoproteins guarantee the viability of spermatozoa and provide protection against ROS. One of the most important selenoproteins is glutathione peroxidase 4 (GPX4) [93, 94]. GPX4 is a selenium protein that contains a selenocysteine at the active site. It is known for reducing complex hydroperoxides in cell membranes and lipoproteins. In spermatozoa, it is also crucial to the normal morphology of the midpiece [94]. In fact, GPX4 firstly appears in pachytene spermatocytes and its expression gradually increases during spermatogenesis. Mature spermatozoa use protein thiols as an alternative donor substrate to glutathione [95]. GPX4 forms covalent cross-links with itself and other proteins that eventually build up as a keratin-like material, which is incorporated into the helix of mitochondria in the midpiece that forms the majority of the mitochondrial capsule [96]. The development of spermatocyte-specific GPx4 knock-out mice show that spermatozoa from these animals were not able to fertilize oocytes *in vitro*. Moreover, those spermatozoa had significant reductions in forward motility and on mitochondrial membrane potential. They also presented structural problems, namely a hairpin-like flagella bend at the midpiece and swelling of mitochondria in the spermatozoa [93]. In humans, it was found that sperm cells of many males diagnosed with infertility (due to a decrease in both sperm count and quality) had significant decreases in polymerized GPX4. In addition, the loss of GPX4 is mostly obvious in oligoasthenozoospermic individuals [97]. In sum, and due to its impact to male reproductive function in several ways, selenium is an essential micronutrient for male fertility potential.

Zinc

Zinc is a cofactor for many enzymes and can be obtained in diet mainly through wheat and seeds [44]. It is involved in several biological processes, including DNA transcription, protein translation, cell proliferation and even apoptosis [45]. Concerning male reproduction, zinc is found in high concentrations within all male reproductive tract, especially in Leydig cells, late type B spermatogonia, spermatids and prostate [98]. In fact, zinc plays a crucial role in steroidogenesis and testicular development, acrosome reaction and sperm chromatin stabilization [45]. Zinc is needed in high concentrations in developing spermatocytes for DNA condensation and meiosis [99]. In the same way, it is also necessary for DNA packaging in spermatids [100]. Besides this role of zinc, it also counteracts oxidation through the occupation of binding sites for cooper and iron in proteins, lipids, and DNA and by binding to sulfhydryl groups in proteins [101]. Although not much is known concerning how zinc reaches developing germ cells, it is hypothesized that it can be through Sertoli cells, since they have one member of zinc importers family, Zip5 [98]. Still, zinc deficiency is difficult to find in industrialized countries, since it is added to several processed food products [102]. However, a deficiency in zinc transport may lead to the same clinical manifestations as zinc intake deficiency [98]. The latter is associated with oligospermia and decreased Leydig cell function, leading to decreased testosterone levels [103, 104]. Moreover, there is a positive correlation between seminal zinc levels and sperm count and morphology [105]. On the contrary, supplementation with 400 mg of zinc sulfate leads to a 100% increase in sperm motility [61]. However, the excessive intake of zinc may lead to loss of appetite, dehydration or even reduced immune function [106].

Coenzyme Q10

Coenzyme Q10 is a lipid-soluble antioxidant that can be either naturally produced in the body or obtained through diet, namely in whole grains, soybeans, nuts, cabbage and others [107]. It is significantly involved in mitochondrial respiratory chain, as it transports electrons thus having a crucial role in sperm midpiece [26]. Coenzyme Q10 also acts as an antioxidant, showing beneficial effects for lipoprotein-rich cell membranes, stabilizing and protecting it from OS [26]. In fact, there is a direct link between coenzyme Q10 concentrations in the seminal fluid and sperm count and motility [108]. It is known that coenzyme Q10 helps to decrease the number of apoptotic cells and DNA fragmentation [109]. Moreover, it inhibits mitochondrial ROS generation and inner mitochondrial depolarization and increases plasma membrane protection against OS [110]. However, the specific mechanisms by which coenzyme Q10 exerts its beneficial effects in the male reproductive tract remain unknown.

Polyunsaturated Fatty Acids

Fatty acids are hydrocarbon chains with a methyl group at one end and a carboxyl group at the other. Its biological reactivity is defined by the length of the chain and by the number and position of double bonds that could be present [111]. Fatty acids are divided in saturated and unsaturated if they contain no double bonds or at least one double bond, respectively. When they have two or more double bonds, the unsaturated fatty acids are mentioned as PUFA [112]. These may be subdivided in omega-3 and omega-6 based on the position of the last double bond relative to the terminal methyl end of the molecule [113]. The principal omega-3 fatty acids are α-linolenic acid, docosahexonic acid and eicosapentonic acid, while the main omega-6 fatty acids are arachidonic acid, and linoleic acid [30]. Some omega-3 and omega-6 fatty acids cannot be synthetized de novo in human and animals due to a lack of appropriate fatty acid desaturase enzymes [111]. Although these are not produced in the body, they can be obtained through diet from fish, plants, and nuts. PUFA represent a crucial constituent of cell membranes since they influence membrane fluidity, regulate the activity of different lipid-dependent membrane-bound enzymes and the membrane resistance to physical and chemical stress [114]. Thus, and concerning male fertility, PUFA are essential for both developing germ cells and spermatozoa membranes [115]. In fact, it was shown that the percentage of long-chain PUFA is linked with the normal morphology of spermatozoa [115]. The correct intake of PUFA was proven to improve sperm count, motility, morphology and even semen antioxidant activity [30]. However, the concentration of omega-3 fatty acids should be higher than omega-6 fatty acids [116]. Moreover, it was shown that omega-3 fatty acids content in spermatozoa was positively correlated with both sperm viability and motility parameters before and after freezing, thus being predictors of cryopreservation success [117]. On the contrary, it was shown that an essential fatty acid deficient diet in male rats leads to degeneration of the seminiferous tubules, as well as a progressive reduction in germ cells and consequently, an absence of spermatozoa [118]. In mice, this deficiency led to an absence of acrosomal reaction [119]. Altogether, there is compelling evidence that fatty acids may improve the reproductive potential of males through the modulation of sperm head and tail fatty acid profiles.

BIOCHEMICAL CHANGES ASSOCIATED TO GLUCOSE AND INSULIN DYSFUNCTION THAT COMPROMISE MALE REPRODUCTIVE HEALTH

As discussed in the previous chapters, both glucose and insulin are crucial for the normal occurrence of spermatogenesis. The latter is a tightly controlled biological process and thus, any alteration in both insulin and glucose regulation may lead to harmful effects to the reproductive health. One of the reasons are modifications in crucial molecular steps of cellular processes. For example, normoglycemia in diabetic patients is very difficult to attain, as well as a normal insulin regulation in both diabetic and/or obese individuals [120, 121]. In fact, although there are drugs to control glycemia according to the different stages of insulin resistance, both hypoglycemia and hyperglycemia are very common to occur in diabetic patients [122]. However, as glucose/insulin dysfunction increases, patients become more resistant to insulin and consequently, more vulnerable to the detrimental effects of these conditions. Remarkably, even though the use of insulin or insulin mimetic agents is essential, they do not assure total efficiency. Furthermore, the safety of insulin therapy has been questioned [123, 124]. Thus, it is imperious to discuss the molecular mechanisms that are affected when insulin and/or glucose dysfunction occurs. As the number of diabetic individuals is rapidly increasing among adolescents and young males, one of the systems that should deserve special attention is the reproductive system. This is of great importance since their reproductive potential may be impaired at a very early age. Indeed, there are innumerous alterations in whole body metabolism that can also affect testicular cells [11].

Few studies have been investigating the molecular mechanisms that are impaired in testicular tissue due to insulin and/or glucose dysregulation. Some of these studies reported synergistic effects of insulin and other hormones in testes, but were still unable to establish the importance of the discovery and its influence to fertility potential of males [125]. Later, it was reported that insulin stimulates the uptake and/or phosphorylation of free nucleosides in cultured Sertoli cells, having a preponderant role in RNA synthesis [126]. Moreover, insulin was also found to increase transferrin secretion by these cells [127]. As transferrin is a glycoprotein responsible for the transport of ferric ions to germ cells, insulin dysfunction may lead to a deficiency in this transport [128]. It was also observed that insulin positively affects the production of lactate by Sertoli cells, which is the metabolic fuel of developing germ cells [129], being that this effect was mediated by insulin receptors [130]. It was also purposed that insulin-like growth factor-1 (IGF-1) had a role in regulating specific functions of Sertoli cells [131]. Indeed, it was suggested that both IGF-1 and insulin may promote spermatogonia differentiation due to its interaction with IGF-1 receptor [132]. Besides the effect in hexoses metabolism, insulin was found to play a role in lipids regulation since it controls the biosynthesis of arachidonic acid [133]. More recently, it was suggested that some of the insulin-mediated effects in male reproductive tract occur through modulation of LH and testosterone levels rather than a direct interaction in the testis [134].

While the presence of insulin has many effects, its deprivation has also several consequences to testicular cells. In fact, it was recently described that insulin deprivation caused numerous important metabolic alterations in cultured Sertoli cells [135]. These cells express specific receptors for insulin thus being highly affected by insulin fluctuations. Under insulin deprivation, Sertoli cells consume less glucose and produce less lactate [130]. These effects are accompanied by a down-regulation of genes related with glucose metabolism, namely with lactate production and glucose import to the cell [135]. Importantly, this condition led to a complete suppression of acetate production. This may compromise the normal course of spermatogenesis since acetate is needed for membrane remodeling of developing germ cells [12]. Notably, insulin plays a role not only in testicular cells but also in the developing germ cells. The first studies date back to the 70s, when it was proposed that insulin played a role in sperm hexoses metabolism [136]. After a study reporting that spermatozoa motility and glucose metabolism could be independent from insulin action [137], it was found that both acrosome and spermatozoa membrane are targets for insulin action [138]. Moreover, the intratesticular injection of insulin led to a decrease of approximately 50% in spermatozoa motility in vas deferens but led to a 70% increase in motile spermatozoa after incubation with a saline solution [139]. Furthermore, defects in insulin secretion may lead to alterations in both pituitary and gonadal functions [140]. Remarkably, a study has shown that a vast majority of men with erectile dysfunction also present insulin resistance, showing a link between insulin and the reproductive health of male individuals [141]. Insulin resistance may also lead to a decrease in testosterone secretion by Leydig cells thus promoting male reproductive dysfunction [142]. More recently, it was found that ejaculated spermatozoa secrete insulin and that this hormone even possesses a physiological role in the autocrine glucose metabolism regulation, being related with capacitation [143]. In line with this finding, other authors described that insulin treatment led to an increase in motility and acrosome reaction, as well as nitric oxide production by washed human spermatozoa from normozoospermic donors [144]. In fact, there was already identified a mitochondrial citrate carrier in human ejaculated sperm and its inhibition leads to reduction of glucose-stimulated insulin secretion and autocrine insulin secretion by sperm. This inhibition has consequences for capacitation and acrosome reaction that contribute to sperm fertilizing ability [145]. This presents a new mechanism by which insulin may affect sperm acquisition of fertilizing ability.

Thus, glucose and insulin dysfunction have a crucial role in male subfertility or infertility, being that these conditions are frequently associated to metabolic disorders. It is crucial to study how therapy with insulin and/or insulin analogs may help to sustain the glycemic control. Furthermore, insulin-induced hypoglycemia, a condition that is recurrent and may be even fatal in some rare cases, has unpredictable effects in overall metabolism of testicular cells. The magnitude of insulin dysfunction and the mechanisms by which insulin controls testicular cells and sperm metabolism are not fully disclosed. This issue should deserve more attention in the future.

IMPLICATIONS OF METABOLIC DISEASES ON SPERM QUALITY

As discussed in other chapters, there is a worldwide very significant percentage of couples with fertility problems. It has been shown that many aspects related to lifestyle may be implicated in their reproductive potential. Some metabolic disorders are intimately linked with wrong dietary habits, as is the case of obesity, type 2 DM and hypertension, which already have been shown to have negative effects on male reproductive function, namely on sperm quality.

Obesity

Obesity is a metabolic disease characterized by excessive body fat and is closely linked with insulin resistance. It is defined as a body mass index (BMI) $\geq$ 30 kg/m^2, while overweight is defined as a BMI between 25.0 and 29.9 kg/m^2 [146]. According to the World Health Organization, in 2014 about 13% of the world's adult population aged 18 years and over were obese and 39% were overweight. In addition, the prevalence of obesity has more than doubled in the last thirty years, thus being a major public health concern [147]. However, and in contrast with other systems of the human body, only recently attention has been given to the effects of obesity on male reproductive system. Nowadays it is known that obesity may harmfully affect male reproductive function due to thermal, endocrine, and genetic mechanisms [148]. For once, obese men have compromised testicular thermoregulation due to a sedentary lifestyle and to increased fat deposition in the abdominal, suprapubic, spermatic cord and upper thigh areas [149]. Although it is known for several years that this leads to suppressed spermatogenesis, the mechanisms are yet fully clarified [149]. However, it is possible that the suppressed spermatogenesis may be also due to increased OS, leading to the apoptosis of developing germ cells [150]. They can undergo apoptosis via either intrinsic or extrinsic mechanisms. The intrinsic pathway is reliant on the mitochondria were Bax, a pro-apoptotic protein, responds to heat stress and accumulates in the mitochondria [151]. On the contrary, Bcl-2, an anti-apoptotic protein, is phosphorylated and becomes inactive. Bax is then introduced into the outer mitochondrial membrane leading to the release of cytochrome C to the cytosol due to conformational changes [152]. Then, cytochrome C forms a complex with apoptotic protease activating factor 1 (Fig. **12.2**). The latter binds to caspase 9 and proteolytically activates the caspase cascade via executioner caspases 3, 6 and 7. The extrinsic pathway, after heat stress exposure, begins when death receptor Fas ligates to its ligand FasL. Fas then recruits Fas-associated death domain through shared death domains. When the Fas/Fas-associated death domain complex binds to initiator caspases 8 or 10 with its N-terminal death effector domain, activated death domains trigger the caspase cascade, leading to its activation via executioner caspases 3, 6 and 7 [152]. Moreover, during heat exposure, p53, a tumor suppressor that increases the expression of pro-apoptotic genes, is moved from the nuclear envelope to the nucleus. Here, it binds to DNA causing cell cycle arrest. Although p53 is part of the extrinsic pathway, it also acts as interveners of the intrinsic pathway, upregulating Bax and downregulating Bcl-2, which are a part of the intrinsic pathway [153] (Fig. **12.2**). Thus, both the pathways converge at the executioner caspase cascade, which results in germ cell death. Autophagy may also be responsible for germ cell death as a back up to apoptosis [149]. Still, despite the attempts to create a treatment to this condition, either scrotal hypothermia, that was designed to lower scrotal temperature, or removal of scrotal adipose tissue proved to be infeasible [154, 155].

Additionally, adipose tissue is now known as an important organ of hormone production and metabolism, thus accumulation of increasing quantities of body fat may interfere with the hormonal regulation of testicular function. Numerous studies observed that metabolic parameters linked with obesity, namely high levels of plasma cholesterol and triglycerides, impair testicular function, leading to decreased semen quality and thus infertility [156].

Moreover, due to a higher percentage of body fat, obese men have reduced levels of total and bioavailable testosterone, as well as decreased inhibin B, that are accompanied by a decrease in LH pulse amplitude [157]. These hormonal changes are suggested to be caused by an estrogen negative-feedback inhibition, due to increased adipose-derived aromatase activity [158, 159], along with decreased formation of inactive 2-hydroxyestrogens [159, 160]. Therefore, Leydig cells in obese men secrete less testosterone, and these levels are negatively correlated with leptin [161] and fasting insulin levels [162]. Along with this, sex hormone-binding globulin (SHBG) has also a preponderant role in obesity-related male infertility. SHBG is produced in the liver and then secreted into the blood, where it binds androgens and estrogens, regulating their bioavailability. However, SHBG production and secretion is under the control of hormones and nutritional factors in human liver [163]. In fact, both *in vitro* and *in vivo* studies suggest that insulin lowers SHBG production [164, 165]. These findings indicate that insulin resistance, directly or indirectly through hyperinsulinemia, may have a role in the regulation of SHBG production. BMI is considered a major determinant of SHBG plasma concentrations and it is known that obese individuals have low levels of this globulin [166]. Thus, in obese males, the decrease in SHBG results in less estrogen bound, ending up in more biologically active, free estrogen. In addition to the conversion of testosterone to estrogen in obese patients, the decreased ability of SHBG to sustain homeostatic levels of free testosterone also contributes to abnormal testosterone levels [167, 168]. This failure to maintain the normal levels of testosterone may magnify the negative feedback of elevated total estrogen levels. Thus, obese men present higher levels of estrogens and decreased levels of total testosterone. Furthermore, it has already been shown that obesity and infertility are genetically related. In fact, twenty-one genes linked with this metabolic disorder were also associated with human infertility and reproduction [146]. However, if we have a closer look to the identified genes, it is not surprising that most of them is related with endocrine regulation. In fact, between these genes it is possible to identify androgens, leptin, FSH and IGF-1 receptors [146].

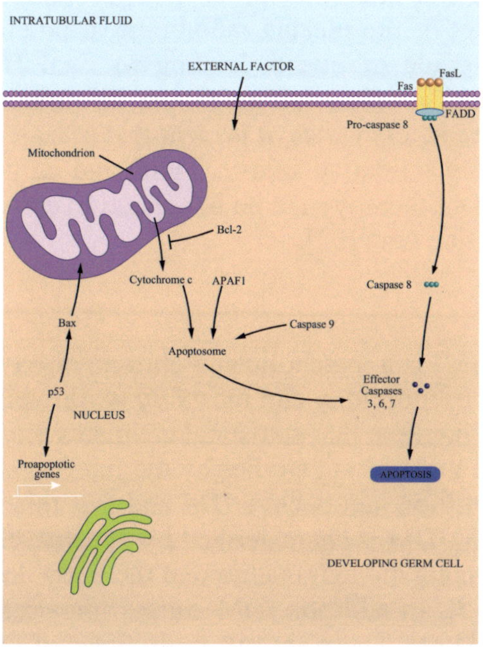

Fig. (12.2). Schematic representation of intrinsic and extrinsic pathways of cellular apoptosis. The intrinsic pathway is reliant on mitochondria were Bax responds to external factor and accumulates in that organelle. On the contrary, Bcl-2 is phosphorylated and becomes inactive. Bax is then introduced into the outer mitochondrial membrane leading to the release of cytochrome c. Then, cytochrome c forms a complex with apoptotic protease activating factor 1 (APAF1). This binds to caspase 9 forming the apoptosome which proteolytically activates the caspase cascade via executioner caspases 3, 6 and 7. The extrinsic pathway after external factors begins when death receptor Fas links to its ligand FasL. Fas recruits Fas-associated death domain (FADD). When this complex binds to initiator caspase 8, activated death domains trigger the caspase cascade, leading to its activation via executioner caspases 3, 6 and 7. Thus, both pathways converge at the executioner caspase cascade, which results in germ cell death. Moreover, p53 is moved from the nuclear envelope to the nucleus. It can also bind to DNA causing cell cycle arrest. ↓- activation; ⊥ - inactivation. Abbreviations: APAF1 - apoptotic protease activating factor 1; FADD - Fas-associated death domain.

Obesity is also intimately linked with the consumption of high energy diets. Due to a fatty acid overload, testicular glycolysis is disrupted, leading to a deficient nurture of developing germ cells. Besides, lipid metabolism is also compromised in Sertoli cells, inducing a deficient germ cell membrane remodeling and structure. All of these effects in testicular environment, due to high energy diet consumption, lead to a decrease in semen quality (for review see [169]). Moreover, a major factor that contributes to obesity-related sperm quality problems is the increased OS and lipid peroxidation [156]. Indeed, it was observed that spermatozoa from infertile obese man presented increased oxidative injury and DNA fragmentation, which reflect the abnormal oxidative state of the testicular microenvironment and efferent duct system [170, 171]. Moreover, it was found that sperm cells from obese individuals have decreased mitochondrial membrane potential. This alteration anticipates phosphatidylserine externalization to the external leaflet of the plasma membrane, a potentially reversible signal, which starts the cascade of events leading to final DNA fragmentation and possibly apoptosis [172]. Thus, although the information about the effects of obesity on sperm parameters varies, it is clear that at least increases the possibility of sperm cells having oxidative injury. Thus, and as previously stated in this chapter, the antioxidant therapy may be beneficial in cases of obesity-induced OS in the male reproductive tract [62].

Diabetes *Mellitus*

Diabetes *mellitus* (DM) is a metabolic and chronic disease, being considered one of the leading cause of morbidity and mortality worldwide. This burden is having such an exponential increase that statistical estimates are outdated years ahead of schedule. One of the most recent studies by the International Diabetes Federation estimates that 415 million adults have DM and that this number will rise to 642 million by 2040 [173]. DM is characterized by hyperglycemia because pancreatic β-cells are not producing enough insulin and the body does not respond properly to insulin, or both [5]. In addition, DM causes impaired carbohydrate, fat, and protein metabolism [174]. There are two main types of DM: type 1 DM and type 2 DM. The first one is an autoimmune disease that leads to the destruction of insulin-producing β-cells. Consequently, there is a dramatic reduction or even elimination of insulin production and patients need exogenous insulin to survive thus being also called insulin dependent diabetes. On the other hand, hyperglycemia in type 2 DM results from insulin resistance along with variable degrees of inadequate insulin secretion. However, the complexity of T2DM led to the establishment of a prodromal stage often called as prediabetes [175]. Here, the patients present glycemic values lower than type 2 DM thresholds but are still higher than normal [176]. Due to the involvement of all body metabolism, DM can lead to a variety of comorbidities, including sexual disorders and impaired fertility [177].

In the last years, and due to the increase of both DM and infertility, the attention given to the mechanisms that may interconnect these disorders has increased. It is now widely accepted that diabetic individuals have a significant decrease in sperm quality [178]. This may be due to several factors, namely increased sperm nuclear DNA fragmentation or mtDNA damage [179]; impairment of sperm viability, motility and morphology [11, 29]; or even to decreased fecundity capacity [180]. In fact, several studies reported damages in both sperm nuclear and mitochondrial DNA. These are, at least in part, due to increased OS in the testis [181]. It was shown that prediabetes, a prodromal stage of DM, decreases the antioxidant potential of testicular tissue, while increases lipid peroxidation and protein carbonylation [29, 182]. Likewise, prediabetic individuals showed a decrease in testicular peroxisome proliferator-activated receptor gamma coactivator-1α (PGC-1α) and sirtuin 3 levels [182]. The decrease of PGC-1α and sirtuin 3 is known to favor OS, due to a disproportion between antioxidant defenses and ROS [183]. Thus, this may lead to the observed DNA damage. Moreover, DM also affects hormonal levels. Indeed, a significant decrease in both LH and FSH levels was described in the plasma of diabetic individuals [180]. Remarkably, insulin injections can restore LH to normal levels [184, 185].

Type 2 DM also induces a decrease in both serum and intratesticular testosterone levels [186]. As testosterone is produced by Leydig cells, this may be related with the finding that Leydig cells presented abnormal morphology in diabetic individuals, with lipid droplets in their cytoplasm [187]. In the same study, it was also reported that Sertoli cells presented an extensive vacuolization and a high degree of degeneration [187]. Although sperm morphology was normal, these modifications have drastic consequences on testicular cells metabolism and consequently, on the adequate nurture of germ cells. In fact, DM led to a reduction in the production of lactate by testicular cells through a decrease in lactate dehydrogenase activity [186]. Furthermore, DM was also found to be related with ionic modifications in both testis and epididymis [188]. In the testis, there was an increase in the transcript levels of several bicarbonate transporters in prediabetic rats. On the other hand, prediabetes also altered the protein expression of some bicarbonate transporters in the epididymis, suggesting an alteration in bicarbonate homeodynamics which may lead to an inadequate environment for sperm storage [188]. Thus, DM impacts sperm viability and, consequently, male reproductive potential. There are several studies indicating that different diabetic animal models present a marked reduction in both fecundity [189 - 191] and sperm quality [180]. Furthermore, diabetic patients were shown to have impaired sperm parameters, namely decreased motility [192]. Concerning assisted reproduction techniques, fertilization rates and embryo quality did not differ from non-diabetic couples, but pregnancy rates were lower in couples with a diabetic male [192]. Of note, diabetic male individuals also present sexual disorders, such as retrograde ejaculation, decreased libido and erectile dysfunction [177]. Despite all that is already known, further studies are needed to deeply understand the molecular mechanisms that interconnect DM and infertility.

TESTICULAR CELLS METABOLIC FUNCTIONING AND GLUCOSE HOMEOSTASIS

As described above, glucose is crucial for spermatogenesis, since it is the precursor for the lactate produced by Sertoli cells that is then used by developing germ cells to suppress their energetic needs [193, 194]. It has been described that glucose deprivation led mammalian cells to increase glucose uptake, showing that glucose may regulate its own transport and metabolism [195, 196]. This regulation includes altered expression of glucose transporters, which is increased in response to glucose deprivation. Glucose transporters 1 and 3 expression was found to be increased through the activation of phosphatidylinositol 3-kinase/protein kinase B, AMP-activated protein kinase and p38 mitogen-activated protein kinase dependent pathways [193]. Besides these, insulin, and some cytokines and growth factors differentially modulate the expression of those glucose transporters [135, 197]. Consequently, Sertoli cells are able to increase the uptake of glucose in order to produce the adequate amounts of lactate. This will fulfill the needs of developing germ cells even though there is a condition of glucose deprivation [193]. These fluctuations in glucose and insulin concentration lead to alterations in Sertoli cells metabolism that can impair the development of germ cells and consequently male fertility. However, besides the relation between insulin and glucose, IGF-1 influences glucose transport in testicular cells. In fact, an overexpression of IGF-1 results in increased developing germ cells apoptosis and thus, abnormal spermatogenesis and reduced male fertility potential [198]. In sum, glucose homeostasis is essential for male fertility, or else may end-up in infertility. There are several homeostasis pathways that cause alterations in testicular cells metabolism. Yet, these cells present some important compensatory mechanisms that allow the preservation of energy necessities of germ cells.

CONCLUDING REMARKS

The prevalence of metabolic disorders is worrying and the number of individuals suffering with them is expected to increase for the next years. This is a major problem at several levels since these diseases are associated with numerous co-morbidities that need endless monitoring and pharmacological management. Connected with this, there is an increasing social problem related with fertility trends. The decrease in fertility rates are in part suggested to be associated with the increase of metabolic disorders. As discussed, men with metabolic diseases present numerous dysfunctions in their reproductive system that can lead to infertility or, at least, subfertility. Therefore, it is of great importance to unveil the mechanisms induced by metabolic disorders that result in the impairment of the male reproductive tract. Within the seminiferous tubules, insulin regulation and glucose metabolism are crucial for male reproductive function since several essential metabolites for developing germ cells, as lactate or acetate, are produced from glucose. Moreover, these metabolic disorders are normally linked with wrong dietary habits. Besides the increase in carbohydrate consumption, normally a deficit of micronutrients also occurs. Some of these are essential for a normal spermatogenesis since they may be intermediates for germ cell development. Some micronutrients are needed not only for germ cells, but also to maintain the antioxidant defenses of the testicular tissue and spermatozoa. As discussed, individuals with metabolic disorders present impaired testicular metabolism that may end-up in reduced sperm quality and consequently in male subfertility/infertility. Thus, it is imperious to further unveil these mechanisms to develop new treatment strategies against metabolic disorders-induced male subfertility/infertility. The information concerning metabolic diseases and their underlying mechanisms in whole body glucose/insulin homeostasis is rapidly shifting. Regrettably, the knowledge in what concerns to testicular metabolism remains scarce. It is pivotal to unveil the way whole body metabolic state may influence testicular metabolic status.

Box 12.1 | Summary

- The prevalence of metabolic disorders and fertility trends are interconnected;
- Oxidative stress, one of the main features of metabolic disorders, highly impairs male reproductive potential as a result of decreased antioxidant defenses or increased free radicals in the intratubular fluid;
- Dietary habits have a major impact on male reproductive function, particularly the deficiency of specific micronutrients;
- As glucose and insulin are extremely important for the normal occurrence of spermatogenesis, their dysregulation has profound consequences on testicular

CONFLICT OF INTEREST

The authors confirm that they have no conflict of interest to declare for this publication.

ACKNOWLEDGEMENTS

This work was supported by the "Fundação para a Ciência e a Tecnologia"–FCT (PTDC/BIM-MET/4712/2014), UMIB (PEst-OE/SAU/UI0215/2014). M. J. Meneses (PD/BD/114256/2016) was also funded by FCT.

REFERENCES

[1] World Health Organization. A Global Brief on Hypertension: Silent Killer, Global Public Health Crisis [Online]. http://www.who.int/cardiovascular_diseases/publications/global_brief_hypertension/en/2013

[2] Guariguata L, Whiting DR, Hambleton I, Beagley J, Linnenkamp U, Shaw JE. Global estimates of diabetes prevalence for 2013 and projections for 2035. Diabetes Res Clin Pract 2014; 103(2): 137-49. [http://dx.doi.org/10.1016/j.diabres.2013.11.002] [PMID: 24630390]

[3] World Health Organization. Obesity: preventing and managing the global epidemic. 2000.

[4] Guh DP, Zhang W, Bansback N, Amarsi Z, Birmingham CL, Anis AH. The incidence of co-morbidities related to obesity and overweight: a systematic review and meta-analysis. BMC Public Health 2009; 9: 88.
[http://dx.doi.org/10.1186/1471-2458-9-88] [PMID: 19320986]

[5] American Diabetes Association. Classification and Diagnosis of Diabetes. Diabetes Care 2016; 39 (Suppl. 1): S13-22.
[http://dx.doi.org/10.2337/dc16-S005] [PMID: 26696675]

[6] Lehuen A, Diana J, Zaccone P, Cooke A. Immune cell crosstalk in type 1 diabetes. Nat Rev Immunol 2010; 10(7): 501-13.
[http://dx.doi.org/10.1038/nri2787] [PMID: 20577267]

[7] Hu FB, Manson JE, Stampfer MJ, *et al.* Diet, lifestyle, and the risk of type 2 diabetes mellitus in women. N Engl J Med 2001; 345(11): 790-7.
[http://dx.doi.org/10.1056/NEJMoa010492] [PMID: 11556298]

[8] Van Waeleghem K, De Clercq N, Vermeulen L, Schoonjans F, Comhaire F. Deterioration of sperm quality in young healthy Belgian men. Hum Reprod 1996; 11(2): 325-9.
[http://dx.doi.org/10.1093/HUMREP/11.2.325] [PMID: 8671218]

[9] Slama R, Kold-Jensen T, Scheike T, Ducot B, Spira A, Keiding N. How would a decline in sperm concentration over time influence the probability of pregnancy? Epidemiology 2004; 15(4): 458-65. [http://dx.doi.org/10.1097/01.ede.0000129520.84568.87] [PMID: 15232407]

[10] Delfino M, Imbrogno N, Elia J, Capogreco F, Mazzilli F. Prevalence of diabetes mellitus in male partners of infertile couples. Minerva Urol Nefrol 2007; 59(2): 131-5.
[PMID: 17571048]

[11] Rato L, Alves MG, Dias TR, *et al.* High-energy diets may induce a pre-diabetic state altering testicular glycolytic metabolic profile and male reproductive parameters. Andrology 2013; 1(3): 495-504. [http://dx.doi.org/10.1111/j.2047-2927.2013.00071.x] [PMID: 23495257]

[12] Alves MG, Socorro S, Silva J, *et al.* *in vitro* cultured human Sertoli cells secrete high amounts of acetate that is stimulated by 17beta-estradiol and suppressed by insulin deprivation. Biochim Biophys Acta 2012; 1823: 1389-94.
[http://dx.doi.org/10.1016/j.bbamcr.2012.06.002] [PMID: 22705155]

[13] Bayir H. Reactive oxygen species. Crit Care Med 2005; 33(12) (Suppl.): S498-501.
[http://dx.doi.org/10.1097/01.CCM.0000186787.64500.12] [PMID: 16340433]

[14] Dormandy TL. Free-radical oxidation and antioxidants. Lancet 1978; 1(8065): 647-50.
[http://dx.doi.org/10.1016/S0140-6736(78)91148-0] [PMID: 76178]

[15] OFlaherty C, de Lamirande E, Gagnon C. Positive role of reactive oxygen species in mammalian sperm capacitation: triggering and modulation of phosphorylation events. Free Radic Biol Med 2006; 41(4): 528-40.
[http://dx.doi.org/10.1016/j.freeradbiomed.2006.04.027] [PMID: 16863985]

[16] Conrad M, Ingold I, Buday K, Kobayashi S, Angeli JP. ROS, thiols and thiol-regulating systems in male gametogenesis. Biochim Biophys Acta 2015; 1850: 1566-74.
[http://dx.doi.org/10.1016/j.bbagen.2014.10.020] [PMID: 25450170]

[17] de Lamirande E, O'Flaherty C. Sperm activation: role of reactive oxygen species and kinases. Biochim Biophys Acta 2008; 1784: 106-5.
[http://dx.doi.org/10.1016/j.bbapap.2007.08.024] [PMID: 17920343]

[18] de Lamirande E, Gagnon C. Human sperm hyperactivation and capacitation as parts of an oxidative process. Free Radic Biol Med 1993; 14(2): 157-66.
[http://dx.doi.org/10.1016/0891-5849(93)90006-G] [PMID: 8381103]

[19] Aitken RJ, Clarkson JS. Cellular basis of defective sperm function and its association with the genesis of reactive oxygen species by human spermatozoa. J Reprod Fertil 1987; 81(2): 459-69.
[http://dx.doi.org/10.1530/jrf.0.0810459] [PMID: 2828610]

[20] Bromfield EG, Aitken RJ, Anderson AL, McLaughlin EA, Nixon B. The impact of oxidative stress on chaperone-mediated human sperm-egg interaction. Hum Reprod 2015; 30(11): 2597-613.
[http://dx.doi.org/10.1093/humrep/dev214] [PMID: 26345691]

[21] Lenzi A, Picardo M, Gandini L, *et al.* Glutathione treatment of dyspermia: effect on the lipoperoxidation process. Hum Reprod 1994; 9(11): 2044-50.
[http://dx.doi.org/10.1093/oxfordjournals.humrep.a138391] [PMID: 7868672]

[22] Ayala A, Munoz MF, Argüelles S. Lipid Peroxidation: Production, Metabolism, and Signaling Mechanisms of Malondialdehyde and 4-Hydroxy-2-Nonenal. Oxid Med Cell Longev 2014; 2014: 31.
[http://dx.doi.org/10.1155/2014/360438]

[23] Moazamian R, Polhemus A, Connaughton H, *et al.* Oxidative stress and human spermatozoa: diagnostic and functional significance of aldehydes generated as a result of lipid peroxidation. Mol Hum Reprod 2015; 21(6): 502-15.
[http://dx.doi.org/10.1093/molehr/gav014] [PMID: 25837702]

[24] Aitken RJ, Gibb Z, Baker MA, Drevet J, Gharagozloo P. Causes and consequences of oxidative stress in spermatozoa. Reprod Fertil Dev 2016; 28(1-2): 1-10.
[http://dx.doi.org/10.1071/RD15325] [PMID: 27062870]

[25] Wong WY, Thomas CM, Merkus JM, Zielhuis GA, Steegers-Theunissen RP. Male factor subfertility: possible causes and the impact of nutritional factors. Fertil Steril 2000; 73(3): 435-42.
[http://dx.doi.org/10.1016/S0015-0282(99)00551-8] [PMID: 10688992]

[26] Balercia G, Buldreghini E, Vignini A, *et al.* Coenzyme Q10 treatment in infertile men with idiopathic asthenozoospermia: a placebo-controlled, double-blind randomized trial. Fertil Steril 2009; 91(5): 1785-92.
[http://dx.doi.org/10.1016/j.fertnstert.2008.02.119] [PMID: 18395716]

[27] Camejo MI, Abdala L, Vivas-Acevedo G, Lozano-Hernández R, Angeli-Greaves M, Greaves ED. Selenium, copper and zinc in seminal plasma of men with varicocele, relationship with seminal parameters. Biol Trace Elem Res 2011; 143(3): 1247-54.
[http://dx.doi.org/10.1007/s12011-011-8957-5] [PMID: 21240565]

[28] Durairajanayagam D, Agarwal A, Ong C, Prashast P. Lycopene and male infertility. Asian J Androl 2014; 16(3): 420-5.
[http://dx.doi.org/10.4103/1008-682X.126384] [PMID: 24675655]

[29] Oliveira PF, Tomás GD, Dias TR, *et al.* White tea consumption restores sperm quality in prediabetic rats preventing testicular oxidative damage. Reprod Biomed Online 2015; 31(4): 544-56.
[http://dx.doi.org/10.1016/j.rbmo.2015.06.021] [PMID: 26276042]

[30] Safarinejad MR, Hosseini SY, Dadkhah F, Asgari MA. Relationship of omega-3 and omega-6 fatty acids with semen characteristics, and anti-oxidant status of seminal plasma: a comparison between fertile and infertile men. Clin Nutr 2010; 29(1): 100-5.
[http://dx.doi.org/10.1016/j.clnu.2009.07.008] [PMID: 19666200]

[31] Vézina D, Mauffette F, Roberts KD, Bleau G. Selenium-vitamin E supplementation in infertile men. Effects on semen parameters and micronutrient levels and distribution. Biol Trace Elem Res 1996; 53(1-3): 65-83.
[http://dx.doi.org/10.1007/BF02784546] [PMID: 8862739]

[32] Bonet ML, Ribot J, Felipe F, Palou A. Vitamin A and the regulation of fat reserves. Cell Mol Life Sci 2003; 60(7): 1311-21.
[http://dx.doi.org/10.1007/s00018-003-2290-x] [PMID: 12943220]

[33] Ko EY, Sabanegh ES. The role of nutraceuticals in male fertility. Urol Clin North Am 2014; 41(1): 181-93.
[http://dx.doi.org/10.1016/j.ucl.2013.08.003] [PMID: 24286776]

[34] Hogarth CA, Griswold MD. The key role of vitamin A in spermatogenesis. J Clin Invest 2010; 120(4): 956-62.
[http://dx.doi.org/10.1172/JCI41303] [PMID: 20364093]

[35] Buhling KJ, Laakmann E. The effect of micronutrient supplements on male fertility. Curr Opin Obstet Gynecol 2014; 26(3): 199-209.
[http://dx.doi.org/10.1097/GCO.0000000000000063] [PMID: 24759120]

[36] Theodosiou M, Laudet V, Schubert M. From carrot to clinic: an overview of the retinoic acid signaling pathway. Cell Mol Life Sci 2010; 67(9): 1423-45.
[http://dx.doi.org/10.1007/s00018-010-0268-z] [PMID: 20140749]

[37] Livera G, Rouiller-Fabre V, Pairault C, Levacher C, Habert R. Regulation and perturbation of testicular functions by vitamin A. Reproduction 2002; 124(2): 173-80.
[http://dx.doi.org/10.1530/rep.0.1240173] [PMID: 12141930]

[38] Koubova J, Menke DB, Zhou Q, Capel B, Griswold MD, Page DC. Retinoic acid regulates sex-specific timing of meiotic initiation in mice. Proc Natl Acad Sci USA 2006; 103(8): 2474-9.
[http://dx.doi.org/10.1073/pnas.0510813103] [PMID: 16461896]

[39] Morales A, Cavicchia JC. Spermatogenesis and blood-testis barrier in rats after long-term Vitamin A deprivation. Tissue Cell 2002; 34(5): 349-55.
[http://dx.doi.org/10.1016/S0040816602000356] [PMID: 12270261]

[40] Amory JK, Muller CH, Shimshoni JA, *et al.* Suppression of spermatogenesis by bisdichloroacetyldiamines is mediated by inhibition of testicular retinoic acid biosynthesis. J Androl 2011; 32(1): 111-9.
[http://dx.doi.org/10.2164/jandrol.110.010751] [PMID: 20705791]

[41] Griswold MD. Spermatogenesis: The Commitment to Meiosis. Physiol Rev 2016; 96(1): 1-17.
[http://dx.doi.org/10.1152/physrev.00013.2015] [PMID: 26537427]

[42] Al-Azemi MK, Omu AE, Fatinikun T, Mannazhath N, Abraham S. Factors contributing to gender differences in serum retinol and alpha-tocopherol in infertile couples. Reprod Biomed Online 2009; 19(4): 583-90.
[http://dx.doi.org/10.1016/j.rbmo.2009.05.005] [PMID: 19909602]

[43] Paradiso Galatioto G, Gravina GL, Angelozzi G, *et al.* May antioxidant therapy improve sperm parameters of men with persistent oligospermia after retrograde embolization for varicocele? World J Urol 2008; 26(1): 97-102.
[http://dx.doi.org/10.1007/s00345-007-0218-z] [PMID: 17982752]

[44] Alpers DH. Manual of nutritional therapeutics. Philadelphia: Lippincott Williams & Wilkins 2008.

[45] Ebisch IM, Thomas CM, Peters WH, Braat DD, Steegers-Theunissen RP. The importance of folate, zinc and antioxidants in the pathogenesis and prevention of subfertility. Hum Reprod Update 2007; 13(2): 163-74.
[http://dx.doi.org/10.1093/humupd/dml054] [PMID: 17099205]

[46] Wong WY, Merkus HM, Thomas CM, Menkveld R, Zielhuis GA, Steegers-Theunissen RP. Effects of folic acid and zinc sulfate on male factor subfertility: a double-blind, randomized, placebo-controlled trial. Fertil Steril 2002; 77(3): 491-8.
[http://dx.doi.org/10.1016/S0015-0282(01)03229-0] [PMID: 11872201]

[47] Young SS, Eskenazi B, Marchetti FM, Block G, Wyrobek AJ. The association of folate, zinc and antioxidant intake with sperm aneuploidy in healthy non-smoking men. Hum Reprod 2008; 23(5): 1014-22.
[http://dx.doi.org/10.1093/humrep/den036] [PMID: 18353905]

[48] Boxmeer JC, Smit M, Weber RF, *et al.* Seminal plasma cobalamin significantly correlates with sperm concentration in men undergoing IVF or ICSI procedures. J Androl 2007; 28(4): 521-7.
[http://dx.doi.org/10.2164/jandrol.106.001982] [PMID: 17287458]

[49] Solomon LR. Disorders of cobalamin (vitamin B12) metabolism: emerging concepts in pathophysiology, diagnosis and treatment. Blood Rev 2007; 21(3): 113-30.
[http://dx.doi.org/10.1016/j.blre.2006.05.001] [PMID: 16814909]

[50] Kefer JC, Agarwal A, Sabanegh E. Role of antioxidants in the treatment of male infertility. Int J Urol 2009; 16(5): 449-57.
[http://dx.doi.org/10.1111/j.1442-2042.2009.02280.x] [PMID: 19383039]

[51] Fraga CG, Motchnik PA, Shigenaga MK, Helbock HJ, Jacob RA, Ames BN. Ascorbic acid protects against endogenous oxidative DNA damage in human sperm. Proc Natl Acad Sci USA 1991; 88(24): 11003-6.
[http://dx.doi.org/10.1073/pnas.88.24.11003] [PMID: 1763015]

[52] Greco E, Iacobelli M, Rienzi L, Ubaldi F, Ferrero S, Tesarik J. Reduction of the incidence of sperm DNA fragmentation by oral antioxidant treatment. J Androl 2005; 26(3): 349-53.
[http://dx.doi.org/10.2164/jandrol.04146] [PMID: 15867002]

[53] Sen Gupta R, Sen Gupta E, Dhakal BK, Thakur AR, Ahnn J. Vitamin C and vitamin E protect the rat testes from cadmium-induced reactive oxygen species. Mol Cells 2004; 17(1): 132-9.
[PMID: 15055539]

[54] Packer JE, Slater TF, Willson RL. Direct observation of a free radical interaction between vitamin E and vitamin C. Nature 1979; 278(5706): 737-8.
[http://dx.doi.org/10.1038/278737a0] [PMID: 431730]

[55] Lewis SE, Sterling ES, Young IS, Thompson W. Comparison of individual antioxidants of sperm and seminal plasma in fertile and infertile men. Fertil Steril 1997; 67(1): 142-7.
[http://dx.doi.org/10.1016/S0015-0282(97)81871-7] [PMID: 8986699]

[56] Biswas NM, Chaudhuri A, Sarkar M, Biswas R. Effect of ascorbic acid on *in vitro* synthesis of testosterone in rat testis. Indian J Exp Biol 1996; 34(6): 612-3. [PMID: 8792655]

[57] Okon UA, Utuk II. Ascorbic acid treatment elevates follicle stimulating hormone and testosterone plasma levels and enhances sperm quality in albino Wistar rats. Niger Med J 2016; 57(1): 31-6. [http://dx.doi.org/10.4103/0300-1652.180570] [PMID: 27185976]

[58] Fernandes GS, Gerardin DC, Assumpção TA, *et al.* Can vitamins C and E restore the androgen level and hypersensitivity of the vas deferens in hyperglycemic rats? Pharmacol Rep 2011; 63(4): 983-91. [http://dx.doi.org/10.1016/S1734-1140(11)70614-4] [PMID: 22001986]

[59] Colagar AH, Marzony ET. Ascorbic Acid in human seminal plasma: determination and its relationship to sperm quality. J Clin Biochem Nutr 2009; 45(2): 144-9. [http://dx.doi.org/10.3164/jcbn.08-251] [PMID: 19794921]

[60] Dawson EB, Harris WA, Rankin WE, Charpentier LA, McGanity WJ. Effect of ascorbic acid on male fertility. Ann N Y Acad Sci 1987; 498: 312-23. [http://dx.doi.org/10.1111/j.1749-6632.1987.tb23770.x] [PMID: 3476000]

[61] Omu AE, Al-Azemi MK, Kehinde EO, Anim JT, Oriowo MA, Mathew TC. Indications of the mechanisms involved in improved sperm parameters by zinc therapy. Med Princ Pract 2008; 17(2): 108-16. [http://dx.doi.org/10.1159/000112963] [PMID: 18287793]

[62] Ross C, Morriss A, Khairy M, *et al.* A systematic review of the effect of oral antioxidants on male infertility. Reprod Biomed Online 2010; 20(6): 711-23. [http://dx.doi.org/10.1016/j.rbmo.2010.03.008] [PMID: 20378409]

[63] Allgrove J. Physiology of Calcium, Phosphate, Magnesium and Vitamin D. Endocr Dev 2015; 28: 7-32. [http://dx.doi.org/10.1159/000380990] [PMID: 26138833]

[64] Bikle DD, Vitamin D. Vitamin D metabolism, mechanism of action, and clinical applications. Chem Biol 2014; 21(3): 319-29. [http://dx.doi.org/10.1016/j.chembiol.2013.12.016] [PMID: 24529992]

[65] Oh YS, Seo JT, Ahn HS, Gye MC. Expression of cubilin in mouse testes and Leydig cells. Andrologia 2016; 48(3): 325-32. [http://dx.doi.org/10.1111/and.12450] [PMID: 26148765]

[66] Blomberg Jensen M, Nielsen JE, Jørgensen A, *et al.* Vitamin D receptor and vitamin D metabolizing enzymes are expressed in the human male reproductive tract. Hum Reprod 2010; 25(5): 1303-11. [http://dx.doi.org/10.1093/humrep/deq024] [PMID: 20172873]

[67] Christakos S, Dhawan P, Verstuyf A, Verlinden L, Carmeliet G, Vitamin D. Vitamin D: Metabolism, Molecular Mechanism of Action, and Pleiotropic Effects. Physiol Rev 2016; 96(1): 365-408. [http://dx.doi.org/10.1152/physrev.00014.2015] [PMID: 26681795]

[68] Zanello LP, Norman AW. Rapid modulation of osteoblast ion channel responses by 1α,25(OH)2-vitamin D_3 requires the presence of a functional vitamin D nuclear receptor. Proc Natl Acad Sci USA 2004; 101(6): 1589-94. [http://dx.doi.org/10.1073/pnas.0305802101] [PMID: 14757825]

[69] Haussler MR, Jurutka PW, Mizwicki M, Norman AW. Vitamin D receptor (VDR)-mediated actions of 1α,25(OH)□vitamin D□: genomic and non-genomic mechanisms. Best Pract Res Clin Endocrinol Metab 2011; 25(4): 543-59. [http://dx.doi.org/10.1016/j.beem.2011.05.010] [PMID: 21872797]

[70] Nandi A, Sinha N, Ong E, Sonmez H, Poretsky L. Is there a role for vitamin D in human reproduction? Horm Mol Biol Clin Investig 2016; 25(1): 15-28. [http://dx.doi.org/10.1515/hmbci-2015-0051] [PMID: 26943610]

[71] Kinuta K, Tanaka H, Moriwake T, Aya K, Kato S, Seino Y. Vitamin D is an important factor in estrogen biosynthesis of both female and male gonads. Endocrinology 2000; 141(4): 1317-24. [PMID: 10746634]

[72] Mordan-McCombs S, Brown T, Wang W-L, Gaupel A-C, Welsh J, Tenniswood M. Tumor progression in the LPB-Tag transgenic model of prostate cancer is altered by vitamin D receptor and serum testosterone status. J Steroid Biochem Mol Biol 2010; 121(1-2): 368-71. [http://dx.doi.org/10.1016/j.jsbmb.2010.03.062] [PMID: 20347977]

[73] Blomberg Jensen M, Lieben L, Nielsen JE, *et al.* Characterization of the testicular, epididymal and endocrine phenotypes in the Leuven Vdr-deficient mouse model: targeting estrogen signalling. Mol Cell Endocrinol 2013; 377(1-2): 93-102. [http://dx.doi.org/10.1016/j.mce.2013.06.036] [PMID: 23850520]

[74] Blomberg Jensen M, Jørgensen A, Nielsen JE, *et al.* Expression of the vitamin D metabolizing enzyme CYP24A1 at the annulus of human spermatozoa may serve as a novel marker of semen quality. Int J Androl 2012; 35(4): 499-510. [http://dx.doi.org/10.1111/j.1365-2605.2012.01256.x] [PMID: 22404291]

[75] Naaby-Hansen S, Wolkowicz MJ, Klotz K, *et al.* Co-localization of the inositol 1,4,5-trisphosphate receptor and calreticulin in the equatorial segment and in membrane bounded vesicles in the cytoplasmic droplet of human spermatozoa. Mol Hum Reprod 2001; 7(10): 923-33. [http://dx.doi.org/10.1093/molehr/7.10.923] [PMID: 11574661]

[76] Aquila S, Guido C, Middea E, *et al.* Human male gamete endocrinology: 1alpha, 25-dihydroxyvitamin D_3 (1,25(OH)2D_3) regulates different aspects of human sperm biology and metabolism. Reprod Biol Endocrinol 2009; 7: 140. [http://dx.doi.org/10.1186/1477-7827-7-140] [PMID: 19948036]

[77] Blomberg Jensen M, Bjerrum PJ, Jessen TE, *et al.* Vitamin D is positively associated with sperm motility and increases intracellular calcium in human spermatozoa. Hum Reprod 2011; 26(6): 1307-17. [http://dx.doi.org/10.1093/humrep/der059] [PMID: 21427118]

[78] OToole CM, Arnoult C, Darszon A, Steinhardt RA, Florman HM. Ca(2+) entry through store-operated channels in mouse sperm is initiated by egg ZP3 and drives the acrosome reaction. Mol Biol Cell 2000; 11(5): 1571-84. [http://dx.doi.org/10.1091/mbc.11.5.1571] [PMID: 10793136]

[79] Aquila S, Guido C, Perrotta I, Tripepi S, Nastro A, Andò S. Human sperm anatomy: ultrastructural localization of 1alpha,25-dihydroxyvitamin D receptor and its possible role in the human male gamete. J Anat 2008; 213(5): 555-64. [http://dx.doi.org/10.1111/j.1469-7580.2008.00975.x] [PMID: 19014363]

[80] Palamanda JR, Kehrer JP. Involvement of vitamin E and protein thiols in the inhibition of microsomal lipid peroxidation by glutathione. Lipids 1993; 28(5): 427-31. [http://dx.doi.org/10.1007/BF02535941] [PMID: 8316051]

[81] Schmölz L, Birringer M, Lorkowski S, Wallert M. Complexity of vitamin E metabolism. World J Biol Chem 2016; 7(1): 14-43. [http://dx.doi.org/10.4331/wjbc.v7.i1.14] [PMID: 26981194]

[82] Neubauer O, Yfanti C. Antioxidants in Athlete's Basic Nutrition: Considerations towards a Guideline for the Intake of Vitamin C and Vitamin E. In: Lamprecht M, Ed. Antioxidants in Sport Nutrition. Boca Raton, FL: CRC Press/Taylor & Francis 2015.

[83] Walczak-Jedrzejowska R, Wolski JK, Slowikowska-Hilczer J. The role of oxidative stress and antioxidants in male fertility. Cent European J Urol 2013; 66(1): 60-7. [http://dx.doi.org/10.5173/ceju.2013.01.art19] [PMID: 24578993]

[84] Kessopoulou E, Powers HJ, Sharma KK, *et al.* A double-blind randomized placebo cross-over controlled trial using the antioxidant vitamin E to treat reactive oxygen species associated male infertility. Fertil Steril 1995; 64(4): 825-31.
[http://dx.doi.org/10.1016/S0015-0282(16)57861-3] [PMID: 7672157]

[85] Eskenazi B, Kidd SA, Marks AR, Sloter E, Block G, Wyrobek AJ. Antioxidant intake is associated with semen quality in healthy men. Hum Reprod 2005; 20(4): 1006-12.
[http://dx.doi.org/10.1093/humrep/deh725] [PMID: 15665024]

[86] Suleiman SA, Ali ME, Zaki ZM, el-Malik EM, Nasr MA. Lipid peroxidation and human sperm motility: protective role of vitamin E. J Androl 1996; 17(5): 530-7.
[PMID: 8957697]

[87] Miller ER III, Pastor-Barriuso R, Dalal D, Riemersma RA, Appel LJ, Guallar E. Meta-analysis: high-dosage vitamin E supplementation may increase all-cause mortality. Ann Intern Med 2005; 142(1): 37-46.
[http://dx.doi.org/10.7326/0003-4819-142-1-200501040-00110] [PMID: 15537682]

[88] Boitani C, Puglisi R. Selenium, a key element in spermatogenesis and male fertility. Adv Exp Med Biol 2008; 636: 65-73.
[http://dx.doi.org/10.1007/978-0-387-09597-4_4] [PMID: 19856162]

[89] Graupner A, Instanes C, Andersen JM, *et al.* Genotoxic effects of two-generational selenium deficiency in mouse somatic and testicular cells. Mutagenesis 2015; 30(2): 217-25.
[http://dx.doi.org/10.1093/mutage/geu059] [PMID: 25358475]

[90] Ursini F, Heim S, Kiess M, *et al.* Dual function of the selenoprotein PHGPx during sperm maturation. Science 1999; 285(5432): 1393-6.
[http://dx.doi.org/10.1126/science.285.5432.1393] [PMID: 10464096]

[91] Scott R, MacPherson A, Yates RW, Hussain B, Dixon J. The effect of oral selenium supplementation on human sperm motility. Br J Urol 1998; 82(1): 76-80.
[http://dx.doi.org/10.1046/j.1464-410x.1998.00683.x] [PMID: 9698665]

[92] Messaoudi I, Banni M, Saïd L, Saïd K, Kerkeni A. Involvement of selenoprotein P and GPx4 gene expression in cadmium-induced testicular pathophysiology in rat. Chem Biol Interact 2010; 188(1): 94-101.
[http://dx.doi.org/10.1016/j.cbi.2010.07.012] [PMID: 20643113]

[93] Imai H, Hakkaku N, Iwamoto R, *et al.* Depletion of selenoprotein GPx4 in spermatocytes causes male infertility in mice. J Biol Chem 2009; 284(47): 32522-32.
[http://dx.doi.org/10.1074/jbc.M109.016139] [PMID: 19783653]

[94] Imai H, Nakagawa Y. Biological significance of phospholipid hydroperoxide glutathione peroxidase (PHGPx, GPx4) in mammalian cells. Free Radic Biol Med 2003; 34(2): 145-69.
[http://dx.doi.org/10.1016/S0891-5849(02)01197-8] [PMID: 12521597]

[95] Beckett GJ, Arthur JR. Selenium and endocrine systems. J Endocrinol 2005; 184(3): 455-65.
[http://dx.doi.org/10.1677/joe.1.05971] [PMID: 15749805]

[96] Schneider M, Förster H, Boersma A, *et al.* Mitochondrial glutathione peroxidase 4 disruption causes male infertility. FASEB J 2009; 23(9): 3233-42.
[http://dx.doi.org/10.1096/fj.09-132795] [PMID: 19417079]

[97] Foresta C, Flohé L, Garolla A, Roveri A, Ursini F, Maiorino M. Male fertility is linked to the selenoprotein phospholipid hydroperoxide glutathione peroxidase. Biol Reprod 2002; 67(3): 967-71.
[http://dx.doi.org/10.1095/biolreprod.102.003822] [PMID: 12193409]

[98] Croxford TP, McCormick NH, Kelleher SL. Moderate zinc deficiency reduces testicular Zip6 and Zip10 abundance and impairs spermatogenesis in mice. J Nutr 2011; 141(3): 359-65.
[http://dx.doi.org/10.3945/jn.110.131318] [PMID: 21248196]

[99] Kundu TK, Rao MR. Zinc dependent recognition of a human CpG island sequence by the mammalian spermatidal protein TP2. Biochemistry 1996; 35(49): 15626-32.
[http://dx.doi.org/10.1021/bi961271i] [PMID: 8961924]

[100] Pradeepa MM, Rao MR. Chromatin remodeling during mammalian spermatogenesis: role of testis specific histone variants and transition proteins. Soc Reprod Fertil Suppl 2007; 63: 1-10.
[PMID: 17566256]

[101] Zago MP, Oteiza PI. The antioxidant properties of zinc: interactions with iron and antioxidants. Free Radic Biol Med 2001; 31(2): 266-74.
[http://dx.doi.org/10.1016/S0891-5849(01)00583-4] [PMID: 11440839]

[102] Trumbo P, Yates AA, Schlicker S, Poos M. Dietary reference intakes: vitamin A, vitamin K, arsenic, boron, chromium, copper, iodine, iron, manganese, molybdenum, nickel, silicon, vanadium, and zinc. J Am Diet Assoc 2001; 101(3): 294-301.
[http://dx.doi.org/10.1016/S0002-8223(01)00078-5] [PMID: 11269606]

[103] Prasad AS. Zinc in human health: effect of zinc on immune cells. Mol Med 2008; 14(5-6): 353-7.
[http://dx.doi.org/10.2119/2008-00033.Prasad] [PMID: 18385818]

[104] Abbasi AA, Prasad AS, Rabbani PR. Experimental zinc deficiency in man: effect on spermatogenesis. Trans Assoc Am Physicians 1979; 92: 292-302.
[PMID: 549254]

[105] Colagar AH, Marzony ET, Chaichi MJ. Zinc levels in seminal plasma are associated with sperm quality in fertile and infertile men. Nutr Res 2009; 29(2): 82-8.
[http://dx.doi.org/10.1016/j.nutres.2008.11.007] [PMID: 19285597]

[106] Maret W, Sandstead HH. Zinc requirements and the risks and benefits of zinc supplementation. J Trace Elem Med Biol 2006; 20(1): 3-18.
[http://dx.doi.org/10.1016/j.jtemb.2006.01.006] [PMID: 16632171]

[107] Ferrari CK. Functional foods, herbs and nutraceuticals: towards biochemical mechanisms of healthy aging. Biogerontology 2004; 5(5): 275-89.
[http://dx.doi.org/10.1007/s10522-004-2566-z] [PMID: 15547316]

[108] Mancini A, De Marinis L, Oradei A, *et al.* Coenzyme Q10 concentrations in normal and pathological human seminal fluid. J Androl 1994; 15(6): 591-4.
[PMID: 7721661]

[109] Moreira PI, Santos MS, Sena C, Nunes E, Seiça R, Oliveira CR. CoQ10 therapy attenuates amyloid β-peptide toxicity in brain mitochondria isolated from aged diabetic rats. Exp Neurol 2005; 196(1): 112-9.
[http://dx.doi.org/10.1016/j.expneurol.2005.07.012] [PMID: 16126199]

[110] Gómez-Díaz C, Burón MI, Alcaín FJ, *et al.* Effect of dietary coenzyme Q and fatty acids on the antioxidant status of rat tissues. Protoplasma 2003; 221(1-2): 11-7.
[http://dx.doi.org/10.1007/s00709-002-0067-y] [PMID: 12768337]

[111] Esmaeili V, Shahverdi AH, Moghadasian MH, Alizadeh AR. Dietary fatty acids affect semen quality: a review. Andrology 2015; 3(3): 450-61.
[http://dx.doi.org/10.1111/andr.12024] [PMID: 25951427]

[112] Calder PC. Polyunsaturated fatty acids, inflammatory processes and inflammatory bowel diseases. Mol Nutr Food Res 2008; 52(8): 885-97.
[http://dx.doi.org/10.1002/mnfr.200700289] [PMID: 18504706]

[113] Wall R, Ross RP, Fitzgerald GF, Stanton C. Fatty acids from fish: the anti-inflammatory potential of long-chain omega-3 fatty acids. Nutr Rev 2010; 68(5): 280-9.
[http://dx.doi.org/10.1111/j.1753-4887.2010.00287.x] [PMID: 20500789]

[114] Shaikh SR, Kinnun JJ, Leng X, Williams JA, Wassall SR. How polyunsaturated fatty acids modify molecular organization in membranes: insight from NMR studies of model systems. Biochim Biophys Acta 2015; 1848: 211-9.
[http://dx.doi.org/10.1016/j.bbamem.2014.04.020] [PMID: 24820775]

[115] Lenzi A, Gandini L, Maresca V, *et al.* Fatty acid composition of spermatozoa and immature germ cells. Mol Hum Reprod 2000; 6(3): 226-31.
[http://dx.doi.org/10.1093/molehr/6.3.226] [PMID: 10694269]

[116] Aksoy Y, Aksoy H, Altinkaynak K, Aydin HR, Ozkan A. Sperm fatty acid composition in subfertile men. Prostaglandins Leukot Essent Fatty Acids 2006; 75(2): 75-9.
[http://dx.doi.org/10.1016/j.plefa.2006.06.002] [PMID: 16893631]

[117] Martínez-Soto JC, Landeras J, Gadea J. Spermatozoa and seminal plasma fatty acids as predictors of cryopreservation success. Andrology 2013; 1(3): 365-75.
[http://dx.doi.org/10.1111/j.2047-2927.2012.00040.x] [PMID: 23596043]

[118] Leat WM, Northrop CA, Harrison FA, Cox RW. Effect of dietary linoleic and linolenic acids on testicular development in the rat. Q J Exp Physiol 1983; 68(2): 221-31.
[http://dx.doi.org/10.1113/expphysiol.1983.sp002714] [PMID: 6856750]

[119] Roqueta-Rivera M, Abbott TL, Sivaguru M, Hess RA, Nakamura MT. Deficiency in the omega-3 fatty acid pathway results in failure of acrosome biogenesis in mice. Biol Reprod 2011; 85(4): 721-32.
[http://dx.doi.org/10.1095/biolreprod.110.089524] [PMID: 21653892]

[120] Ling SH, San PP, Nguyen HT. Non-invasive hypoglycemia monitoring system using extreme learning machine for Type 1 diabetes. ISA Trans 2016; 64: 440-6.
[http://dx.doi.org/10.1016/j.isatra.2016.05.008] [PMID: 27311357]

[121] Jia L, Vianna CR, Fukuda M, *et al.* Hepatocyte Toll-like receptor 4 regulates obesity-induced inflammation and insulin resistance. Nat Commun 2014; 5: 3878.
[http://dx.doi.org/10.1038/ncomms4878] [PMID: 24815961]

[122] Giorda CB, Ozzello A, Gentile S, *et al.* Incidence and risk factors for severe and symptomatic hypoglycemia in type 1 diabetes. Results of the HYPOS-1 study. Acta Diabetol 2015; 52(5): 845-53.
[http://dx.doi.org/10.1007/s00592-015-0713-4] [PMID: 25670242]

[123] Fadini GP, Albiero M, Vigili de Kreutzenberg S, Avogaro A. Hypoglycemia affects the changes in endothelial progenitor cell levels during insulin therapy in type 2 diabetic patients. J Endocrinol Invest 2015; 38(7): 733-8.
[http://dx.doi.org/10.1007/s40618-015-0247-1] [PMID: 25722222]

[124] McNay EC, Teske JA, Kotz CM, *et al.* Long-term, intermittent, insulin-induced hypoglycemia produces marked obesity without hyperphagia or insulin resistance: a model for weight gain with intensive insulin therapy. Am J Physiol Endocrinol Metab 2013; 304(2): E131-8.
[http://dx.doi.org/10.1152/ajpendo.00262.2012] [PMID: 23169787]

[125] Karl AF, Griswold MD. Actions of insulin and vitamin A on Sertoli cells. Biochem J 1980; 186(3): 1001-3.
[http://dx.doi.org/10.1042/bj1861001] [PMID: 6249257]

[126] Griswold MD, Merryweather J. Insulin stimulates the incorporation of 32Pi into ribonucleic acid in cultured sertoli cells. Endocrinology 1982; 111(2): 661-7.
[http://dx.doi.org/10.1210/endo-111-2-661] [PMID: 6178581]

[127] Skinner MK, Griswold MD. Secretion of testicular transferrin by cultured Sertoli cells is regulated by hormones and retinoids. Biol Reprod 1982; 27(1): 211-21.
[http://dx.doi.org/10.1095/biolreprod27.1.211] [PMID: 6810965]

[128] Sylvester SR, Griswold MD. The testicular iron shuttle: a nurse function of the Sertoli cells. J Androl 1994; 15(5): 381-5.
[PMID: 7860417]

[129] Oonk RB, Grootegoed JA, van der Molen HJ. Comparison of the effects of insulin and follitropin on glucose metabolism by Sertoli cells from immature rats. Mol Cell Endocrinol 1985; 42(1): 39-48. [http://dx.doi.org/10.1016/0303-7207(85)90005-X] [PMID: 3928417]

[130] Oonk RB, Grootegoed JA. Identification of insulin receptors on rat Sertoli cells. Mol Cell Endocrinol 1987; 49(1): 51-62. [http://dx.doi.org/10.1016/0303-7207(87)90063-3] [PMID: 3549388]

[131] Mita M, Borland K, Price JM, Hall PF. The influence of insulin and insulin-like growth factor-I on hexose transport by Sertoli cells. Endocrinology 1985; 116(3): 987-92. [http://dx.doi.org/10.1210/endo-116-3-987] [PMID: 3882401]

[132] Nakayama Y, Yamamoto T, Abé SI. IGF-I, IGF-II and insulin promote differentiation of spermatogonia to primary spermatocytes in organ culture of newt testes. Int J Dev Biol 1999; 43(4): 343-7. [PMID: 10470651]

[133] Hurtado de Catalfo GE, De Gómez Dumm IN. Lipid dismetabolism in Leydig and Sertoli cells isolated from streptozotocin-diabetic rats. Int J Biochem Cell Biol 1998; 30(9): 1001-10. [http://dx.doi.org/10.1016/S1357-2725(98)00055-7] [PMID: 9785463]

[134] Schoeller EL, Albanna G, Frolova AI, Moley KH. Insulin rescues impaired spermatogenesis *via* the hypothalamic-pituitary-gonadal axis in Akita diabetic mice and restores male fertility. Diabetes 2012; 61(7): 1869-78. [http://dx.doi.org/10.2337/db11-1527] [PMID: 22522616]

[135] Oliveira PF, Alves MG, Rato L, *et al.* Effect of insulin deprivation on metabolism and metabolism-associated gene transcript levels of *in vitro* cultured human Sertoli cells. Biochim Biophys Acta 2012; 1820: 84-9. [http://dx.doi.org/10.1016/j.bbagen.2011.11.006] [PMID: 22146232]

[136] Hicks JJ, Rojas L, Rosado A. Insulin regulation of spermatozoa metabolism. Endocrinology 1973; 92(3): 833-9. [http://dx.doi.org/10.1210/endo-92-3-833] [PMID: 4701485]

[137] Gorus FK, Pipeleers DG. Glucose metabolism in human spermatozoa: lack of insulin effects and dissociation from alloxan handling. J Cell Physiol 1986; 127(2): 261-6. [http://dx.doi.org/10.1002/jcp.1041270211] [PMID: 3517012]

[138] Silvestroni L, Modesti A, Sartori C. Insulin-sperm interaction: effects on plasma membrane and binding to acrosome. Arch Androl 1992; 28(3): 201-11. [http://dx.doi.org/10.3109/01485019208987699] [PMID: 1530369]

[139] Sliwa L. Effects of selected hormones on the motility of spermatozoa in the mouse vas deferens. Arch Androl 1994; 33(3): 145-9. [http://dx.doi.org/10.3109/01485019408987817] [PMID: 7857164]

[140] Chandrashekar V, Bartke A. The role of insulin-like growth factor-I in neuroendocrine function and the consequent effects on sexual maturation: inferences from animal models. Reprod Biol 2003; 3(1): 7-28. [PMID: 14666141]

[141] Bansal TC, Guay AT, Jacobson J, Woods BO, Nesto RW. Incidence of metabolic syndrome and insulin resistance in a population with organic erectile dysfunction. J Sex Med 2005; 2(1): 96-103. [http://dx.doi.org/10.1111/j.1743-6109.2005.20120.x] [PMID: 16422911]

[142] Pitteloud N, Hardin M, Dwyer AA, *et al.* Increasing insulin resistance is associated with a decrease in Leydig cell testosterone secretion in men. J Clin Endocrinol Metab 2005; 90(5): 2636-41. [http://dx.doi.org/10.1210/jc.2004-2190] [PMID: 15713702]

[143] Aquila S, Gentile M, Middea E, Catalano S, Andò S. Autocrine regulation of insulin secretion in human ejaculated spermatozoa. Endocrinology 2005; 146(2): 552-7.
[http://dx.doi.org/10.1210/en.2004-1252] [PMID: 15550513]

[144] Lampiao F, du Plessis SS. Insulin and leptin enhance human sperm motility, acrosome reaction and nitric oxide production. Asian J Androl 2008; 10(5): 799-807.
[http://dx.doi.org/10.1111/j.1745-7262.2008.00421.x] [PMID: 18645684]

[145] Cappello AR, Guido C, Santoro A, *et al.* The mitochondrial citrate carrier (CIC) is present and regulates insulin secretion by human male gamete. Endocrinology 2012; 153(4): 1743-54.
[http://dx.doi.org/10.1210/en.2011-1562] [PMID: 22355067]

[146] Butler MG, McGuire A, Manzardo AM. Clinically relevant known and candidate genes for obesity and their overlap with human infertility and reproduction. J Assist Reprod Genet 2015; 32(4): 495-508.
[http://dx.doi.org/10.1007/s10815-014-0411-0] [PMID: 25631154]

[147] World Health Organization. A Obesity and overweight: World Health Organization. Available from: http://www.who.int/mediacentre/factsheets/fs311/en/ 2016.

[148] Obesity and reproduction: a committee opinion. Fertil Steril 2015; 104(5): 1116-26.
[http://dx.doi.org/10.1016/j.fertnstert.2015.08.018] [PMID: 26434804]

[149] Durairajanayagam D, Agarwal A, Ong C. Causes, effects and molecular mechanisms of testicular heat stress. Reprod Biomed Online 2015; 30(1): 14-27.
[http://dx.doi.org/10.1016/j.rbmo.2014.09.018] [PMID: 25456164]

[150] Shiraishi K, Takihara H, Matsuyama H. Elevated scrotal temperature, but not varicocele grade, reflects testicular oxidative stress-mediated apoptosis. World J Urol 2010; 28(3): 359-64.
[http://dx.doi.org/10.1007/s00345-009-0462-5] [PMID: 19655149]

[151] Vera Y, Diaz-Romero M, Rodriguez S, *et al.* Mitochondria-dependent pathway is involved in heat-induced male germ cell death: lessons from mutant mice. Biol Reprod 2004; 70(5): 1534-40.
[http://dx.doi.org/10.1095/biolreprod.103.024661] [PMID: 14749299]

[152] Miura M, Sasagawa I, Suzuki Y, Nakada T, Fujii J. Apoptosis and expression of apoptosis-related genes in the mouse testis following heat exposure. Fertil Steril 2002; 77(4): 787-93.
[http://dx.doi.org/10.1016/S0015-0282(01)03255-1] [PMID: 11937135]

[153] Yin Y, Stahl BC, DeWolf WC, Morgentaler A. p53-mediated germ cell quality control in spermatogenesis. Dev Biol 1998; 204(1): 165-71.
[http://dx.doi.org/10.1006/dbio.1998.9074] [PMID: 9851850]

[154] Zorgniotti AW, Sealfon AI. Scrotal hypothermia: new therapy for poor semen. Urology 1984; 23(5): 439-41.
[http://dx.doi.org/10.1016/S0090-4295(84)80006-0] [PMID: 6372197]

[155] Shafik A, Olfat S. Lipectomy in the treatment of scrotal lipomatosis. Br J Urol 1981; 53(1): 55-61.
[http://dx.doi.org/10.1111/j.1464-410X.1981.tb03129.x] [PMID: 7470804]

[156] Jones R, Mann T, Sherins R. Peroxidative breakdown of phospholipids in human spermatozoa, spermicidal properties of fatty acid peroxides, and protective action of seminal plasma. Fertil Steril 1979; 31(5): 531-7.
[http://dx.doi.org/10.1016/S0015-0282(16)43999-3] [PMID: 446777]

[157] Vermeulen A, Kaufman JM, Deslypere JP, Thomas G. Attenuated luteinizing hormone (LH) pulse amplitude but normal LH pulse frequency, and its relation to plasma androgens in hypogonadism of obese men. J Clin Endocrinol Metab 1993; 76(5): 1140-6.
[PMID: 8496304]

[158] Roth MY, Amory JK, Page ST. Treatment of male infertility secondary to morbid obesity. Nat Clin Pract Endocrinol Metab 2008; 4(7): 415-9.
[http://dx.doi.org/10.1038/ncpendmet0844] [PMID: 18523426]

[159] Wake DJ, Strand M, Rask E, *et al.* Intra-adipose sex steroid metabolism and body fat distribution in idiopathic human obesity. Clin Endocrinol (Oxf) 2007; 66(3): 440-6.
[http://dx.doi.org/10.1111/j.1365-2265.2007.02755.x] [PMID: 17302881]

[160] Palmer NO, Bakos HW, Fullston T, Lane M. Impact of obesity on male fertility, sperm function and molecular composition. Spermatogenesis 2012; 2(4): 253-63.
[http://dx.doi.org/10.4161/spmg.21362] [PMID: 23248766]

[161] Isidori AM, Caprio M, Strollo F, *et al.* Leptin and androgens in male obesity: evidence for leptin contribution to reduced androgen levels. J Clin Endocrinol Metab 1999; 84(10): 3673-80.
[http://dx.doi.org/10.1210/jcem.84.10.6082] [PMID: 10523013]

[162] Hofny ER, Ali ME, Abdel-Hafez HZ, *et al.* Semen parameters and hormonal profile in obese fertile and infertile males. Fertil Steril 2010; 94(2): 581-4.
[http://dx.doi.org/10.1016/j.fertnstert.2009.03.085] [PMID: 19423100]

[163] Pugeat M, Nader N, Hogeveen K, Raverot G, Déchaud H, Grenot C. Sex hormone-binding globulin gene expression in the liver: drugs and the metabolic syndrome. Mol Cell Endocrinol 2010; 316(1): 53-9.
[http://dx.doi.org/10.1016/j.mce.2009.09.020] [PMID: 19786070]

[164] Kalme T, Koistinen H, Loukovaara M, Koistinen R, Leinonen P. Comparative studies on the regulation of insulin-like growth factor-binding protein-1 (IGFBP-1) and sex hormone-binding globulin (SHBG) production by insulin and insulin-like growth factors in human hepatoma cells. J Steroid Biochem Mol Biol 2003; 86(2): 197-200.
[http://dx.doi.org/10.1016/S0960-0760(03)00268-1] [PMID: 14568572]

[165] Peiris AN, Stagner JI, Plymate SR, Vogel RL, Heck M, Samols E. Relationship of insulin secretory pulses to sex hormone-binding globulin in normal men. J Clin Endocrinol Metab 1993; 76(2): 279-82.
[http://dx.doi.org/10.1210/jcem.76.2.8432769] [PMID: 8432769]

[166] Kopelman PG, Pilkington TR, White N, Jeffcoate SL. Abnormal sex steroid secretion and binding in massively obese women. Clin Endocrinol (Oxf) 1980; 12(4): 363-9.
[http://dx.doi.org/10.1111/j.1365-2265.1980.tb02721.x] [PMID: 6769612]

[167] Jensen TK, Andersson AM, Jørgensen N, *et al.* Body mass index in relation to semen quality and reproductive hormones among 1,558 Danish men. Fertil Steril 2004; 82(4): 863-70.
[http://dx.doi.org/10.1016/j.fertnstert.2004.03.056] [PMID: 15482761]

[168] Du Plessis SS, Cabler S, McAlister DA, Sabanegh E, Agarwal A. The effect of obesity on sperm disorders and male infertility. Nat Rev Urol 2010; 7(3): 153-61.
[http://dx.doi.org/10.1038/nrurol.2010.6] [PMID: 20157305]

[169] Rato L, Alves MG, Cavaco JE, Oliveira PF. High-energy diets: a threat for male fertility? Obes Rev 2014; 15(12): 996-1007.
[http://dx.doi.org/10.1111/obr.12226] [PMID: 25346452]

[170] Aitken RJ, Gordon E, Harkiss D, *et al.* Relative impact of oxidative stress on the functional competence and genomic integrity of human spermatozoa. Biol Reprod 1998; 59(5): 1037-46.
[http://dx.doi.org/10.1095/biolreprod59.5.1037] [PMID: 9780307]

[171] Kort HI, Massey JB, Elsner CW, *et al.* Impact of body mass index values on sperm quantity and quality. J Androl 2006; 27(3): 450-2.
[http://dx.doi.org/10.2164/jandrol.05124] [PMID: 16339454]

[172] La Vignera S, Condorelli RA, Vicari E, Calogero AE. Negative effect of increased body weight on sperm conventional and nonconventional flow cytometric sperm parameters. J Androl 2012; 33(1): 53-8.
[http://dx.doi.org/10.2164/jandrol.110.012120] [PMID: 21273503]

[173] International Diabetes Federation. IDF Diabetes Atlas 7th ed. http://www.diabetesatlas.org 2016.

[174] Tay J, Luscombe-Marsh ND, Thompson CH, *et al.* Comparison of low- and high-carbohydrate diets for type 2 diabetes management: a randomized trial. Am J Clin Nutr 2015; 102(4): 780-90.
[http://dx.doi.org/10.3945/ajcn.115.112581] [PMID: 26224300]

[175] Meneses MJ, Bernardino RL, Sousa M, *et al.* Regulation of testicular glucose metabolism in (pre)diabetes and its implications to male reproductive health. In: Berhardt LV, Ed. Advances in Medicine and Biology. New York: Nova Science Publishers 2015; pp. 29-56.

[176] Tabák AG, Herder C, Rathmann W, Brunner EJ, Kivimäki M. Prediabetes: a high-risk state for diabetes development. Lancet 2012; 379(9833): 2279-90.
[http://dx.doi.org/10.1016/S0140-6736(12)60283-9] [PMID: 22683128]

[177] Meneses MJ, Sousa M, Alves MG, Oliveira PF. The Antidiabetic Drug Metformin and Male Reproductive Function: An Overview. Int J Diabetol Vasc Disease Res 2015; 3: 1-2.

[178] La Vignera S, Calogero AE, Condorelli R, Lanzafame F, Giammusso B, Vicari E. Andrological characterization of the patient with diabetes mellitus. Minerva Endocrinol 2009; 34(1): 1-9.
[PMID: 19209124]

[179] Agbaje IM, Rogers DA, McVicar CM, *et al.* Insulin dependant diabetes mellitus: implications for male reproductive function. Hum Reprod 2007; 22(7): 1871-7.
[http://dx.doi.org/10.1093/humrep/dem077] [PMID: 17478459]

[180] Scarano WR, Messias AG, Oliva SU, Klinefelter GR, Kempinas WG. Sexual behaviour, sperm quantity and quality after short-term streptozotocin-induced hyperglycaemia in rats. Int J Androl 2006; 29(4): 482-8.
[http://dx.doi.org/10.1111/j.1365-2605.2006.00682.x] [PMID: 16524366]

[181] Alves MG, Martins AD, Rato L, Moreira PI, Socorro S, Oliveira PF. Molecular mechanisms beyond glucose transport in diabetes-related male infertility. Biochim Biophys Acta 2013; 1832: 626-35.
[http://dx.doi.org/10.1016/j.bbadis.2013.01.011] [PMID: 23348098]

[182] Rato L, Duarte AI, Tomas GD, *et al.* Pre-diabetes alters testicular PGC1-alpha/SIRT3 axis modulating mitochondrial bioenergetics and oxidative stress. Biochim Biophys Acta 2014; 1837: 335-44.
[http://dx.doi.org/110.1016/j.bbabio.2013.12.008] [PMID: 24361842]

[183] Jing E, Emanuelli B, Hirschey MD, *et al.* Sirtuin-3 (Sirt3) regulates skeletal muscle metabolism and insulin signaling *via* altered mitochondrial oxidation and reactive oxygen species production. Proc Natl Acad Sci USA 2011; 108(35): 14608-13.
[http://dx.doi.org/10.1073/pnas.1111308108] [PMID: 21873205]

[184] Benitez A, Perez Diaz J. Effect of streptozotocin-diabetes and insulin treatment on regulation of Leydig cell function in the rat. Horm Metab Res 1985; 17(1): 5-7.
[http://dx.doi.org/10.1055/s-2007-1013433] [PMID: 2981762]

[185] Hutson JC, Stocco DM, Campbell GT, Wagoner J. Sertoli cell function in diabetic, insulin-treated diabetic, and semi-starved rats. Diabetes 1983; 32(2): 112-6.
[http://dx.doi.org/10.2337/diab.32.2.112] [PMID: 6219025]

[186] Rato L, Alves MG, Dias TR, Cavaco JE, Oliveira PF. Testicular Metabolic Reprogramming in Neonatal Streptozotocin-Induced Type 2 Diabetic Rats Impairs Glycolytic Flux and Promotes Glycogen Synthesis. J Diabetes Res 2015; 2015: 13.
[http://dx.doi.org/10.1155/2015/973142] [PMID: 26064993]

[187] Cameron DF, Murray FT, Drylie DD. Interstitial compartment pathology and spermatogenic disruption in testes from impotent diabetic men. Anat Rec 1985; 213(1): 53-62. [http://dx.doi.org/10.1002/ar.1092130108] [PMID: 4073561]

[188] Bernardino RL, Martins AD, Socorro S, Alves MG, Oliveira PF. Effect of prediabetes on membrane bicarbonate transporters in testis and epididymis. J Membr Biol 2013; 246(12): 877-83. [http://dx.doi.org/10.1007/s00232-013-9601-4] [PMID: 24105628]

[189] Frenkel GP, Homonnai ZT, Drasnin N, Sofer A, Kaplan R, Kraicer PF. Fertility of the streptozotocin-diabetic male rat. Andrologia 1978; 10(2): 127-36. [http://dx.doi.org/10.1111/j.1439-0272.1978.tb01327.x] [PMID: 646142]

[190] Murray FT, Cameron DF, Orth JM. Gonadal dysfunction in the spontaneously diabetic BB rat. Metabolism 1983; 32(7) (Suppl. 1): 141-7. [http://dx.doi.org/10.1016/S0026-0495(83)80028-6] [PMID: 6865764]

[191] Cameron DF, Rountree J, Schultz RE, Repetta D, Murray FT. Sustained hyperglycemia results in testicular dysfunction and reduced fertility potential in BBWOR diabetic rats. Am J Physiol 1990; 259(6 Pt 1): E881-9. [PMID: 2260654]

[192] Mulholland J, Mallidis C, Agbaje I, McClure N. Male diabetes mellitus and assisted reproduction treatment outcome. Reprod Biomed Online 2011; 22(2): 215-9. [http://dx.doi.org/10.1016/j.rbmo.2010.10.005] [PMID: 21227754]

[193] Riera MF, Galardo MN, Pellizzari EH, Meroni SB, Cigorraga SB. Molecular mechanisms involved in Sertoli cell adaptation to glucose deprivation. Am J Physiol Endocrinol Metab 2009; 297(4): E907-14. [http://dx.doi.org/10.1152/ajpendo.00235.2009] [PMID: 19638510]

[194] Mita M, Hall PF. Metabolism of round spermatids from rats: lactate as the preferred substrate. Biol Reprod 1982; 26(3): 445-55. [http://dx.doi.org/10.1095/biolreprod26.3.445] [PMID: 7082719]

[195] Klip A, Tsakiridis T, Marette A, Ortiz PA. Regulation of expression of glucose transporters by glucose: a review of studies *in vivo* and in cell cultures. FASEB J 1994; 8(1): 43-53. [PMID: 8299889]

[196] Dias TR, Martins AD, Reis VP, *et al.* Glucose transport and metabolism in sertoli cell: relevance for male fertility. Curr Chem Biol 2013; 7: 282-93. [http://dx.doi.org/10.2174/2212796807999131128125510] [PMID: 25486098]

[197] Berg JM, Tymoczko JL, Stryer L. Glycolysis and gluconeogenesis 2002.

[198] Froment P, Staub C, Hembert S, *et al.* Reproductive abnormalities in human insulin-like growth factor-binding protein-1 transgenic male mice. Endocrinology 2004; 145(4): 2080-91. [http://dx.doi.org/10.1210/en.2003-0956] [PMID: 14726451]

CHAPTER 13

Environmental Cues and Sperm Quality

Ana M. Cardoso and **Luís Rato***

Health Sciences Research Centre, University of Beira Interior, Rua Marquês d'Ávila e Bolama, 6201-001, Covilhã, Portugal

Abstract: The increase in the occurrence of defective spermatogenesis and other important fertility issues in males evidenced over the past few decades have prompted the research on the possible contribution of environmental factors to this adverse trend. Environmental contaminants may act through different molecular targets in male reproductive system, being able to disrupt the functioning of reproductive axis and, consequently, testicular physiology and metabolism. In addition, endocrine disruptors and environmental compounds that favor adipogenesis, namely obesogens, are also related to the imbalance of tightly regulated metabolic processes and to a host of other adverse reproductive outcomes. Such effects may result from an exposure during gestation, prepubertal age or adulthood, emphasizing the importance of different environmental impacts throughout the life course. Environmental contaminants may also promote disturbances in the metabolic performance of the following generations, through epigenetic modifications passed by male gametes. As society increasingly introduces new potentially toxic substances into daily life, unveiling the molecular pathways by which environmental contaminants induce toxicity that may end-up in epigenetic modifications is imperative. Otherwise, a transgenerational susceptibility to metabolic diseases may be favored. Herein, we discuss the suggested molecular targets and potential mechanisms for environmental contaminants action and the subsequent effects of exposure during different life stages of the male. We also present an up-to-date overview about the impact of endocrine disruptors and obesogens on male reproductive health, as well as the epigenetic modifications induced by these environmental cues.

Keywords: Environmental contaminants, Endocrine disruptors, Epigenetic modifications, Glucose metabolism, Lipid metabolism, Male fertility, Molecular toxicology, Obesogens, Spermatogenesis, Sertoli cells, Sperm quality, Transgenerational effects.

INTRODUCTION

Nearly 50% of infertility cases, affecting millions of couples worldwide, are

* **Corresponding author Luís Rato:** Centro de Investigação em Ciências da Saúde (CICS-UBI), Av. Infante D. Henrique, 6201-506, Covilhã, Portugal; Tel: +351 275 329 002; Fax: +351 275 329 099; E-mail: luis.pedro.rato@gmail.com

Marco G. Alves and Pedro F. Oliveira (Eds.)

exclusively attributed to the male factor [1]. As in these cases treatment is not usually directed at a specific identified cause, it becomes difficult to establish an accurate diagnosis for the observed anomalies in male reproductive health. Moreover, men apparently normal may suffer abnormalities in the quality of spermatozoa [2]. Treatment is usually associated with assisted reproductive technologies, which are applied to increase the chances of conception. Indeed, a negative correlation has been suggested in this context: while life expectancy increases, the quality of spermatozoa substantially declines, thus becoming a matter of great concern specially in most developed societies [3]. Although the etiology of this adverse trend remains a subject of great debate, there has been a consensual awareness regarding the contribution of external factors, such as lifestyle habits and its associated factors, as is the case of permanent exposure to environmental contaminants. These contaminants can be found virtually everywhere, with exposures throughout lifespan, from gestation to adulthood, emerging as an important health issue. Male reproductive function is highly susceptible to the effects of environmental contaminants, such as pesticides, plasticizers, heavy metals, food additives and others [4]. Most of these environmental contaminants exhibit lipophilic characteristics and can mimic naturally occurring hormones acting as endocrine disruptors (EDCs). EDCs are defined as exogenous agents that interfere with the production, release, transport, metabolism, binding, action, or elimination of natural hormones in the body, which are responsible for the maintenance of homeostasis and the regulation of developmental processes [5]. Considering reproductive function, most of the effects are exerted through disturbance of estrogens-, anti-estrogens-, androgens- and anti-androgens-mediated processes [6, 7]. The majority of these substances act by interfering with the receptors of endogenous hormones and impairing the usual gene transcription response [8]. However, some EDCs are also capable of modifying hormone bioavailability by interfering with its secretion and transport or by disrupting the enzymatic pathways involved in hormone synthesis and metabolism [9, 10]. EDCs are a heterogeneous group of substances and several harmful effects were already associated to their exposure in healthy individuals. This is extremely important concerning male reproduction, which is highly dependent on endocrine regulation, specially reproductive events (such as steroidogenesis and spermatogenesis) that are dependent on Leydig and Sertoli cells, respectively [11]. However, the molecular mechanisms by which the environmental cues affect male reproductive health are not entirely dissected yet. Besides, the adverse effects of an exposure to these compounds was mainly studied at an occupational context and not applied to the general population [12], making people less concerned about their effects. Information regarding human data is scarce. Furthermore, humans are exposed to at least hundreds of environmental chemicals of which dozens are classified as EDCs. One limitation of epidemiological studies is that they only evaluate human exposure to a single environmental contaminant, or at best to a set of isomers or congeners within a family of EDCs. Understanding the potential human health risks requires the study of the complex mixtures to which we are permanently exposed. In this context, animal studies have suggested that environmental cues play a significant role in spermatozoa quality and thus, in male fertility [13 - 15].

Spermatogenesis is an exclusive function of mature testes, since it begins during puberty and continues spanning through the entire reproductive life [16]. This event is extremely complex and its function becomes easily vulnerable to the effects of environmental contaminants [17]. However, it is important to highlight that the effects of insults from these environmental contaminants occurring at early ages, even gestational, may be manifested only at adulthood [18]. In this chapter, the impact of environmental contaminants on male reproductive health and testis physiology will be discussed from a biochemical point of view. It will also explore the putative effects of environmental contaminants on sperm parameters and the subsequent consequences to overall male fertility potential.

MOLECULAR TARGETS OF ENVIRONMENTAL CONTAMINANTS

The impact of environmental compounds on male fertility has been under discussion for more than 50 years, when Ratcliffe [19] associated the dramatic decline in the population of certain bird species to a persistent pesticide exposure. Pesticides, heavy metals, chemicals in plastics, phytoestrogens and other environmental chemicals have been described since then to act like "uncontrolled medicines" for humans [20], being capable of affecting their health. Originally it was thought that environmental contaminants, in particular those acting as EDCs, exerted its effects through nuclear hormone receptors, including estrogen receptors, androgen receptors, progesterone receptors, thyroid receptors and others [21]. However, today it is known that those mechanisms are much broader than was initially postulated. The group of molecules classified as EDCs is very heterogeneous and includes industrially produced chemicals, such as polychlorinated biphenyls (PCBs), polybrominated biphenyls (PBBs), dioxins, bisphenol A (BPA), phthalates, pesticides (methoxychlor, chlorpyrifos, dichlorodiphenyltrchloroethane (DDT)), fungicides and pharmaceutical drugs. Likewise, natural chemicals found in human and animal diets (e.g. phytoestrogens, such as genistein) can also act as EDCs. Individuals are mainly exposed to these contaminants through ingestion, inhalation and/or dermal absorption. EDCs such as dioxins, PCBs, PBBs and pesticides often contain a phenolic moiety that is thought to mimic natural steroid hormones and enable EDCs to interact with steroid hormones receptors as agonists or antagonists. Furthermore, the majority of these compounds are lipophilic and this is particularly relevant from a physiologic point of view, since reproductive organs, due to their high lipid content, may serve as "hot spot" for the storage of environmental contaminants [22]. On the other hand, some of these contaminants easily cross the biological barriers (blood-brain and blood-testis barriers) disrupting male reproductive function at either central and/or gonadal levels through multiple mechanisms of action [23].

Hypothalamic-pituitary-testicular Axis

Male fertility is tightly controlled by neuroendocrine network. These processes are initiated in central nervous system, specifically at hypothalamus being firstly conveyed by neural and then by endocrine effectors (see Chapter **5**). Disruption of these neuroendocrine pathways by environmental chemicals can ensure several perturbations in the reproductive function, particularly when endocrine disruption occurs during critical development periods. There has been an increased research interest on the effects of EDCs on neuroendocrine signaling pathways. Several studies have focused on the hypothalamus-pituitary-testicular (HPT) axis, since this system is on the frontline of the targets for environmental contaminants. In fact, different environmental compounds may target HPT axis at different sites with different intensities, disrupting its regulation. Among the several environmental toxicants, bisphenol A (BPA) has arisen as an EDC that acts through a variety of physiological receptors. BPA molecules are linked by ester bonds that are subject to hydrolysis when exposed to high temperatures or to acidic or basic substances [24]. BPA was thought to exhibit a weak estrogenic activity, based on the relative binding affinity of BPA for the nuclear estrogen receptors (ERs) α and β, which were estimated to be over 1000-10000 fold lower when compared to 17β-Estradiol (E2) [25]. In fact, BPA binds to both ERα and ERβ [26, 27] and plasma membrane-bound ERs [28], as well as to the G-protein-coupled receptor 30, thus illustrating that beyond the genomic actions, BPA may also act by non-genomic pathways. Rodents exposed to BPA during the perinatal and postnatal periods exhibited an upregulation of kisspeptin (KiSS-1) expression levels, gonadotropin-releasing hormone (GnRH) and mRNA of FSH [29]. KiSS-1 acts as a guardian to the onset of puberty and for the regulation of gene expression in the HPT axis. The upregulation of KiSS-1 expression stimulated the synthesis and release of GnRH and gonadotropins in the hypothalamus and pituitary, respectively [29]. However, it was later showed that the hypothalamus is not involved in the disruption caused on the HPT axis by an adult exposure to BPA. In this study, the relative levels of GnRH receptor mRNA, the gene which encodes the receptor for type 1 GnRH was increased by five-fold in pituitary of BPA-exposed groups [30]. Since GnRH is responsible for the release of follicle-stimulating hormone (FSH) and luteinizing hormone (LH) from the anterior pituitary, as expected both relative levels of LHb mRNA and FSHb mRNA, the corresponding genes, were also increased. Although the increased GnRH receptor expression may correspond to augmented testosterone (T) levels, this increase in androgen and E2 receptors suggests the stimulation of negative feedback mechanisms [31]. The same compound was also related to an imbalance in the ratio T/E2 due to an enhanced aromatase activity that increases E2 levels [32]. As a result, the release of gonadotropins at the hypothalamic-pituitary axis is inhibited, compromising all downstream events of the HPT axis, namely spermatogenesis.

The environmental toxicant tributyltin (TBT) is also involved in the dysregulation of HPT axis. TBT belongs to the organotin family and presents three organic groups covalently bonded to a tin atom [33]. TBT leads to a dysfunctional HPT axis by inducing leptin resistance and increasing plasma insulin levels, accounting for reduced gonadotropin secretion at hypothalamic–pituitary level [34]. In parallel with this, also several phthalates [35] may promote insulin resistance, accounting for reduced gonadotropin secretion at hypothalamic–pituitary level. Insulin may directly act through its receptors located in the hypothalamus and pituitary [36], being pivotal for a normal function of HPT axis [37]. From the perspective of reproductive potential onset, puberty can be defined as activation of the HPT axis, leading to steroidogenesis, gametogenesis and the development of secondary sexual characteristics. Thus, many aspects resultant from the functioning of this complex system are also susceptible to the exposure of environmental contaminants and modulation of the HPT axis.

Leydig Cells

Leydig cells are the primordial site of steroidogenesis and well-known targets for environmental contaminants. Certain EDCs may inhibit enzymes involved in steroidogenesis, leading to the reduction of hormone synthesis (Fig. **13.1**). Since synthesis of steroids is highly dependent on cholesterol and lipids, it would be expectable that any dysregulation in the homeostasis of these components may compromise the synthesis of steroids hormones. Indeed, 2,4-dichlorophenoxyacetic acid (2,4-D), a worldwide used pesticide, downregulated the expression of 3-hydroxy-3-methylglutaryl coenzyme A synthase (HMG-CoA synthase) and reductase (HMG-CoA reductase) in Leydig cells of mice [38]. These enzymes are pivotal for cholesterol synthesis, where HMG-CoA synthase is responsible for the condensation of acetyl-CoA with acetoacetyl-CoA to form HMG-CoA, which is reduced to mevalonate for the synthesis of cholesterol.

Importantly, the synthesis of mevalonate is the commitment step in cholesterol formation and the enzyme catalyzing this irreversible step is HMG-CoA reductase, an important control point in cholesterol biosynthesis. Exposure to 2,4-

D disrupted the expression of these genes impairing the synthesis of cholesterol, the main precursor of sexual steroid hormones, which therefore disturb T synthesis. Once synthesized, cholesterol is then carried from outer mitochondrial membrane by steroid acute regulatory protein (StAR), where it is converted to pregnenolone *via* P450 side chain cleavage enzyme (P450scc). This intermediate metabolite is transported to the smooth endoplasmic reticulum where 3β-hydroxysteroid dehydrogenase (3β-HSD) will convert it into progesterone. Afterwards, P450c17 converts progesterone in 17-hydroxyprogesterone and in androstenedione, which is converted to T by 17β-hydroxysteroid dehydrogenase.

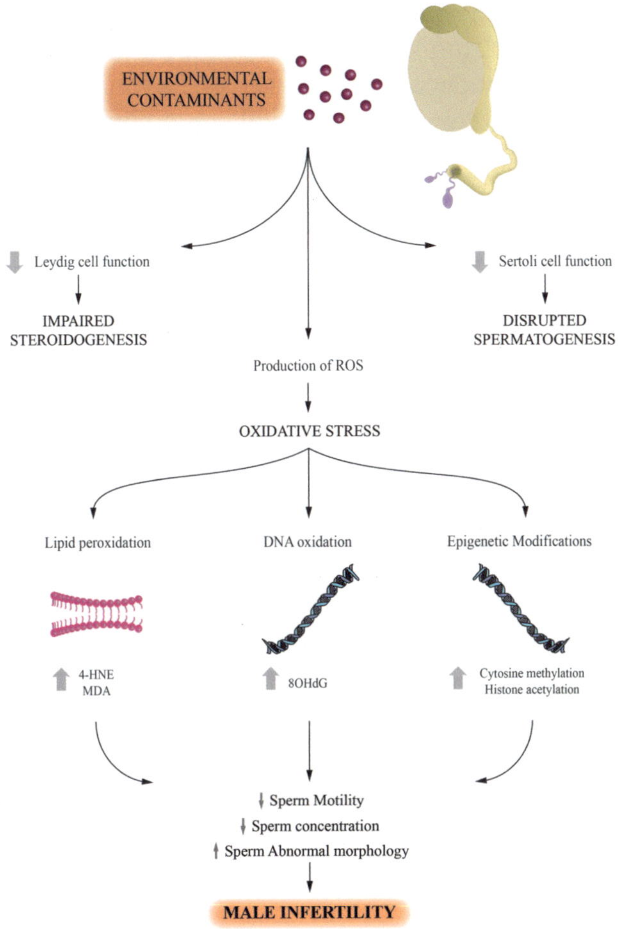

Fig. (13.1). Effects of environmental chemicals in male reproductive health. The increased storage of environmental chemicals impairs testicular function by disrupting both steroidogenesis and spermatogenesis, which depend of Leydig cells and Sertoli cells, respectively. Furthermore, environmental chemicals also impair male reproductive potential by declining sperm reproductive parameters, due to increased oxidative stress. Abbreviations: 4HNE: 4-hydroxynonenal; 8OHdG: 8-hydroxydeoxyguanosine; MDA: malondialdehyde; Up arrows (grey): increased; Down arrows (grey): decreased.

The exposure to di(n-butyl)phthalate decreased the expression of cholesterol transport genes such as the high-density lipoprotein receptor, also known as SRB1 and StAR [39]. Furthermore, the expression of genes involved in T biosynthesis, namely P450scc, 3β-HSD and P450c17 was downregulated, which probably contributed to the lower T levels [40]. In line with this, Bis(2-ethylhexyl) phthalate (DEHP) also exerts anti-androgenic action by directly inhibiting T synthesis in Leydig cells, probably inducing dysfunction in CYP17 [41].

Moreover, its metabolite mono-(2-ethylhexyl) phthalate (MEHP) inhibited all expression of steroidogenic enzymes, as well as all T precursors, in both the Δ4 and Δ5 steroidogenic pathways, leading to a deficient T synthesis [41]. Besides, a continuous exposure to 200 mg/kg/day of BPA during 6 weeks, not only reveal the same effects, but also reduced the number of Leydig cells, highlighting the possible cytotoxic effects of this environmental contaminant in testicular function [42]. Likewise, a recent study showed that oral administration of 2 μg/kg of BPA for 14 consecutive days to adult rats decreased the expression of steroidogenic enzymes, thus leading to a deficient T synthesis [43].

An in utero exposure to linuron, an urea-based herbicide, reveals to affect fetal testis gene expression and to reduce T production in adult male rat offspring [44]. Curiously, unlike phthalate esters that reduce T production, linuron did not affect the expression of steroidogenic genes [44]. Linuron seems to bind to the androgen receptor but, interestingly, the set of malformations displayed after an in utero exposure to this compound [45] differs from other androgen receptor antagonists [46]. Thus, it is suggested that decreased T production induced by linorun may be due to an alternative mechanism in the absence of cytotoxicity. Linuron is also causally related to changes in sex differentiation of the male reproductive tract [47], which allow to hypothesize that the inhibition of T synthesis along with androgen receptor antagonism may contribute to impact the androgen signaling pathway.

Alterations in sex differentiation were also found after an exposure to vinclozolin, a fungicide with anti-androgenic properties as well [48]. Indeed, female-like anogenital distance at birth, retained nipples, undescended testes, and small sex accessory glands were associated to an in utero vinclozolin exposure in male rat offspring [48]. The anti-androgen effects of vinclozolin were already related to increased levels of LH and T [49] and to inhibited DHT-induced transcriptional activation, through a blockage of the androgen receptor-bind to androgen response elements in DNA [50].

Sertoli Cells

Typically known as "nurse cells", Sertoli cells present an important role in male reproductive function, since the glycolytic pathway that occurs in these cells is crucial for the development of the germ cell line. Notably, this mechanism is under strict control of hormonal and/or endogenous factors (Table **13.1**) [51, 52]. Sertoli cells are well-known targets for numerous toxic substances, thus being highly susceptible to alterations that may arrest spermatogenesis and compromise male fertility [53]. It has been reported that adult rats exposed to BPA reveal a blockage in glucose movement in Sertoli cells glycolytic metabolism, by binding to the intracellular transporters in the pore region and an impairment of insulin signaling [54]. BPA also decreases testicular insulin signaling molecules, particularly insulin receptor substrate 1, insulin receptor substrate 2 and phosphatidylinositol 3 kinase (PI3K) [54]. Since PI3K is involved in the control of glucose uptake, namely in the translocation of glucose transporter 1 (GLUT1) to cell surface [55], this leads to major alterations on the glycolytic flux of Sertoli cells. In normal conditions, glucose enters in Sertoli cells and is readily converted to pyruvate through the glycolytic pathway, where phosphofructokinase 1 (PFK1) is the first rate-limiting step [56]. The majority of this cytosolic pyruvate will be converted to lactate by the action of lactate dehydrogenase (LDH), with a part being also converted to alanine. Previous reports showed that plasmatic concentrations detected in men exposed to 2,4-D are enough to decrease not only the intracellular levels of glucose but also the transcript levels of glucose transporter 3 (GLUT3), PFK1 and LDH [57]. Similarly, lactate, alanine and monocarboxylate transporter 4 (MCT4), the transporter through which lactate is exported to the luminal fluid to be used as a metabolic fuel by the developing germ cells, were decreased as well. In addition to compromise the intracellular levels of lactate, the exposure to these doses of 2,4-D also reduced the lactate/alanine ratio, which is an indicator of a reduced cytosolic state, and thus hamper the glycolytic metabolism of rat Sertoli cells [57, 58]. The decrease on PI3K also downregulates the stimulation of lactate production and LDH activity, illustrating the impact of PI3K/Protein kinase B signaling pathway in Sertoli cells metabolism [55]. Besides, these changes are also closely related with the apoptotic process [59], suggesting that these metabolic alterations may lead to abnormal apoptosis in Sertoli cells and thus induce problems on spermatogenesis and male fertility.

Table 13.1. Summary the main environmental compounds and their proposed effects in both glucose and lipid metabolism and their toxic effects in reproductive system.

Environmental Contaminant	Glycolytic Metabolism Effects	Lipid Metabolism Effects	Reproductive Toxic Effects
2,4-D	↓GLUT3, PFK1 and LDH mRNA, ↓Lactate production [57]	↑MDA, ↑LDL/HDL index, ↓PUFAs ratio, ↑Lipid peroxidation [71]	↑ Spermatogenic disorders, ↑Sterility [72], Delayed preputial separation [73]

(Table 13.1) contd.....

Environmental Contaminant	Glycolytic Metabolism Effects	Lipid Metabolism Effects	Reproductive Toxic Effects
BPA	↓IRS-1, ↓GLUT2 [54] ↓HEX, ↓PFK [74]	↑ACC and FAS mRNA, ↑LPL [75]	↓Sperm count and motility [76], Erectile dysfunction [77]
CPYF	↑LDH [78]	↑Lipid peroxidation, ↑MDA, ↑4-HNE [79]	↑Abnormal spermatozoa, ↓Sperm motility and count [13]
DES	↑LDH activity [80]	↑Lipid deposition [81]	Penis morphological abnormalities [81]
GES	↓Glucose uptake [82]	↑MCAD mRNA, ↓MDA, ↑GSH [13]	↓Sperm counts, ↑Sperm motility, LCs hyperplasia [80]
Lead	↑Lactate production [83]	↑Lipid peroxidation, ↑CAT activity, ↑GSH, ↓SOD activity [83]	↓Semen volume, ↓Sperm concentration and viability [67]
PCBs	↑Lactate production [84]	↓Fatty acids, ↑Fatty acid degradation related genes [85]	↓Sperm quality and integrity, ↓Reproductive hormones [86]
PIO	↑Glycolysis, ↓Insulin secretion [87]	↓Free fatty acids, ↑HDL, ↓Triglycerides [88]	↑Sperm motility and viability [89]
PTLs	↑Pyruvate production, ↑Lactate production [90]	↓ACC, ↑LCAD, ↑TP-beta [91]	Affected male maturity, ↓Sperm motility and concentration [92]
TBT	↓G6P, ↓F6P, ↓GLUT1 [93]	↑Lipid accumulation [94]	↑Apoptotic germ cells, ↓T production [95]

Legend: Abbreviations: 2,4-D, 2,4-dichlorophenoxyacetic; 4-HNE, 4-hydroxy-2-nonanal; ACC, Acetyl CoA carboxylase; BPA, Bisphenol A; CAT, chloramphenicol acetyltransferase; CPYF, chlorpyrifos; DES, diethylstilbestrol; F6P, fructose 6-phosphate; FAS, fatty acid synthase; G6P, glucose 6-phosphate; GES, genistein; GLUT1, glucose transporter 1; GLUT2, glucose transporter 2; GLUT3, glucose transporter 3; GSH, glutathione; HDL, high-density lipoprotein; HEX, hexokinase; IRS-1, insulin receptor substrate 1; LCAD, long-chain acyl-CoA dehydrogenase; LCs, Leydig cells; LDH, lactate dehydrogenase; LPL, lipoprotein lipase; MCAD, medium-chain acyl-CoA dehydrogenase; MDA, malondialdehyde; PCBs, polychlorinated biphenyls; PFK, phosphofructokinase; PFK1, phosphofructokinase 1; PIO, pioglitazone; PTLs, phthalates; PUFAS, polyunsaturated fatty acids; SOD, superoxide dismutase; T, testosterone; TBT, tributyltin; TP-beta, 3-ketoacyl-CoA thiolase.

Germ Cells

Compelling evidence shows that the toxicity of the environmental contaminants induces several dysfunctions associated with the testicular dysgenesis syndrome, including seminiferous tubules atrophy and germ cell degeneration [60]. Furthermore, lipids are essential components of the membranes of germ cells. A deficient lipid incorporation into these cells leads to a deficient germ cell structure and contributes to the impairment of sperm parameters and consequently to alterations of sperm functionality.

The oral administration of TBT has also been associated with induced apoptosis in testicular germ cells in prepubertal mice [22]. In other study, activation of caspase-3 and phosphorylation of c-Jun N-terminal kinase and mitogen-activated protein kinase p-38 in germ cells was also associated to an exposure of TBT [61]. These works did not explore the molecular mechanisms by which germ cell apoptosis was induced, but it seems that environmental contaminants activate both intrinsic and extrinsic pathways of apoptosis. Interestingly, germ cells are also targeted by diethylstilbestrol (DES), since apoptosis of spermatogenic cells was also reported in prenatal and/or neonatal mice exposed to this compound from gestational day 12 to postnatal day 20 [62].

In healthy individuals, germ cells present high levels of polyunsaturated fatty acids (PUFAs), which are crucial to their membrane fluidity and flexibility and thus for fertilization. Since these cells are, however, unable to synthesize PUFAs, they take these fatty acids from Sertoli cells and incorporate them into phospholipids, *via* lysophosphatidic acid acyltransferase 3 [63]. Several data had already suggested that the current dietary habits, particularly the excessive consumption of high-energy diets (HEDs) with high content in saturated fats and trans fatty acids, decreases Δ5 and Δ6 desaturases activity [64]. In fact, it was proposed that the limitation of PUFAs incorporation in membranes of germ cells adversely affects testicular lipid metabolism and thus contributes to impaired production of spermatozoa [65].

Spermatozoa as a Target for Environmental Chemicals

The development of germ cells into spermatozoa is also a pathway of great relevance for a proper fertility, which is easily targeted by environmental contaminants as well. As aforementioned, diet is one of the main routes by which humans are exposed to environmental contaminants because they are present in foods, even in a very small percentage. A recent study showed that men who consumed fruits and vegetables rich in pesticide residues presented 49% lower sperm count and 32% lower normal sperm than men who had not been exposed to the same substances [66]. Recent studies also showed that men chronically exposed to lead exhibited decreased semen volume, concentration, morphology and viability of spermatozoa [67]. Similarly, men who consumed fruits and vegetables rich in pesticide residues presented 49% lower sperm count and 32% lower normal sperm than men who had not been exposed to the same substances [66]. In molecular terms, recent data suggests that the anti-androgenic effects of DEHP may cause reactive oxygen species (ROS) production, lipid peroxidation and apoptosis of spermatocytes [68]. The production of these ROS is related with Ca^{2+} mediated activation of the nicotinamide adenine dinucleotide phosphate (NADPH) complex, which may correlate with DEHP-induced Ca^{2+} entry.

Similarly, BPA can induce oxidative stress in fish spermatozoa *in vitro*, which results in decreased spermatozoa motility and velocity [69]. BPA also induce DNA damage in human spermatozoa, with a direct relationship between urinary concentrations of the compound and increased single-strand breaks DNA damage of spermatozoa (Fig. **13.1**) [70]. There is a need for further evaluation concerning the properties of these contaminants and their reproductive toxicity to establish safety thresholds and protocols. This might be important to confirm which of environmental contaminants are contributing to current the decline of male fertility.

ENDOCRINE DISRUPTORS AND OBESOGENS

Excess of release of environmental contaminants due to agricultural and industrial activities has been concurrent with infertility rates [96]. Moreover, there is a cumulative noxious effect on human health resultant from the inevitable contact with these compounds. In addition, their effect as EDCs is intimately associated with several neurodegenerative disease [97] and obesity [98]. Since obesity epidemic occurred very quickly, it was suggested that it cannot be explained only by lifestyle habits, but also by environmental cues, more than genetic factors, that are possibly exacerbating or even being the main cause for the development of the disease. This rises the hypothesis that some EDCs are able to enhance adipogenesis, increasing the complexity of obesity's etiology and leading to the concept of obesogens [99].

Obesogens are chemical compounds present either in the environment as in foods, which are able to predispose to weight gain by increasing the number of fat cells and/or the storage of fat-soluble toxicants into existing fat cells [100], changing the amount of stored calories or affecting the biochemical mechanisms by which the body regulates satiety and appetite [101]. Previous evidence proposed a dose-response relationship between body mass index and infertility, since even subtle increases in male weight were suggested to affect fertility [102]. The normal reproductive function requires an appropriate nutritional state, thus it is expectable that metabolic disturbances promoted by obesogens will affect the reproductive potential. Obesogens can be found virtually everywhere, including in HEDs or in the surrounding environment. Regarding agricultural and industrial chemicals, TBT, for example, arises as the "obesogenic" model, being considered one of the most toxic substances ever deliberately introduced into the environment [33] and the most abundantly investigated obesogenic compound evidencing effects on lipid metabolism.

Lipid metabolism was the first to be evidenced as primarily affected by obesogens and thus associated with the promotion of adipogenesis and obesity [103].

Environmental contaminants can interact with the peroxisome proliferator-activated receptors (PPARs), particularly the peroxisome proliferator-activated receptor γ (PPARγ) that governs lipid metabolism, adipocyte function and differentiation [104]. Thus, PPARs, and mainly PPARγ, are master regulators of adipogenesis [103]. In order to respond to peroxisome proliferators, PPARs need to co-operate with another member of the steroid hormone receptor family, the retinoid X receptor (RXR) [105]. Indeed, TBT was suggested to be a RXR-PPARγ agonist, since it promotes adipogenic gene expression, adipocyte differentiation and lipid accumulation in preadipocytes [106]. The activation of RXR-PPARγ signaling by TBT represents an example of an obesogen capable of impact both lipid and glycolytic metabolism, with long-term metabolic effects [103]. Indeed, it was shown that, in addition to promote lipid accumulation, TBT also increased adipocyte glucose uptake in preadipocytes, promoting glycolysis [94].

There are, however, several options through which environmental contaminants may promote obesity through PPARγ. A ligand is usually needed in order to allow this receptor to bind co-activators, release co-repressors, decondensate the chromatin and activate transcription [101]. Nevertheless, post-translational modifications, such as phosphorylations, may activate PPARγ in the absence of a ligand as well [107]. Additionally, obesogens may also induce the production of multipotent stromal cells, which predominantly differentiate into adipose tissue that express PPARγ [101].

Other environmental contaminants had already revealed an obesogenic action, namely BPA, a chemical present in plastics that predisposes murine preadipocytes differentiation, not acting only on nuclear estrogen receptors [108], but also *via* cell membrane associated estrogen receptors in a nongenomic manner [109]. This action directly modulates insulin dependent PI3K/AKT kinase pathway and enhances glucose uptake [110]. Similarly, metabolites of the potent PPARα agonist DEHP, such as MEHP, also activate PPARγ, promoting the differentiation of preadipocytes and subsequent lipid accumulation and thus providing a suggested obesogenic response [111, 112].

The pharmacological route can also be pointed out regarding the exposure to obesogens, for example, through the use of antidiabetic drugs. Thiazolidinediones (TZDs) belong to the class of oral antidiabetic drugs that improve insulin sensitivity. These drugs exert their antidiabetic effects through a mechanism involving the activation of PPARγ and had been already associated with a persistent weight gain [89, 113]. Pioglitazone, the main thiazolidinedione, is a potent PPARγ agonist, modulating its activity [104]. The activation of this heterodimer promotes insulin-stimulated uptake of glucose in peripheral tissues as well as insulin sensitivity in adipose tissue [114]. Still, it seems that pioglitazone exerts positive effects in male reproductive health. Recent data evidenced that pioglitazone improved sperm motility and morphology in diabetic rats [115, 116].

Other environmental contaminants, such as the heavy metals lead and cadmium and some phytoestrogens, also exhibit obesogenic effects, however one should note that the effects vary with the time of the exposure and that compounds present also a non-monotonic dose-response, with results for higher doses often being opposite from what was observed for lower doses. Genistein for example, and in contrast to its effects in adults [117], may produce obesogenic effects in animals exposed at critical periods of development. Interestingly, mice exposed to lower doses of phytoestrogen during gestation and lactation present a lower birth weight, but develop obesity, high leptin and E2 levels, and impaired glucose responses [118]. A couple of studies also proposed that obesogens affect testicular metabolism, which is highly dependent on glucose [54, 57, 90]. However, it becomes necessary to deepen the knowledge on how these compounds may affect testicular metabolism, since disruption of the cooperation between testicular cells can lead to an arrest of spermatogenesis, and therefore compromise male fertility. Furthermore, some data suggested that harmful lipophilic compounds that accumulate in the fat of expecting mothers can be delivered to the fetus [119]. Similarly, it seems that some of these compounds are appearing in human breast milk, thus probably transferring their effects to children who are breastfed [120]. These evidence must serve as an alarming signal that even early in utero developmental events might be affected by environmental contaminants, which can influence testicular development and the quality of spermatozoa in the adult offspring and thus determine the reproductive health of individuals for the rest of their lives.

EPIGENETIC CHANGES IN GERM CELLS

The permanent exposure to environmental chemicals may induce modifications in the genome without altering the DNA sequence (known as epigenetic modifications). In molecular terms, epigenetics refers to a range of mechanisms, such as DNA methylation, histone and long non-coding RNAs modifications, remodeling of nucleosomes and higher order chromatin reorganization, that define cellular identity by regulating gene expression [121]. This is of great physiological relevance, since germ cells act as "vehicles" in the transmission of genetic information to the next generation. Besides constituting a unique profile in each cell, epigenetics also ensures that daughter cells have the same phenotype as the parental cell, controlling gene function from one generation to the next [121]. Indeed, the role of epigenetics varies between somatic and germ cells, as these last undergo meiosis, which is of particular importance to maintain genomic integrity

[122]. The epigenetic programming of germline arises during early embryonic development, particularly at the migration of primordial germ cells in the embryo [123]. After determination of gonadal sex being initiated, the primordial germ cells remethylate DNA and develop the germ cell lineage in a gender-specific manner [123]. During the period of gonadal sex determination, which occurs between 12th and 15th days of embryonic development [124], the fetal testes starts expressing steroid receptors, which become potential targets for external compounds with endocrine activity [125]. Thus, EDCs acting inappropriately at the time of gonadal sex determination potentially could reprogram germ line through DNA methylation, an epigenetic mechanism, to cause the transgenerational transmission of an altered phenotype or genetic characteristic [126]. Because of the possible time span between the occurrence of the exposure to the contaminants and the detectable impacts in offspring (mainly at their adulthood), animal models have been very helpful to study those mechanisms. Data from animal studies supported that such exposure may affect the male reproductive function of offspring, determining the success of fertility.

Two different studies showed that exposure to vinclozolin or methoxyclor during the remethylation programming of the germ line in rats, induced aberrant sexual differentiation, gonad formation, and reproductive functions of the following generation [127, 128]. Interestingly, increased spermatogenic cell apoptosis and reduced number and motility of spermatozoa in the same conditions had already been noticed until the fourth filial (F4) generation [124]. This transmission of the exposure–induced phenotype in a transgenerational manner suggests an epigenetic alteration in DNA methylation pattern of the male germ line, namely an epigenetic mechanism involving reprogramming of the germ line. Similarly, exposure of rats to the anti-androgenic fungicide vinclozolin at the time of gonadal sex development originated male offspring with testicular abnormalities and reduced spermatogenic capacity, which persisted in male offspring until the F4 generation [129]. It has been suggested that these transgenerational effects were caused by epigenetic changes, involving the abnormal regulation of DNA (cytosine-5)-methyltransferase 3 alpha (DNMT3A) and DNA (cytosine-5- -methyltransferase 3-like (DNMT3L), methyltransferases required for methylation of most imprinted loci in germ cells [130]. Thus, male fertility problems were suggested to be caused by a change in genome-wide methylation and, consequently, in gene expression. In accordance, it was shown that individuals with oligospermia reveal an increased frequency of defective methylation compared with normospermic males, suggesting that spermatozoa from men with fertility problems may carry a higher risk of transmitting incorrect primary imprints to their offspring [131]. Deleterious effects on male fertility not limited to the generation directly exposed to environmental contaminants were also confirmed by maternal rat exposure to BPA, which modified methylation of the metastable loci Avy and CapbIAP [132]. Interestingly, this effect on DNA methylation was avoided by maternal dietary supplementation with a source of methyl groups such as the phytoestrogen genistein, also a proven endocrine disruptor [132]. As regarding phthalates, namely DEHP, it was reported that when given to outbred mice between 7-14 days of embryonic development, reduced both counts and motility of spermatozoa in male offspring beyond F3 generation [133]. Accordingly, it was suggested that DNA methylation was the potential epigenetic mechanism underlying these alterations, since 16 differentially methylated and expressed genes were identified in newborn pups. Thus, this group of genes is suggested to hold clues on how DEHP transgenerationally acts. On the other hand, some studies in humans were already performed in the field of the environmental influence in epigenetics as well. DES, which has been associated decades ago to the presence of hypospadias in human males exposed in utero [134] or whose mothers had been exposed in utero [135], was also reported among unexposed grandsons of women who had been exposed in utero [136]. The exposure occurred during the development of reproductive system in primordial germ cells of the fetuses, being subsequently transmitted across generations to affected sons and grandsons [136]. The suggested mechanism to sustain these results is not well understood at molecular level, but relies on an epigenetic alteration in the androgen receptor gene.

Besides DNA methylation, the role of histone modifications is also of major importance in epigenetics, since the establishment of embryo constitutive heterochromatin may be defined by the placement of histone modifications in sperm [137]. Indeed, histone modifications have been shown to be pivotal in changing chromatin structure and, therefore, DNA accessibility [138], being able to regulate gene expression, chromatin remodeling, cell survival and cell death [138]. Histone modifications include methylation, acetylation, phosphorylation, ubiquitination, ribosylation, and sumoylation, which can be easily induced and removed by a wide range of enzymes [138]. The functional effects of these modifications depend both on the modified amino acid and on the specific covalently attached group [139]. Acetylation patterns may direct histone assembly and help regulate the unfolding and activate gene expression, while a methylation tights DNA and restricts its access to the transcription machinery [139]. It has been suggested that two xenobiotics, valproic acid, a commonly prescribed anticonvulsant and mood stabilizer [140], and methoxyacetic acid, a solvent usually used in paints, dyes and fuel additives, can exert wide effects on DNA by inhibiting histone deacetylases [141]. Additionally, paternal dietary folate seems also to improve offspring's susceptibility to birth defects through changes in histone methylation [142]. Interestingly, it has been observed that fathers fed with a high-fat diet evidenced changes in sperm histone composition, although DNA methylation of several imprinted loci appears to remain static [143]. These findings suggest that individuals who are exposed to these contaminants are more likely to experience histone modifications, which represent a relevant pathway into the 'hidden' programming of endocrine disruption to offspring.

Long non-coding RNAs (lncRNAs) modifications are another epigenetic-related mechanisms that can be pointed out as an effect of the exposure to environmental contaminants. The role of lncRNAs in epigenetic processes has been more recently highlighted and several data have suggested that lncRNAs are involved in the cellular stress response [144]. LncRNAs are defined as transcribed RNA molecules greater than 200 nucleotides in length with little or no protein-coding competence. It is known that lncRNAs regulate gene expression although the mechanisms need to be fully clarified [145, 146]. A few works have showed that lncRNAs control gene regulation at every level including transcriptional gene silencing *via* DNA methylation and regulation of the chromatin structure [146, 147]. So in this context, it is likely that lncRNAs drive important exposure-disease associations and may also function as biomarkers of environmental exposure. Studies have reported an increased transcription of telomeric repeat-containing RNA and satellite sequences (Sat III) in humans, following physiological stress induced by heat or ethanol [148, 149]. Furthermore it has been showed that long non-coding transcripts resultant from highly repetitive sequences are overexpressed after exposure to BPA and cadmium [150]. A drastic and sudden activation of telomeric non-coding RNA and an increased transcription of Cla sequences that are mainly located in the centromeric regions were evidenced after an exposure to both compounds [150]. Although Cla sequences are dispersed in the genome and other chromosomal regions, the centromeres appeared highly labelled for DNA/RNA hybrids after exposures to BPA and cadmium, which suggest a preferential effect of these chemicals in the centromere. Interestingly, this appears to be a toxicant-specific response and not a generic one, since the exposure to benzyl butyl phthalate did not affect the transcription of these sequences [150].

Overall, these results strongly suggest a link between specific stressors and altered long non-coding RNA expression. The upregulation of telomeric RNA and RNA from centromeric Cla sequences may reflect a cellular adaptation to the effects induced by BPA and cadmium. This may indicate that lncRNAs have a regulatory transcriptional role, as suggested for other similar RNAs such as telomeric repeat-containing RNA and Sat III [148, 149]. Likewise, satellite DNA transcription appears also to be regulated by environmental cues such as temperature [151]. In addition to these observations, lncRNAs and piwi-interacting RNAs (piRNAs) seem to be involved in mechanisms of histone modification. lncRNAs recruit modifying enzymes to specific genomic loci that are able to change the chromatin state. Indeed, it has been observed that lncRNAs and piRNAs in the landscape of epigenetic modifications of chromatin state and histone codes is the production of piRNAs by the lncRNAs that induce up-regulation of the tumor necrosis factor-related apoptosis-inducing ligand protein *via* H3K4/H3K27 methylation/ demethylation [152].

Since the knowledge of the biological functions of lncRNAs is increasing, it is important to analyse their response to a wider spectrum of contaminants. This is pivotal not only to identify the potential inducers that may help to explain the underlying mechanism of action of many toxicants, but also the functional role of lncRNAs in the toxic response of eukaryotic cells.

Although some mechanisms of toxicity and responses to certain environmental chemicals remains to be completely elucidated, there is consistent data which allow to link epigenetic changes both in experimental and epidemiological studies to an environmental contamination and subsequent effects in spermatozoa quality. Because these epigenetic changes are small, potentially cumulative, and they may develop over time, it may be difficult to establish concrete cause-effect relationships among environmental contaminants, epigenetic changes and diseases etiology. However, knowing the relevance of the transgenerational epigenetic inheritance to many human diseases will certainly become an exciting area, for which research on germ cells is particularly important.

CONCLUDING REMARKS

There is an intense debate concerning the contribution of environmental cues to spermatozoa quality. Several studies concerning this topic reveal a negative impact of external compounds in the reproductive function of individuals exposed from a very early age (even in prenatal period), not only through indirect effects mediated by changes in hormonal levels and HPT axis, but also by direct changes in testicular cells. Such effects may compromise the spermatogenic event and end-up in impairment of the molecular composition of spermatozoa, quality and function. Definitive conclusions on how each compound affects the molecular and cellular mechanisms involved in the production and function of spermatozoa are, however, very hard to establish. First, when exposure occurs it is often through a combined mixture of environmental chemicals and not due to a single compound. Besides, sometimes there is also a long latency period between the exposure and the noticed effects, which further hampers the association to a specific agent.

Recent studies started to examine the relationship between the exposure to environmental contaminants and epigenetics, and identified several toxicants that modify epigenetic marks, particularly regarding DNA methylation. This field reveals a huge potential for a precocious disease diagnosis, since future research may allow to predict which contaminants would put exposed individuals at risk, which individuals will be more susceptible to develop disease and whether such epigenetic alterations increase the risk of disease.

Since we are permanently exposed to environmental contaminants that may induce a myriad of effects that persist through the generations, this topic will certainly become a hot research topic for those who are interested in environmental toxicology and male fertility. The effect of environmental cues in the quality of spermatozoa raises new questions concerning to where human evolution is heading. We are all combinations of what we inherit and what we are exposed to during our fetal and adult lives.

Box 13.1 | Summary

- HPT axis, Leydig cells, Sertoli cells and spermatogenesis constitute important molecular targets of environmental contaminants.
- Environmental chemicals affect male reproductive function by acting as EDCs interfering with the regulation of endogenous hormones.
- Some EDCs are also able to enhance adipogenesis, being defined as "obesogens".
- Environmental contaminants induce epigenetic changes in germ cells mainly DNA methylation, and cause the transmission of an altered phenotype or genetic characteristics.

CONFLICT OF INTEREST

The authors confirm that they have no conflict of interest to declare for this publication.

ACKNOWLEDGEMENTS

This work was supported by the "Fundação para a Ciência e a Tecnologia"–FCT (PTDC/BBB-BQB/1368/2014), CICS (UID/Multi/00709/2013), and of FEDER through the POPH and POCI - COMPETE 2020 (POCI-01-0145-FE-ER-007491) and National Funds by FCT - Foundation for Science and Technology (Project UID/Multi /00709). Luís Rato is funded by Santader-Totta/University of Beira Interior (BIPD/ICI-CICS-BST-UBI).

REFERENCES

[1] Lutz W. Fertility rates and future population trends: will Europes birth rate recover or continue to decline? Int J Androl 2006; 29(1): 25-33.
[http://dx.doi.org/10.1111/j.1365-2605.2005.00639.x] [PMID: 16466521]

[2] Pacey AA. Male fertility and infertility. Obstetrics, Gynaecol Reprod Med 2009; 19: 42-7.
[http://dx.doi.org/10.1016/j.ogrm.2008.11.006]

[3] Merzenich H, Zeeb H, Blettner M. Decreasing sperm quality: a global problem? BMC Public Health 2010; 10: 24.
[http://dx.doi.org/10.1186/1471-2458-10-24] [PMID: 20085639]

[4] Wong EW, Cheng CY. Impacts of environmental toxicants on male reproductive dysfunction. Trends Pharmacol Sci 2011; 32(5): 290-9.
[http://dx.doi.org/10.1016/j.tips.2011.01.001] [PMID: 21324536]

[5] Kavlock RJ, Daston GP, DeRosa C, *et al.* Research needs for the risk assessment of health and environmental effects of endocrine disruptors: a report of the U.S. EPA-sponsored workshop. Environ Health Perspect 1996; 104 (Suppl. 4): 715-40.
[http://dx.doi.org/10.1289/ehp.96104s4715] [PMID: 8880000]

[6] Kelce WR, Wilson EM. Environmental antiandrogens: developmental effects, molecular mechanisms, and clinical implications. J Mol Med 1997; 75(3): 198-207.
[http://dx.doi.org/10.1007/s001090050104] [PMID: 9106076]

[7] Sohoni P, Sumpter JP. Several environmental oestrogens are also anti-androgens. J Endocrinol 1998; 158(3): 327-39.
[http://dx.doi.org/10.1677/joe.0.1580327] [PMID: 9846162]

[8] De Coster S, van Larebeke N. Endocrine-disrupting chemicals: associated disorders and mechanisms of action. J Environ Public Health 2012; 2012: 1-52.
[http://dx.doi.org/10.1155/2012/713696] [PMID: 22991565]

[9] Phillips KP, Foster WG. Key developments in endocrine disrupter research and human health. J Toxicol Environ Health B Crit Rev 2008; 11(3-4): 322-44.
[http://dx.doi.org/10.1080/10937400701876194] [PMID: 18368559]

[10] Whitehead SA, Rice S. Endocrine-disrupting chemicals as modulators of sex steroid synthesis. Best Pract Res Clin Endocrinol Metab 2006; 20(1): 45-61.
[http://dx.doi.org/10.1016/j.beem.2005.09.003] [PMID: 16522519]

[11] Mathur PP, DCruz SC. The effect of environmental contaminants on testicular function. Asian J Androl 2011; 13(4): 585-91.
[http://dx.doi.org/10.1038/aja.2011.40] [PMID: 21706039]

[12] Kirkhus NE, Thomassen Y, Ulvestad B, Woldbæk T, Ellingsen DG. Occupational exposure to airborne contaminants during offshore oil drilling. Environ Sci Process Impacts 2015; 17(7): 1257-64.
[http://dx.doi.org/10.1039/C5EM00081E] [PMID: 26020723]

[13] Farag AT, Radwan AH, Sorour F, El Okazy A, El-Agamy S, El-Sebae Ael-K. Chlorpyrifos induced reproductive toxicity in male mice. Reprod Toxicol 2010; 29(1): 80-5.
[http://dx.doi.org/10.1016/j.reprotox.2009.10.003] [PMID: 19850121]

[14] Han XD, Tu ZG, Gong Y, *et al.* The toxic effects of nonylphenol on the reproductive system of male rats. Reprod Toxicol 2004; 19(2): 215-21.
[http://dx.doi.org/10.1016/j.reprotox.2004.06.014] [PMID: 15501387]

[15] Lee B-J, Jung E-Y, Yun Y-W, *et al.* Effects of exposure to genistein during pubertal development on the reproductive system of male mice. J Reprod Dev 2004; 50(4): 399-409.
[http://dx.doi.org/10.1262/jrd.50.399] [PMID: 15329471]

[16] Cheng C, Mruk D. Spermatogenesis, Mammals. In: Maloy S, Hughes K, Eds. Brenner's Encyclopedia of Genetics. San Diego: Elsevier/Academic Press 2013; pp. 525-8. [http://dx.doi.org/10.1016/B978-0-12-374984-0.01459-5]

[17] Sharpe RM. Environmental/lifestyle effects on spermatogenesis. Philos Trans R Soc Lond B Biol Sci 2010; 365(1546): 1697-712. [http://dx.doi.org/10.1098/rstb.2009.0206] [PMID: 20403879]

[18] Perera F, Herbstman J. Prenatal environmental exposures, epigenetics, and disease. Reprod Toxicol 2011; 31(3): 363-73. [http://dx.doi.org/10.1016/j.reprotox.2010.12.055] [PMID: 21256208]

[19] Ratcliffe DA. Decrease in eggshell weight in certain birds of prey. Nature 1967; 215(5097): 208-10. [http://dx.doi.org/10.1038/215208a0] [PMID: 6049131]

[20] Birnbaum LS. When environmental chemicals act like uncontrolled medicine. Trends Endocrinol Metab 2013; 24(7): 321-3. [http://dx.doi.org/10.1016/j.tem.2012.12.005] [PMID: 23660158]

[21] Diamanti-Kandarakis E, Bourguignon J-P, Giudice LC, *et al.* Endocrine-disrupting chemicals: an Endocrine Society scientific statement. Endocr Rev 2009; 30(4): 293-342. [http://dx.doi.org/10.1210/er.2009-0002] [PMID: 19502515]

[22] Reame V, Pytlowanciv EZ, Ribeiro DL, *et al.* Obesogenic environment by excess of dietary fats in different phases of development reduces spermatic efficiency of wistar rats at adulthood: correlations with metabolic status. Biol Reprod 2014; 91(6): 151-61. [http://dx.doi.org/10.1095/biolreprod.114.121962] [PMID: 25339108]

[23] Colborn T, vom Saal FS, Soto AM. Developmental effects of endocrine-disrupting chemicals in wildlife and humans. Environ Health Perspect 1993; 101(5): 378-84. [http://dx.doi.org/10.1289/ehp.93101378] [PMID: 8080506]

[24] Welshons WV, Nagel SC, vom Saal FS. Large effects from small exposures. III. Endocrine mechanisms mediating effects of bisphenol A at levels of human exposure. Endocrinology 2006; 147(6) (Suppl.): S56-69. [http://dx.doi.org/10.1210/en.2005-1159] [PMID: 16690810]

[25] Rubin BS. Bisphenol A: an endocrine disruptor with widespread exposure and multiple effects. J Steroid Biochem Mol Biol 2011; 127(1-2): 27-34. [http://dx.doi.org/10.1016/j.jsbmb.2011.05.002] [PMID: 21605673]

[26] Kuiper GG, Lemmen JG, Carlsson B, *et al.* Interaction of estrogenic chemicals and phytoestrogens with estrogen receptor beta. Endocrinology 1998; 139: 4252-63. [http://dx.doi.org/10.1210/endo.139.10.6216] [PMID: 9751507]

[27] Gould JC, Leonard LS, Maness SC, *et al.* Bisphenol A interacts with the estrogen receptor alpha in a distinct manner from estradiol. Mol Cell Endocrinol 1998; 142(1-2): 203-14. [http://dx.doi.org/10.1016/S0303-7207(98)00084-7] [PMID: 9783916]

[28] Wozniak AL, Bulayeva NN, Watson CS. Xenoestrogens at picomolar to nanomolar concentrations trigger membrane estrogen receptor-α-mediated Ca^{2+} fluxes and prolactin release in GH3/B6 pituitary tumor cells. Environ Health Perspect 2005; 113(4): 431-9. [http://dx.doi.org/10.1289/ehp.7505] [PMID: 15811834]

[29] Xi W, Lee CK, Yeung WS, *et al.* Effect of perinatal and postnatal bisphenol A exposure to the regulatory circuits at the hypothalamus-pituitary-gonadal axis of CD-1 mice. Reprod Toxicol 2011; 31(4): 409-17. [http://dx.doi.org/10.1016/j.reprotox.2010.12.002] [PMID: 21182934]

[30] Wisniewski P, Romano RM, Kizys MM, *et al.* Adult exposure to bisphenol A (BPA) in Wistar rats reduces sperm quality with disruption of the hypothalamic-pituitary-testicular axis. Toxicology 2015; 329: 1-9.
[http://dx.doi.org/10.1016/j.tox.2015.01.002] [PMID: 25575453]

[31] Jeong K, Kaiser U. Gonadotropin-releasing hormone regulation of gonadotropin biosynthesis and secretion. In: Neill JD, Ed. Knobil and Neill's Physiology of reproduction. San Diego: Elsevier 2006.
[http://dx.doi.org/10.1016/B978-012515400-0/50036-1]

[32] Arase S, Ishii K, Igarashi K, *et al.* Endocrine disrupter bisphenol A increases *in situ* estrogen production in the mouse urogenital sinus. Biol Reprod 2011; 84(4): 734-42.
[http://dx.doi.org/10.1095/biolreprod.110.087502] [PMID: 21123812]

[33] Goldberg ED. TBT: an environmental dilemma. Environ Sci Policy Sustainable Develop 1986; 28: 17-44.
[http://dx.doi.org/10.1080/00139157.1986.9928814]

[34] Zuo Z, Chen S, Wu T, *et al.* Tributyltin causes obesity and hepatic steatosis in male mice. Environ Toxicol 2011; 26(1): 79-85.
[http://dx.doi.org/10.1002/tox.20531] [PMID: 19760618]

[35] Stahlhut RW, van Wijngaarden E, Dye TD, Cook S, Swan SH. Concentrations of urinary phthalate metabolites are associated with increased waist circumference and insulin resistance in adult U.S. males. Environ Health Perspect 2007; 115(6): 876-82.
[http://dx.doi.org/10.1289/ehp.9882] [PMID: 17589594]

[36] Havrankova J, Schmechel D, Roth J, Brownstein M. Identification of insulin in rat brain. Proc Natl Acad Sci USA 1978; 75(11): 5737-41.
[http://dx.doi.org/10.1073/pnas.75.11.5737] [PMID: 364489]

[37] Schoeller EL, Albanna G, Frolova AI, Moley KH. Insulin rescues impaired spermatogenesis *via* the hypothalamic-pituitary-gonadal axis in Akita diabetic mice and restores male fertility. Diabetes 2012; 61(7): 1869-78.
[http://dx.doi.org/10.2337/db11-1527] [PMID: 22522616]

[38] Harada Y, Tanaka N, Ichikawa M, *et al.* PPARα-dependent cholesterol/testosterone disruption in Leydig cells mediates 2,4-dichlorophenoxyacetic acid-induced testicular toxicity in mice. Arch Toxicol 2016; 90(12): 3061-71.
[http://dx.doi.org/10.1007/s00204-016-1669-z] [PMID: 26838045]

[39] Barlow NJ, Phillips SL, Wallace DG, Sar M, Gaido KW, Foster PM. Quantitative changes in gene expression in fetal rat testes following exposure to di(n-butyl) phthalate. Toxicol Sci 2003; 73(2): 431-41.
[http://dx.doi.org/10.1093/toxsci/kfg087] [PMID: 12700402]

[40] Hu J, Zhang Z, Shen W-J, Azhar S. Cellular cholesterol delivery, intracellular processing and utilization for biosynthesis of steroid hormones. Nutr Metab (Lond) 2010; 7: 47.
[http://dx.doi.org/10.1186/1743-7075-7-47] [PMID: 20515451]

[41] Desdoits-Lethimonier C, Albert O, Le Bizec B, *et al.* Human testis steroidogenesis is inhibited by phthalates. Hum Reprod 2012; 27(5): 1451-9.
[http://dx.doi.org/10.1093/humrep/des069] [PMID: 22402212]

[42] Nakamura D, Yanagiba Y, Duan Z, *et al.* Bisphenol A may cause testosterone reduction by adversely affecting both testis and pituitary systems similar to estradiol. Toxicol Lett 2010; 194(1-2): 16-25.
[http://dx.doi.org/10.1016/j.toxlet.2010.02.002] [PMID: 20144698]

[43] Jin P, Wang X, Chang F, *et al.* Low dose bisphenol A impairs spermatogenesis by suppressing reproductive hormone production and promoting germ cell apoptosis in adult rats. J Biomed Res 2013; 27(2): 135-44.
[http://dx.doi.org/10.7555%2FJBR.27.20120076] [PMID: 23554804]

[44] Wilson VS, Lambright CR, Furr JR, Howdeshell KL, Earl Gray L Jr. The herbicide linuron reduces testosterone production from the fetal rat testis during both in utero and *in vitro* exposures. Toxicol Lett 2009; 186(2): 73-7.
[http://dx.doi.org/10.1016/j.toxlet.2008.12.017] [PMID: 19167474]

[45] Lambright C, Ostby J, Bobseine K, *et al.* Cellular and molecular mechanisms of action of linuron: an antiandrogenic herbicide that produces reproductive malformations in male rats. Toxicol Sci 2000; 56(2): 389-99.
[http://dx.doi.org/10.1093/toxsci/56.2.389] [PMID: 10910998]

[46] Wolf C Jr, Lambright C, Mann P, *et al.* Administration of potentially antiandrogenic pesticides (procymidone, linuron, iprodione, chlozolinate, p,p-DDE, and ketoconazole) and toxic substances (dibutyl- and diethylhexyl phthalate, PCB 169, and ethane dimethane sulphonate) during sexual differentiation produces diverse profiles of reproductive malformations in the male rat. Toxicol Ind Health 1999; 15(1-2): 94-118.
[http://dx.doi.org/10.1177/074823379901500109] [PMID: 10188194]

[47] Hotchkiss AK, Parks-Saldutti LG, Ostby JS, *et al.* A mixture of the antiandrogens linuron and butyl benzyl phthalate alters sexual differentiation of the male rat in a cumulative fashion. Biol Reprod 2004; 71(6): 1852-61.
[http://dx.doi.org/10.1095/biolreprod.104.031674] [PMID: 15286035]

[48] Gray LE Jr, Ostby J, Monosson E, Kelce WR. Environmental antiandrogens: low doses of the fungicide vinclozolin alter sexual differentiation of the male rat. Toxicol Ind Health 1999; 15(1-2): 48-64.
[http://dx.doi.org/10.1191/074823399678846646] [PMID: 10188191]

[49] Monosson E, Kelce WR, Lambright C, Ostby J, Gray LE Jr. Peripubertal exposure to the antiandrogenic fungicide, vinclozolin, delays puberty, inhibits the development of androgen-dependent tissues, and alters androgen receptor function in the male rat. Toxicol Ind Health 1999; 15(1-2): 65-79.
[http://dx.doi.org/10.1177/074823379901500107] [PMID: 10188192]

[50] Wong C, Kelce WR, Sar M, Wilson EM. Androgen receptor antagonist *versus* agonist activities of the fungicide vinclozolin relative to hydroxyflutamide. J Biol Chem 1995; 270(34): 19998-20003.
[http://dx.doi.org/10.1074/jbc.270.34.19998] [PMID: 7650017]

[51] Alves MG, Rato L, Carvalho RA, Moreira PI, Socorro S, Oliveira PF. Hormonal control of Sertoli cell metabolism regulates spermatogenesis. Cell Mol Life Sci 2013; 70(5): 777-93.
[http://dx.doi.org/10.1007/s00018-012-1079-1] [PMID: 23011766]

[52] Rato L, Meneses MJ, Silva BM, Sousa M, Alves MG, Oliveira PF. New insights on hormones and factors that modulate Sertoli cell metabolism. Histol Histopathol 2016; 31(5): 499-513.
[http://dx.doi.org/10.14670/HH-11-717] [PMID: 26711246]

[53] Cardoso AM, Alves MG, Mathur PP, Oliveira PF, Cavaco JE, Rato L. Obesogens and male fertility. Obes Rev 2017; 18(1): 109-25.
[http://dx.doi.org/10.1111/obr.12469] [PMID: 27776203]

[54] DCruz SC, Jubendradass R, Jayakanthan M, Rani SJ, Mathur PP. Bisphenol A impairs insulin signaling and glucose homeostasis and decreases steroidogenesis in rat testis: an *in vivo* and in silico study. Food Chem Toxicol 2012; 50(3-4): 1124-33.
[http://dx.doi.org/10.1016/j.fct.2011.11.041] [PMID: 22142692]

[55] Meroni SB, Riera MF, Pellizzari EH, Cigorraga SB. Regulation of rat Sertoli cell function by FSH: possible role of phosphatidylinositol 3-kinase/protein kinase B pathway. J Endocrinol 2002; 174(2): 195-204.
[http://dx.doi.org/10.1677/joe.0.1740195] [PMID: 12176658]

[56] Chehtane M, Khaled AR. Interleukin-7 mediates glucose utilization in lymphocytes through transcriptional regulation of the hexokinase II gene. Am J Physiol Cell Physiol 2010; 298(6): C1560-71.
[http://dx.doi.org/10.1152/ajpcell.00506.2009] [PMID: 20200205]

[57] Alves MG, Neuhaus-Oliveira A, Moreira PI, Socorro S, Oliveira PF. Exposure to 2,4-dichlorophenoxyacetic acid alters glucose metabolism in immature rat Sertoli cells. Reprod Toxicol 2013; 38: 81-8.
[http://dx.doi.org/10.1016/j.reprotox.2013.03.005] [PMID: 23538319]

[58] Rato L, Alves MG, Socorro S, Carvalho RA, Cavaco JE, Oliveira PF. Metabolic modulation induced by oestradiol and DHT in immature rat Sertoli cells cultured *in vitro*. Biosci Rep 2012; 32(1): 61-9.
[http://dx.doi.org/10.1042/BSR20110030] [PMID: 21671886]

[59] Majors BS, Betenbaugh MJ, Chiang GG. Links between metabolism and apoptosis in mammalian cells: applications for anti-apoptosis engineering. Metab Eng 2007; 9(4): 317-26.
[http://dx.doi.org/10.1016/j.ymben.2007.05.003] [PMID: 17611135]

[60] Skakkebaek NE, Rajpert-De Meyts E, Main KM. Testicular dysgenesis syndrome: an increasingly common developmental disorder with environmental aspects. Hum Reprod 2001; 16(5): 972-8.
[http://dx.doi.org/10.1093/humrep/16.5.972] [PMID: 11331648]

[61] Mitra S, Srivastava A, Khanna S, Khandelwal S. Consequences of tributyltin chloride induced stress in Leydig cells: an ex-vivo approach. Environ Toxicol Pharmacol 2014; 37(2): 850-60.
[http://dx.doi.org/10.1016/j.etap.2014.02.018] [PMID: 24657357]

[62] Fielden MR, Halgren RG, Fong CJ, *et al.* Gestational and lactational exposure of male mice to diethylstilbestrol causes long-term effects on the testis, sperm fertilizing ability *in vitro*, and testicular gene expression. Endocrinology 2002; 143(8): 3044-59.
[http://dx.doi.org/10.1210/endo.143.8.8968] [PMID: 12130571]

[63] Koeberle A, Shindou H, Harayama T, Yuki K, Shimizu T. Polyunsaturated fatty acids are incorporated into maturating male mouse germ cells by lysophosphatidic acid acyltransferase 3. FASEB J 2012; 26(1): 169-80.
[http://dx.doi.org/10.1096/fj.11-184879] [PMID: 21968070]

[64] Saether T, Tran TN, Rootwelt H, Christophersen BO, Haugen TB. Expression and regulation of delta5-desaturase, delta6-desaturase, stearoyl-coenzyme A (CoA) desaturase 1, and stearoyl-CoA desaturase 2 in rat testis. Biol Reprod 2003; 69(1): 117-24.
[http://dx.doi.org/10.1095/biolreprod.102.014035] [PMID: 12606372]

[65] Rato L, Alves MG, Dias TR, *et al.* High-energy diets may induce a pre-diabetic state altering testicular glycolytic metabolic profile and male reproductive parameters. Andrology 2013; 1(3): 495-504.
[http://dx.doi.org/10.1111/j.2047-2927.2013.00071.x] [PMID: 23495257]

[66] Chiu YH, Afeiche MC, Gaskins AJ, *et al.* Fruit and vegetable intake and their pesticide residues in relation to semen quality among men from a fertility clinic. Hum Reprod 2015; 30(6): 1342-51.
[http://dx.doi.org/10.1093/humrep/dev064] [PMID: 25824023]

[67] Morán-Martínez J, Carranza-Rosales P, Morales-Vallarta M, *et al.* Chronic environmental exposure to lead affects semen quality in a Mexican men population. Iran J Reprod Med 2013; 11(4): 267-74.
[PMID: 24639755]

[68] Palleschi S, Rossi B, Diana L, Silvestroni L. Di(2-ethylhexyl)phthalate stimulates Ca(2+) entry, chemotaxis and ROS production in human granulocytes. Toxicol Lett 2009; 187(1): 52-7.
[http://dx.doi.org/10.1016/j.toxlet.2009.01.031] [PMID: 19429244]

[69] Hulak M, Gazo I, Shaliutina A, Linhartova P. *In vitro* effects of bisphenol A on the quality parameters, oxidative stress, DNA integrity and adenosine triphosphate content in sterlet (Acipenser ruthenus) spermatozoa. Comp Biochem Physiol C Toxicol Pharmacol 2013; 158(2): 64-71.
[http://dx.doi.org/10.1016/j.cbpc.2013.05.002] [PMID: 23680852]

[70] Meeker JD, Ehrlich S, Toth TL, *et al.* Semen quality and sperm DNA damage in relation to urinary bisphenol A among men from an infertility clinic. Reprod Toxicol 2010; 30(4): 532-9. [http://dx.doi.org/10.1016/j.reprotox.2010.07.005] [PMID: 20656017]

[71] Tayeb W, Nakbi A, Cheraief I, Miled A, Hammami M. Alteration of lipid status and lipid metabolism, induction of oxidative stress and lipid peroxidation by 2,4-dichlorophenoxyacetic herbicide in rat liver. Toxicol Mech Methods 2013; 23(6): 449-58. [http://dx.doi.org/10.3109/15376516.2013.780275] [PMID: 23464821]

[72] Galimov ShN, Valeeva GR. Effect of 2,4-D ecotoxicants on spermatogenesis and fertility of albino rats. Aviakosm Ekolog Med 1999; 33(1): 32-4. [PMID: 10330569]

[73] Marty MS, Neal BH, Zablotny CL, *et al.* An F1-extended one-generation reproductive toxicity study in Crl:CD(SD) rats with 2,4-dichlorophenoxyacetic acid. Toxicol Sci 2013; 136(2): 527-47. [http://dx.doi.org/10.1093/toxsci/kft213] [PMID: 24072463]

[74] DCruz SC, Jubendradass R, Mathur PP. Bisphenol A induces oxidative stress and decreases levels of insulin receptor substrate 2 and glucose transporter 8 in rat testis. Reprod Sci 2012; 19(2): 163-72. [http://dx.doi.org/10.1177/1933719111415547] [PMID: 22101236]

[75] Park Y, Cho SY, Jeong M. Effects of Bisphenol A and Its Metabolites on Lipid and Glucose Metabolism in Differentiated Murine Adipocytes. FASEB J 2015; 29: LB367.

[76] Chitra KC, Rao KR, Mathur PP. Effect of bisphenol A and co-administration of bisphenol A and vitamin C on epididymis of adult rats: a histological and biochemical study. Asian J Androl 2003; 5(3): 203-8. [PMID: 12937802]

[77] Galloway T, Cipelli R, Guralnik J, *et al.* Daily bisphenol A excretion and associations with sex hormone concentrations: results from the InCHIANTI adult population study. Environ Health Perspect 2010; 118(11): 1603-8. [http://dx.doi.org/10.1289/ehp.1002367] [PMID: 20797929]

[78] Sai L, Li X, Liu Y, *et al.* Effects of chlorpyrifos on reproductive toxicology of male rats. Environ Toxicol 2014; 29(9): 1083-8. [http://dx.doi.org/10.1002/tox.21838] [PMID: 23364943]

[79] Mehta A, Verma RS, Srivastava N. Chlorpyrifos-induced alterations in rat brain acetylcholinesterase, lipid peroxidation and ATPases. Indian J Biochem Biophys 2005; 42(1): 54-8. [PMID: 23923582]

[80] Wang W, Zhong X-H, Ma A, Shi W, Zhang X-S, Liu Y. Effects of ginkgo biloba on testicle injury induced by diethylstilbestrol in mice. Am J Chin Med 2008; 36(6): 1135-44. [http://dx.doi.org/10.1142/S0192415X08006478] [PMID: 19051341]

[81] Goyal HO, Braden TD, Williams CS, *et al.* Abnormal morphology of the penis in male rats exposed neonatally to diethylstilbestrol is associated with altered profile of estrogen receptor-α protein, but not of androgen receptor protein: a developmental and immunocytochemical study. Biol Reprod 2004; 70(5): 1504-17. [http://dx.doi.org/10.1095/biolreprod.103.026328] [PMID: 14749301]

[82] Bazuine M, van den Broek PJ, Maassen JA. Genistein directly inhibits GLUT4-mediated glucose uptake in 3T3-L1 adipocytes. Biochem Biophys Res Commun 2005; 326(2): 511-4. [http://dx.doi.org/10.1016/j.bbrc.2004.11.055] [PMID: 15582607]

[83] Batarseh LI, Welsh MJ, Brabec MJ. Effect of lead acetate on Sertoli cell lactate production and protein synthesis *in vitro.* Cell Biol Toxicol 1986; 2(2): 283-92. [http://dx.doi.org/10.1007/BF00122696] [PMID: 3267452]

[84] Raychoudhury SS, Flowers AF, Millette CF, Finlay MF. Toxic effects of polychlorinated biphenyls on cultured rat Sertoli cells. J Androl 2000; 21(6): 964-73. [http://dx.doi.org/10.1002/j.1939-4640.2000.tb03428.x] [PMID: 11105924]

[85] Mojena M, Marcos ML, Monge L, Felíu JE. Effect of sulfonylureas on hepatic glycogen metabolism: activation of glycogen phosphorylase. Metabolism 1989; 38(5): 466-70. [http://dx.doi.org/10.1016/0026-0495(89)90200-X] [PMID: 2725285]

[86] Howard BV, Xiaoren P, Harper I, Foley JE, Cheung MC, Taskinen M-R. Effect of sulfonylurea therapy on plasma lipids and high-density lipoprotein composition in non-insulin-dependent diabetes mellitus. Am J Med 1985; 79(3B): 78-85. [http://dx.doi.org/10.1016/S0002-9343(85)80012-7] [PMID: 4050825]

[87] Lamontagne J, Jalbert-Arsenault E, Pepin E, *et al.* Pioglitazone acutely reduces energy metabolism and insulin secretion in rats. Diabetes 2013; 62(6): 2122-9. [http://dx.doi.org/10.2337/db12-0428] [PMID: 23378607]

[88] Eleftheriadou I, Grigoropoulou P, Katsilambros N, Tentolouris N. The effects of medications used for the management of diabetes and obesity on postprandial lipid metabolism. Curr Diabetes Rev 2008; 4(4): 340-56. [http://dx.doi.org/10.2174/157339908786241133] [PMID: 18991602]

[89] Larsen TM, Toubro S, Astrup A. PPARgamma agonists in the treatment of type II diabetes: is increased fatness commensurate with long-term efficacy? Int J Obes Relat Metab Disord 2003; 27(2): 147-61. [http://dx.doi.org/10.1038/sj.ijo.802223] [PMID: 12586994]

[90] Moss EJ, Cook MW, Thomas LV, Gray TJ. The effect of mono-(2-ethylhexyl) phthalate and other phthalate esters on lactate production by Sertoli cells *in vitro.* Toxicol Lett 1988; 40(1): 77-84. [http://dx.doi.org/10.1016/0378-4274(88)90185-3] [PMID: 3341051]

[91] Itsuki-Yoneda A, Kimoto M, Tsuji H, Hiemori M, Yamashita H. Effect of a hypolipidemic drug, Di (2-ethylhexyl) phthalate, on mRNA-expression associated fatty acid and acetate metabolism in rat tissues. Biosci Biotechnol Biochem 2007; 71(2): 414-20. [http://dx.doi.org/10.1271/bbb.60478] [PMID: 17284823]

[92] Wong L, Chen HM, Lai SQ, Yang HZ, Kuang J, Pei JH. Effects of sulfonylurea as initial treatment on testosterone of middle-aged men with type 2 diabetes: A 16-week, pilot study. J Diabetes Investig 2015; 6(4): 454-9. [http://dx.doi.org/10.1111/jdi.12324] [PMID: 26221524]

[93] Yamada S, Kotake Y, Sekino Y, Kanda Y. AMP-activated protein kinase-mediated glucose transport as a novel target of tributyltin in human embryonic carcinoma cells. Metallomics 2013; 5(5): 484-91. [http://dx.doi.org/10.1039/c3mt20268b] [PMID: 23536109]

[94] Regnier SM, El-Hashani E, Kamau W, Zhang X, Massad NL, Sargis RM. Tributyltin differentially promotes development of a phenotypically distinct adipocyte. Obesity (Silver Spring) 2015; 23(9): 1864-71. [http://dx.doi.org/10.1002/oby.21174] [PMID: 26243053]

[95] Regueira M, Riera MF, Galardo MN, Pellizzari EH, Cigorraga SB, Meroni SB. Activation of PPAR α and PPAR β/δ regulates Sertoli cell metabolism. Mol Cell Endocrinol 2014; 382(1): 271-81. [http://dx.doi.org/10.1016/j.mce.2013.10.006] [PMID: 24128860]

[96] Mnif W, Hassine AI, Bouaziz A, Bartegi A, Thomas O, Roig B. Effect of endocrine disruptor pesticides: a review. Int J Environ Res Public Health 2011; 8(6): 2265-303. [http://dx.doi.org/10.3390/ijerph8062265] [PMID: 21776230]

[97] Cannon JR, Greenamyre JT. The role of environmental exposures in neurodegeneration and neurodegenerative diseases. Toxicol Sci 2011; 124(2): 225-50. [http://dx.doi.org/10.1093/toxsci/kfr239] [PMID: 21914720]

[98] Baillie-Hamilton PF. Chemical toxins: a hypothesis to explain the global obesity epidemic. J Altern Complement Med 2002; 8(2): 185-92. [http://dx.doi.org/10.1089/107555302317371479] [PMID: 12006126]

[99] Grün F, Blumberg B. Endocrine disrupters as obesogens. Mol Cell Endocrinol 2009; 304(1-2): 19-29. [http://dx.doi.org/10.1016/j.mce.2009.02.018] [PMID: 19433244]

[100] Angle BM, Do RP, Ponzi D, *et al.* Metabolic disruption in male mice due to fetal exposure to low but not high doses of bisphenol A (BPA): evidence for effects on body weight, food intake, adipocytes, leptin, adiponectin, insulin and glucose regulation. Reprod Toxicol 2013; 42: 256-68. [http://dx.doi.org/10.1016/j.reprotox.2013.07.017] [PMID: 23892310]

[101] Janesick A, Blumberg B. Obesogens, stem cells and the developmental programming of obesity. Int J Androl 2012; 35(3): 437-48. [http://dx.doi.org/10.1111/j.1365-2605.2012.01247.x] [PMID: 22372658]

[102] Sallmén M, Sandler DP, Hoppin JA, Blair A, Baird DD. Reduced fertility among overweight and obese men. Epidemiology 2006; 17(5): 520-3. [http://dx.doi.org/10.1097/01.ede.0000229953.76862.e5] [PMID: 16837825]

[103] Grün F, Blumberg B. Environmental obesogens: organotins and endocrine disruption *via* nuclear receptor signaling. Endocrinology 2006; 147(6) (Suppl.): S50-5. [http://dx.doi.org/10.1210/en.2005-1129] [PMID: 16690801]

[104] Grün F, Blumberg B. Minireview: the case for obesogens. Mol Endocrinol 2009; 23(8): 1127-34. [http://dx.doi.org/10.1210/me.2008-0485] [PMID: 19372238]

[105] Bardot O, Aldridge TC, Latruffe N, Green S. PPAR-RXR heterodimer activates a peroxisome proliferator response element upstream of the bifunctional enzyme gene. Biochem Biophys Res Commun 1993; 192(1): 37-45. [http://dx.doi.org/10.1006/bbrc.1993.1378] [PMID: 8386511]

[106] Li X, Ycaza J, Blumberg B. The environmental obesogen tributyltin chloride acts *via* peroxisome proliferator activated receptor gamma to induce adipogenesis in murine 3T3-L1 preadipocytes. J Steroid Biochem Mol Biol 2011; 127(1-2): 9-15. [http://dx.doi.org/10.1016/j.jsbmb.2011.03.012] [PMID: 21397693]

[107] Perissi V, Jepsen K, Glass CK, Rosenfeld MG. Deconstructing repression: evolving models of co-repressor action. Nat Rev Genet 2010; 11(2): 109-23. [http://dx.doi.org/10.1038/nrg2736] [PMID: 20084085]

[108] Thomas P, Dong J. Binding and activation of the seven-transmembrane estrogen receptor GPR30 by environmental estrogens: a potential novel mechanism of endocrine disruption. J Steroid Biochem Mol Biol 2006; 102(1-5): 175-9. [http://dx.doi.org/10.1016/j.jsbmb.2006.09.017] [PMID: 17088055]

[109] Watson CS, Bulayeva NN, Wozniak AL, Alyea RA. Xenoestrogens are potent activators of nongenomic estrogenic responses. Steroids 2007; 72(2): 124-34. [http://dx.doi.org/10.1016/j.steroids.2006.11.002] [PMID: 17174995]

[110] Masuno H, Iwanami J, Kidani T, Sakayama K, Honda K. Bisphenol a accelerates terminal differentiation of 3T3-L1 cells into adipocytes through the phosphatidylinositol 3-kinase pathway. Toxicol Sci 2005; 84(2): 319-27. [http://dx.doi.org/10.1093/toxsci/kfi088] [PMID: 15659569]

[111] Feige JN, Gelman L, Rossi D, *et al.* The endocrine disruptor monoethyl-hexyl-phthalate is a selective peroxisome proliferator-activated receptor γ modulator that promotes adipogenesis. J Biol Chem 2007; 282(26): 19152-66. [http://dx.doi.org/10.1074/jbc.M702724200] [PMID: 17468099]

[112] Hurst CH, Waxman DJ. Activation of PPARalpha and PPARgamma by environmental phthalate monoesters. Toxicol Sci 2003; 74(2): 297-308.
[http://dx.doi.org/10.1093/toxsci/kfg145] [PMID: 12805656]

[113] Rubenstrunk A, Hanf R, Hum DW, Fruchart J-C, Staels B. Safety issues and prospects for future generations of PPAR modulators. Biochim Biophys Acta, Lipids Lipid Metab 2007; 1771: 1065-81.
[http://dx.doi.org/10.1016/j.bbalip.2007.02.003] [PMID: 17428730]

[114] Miyazaki Y, Mahankali A, Matsuda M, *et al.* Improved glycemic control and enhanced insulin sensitivity in type 2 diabetic subjects treated with pioglitazone. Diabetes Care 2001; 24(4): 710-9.
[http://dx.doi.org/10.2337/diacare.24.4.710] [PMID: 11315836]

[115] Akinola O, Dosumu O, Sanusi S, Ajayi T, Olajide T. PPAR-γ agonist pioglitazone improves semen quality and testicular histomorphometrics with partial reversal of hyperglycaemia in alloxan-induced diabetic rats. Middle East Fertil Soc J 2015; 20: 271-9.
[http://dx.doi.org/10.1016/j.mefs.2015.04.003]

[116] Rabbani SI, Devi K, Khanam S. Effect of thiazolidinediones on the erythropoeitic and germinal cells in the male wistar rats. Clin Med Oncol 2008; 2: 423-9.
[PMID: 21892311]

[117] Penza M, Montani C, Romani A, *et al.* Genistein affects adipose tissue deposition in a dose-dependent and gender-specific manner. Endocrinology 2006; 147(12): 5740-51.
[http://dx.doi.org/10.1210/en.2006-0365] [PMID: 16959845]

[118] Ruhlen RL, Howdeshell KL, Mao J, *et al.* Low phytoestrogen levels in feed increase fetal serum estradiol resulting in the fetal estrogenization syndrome and obesity in CD-1 mice. Environ Health Perspect 2008; 116(3): 322-8.
[http://dx.doi.org/10.1289/ehp.10448] [PMID: 18335098]

[119] Ramlau-Hansen CH, Nohr EA, Thulstrup AM, Bonde JP, Storgaard L, Olsen J. Is maternal obesity related to semen quality in the male offspring? A pilot study. Hum Reprod 2007; 22(10): 2758-62.
[http://dx.doi.org/10.1093/humrep/dem219] [PMID: 17704100]

[120] Alleva E, Brock J, Brouwer A, *et al.* Statement from the work session on environmental endocrine-disrupting chemicals: neural, endocrine, and behavioral effects. Toxicol Ind Health 1998; 14(1-2): 1-8.
[http://dx.doi.org/10.1177/074823379801400103] [PMID: 9460166]

[121] Sasaki H, Matsui Y. Epigenetic events in mammalian germ-cell development: reprogramming and beyond. Nat Rev Genet 2008; 9(2): 129-40.
[http://dx.doi.org/10.1038/nrg2295] [PMID: 18197165]

[122] Moore DS. The developing genome: An introduction to behavioral epigenetics. Oxford University Press 2015; pp. 1-320.

[123] Skinner MK, Manikkam M, Guerrero-Bosagna C. Epigenetic transgenerational actions of environmental factors in disease etiology. Trends Endocrinol Metab 2010; 21(4): 214-22.
[http://dx.doi.org/10.1016/j.tem.2009.12.007] [PMID: 20074974]

[124] Anway MD, Cupp AS, Uzumcu M, Skinner MK. Epigenetic transgenerational actions of endocrine disruptors and male fertility. Science 2005; 308(5727): 1466-9.
[http://dx.doi.org/10.1126/science.1108190] [PMID: 15933200]

[125] Piprek RP. Genetic mechanisms underlying male sex determination in mammals. J Appl Genet 2009; 50(4): 347-60.
[http://dx.doi.org/10.1007/BF03195693] [PMID: 19875885]

[126] Schug TT, Janesick A, Blumberg B, Heindel JJ. Endocrine disrupting chemicals and disease susceptibility. J Steroid Biochem Mol Biol 2011; 127(3-5): 204-15.
[http://dx.doi.org/10.1016/j.jsbmb.2011.08.007] [PMID: 21899826]

[127] Cupp AS, Uzumcu M, Suzuki H, Dirks K, Phillips B, Skinner MK. Effect of transient embryonic *in vivo* exposure to the endocrine disruptor methoxychlor on embryonic and postnatal testis development. J Androl 2003; 24(5): 736-45.
[http://dx.doi.org/10.1002/j.1939-4640.2003.tb02736.x] [PMID: 12954667]

[128] Uzumcu M, Suzuki H, Skinner MK. Effect of the anti-androgenic endocrine disruptor vinclozolin on embryonic testis cord formation and postnatal testis development and function. Reprod Toxicol 2004; 18(6): 765-74.
[http://dx.doi.org/10.1016/j.reprotox.2004.05.008] [PMID: 15279874]

[129] Anway MD, Leathers C, Skinner MK. Endocrine disruptor vinclozolin induced epigenetic transgenerational adult-onset disease. Endocrinology 2006; 147(12): 5515-23.
[http://dx.doi.org/10.1210/en.2006-0640] [PMID: 16973726]

[130] Kaneda M, Okano M, Hata K, *et al.* Essential role for de novo DNA methyltransferase Dnmt3a in paternal and maternal imprinting. Nature 2004; 429(6994): 900-3.
[http://dx.doi.org/10.1038/nature02633] [PMID: 15215868]

[131] Kobayashi H, Sato A, Otsu E, *et al.* Aberrant DNA methylation of imprinted loci in sperm from oligospermic patients. Hum Mol Genet 2007; 16(21): 2542-51.
[http://dx.doi.org/10.1093/hmg/ddm187] [PMID: 17636251]

[132] Dolinoy DC, Huang D, Jirtle RL. Maternal nutrient supplementation counteracts bisphenol A-induced DNA hypomethylation in early development. Proc Natl Acad Sci USA 2007; 104(32): 13056-61.
[http://dx.doi.org/10.1073/pnas.0703739104] [PMID: 17670942]

[133] Doyle TJ, Bowman JL, Windell VL, McLean DJ, Kim KH. Transgenerational effects of di-(- -ethylhexyl) phthalate on testicular germ cell associations and spermatogonial stem cells in mice. Biol Reprod 2013; 88(5): 112.
[http://dx.doi.org/10.1095/biolreprod.112.106104] [PMID: 23536373]

[134] Whitehead ED, Leiter E. Genital abnormalities and abnormal semen analyses in male patients exposed to diethylstilbestrol in utero. J Urol 1981; 125(1): 47-50.
[PMID: 7463583]

[135] Brouwers MM, Feitz WF, Roelofs LA, Kiemeney LA, de Gier RP, Roeleveld N. Hypospadias: a transgenerational effect of diethylstilbestrol? Hum Reprod 2006; 21(3): 666-9.
[http://dx.doi.org/10.1093/humrep/dei398] [PMID: 16293648]

[136] Kalfa N, Paris F, Soyer-Gobillard M-O, Daures J-P, Sultan C. Prevalence of hypospadias in grandsons of women exposed to diethylstilbestrol during pregnancy: a multigenerational national cohort study. Fertil Steril 2011; 95(8): 2574-7.
[http://dx.doi.org/10.1016/j.fertnstert.2011.02.047] [PMID: 21458804]

[137] van de Werken C, van der Heijden GW, Eleveld C, *et al.* Paternal heterochromatin formation in human embryos is H3K9/HP1 directed and primed by sperm-derived histone modifications. Nat Commun 2014; 5: 5868.
[http://dx.doi.org/10.1038/ncomms6868] [PMID: 25519718]

[138] Kouzarides T. Chromatin modifications and their function. Cell 2007; 128(4): 693-705.
[http://dx.doi.org/10.1016/j.cell.2007.02.005] [PMID: 17320507]

[139] Collotta M, Bertazzi PA, Bollati V. Epigenetics and pesticides. Toxicology 2013; 307: 35-41.
[http://dx.doi.org/10.1016/j.tox.2013.01.017] [PMID: 23380243]

[140] Dansky LV, Finnell RH. Parental epilepsy, anticonvulsant drugs, and reproductive outcome: epidemiologic and experimental findings spanning three decades; 2: Human studies. Reprod Toxicol 1991; 5(4): 301-35.
[http://dx.doi.org/10.1016/0890-6238(91)90091-S] [PMID: 1806139]

[141] Tabb MM, Blumberg B. New modes of action for endocrine-disrupting chemicals. Mol Endocrinol 2006; 20(3): 475-82.
[http://dx.doi.org/10.1210/me.2004-0513] [PMID: 16037129]

[142] Lambrot R, Xu C, Saint-Phar S, *et al.* Low paternal dietary folate alters the mouse sperm epigenome and is associated with negative pregnancy outcomes. Nat Commun 2013; 4: 2889.
[http://dx.doi.org/10.1038/ncomms3889] [PMID: 24326934]

[143] Terashima M, Barbour S, Ren J, Yu W, Han Y, Muegge K. Effect of high fat diet on paternal sperm histone distribution and male offspring liver gene expression. Epigenetics 2015; 10(9): 861-71.
[http://dx.doi.org/10.1080/15592294.2015.1075691] [PMID: 26252449]

[144] Chen L-L, Carmichael GG. Decoding the function of nuclear long non-coding RNAs. Curr Opin Cell Biol 2010; 22(3): 357-64.
[http://dx.doi.org/10.1016/j.ceb.2010.03.003] [PMID: 20356723]

[145] Wang KC, Chang HY. Molecular mechanisms of long noncoding RNAs. Mol Cell 2011; 43(6): 904-14.
[http://dx.doi.org/10.1016/j.molcel.2011.08.018] [PMID: 21925379]

[146] Bernstein E, Allis CD. RNA meets chromatin. Genes Dev 2005; 19(14): 1635-55.
[http://dx.doi.org/10.1101/gad.1324305] [PMID: 16024654]

[147] Whitehead J, Pandey GK, Kanduri C. Regulation of the mammalian epigenome by long noncoding RNAs. Biochim Biophys Acta 2009; 1790: 936-47.
[http://dx.doi.org/10.1016/j.bbagen.2008.10.007] [PMID: 19015002]

[148] Jolly C, Lakhotia SC. Human sat III and Drosophila hsr ω transcripts: a common paradigm for regulation of nuclear RNA processing in stressed cells. Nucleic Acids Res 2006; 34(19): 5508-14.
[http://dx.doi.org/10.1093/nar/gkl711] [PMID: 17020918]

[149] Luke B, Lingner J. TERRA: telomeric repeat-containing RNA. EMBO J 2009; 28(17): 2503-10.
[http://dx.doi.org/10.1038/emboj.2009.166] [PMID: 19629047]

[150] Martínez-Guitarte J-L, Planelló R, Morcillo G. Overexpression of long non-coding RNAs following exposure to xenobiotics in the aquatic midge Chironomus riparius. Aquat Toxicol 2012; 110-111: 84-90.
[http://dx.doi.org/10.1016/j.aquatox.2011.12.013] [PMID: 22277249]

[151] Pezer Ž, Brajković J, Feliciello I, Ugarković Đ. Transcription of satellite DNAs in insects Long Non-Coding RNAs. Springer 2011; pp. 161-78.
[http://dx.doi.org/10.1007/978-3-642-16502-3_8]

[152] He X, Chen X, Zhang X, *et al.* An Lnc RNA (GAS5)/SnoRNA-derived piRNA induces activation of TRAIL gene by site-specifically recruiting MLL/COMPASS-like complexes. Nucleic Acids Res 2015; 43(7): 3712-25.
[http://dx.doi.org/10.1093/nar/gkv214] [PMID: 25779046]

CHAPTER 14

Biochemical Changes in the Reproductive Function of the Aging Male

Susana P. Almeida[1] and **Luís Rato**[2,*]

[1] *Department of Microscopy, Laboratory of Cell Biology, Institute of Biomedical Sciences Abel Salazar and Unit for Multidisciplinary Research in Biomedicine, University of Porto, Rua de Jorge Viterbo Ferreira, 4050-313, Porto, Portugal*

[2] *Health Sciences Research Center, University of Beira Interior, Rua Marquês d'Ávila e Bolama, 6201-001, Covilhã, Portugal*

Abstract: Late-onset hypogonadism (LOH) is a situation where a middle-aged or older man has low serum testosterone in conjunction with diffuse symptoms resembling those of genuine male hypogonadism. Testosterone replacement therapy has become a popular choice for the treatment of LOH. Aging is a process that includes irreversible changes because of a large variety of endogenous and environmental factors. Paternal aging also causes genetic and epigenetic changes in spermatozoa that damage male reproductive functions through adverse effects on sperm quality and count, as well as on sexual organs and also on the hypothalamic-pituitary testicular axis. If on one hand, hormone production, spermatogenesis, and testes undergo changes as a man ages, on the other hand, the offspring of older fathers show high prevalence of genetic abnormalities, childhood cancers, and several disorders. Information on the impact of age on male fertility is of growing importance, therefore, further studies should investigate the onset of changes in the reproductive function and its effects on aging men. The aim of this chapter is to briefly discuss the effects of aging on the male reproductive system and function.

Keywords: Aging, Epigenetics, Infertility, Late-onset hypogonadism, Male fertility, Oxidative stress, Paternal age, Replacement therapy, Semen parameters, Spermatogenesis, Spermatozoa, Testes, Testosterone.

INTRODUCTION

Aging of males exerts effects on reproductive organs and tissues and such changes seem to evolve progressively without a well-marked threshold of age. Among those alterations are the testicular changes that are most often accompanied by variations on the levels of reproductive hormones [1, 2]. In

* **Corresponding author Luís Rato:** Health Sciences Research Centre (CICS-UBI), Av. Infante D. Henrique, 6201-506, Covilhã, Portugal; Tel: +351 275 329 002; Fax: +351 275 329 099; E-mail: luis.pedro.rato@gmail.com

Marco G. Alves and Pedro F. Oliveira (Eds.)

menopausal women, the cessation of ovarian function is due to the inevitable decline and final exhaustion of the oocyte pool, paralleled by increase in the levels of follicle-stimulating hormone (FSH). However, in males, spermatogenesis continues throughout life [2]. As they age, men experience a gradual and progressive decline in reproductive function when compared to women. Also, in contrast to menopause, which is universal and a well characterized timed process related with absolute gonadal failure, this condition in men is characterized by insidious beginning and slow progression [3]. This variability is a trait of male reproductive system aging and of the general male aging process. As reported in several recent studies, androgens play an important role within the development and maintenance of male reproductive and sexual functions. Diminished levels of circulating androgens lead to innate abnormalities of the male reproductive tract. Indeed, testosterone levels decrease as age advances. The symptoms caused by this decline can be regarded as a normal part of aging. At more advanced age, this is reported to be associated with reduced fertility, sexual disorders, decreased muscle formation and bone mineralization, disturbances of metabolism, and psychological feature dysfunction. Moreover, low testosterone levels are also related to many chronic diseases, and symptomatic patients could benefit from testosterone treatment [4] though this remains a matter of intense debate. Though the biochemical changes induced by aging in the male reproductive tract remain largely unknown, we will briefly discuss the mechanisms known so far.

IMPACT OF AGING ON TESTICULAR ANATOMY AND PHYSIOLOGY

Generally, as men grow older, they retain their fertility though some changes may occur. Indeed, they develop certain physiological changes affecting the endocrine system and testicular function (Fig. **14.1**). Notwithstanding individual variations, alterations in testicular morphology are one of the several effects of aging on the reproductive system of males. Testicular function declines with advancing age, but this reduction has a magnitude similar as that of other body organs [5 - 7]. Still, the decreased efficiency in testicular function has been the subject of a great number of studies, which evidenced the relationship between testicular function and age [8 - 12]. During aging there is a thickening of the basal membrane of the seminiferous tubules, accompanied with a reduction in both the height of the seminiferous epithelium and in the vascularization of the testes [13, 14], which are associated with testicular hernia-like protrusions [15]. Sertoli cells and germ cells represent up to 90% of the testicular volume, while Leydig cells contribute to less than 1%. Aging leads to a reduction in the number of Sertoli cells and Leydig cells [2, 16] which could results in a decrease of testicular volume [1]. In fact, a negative association between increasing age and reduction in testicular volume for men over 80 years was already established [17]. In general, the observed mean testicular volume between 20 and 30 years of age is 16.5 cm^3 and the maximal testis volume is observed at 25 years of age, after which there is a slight but significant decline to a mean volume of 14 cm^3 between 80 and 90 years of age [18]. Compared to the age group 18-40 years, men aged over 75 years have a 31% smaller mean testicular volume. This variation in the testes volume is related with higher average serum levels of gonadotropins and lower serum free testosterone [1]. Age-related increment in gonadotropins is mostly due to primary testicular failure. The aforementioned decrease in Leydig cells number is reflected in the observation that older men display a diminished secretory capacity compared with younger men when testes are stimulated with human chorionic gonadotropin or via pulsatile GnRH [19]. In fact, the testicular volume decrease in older men showed strong direct correlation with serum levels of inhibin B and inhibin B/FSH ratio, and indirect correlation with FSH [1] and on LH levels [1, 6]. Serum gonadotropins levels increase due to feedback mechanisms that cause increased secretion of gonadotropins [20, 21]. In fact, testicular androgen metabolism increases between the 11th and 40th year of age and progressively decreases between the age of 40 and 90 [8, 9].

ENDOCRINE DYSFUNCTION IN THE AGING MALE

Aging is related to important alterations in the control of the hormonal axis that regulate male fertility [22]. The hypothalamic-pituitary-testicular (HPT) axis is the key regulator of the male reproductive function and controls the synthesis of sex hormones and the formation and maturation of male germ cells. As referred in previous chapters, it is constituted by three major elements, including the hypothalamus, anterior pituitary, and the testes. In this axis, gonadotropin-releasing hormone (GnRH) secreted from the hypothalamus reaches the anterior pituitary gland via the hypophyseal portal system and stimulates the secretion of luteinizing hormone (LH) and follicle-stimulating hormone (FSH), by the gonadotropic cells, into the bloodstream. In broad terms, LH induces the production of testosterone by the Leydig cells, while FSH stimulates Sertoli cells to secrete androgen-binding protein (ABP) and inhibin and plays a vital role in spermatogenesis [23].

Independent from primary, events that affect the hypothalamic-pituitary axis have a major outcome on the reproductive tract and the reproductive potential of the aging male. Aging causes a decrease in the secretion of GnRH, which in turn leads to smaller LH pulses. In older men, there is an impairment on the response of gonadotropic cells to exogenous GnRH, a decrease of LH pulse size and/or reduction of LH bioactivity [23, 24]. Moreover, it has been reported that serum FSH levels rise more pronouncedly in men after 40 years of age, reflecting a progressive tenacity of the gonadotropic support to the germinal epithelium [25 - 27]. This increase in FSH is concurrent with age-dependent alterations in testicular histology and semen parameters and with the slight but significant decrease in inhibin B. Nevertheless this alteration was also described in men with apparently normal semen parameters [1, 28]. Furthermore, there is a consensus that testicular steroidogenesis decreases with aging [6]. It is well known that androgen levels suffer a decrease in men as they age [29]. As referred in previous chapters, androgens are key hormones in the male reproductive tract, having a major role in the expression of the male phenotype. They have very important roles during male sexual differentiation, development and maintenance of secondary male characteristics, and also during the initiation and maintenance of spermatogenesis [30]. The major circulating androgen in men is testicular testosterone [31], which is also the key sex hormone responsible for regulating masculinization [32]. Testosterone is also directly involved in the development and differentiation of the Wolffian duct derived structures, namely the epididymis, *vas deferens* and seminal vesicles [30, 33], exerting its action by binding to and activating the androgen receptor (AR), affecting intracellular signals and changing the expression of various genes [34]. Approximately half of testosterone is present in the circulation bound to sex hormone-binding globulin (SHBG) and another half to albumin, with only 0.5–3% of testosterone being unbound or free representing the biologically active fraction [7, 35, 36]. Several studies have confirmed the age-related decline of serum testosterone, which is accompanied by a marked decrease of the free and bioavailable testosterone (larger than that of total testosterone), partly due to the concomitant increase of SHBG [6, 37]. A clear decrease in the levels of testosterone precursors (progesterone, 17α-hydroxyprogesterone, 17α-hydroxypregnenolone, androstenedione, pregnenolone, dehydroepiandrosterone, androstenediol and dehydroepiandrosterone sulfate) was also described in the spermatic vein and testicular tissues from older men [38, 39]. With respect to the total testosterone, the decrease becomes evident from the age of 45-50 years, however, for the fraction of free testosterone, this reduction is more pronounced and earlier when compared to total testosterone.

Testicular secretion of testosterone takes place as a result of the secretion of LH by the pituitary, which is stimulated by pulsatile release of GnRH from the hypothalamus and then acts on Leydig cells to stimulate testosterone synthesis and release [32]. Total serum testosterone levels decrease with age particularly due to the decrease in the number of Leydig cells, deterioration of testicular perfusion, and disturbance in diurnal rhythm of GnRH and chorionic gonadotropin secretion [40 - 42]. Increased LH (primary gonadal failure) or inappropriately normal LH (secondary hypogonadism) can also occur in men with low testosterone levels, and can be difficult to differentiate from the dysfunction associated with aging if there is no evidence of a pathological disruption of the HPT axis [32]. In older men, combined forms of primary and secondary hypogonadism are often observed, with a concomitant age-related decline in testosterone levels as a consequence from defects both in testicular as well as hypothalamic-pituitary function. A large part of these men have serum testosterone levels below the lower reference limits in young adults [38, 43 - 45] and this decrease tends to be permanent rather than transient [36], being set above 1% per year in men after the age of 40 [7, 32]. In men between 55 and 68 years of age, total testosterone decrease averages 1.4% per year, while free testosterone decreases as much as 2.7% (concurrently with an increase of SHBG) [46]. In addition, the rate of decline in testosterone levels is also affected by chronic disease, such as obesity, illness, serious emotional stress, and medications, and this decline can be slow down by management of health and lifestyle factors [3]. Still, while this decrease tends to be small in some men, in most it can lead to clinical hypogonadism [47], being also associated with diffuse sexual, physical and psychological symptoms in some of aging men [7, 29, 31].

This condition of general and sexual deterioration in men was firstly described by Hellers and Meyers [48], who associated it with the decreased testosterone levels and used for the first time the term male menopause to denominate it [36]. Other denominations are also used for this condition that includes the combination of low testosterone and an array of the above symptoms, such as male menopause or climacterium, andropause (which are not adequate as the physiological decline of androgen secretion does not stop abruptly, but rather occurs gradually over time), partial androgen deficiency of the aging male (PADAM) and late-onset hypogonadism (LOH), with this last one being the preferred and most widely used [7, 49, 50]. Late-onset hypogonadism, according with a recent definition "*is a clinical and biochemical syndrome associated with advancing age and characterized by symptoms and a deficiency in serum testosterone levels (below the young healthy adult male reference range). This condition may result in significant detriment in the quality of life and adversely affect the function of multiple organ systems*" [51]. However, it is worth mentioning that decreased testosterone levels alone with diffuse symptoms do not justify the diagnosis of LOH neither do sexual symptoms in men with normal testosterone [47]. The diagnostic criteria for LOH has been recently defined by The European Male Ageing Study (EMAS) and includes the simultaneous presence of reproducibly low serum testosterone (total testosterone <11 nmol l^{-1} and free testosterone <220 pmol l^{-1}) and three other sexual symptoms (erectile dysfunction, reduced frequency of sexual thoughts and morning erections) and is said to affect 2% of 40 to 80-year-old men [7].

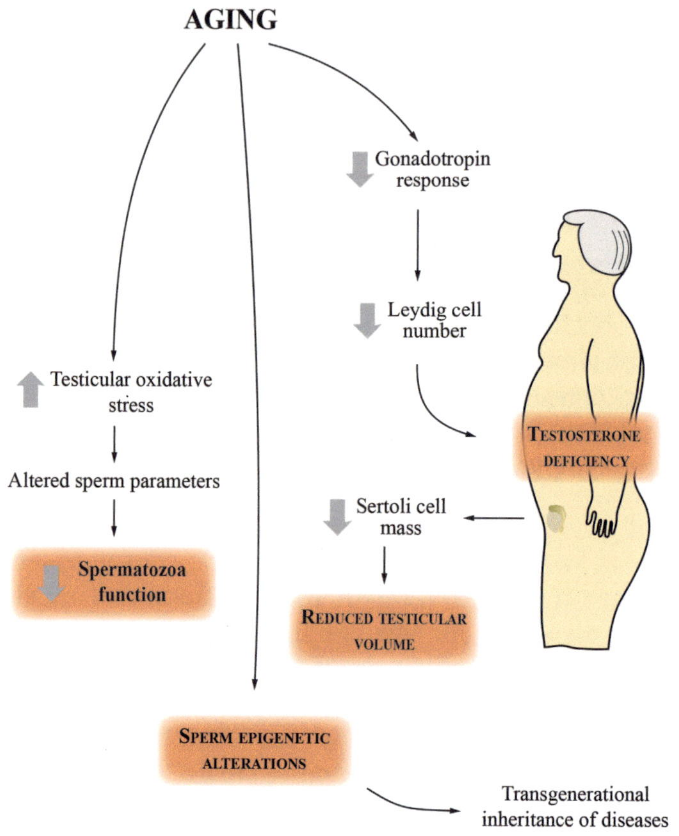

Fig. (14.1). The aging effects in the male reproductive function. As age advances the amount of gonadotropin-releasing hormone secreted from the hypothalamus also decrease and this is reflected in lower luteinizing hormone pulsatile secretion. As a consequence, there is a decrease in the number of Leydig cells and the production of testosterone in hampered, leading to testosterone deficiency. Moreover, the Sertoli cell mass also decreases with aging leading to decreased testicular volume and remarkable alterations in testicular morphology. Advanced paternal age has been associated with a negative impact on the quality of male germ cells and this is attributed mainly due to the aging-induced oxidative stress which impairs several functions of the spermatozoa, as is the case of motility and morphology. Apart from those changes that aging induces in spermatozoa, other molecular alterations may also occur. Epigenetic changes, mainly DNA methylation, have been associated with age-related diseases. These epigenetic modifications may be passed from the father to offspring increasing the susceptibility of the next generations for the development of several diseases. Up-arrows (grey): increased; Down-arrows (grey): decreased.

CONTROVERSIES AND TREATMENT OF LATE-ONSET HYPOGONADISM

Several studies have associated low levels of testosterone with increased mortality, which shows that LOH has a serious impact on health [32, 47, 52]. Severe LOH is directly related with significantly increased risks to all-cause of cardiovascular and cancer-related mortality, for which not only the level of testosterone, but also the presence of sexual symptoms, contributes independently. Therefore, men affected by LOH should be subjected to treatment, since their lives are at risk [47]. There are two types of treatment for LOH: testosterone replacement therapy and lifestyle modification (including weight loss and treatment of comorbidities). Due to the fact that symptoms of hypogonadism in young men are very similar to those of LOH, testosterone replacement therapy has become the most popular choice for the treatment of this aging related condition. Still, although it is tempting to speculate that just by replacing decreased testosterone levels with exogenous hormone administration all problems caused by this decrease will be corrected, this is not absolutely true and is far from being demonstrated in a convincing way [47]. One of the problems in this approach is to set the level of testosterone that causes LOH, to then proceed with the proper doses of testosterone supplementation [53]. Thus, to diagnosis LOH, in addition to testosterone serum levels, clinical symptoms should be considered before proceeding with the therapy. Moreover, possible complications such as benign prostatic hyperplasia, prostate cancer, exacerbation of sleep apnea, gynecomastia, polycythemia and liver toxicity should be also taken into consideration [54].

The main goal of therapy with testosterone is to restore testosterone levels to the physiological range in men with low serum testosterone levels and that also exhibit associated symptoms of androgen deficiency. The purpose of this treatment is to improve the quality of life, well-being, sexual function, muscle strength and bone mineral density [4]. In the initial phase of treatment the preparations more suitable are those, which act at the short term, so that if any adverse effect arises, these can be immediately detected and treatment can be discontinued [55]. There are several preparations available that differ in the method of administration and pharmacokinetics, and the selection should be a joint decision by both the patient and the physician [56]. Testosterone replacement therapy is available in the form of oral preparations, intramuscular injections and transdermal gel or patches [57] (Table **14.1**), namely intramuscular injections of testosterone esters (such as Testoviron™ (Schering, Germany) and Sustanon™ (Organon, The Netherlands), testosterone pellets for subcutaneous implantation and long-acting injectable testosterone esters (such as testosterone-bucyclate or testosterone undecanoate), oral preparations (such as Mesterolon™ (Proviron, Schering, Germany) or testosterone undecanoate (Andriol™, Organon, The Netherlands)). There are also transdermal delivery systems of testosterone, scrotal (Testoderm™, Alza, USA) and non-scrotal (Androderm™, Smithkline Beecham, UK) patches, among other systems that are being constantly developed. In all these options the replacement drug must be given daily to exert and adequate biological effect [29]. Numerous studies have shown the health benefits of testosterone replacement, which include increased strength and durability of erection and improved sexual performance of men with LOH [58]; increased bone density, muscle mass, improved mood, quality of life and cognitive function, as well as increase in stamina [54].

Table 14.1. Testosterone preparations used for replacement therapy.

Preparation	Administration	Advantages	Disadvantages
Testosterone Undecanoate	Oral; 2-6 cps every 6 h	Absorbed through the lymphatic system, with consequent reduction of liver involvement.	Variable levels of testosterone above and below the mid-range. Need for several doses per day with intake of fatty food [59].
	Intramuscular; one injection Every 10-14 weeks	Steady-state testosterone levels without fluctuation.	Long-acting preparation that cannot allow drug withdrawal in case of onset of side effects [29].
Testosterone Cypionate	Intramuscular; one injection every 2-3 weeks	Short-acting preparation that allows drug withdrawal in case of onset of side effects.	Possible variation of testosterone levels [60, 61].
Testosterone Enanthate	Intramuscular; one injection every 2-3 weeks	Short-acting preparation that allows drug withdrawal in case of onset of side effects.	Possible variation of testosterone levels [60, 61].
Transdermal Testosterone	Gel or skin patches; daily application	Steady-state testosterone level without fluctuation.	Skin irritation at the site of application and risk of interpersonal transfer [62, 63].
Sublingual Testosterone	Sublingual; daily doses	Rapid absorption and achievement of physiological serum level of testosterone.	Local irritation [58, 64].
Buccal Testosterone	Buccal tablet; two doses per day.	Rapid absorption and achievement of physiological serum level of testosterone	Irritation and pain at the site of application [58, 64].
Subdermal Depots	Subdermal implant every 5-7 months	Long duration and constant serum testosterone level.	Risk of infection and extrusion of the implants [59, 65, 66].

Moreover, recent EMAS data also showed that weight gain or loss has an evident inverse correlation with circulating testosterone and vice versa. Testosterone replacement treatment had important effects on body composition, resulting in a meaningful increase in lean body mass, and a significant decrease in fat mass without a change in body weight [40]. However, adverse effects caused by testosterone replacement treatment have also been described, such us increased acne, oily skin, gynecomastia, risk of prostate cancer, cardiovascular disease and lipid changes, and also increased hematocrit levels [54, 58, 66, 67]. There are also recent studies that drawn attention concerning cardiovascular complication in ageing men during testosterone replacement therapy [5, 14, 30]. Prostate and breast cancer are absolute contraindications to testosterone replacement therapy, severe lower urinary tract symptoms caused by benign prostatic hypertrophy (as defined by an International Prostate Symptom Score [IPSS]), untreated or poorly controlled congestive heart failure, and untreated sleep apnea are relative contraindications [67]. Nonetheless, the indications and contraindications for testosterone treatment of LOH, including short and long term benefits and risks, still await evidence-based information. The current information about the benefits and risks of testosterone replacement therapy is not yet complete and accurate because it still relies mostly in data derived from studies that are insufficiently powered, poorly controlled and of short duration [7].

BIOCHEMICAL MODIFICATIONS IN SPERMATOZOA OF THE AGING MALE

Spermatogenesis is a continuous process that allows males to produce sperm from the beginning of puberty until late age. Notwithstanding, spermatozoa are continuously produced with advancing age, there is a growing body of evidence indicating that advanced paternal age is linked with a negative impact on the quality of male germ cells [68, 69]. It was reported that males after 40 years of age exhibited a gradual decrease in sperm motility [10]. A negative correlation between advanced age and sperm motility in healthy men has also been reported [9]. Nieschlag and collaborators found a negative correlation between sperm motility and aging after comparing sperm between old (60-88 years of age) and young (24-37 years of age) individuals [70]. Similarly, the values of sperm motility for old individuals were significantly lower in the group of males with 36 to 40 years of age when compared with the group of males with ≤25 years of age [71]. However, it must be taking into account that potential confounders, such as lifestyle factors (*e.g.* smoking) and type of infertility among individuals may contribute for some variability in the results available in literature [72, 73]. Still, it is generally accepted that sperm motility decreases as age increases. Nevertheless, this is not so obvious for other sperm parameters, as is the case of sperm concentration. Daily sperm production decreases more than 30% in men over the age of 50 and is negatively correlated with age of men in general [23] and several studies have reported a decrease in sperm concentration with increased age [6, 74 - 76]. Older men (≥50 years) exhibited nearly half the sperm concentration when compared with young individuals (≤30 years) [12]. This is in line with other reports demonstrating that the number of men exhibiting decreased sperm concentration was 3-fold higher in older men when compared with young men [77]. It must be also considered that such remarkable differences may be due to individuals attending to infertility clinics and for these reason generalizing to the overall male population must be done with some caution, since these individuals represent a small percentage of the general population.

It is also important to highlight that some evidence found little or no association between age and sperm concentration. It has been found an inversed U-shaped curve with youngest age groups (22–30 years) exhibiting lower sperm concentrations than intermediate age groups, but the concentrations were similar to those of the oldest age group (≥50 years) [78]. It would be reasonable to argue that the impaired reproductive health of individuals might be explained since all participants were infertile men. However similar results have been reported from men with apparently normal reproductive health [71]. It is noteworthy that in certain cases these results could be biased, due to the heterogeneity of the individuals. Some studies come from infertile men, but other reports come from men attending to family planning [72, 79] and may represent men with improved fertility due to lifestyle modifications (*e.g.* healthy eating behavior, vitamins and supplements, regular physical exercise). Sperm morphology is also an important parameter to evaluate sperm quality and that is also affected by aging. After 40 years of age the percentage of sperm with normal morphology begins to decrease [25]. A semen comparison between men in younger (≤30 years) and older (≥50 years) age groups revealed that sperm morphology decreased by 0.9% for each year of age [8]. Other studies have also showed a consistency toward decreasing percentage of sperm with normal morphology in old men [12, 71, 79 - 82] illustrating that aging also affects the morphology of sperm and it may be a main reason for decreased sperm quality in older men.

Human studies have several limitations and several external insults (*e.g.* smoking, alcohol, drugs, environmental contaminants) and pathological conditions easily disturb human spermatogenesis being one of the limiting aspects when interpreting the results concerning sperm quality [83]. Conventional semen analysis, including ejaculate volume, sperm concentration, motility, and morphology determined according to World Health Organization criteria [84, 85], are the first step in the evaluation of male infertility. However, this conventional analysis has already been recognized to be of limited value in the determination of sperm quality in part due to the notable biologic variability of conventional sperm parameters and the fact that these parameters are poor predictors of sperm quality.

Aging exerts multiple effects on the acquisition of motility, sperm morphology and sperm number and all alterations in these parameters indicate that the quality of spermatozoa declines over time. However, few works have explored in detail the molecular mechanisms that hamper sperm function in old men. Sperm parameters seem to be significantly affected after 40 years of age, which is coincident with the increased levels of reactive oxygen species (ROS) in semen [86]. It is well known that excessive ROS and oxidative damage in spermatozoa are consequences of aging [69, 87, 88]. Negative correlations between seminal ROS levels and sperm motility have been established, foreseeing that an elevation of seminal ROS levels may be a causative factor for increased incidence of asthenozoospermia in old individuals [86], probably due to defects in sperm plasma membranes, as previously discussed in other chapters. Sperm are devoid of antioxidant defenses. Furthermore, as age advances the efficiency of the antioxidant defense system in male reproductive system decreases. Aging declines the expression of antioxidant defenses, in particular glutathione peroxidase 5 (GPX5) throughout reproductive tract [89]. GPX5 is part of the glutathione peroxidases family, which is one of the most important constituents of the antioxidant system. GPX5 plays a role in protecting the membranes of spermatozoa from the damaging effects of lipid peroxidation. With the diminished antioxidant activity, oxidative stress may occur due to uncontrolled and excessive ROS production and an inefficient ROS-defense system. Sperm are extremely susceptible to ROS attack and this vulnerability is mainly ascribed to the presence of polyunsaturated fatty acids (PUFAs), namely docosahexaenoic acid, in sperm plasma membrane. PUFAs are particularly prone to free radical attack due to the conjugated nature of the double bonds adjacent to methylene group (C-H), making the methylene bond weaker and consequently the hydrogen more susceptible to abstraction. Therefore, the new carbon centered-radical formed in this process is stabilized by conjugated diene, which then combines with oxygen to origin a lipid peroxyl radical. This peroxyl radical is able of subtracting a hydrogen atom from another polyunsaturated fatty acid thus triggering a lipid peroxidation cascade [90]. The lipid peroxidation chain reactions initiated in spermatozoa result in the formation of a cascade of aldehyde by-products that include malondialdehyde, 4-hydroxynonenal (4HNE) and acrolein. Specifically, 4HNE and acrolein, may form adducts with several proteins within the spermatozoa [91], as is the case of dynein heavy chain. Dynein heavy chain is essential to generate the force for the movement of flagellum. The formation of adducts may explain the effect of these aldehydes, for instance in the inhibition of sperm motility [91, 92]. Similarly to what happens with lipids, nuclear DNA of sperm is also targeted by ROS. A growing body of evidence have showed that advanced paternal age is associated with an increased frequency of DNA damage in sperm [93 - 95], which is a consequence of the accumulated damages induced by ROS over time, especially in the structure of sperm chromatin. In fact, it was recently reported an association between DNA fragmentation and chromatin defects in old individuals [96, 97]. The chromatin structure of human sperm is highly condensed and organized. During spermiogenesis, sperm chromatin undergoes a series of modifications in which histones are replaced by protamines 1 and 2 (P1 and P2) to form a tight toroidal structure. This organization is essential to protect sperm DNA from oxidative damage and is particularly resistant to ROS attack [98]. Altered P1:P2 ratio, leads to an abnormal protamination compromising DNA integrity [99 - 101]. As a result, DNA becomes "exposed" to the damages of ROS. The oxidative damages primarily occur at the guanine bases and causes the formation of adducts, the most common of which are 8-hydroxy-2′-deoxyguanosine and 8–oxo-7,8-dihydro-2′-deoxyguanosine. Moreover, sperm are able to produce ROS during the events associated with sperm post-ejaculatory journey. For instance, hydrogen peroxide, superoxide anion and peroxynitrite radical are generated during sperm capacitation. In sperm the majority of these reactive oxygen metabolites are generated due to electron leakage from sperm mitochondria [102]. On the other hand, the nicotinamide adenine dinucleotide phosphate oxidases may also generate ROS [103]. DNA fragmentation associated with advanced paternal age has been implicated in a broad range of abnormal reproductive outcomes, which include declined sperm quality [104] and reduced fertility [104].

PATERNAL AGE AND EPIGENETIC RISKS

The number of couples deciding to become parents later in life has increased in the last few years, not only due to professional and social reasons, but also by the use of several methods of contraception, which contributes to the postponement of parenthood to middle or old age. Later parenthood is considered by many to have advantages and in many cases men have constituted a second family later in life. Consequently, paternal age becomes an issue increasingly discussed and studied that must continue to gain attention for discussion in the next decades [2, 105]. It is well established that children born from older parents are exposed to higher risk for genetic disorders. This fact is well described and supported, especially for women who are mothers at a later age. Advanced paternal age is a risk factor for a wide range of health conditions in the offspring . These may include spontaneous dominant disorders, congenital anomalies, neurological diseases (*e.g.* schizophrenia and autism) and some types of childhood cancers [106 - 113]. Moreover, it was demonstrated that children of older parents have a higher prevalence not only of childhood cancers but also of certain sporadic nervous system cancers [114, 115].

Epigenetic changes, mainly DNA methylation, have been associated with age-related diseases. Furthermore, these modifications are also associated with increased advanced paternal age, along with mutations in DNA and chromosomal aneuploidies. It is important to consider the degree to which sperm are susceptible to epigenetic modifications induced by aging that could lead not only to embryonic dysfunction, but also to diseases in the offspring. Some of these alterations may be passed to the next generations and due to the "plasticity" of epigenetic modifications, sperm epigenetics has become one of the major hot topics for research worldwide. Few studies have been performed and it seems that the pattern of sperm methylation induced by aging show remarkable differences than what was observed in somatic cells [116]. Intriguingly, it has been proposed that there is an increase in the global level of methylation in human sperm from old individuals, while regionally there is a bias toward methylation loss [116]. In fact, it has been demonstrated that specific genomic regions of DNA methylation are commonly altered with age and some regions of the sperm genome are more susceptible than others to age-associated epigenetic alterations [116]. In this context, it has been identified a regional loss of DNA methylation in the sperm of old mice, whilst no global changes were observed [117]. Moreover, the finding that CpG islands (CGI) shores, rather than in the islands themselves, are abnormally methylated in the offspring of old fathers suggests that advanced paternal age has large impact on gene expression and possible implications in the offspring's health. It was recently evidenced that paternal age is associated with reduced methylation and variation of the transcriptional regulator Forkhead Box K1 (FOXK1) and the potassium voltage-gated channel subfamily A member 7 in sperm. It has been showed that paternal age is not only associated with FOXK1 hypomethylation in sperm, but also with reduced methylation of the paternal allele in somatic cells of the offspring. Alarmingly, these age-related genes are associated with neuropsychiatric and other disorders [118]. These evidence indicate that some of the abnormalities in sperm DNA methylation of old fathers are transferred to the offspring, and that epigenetic reprogramming erases some but not all of these modifications. As age advances, sperm DNA become particularly sensitive to demethylation and the residual nucleosomes, resultant from the chromatin dynamics, are specifically retained at unmethylated CpG-dense regions, such as CGI promoters [119]. This may suggest a mechanism by which CGI shores are more susceptible to methylation abnormalities in sperm. Interestingly, the retention of nucleosomes in sperm is associated with the establishment of DNA methylation-free regions in the early embryo [119] and this has been proposed as a possible mechanism for transgenerational inheritance [119, 120].

CONCLUDING REMARKS

The deterioration of testicular endocrine function has been a matter of great debate and this is due to the fact that many of the symptoms involved in the decline of well-being associated with aging (such as frailty, depression and worsened sexual function) have been related to the decline of testicular androgen production. In light of new population-based studies, the existence of the clinical and biochemical syndrome known as LOH has been confirmed, but its incidence appears to be lower than originally estimated. It is generally accepted that LOH constitutes a predictive value for the entire well-being of a man and may identify him as a high risk candidate for multiple diseases. Most authors recommend the use of replacement therapy even at the initial manifestations as testosterone levels decrease and there is a presence of specific sexual clinical manifestations. Nevertheless, there is not yet full agreement on the risk-benefit index in testosterone replacement therapy.

Aging also contributes to the decline of spermatozoa quality, by affecting essential parameters such as sperm motility, morphology and its numbers. This is in part due to the accumulated damages caused by the aging-induced oxidative stress. So it will be essential to explore in depth the underlying mechanisms of aging-induced oxidative since there is compelling evidence that it may hamper the function of spermatozoa. Furthermore, advanced paternal age has been associated with epigenetic alterations in sperm, namely abnormalities in DNA methylation. This is of major relevance, since some of these epigenetic alterations are heritable, which prompts the offspring to develop several congenital disorders, neurological and metabolic diseases and even cancer.

Box 14.1 | Summary

- Aged father is an increasing social phenomenon.
- Increased paternal age is related to decreased fertility.
- There are two types of treatment for LOH: testosterone replacement therapy and lifestyle modification.
- There is a need to improve the knowledge concerning the benefits and risks of testosterone replacement therapy.
- Advanced paternal age is linked with a negative impact on the quality of spermatozoa.
- Epigenetics of sperm seem to be implicated in the offspring disease susceptibility.
- Children of older fathers show increased risk for congenital

CONFLICT OF INTEREST

The authors confirm that they have no conflict of interest to declare for this publication.

ACKNOWLEDGEMENTS

This work was supported by the “Fundação para a Ciência e a Tecnologia”–FCT (PTDC/BBB-BQB/1368/2014), UMIB (PEst-OE/SAU/UI0215/2014); and of FEDER through the POPH and POCI - COMPETE 2020 (POCI-01-01-

5-FEDER-007491) funds. Susana Almeida (SFRH/BD/112012/2015) was also financed by FCT. Luís Rato is funded by Santander Totta/University of Beira Interior (BIPD/ICI-CICS-BST-UBI).

REFERENCES

[1] Mahmoud AM, Goemaere S, El-Garem Y, Van Pottelbergh I, Comhaire FH, Kaufman JM. Testicular volume in relation to hormonal indices of gonadal function in community-dwelling elderly men. J Clin Endocrinol Metab 2003; 88(1): 179-84.
[http://dx.doi.org/10.1210/jc.2002-020408] [PMID: 12519849]

[2] Zitzmann M. Effects of age on male fertility. Best Pract Res Clin Endocrinol Metab 2013; 27(4): 617-28.
[http://dx.doi.org/10.1016/j.beem.2013.07.004] [PMID: 24054934]

[3] Singh P. Andropause: Current concepts. Indian J Endocrinol Metab 2013; 17 (Suppl. 3): S621-9.
[http://dx.doi.org/10.4103/2230-8210.123552] [PMID: 24910824]

[4] Dohle G, Arver S, Bettocchi C, Kliesch S, Punab M, De Ronde W. Guidelines on male hypogonadism. Eur Association Urolo 2015.

[5] Lamberts SW, van den Beld AW, van der Lely AJ. The endocrinology of aging. Science 1997; 278(5337): 419-24.
[http://dx.doi.org/10.1126/science.278.5337.419] [PMID: 9334293]

[6] Perheentupa A, Huhtaniemi I. Aging of the human ovary and testis. Mol Cell Endocrinol 2009; 299(1): 2-13.
[http://dx.doi.org/10.1016/j.mce.2008.11.004] [PMID: 19059459]

[7] Huhtaniemi I. Late-onset hypogonadism: current concepts and controversies of pathogenesis, diagnosis and treatment. Asian J Androl 2014; 16(2): 192-202.
[http://dx.doi.org/10.4103/1008-682X.122336] [PMID: 24407185]

[8] Auger J, Kunstmann JM, Czyglik F, Jouannet P. Decline in semen quality among fertile men in Paris during the past 20 years. N Engl J Med 1995; 332(5): 281-5.
[http://dx.doi.org/10.1056/NEJM199502023320501] [PMID: 7816062]

[9] Centola GM, Eberly S. Seasonal variations and age-related changes in human sperm count, motility, motion parameters, morphology, and white blood cell concentration. Fertil Steril 1999; 72(5): 803-8.
[http://dx.doi.org/10.1016/S0015-0282(99)00395-7] [PMID: 10560981]

[10] Dondero F, Mazzilli F, Giovenco P, Lenzi A, Cerasaro M. Fertility in elderly men. J Endocrinol Invest 1985; 8 (Suppl. 2): 87-91.
[PMID: 4031398]

[11] Fisch H, Goluboff ET, Olson JH, Feldshuh J, Broder SJ, Barad DH. Semen analyses in 1,283 men from the United States over a 25-year period: no decline in quality. Fertil Steril 1996; 65(5): 1009-14.
[http://dx.doi.org/10.1016/S0015-0282(16)58278-8] [PMID: 8612826]

[12] Haidl G, Jung A, Schill W-B. Ageing and sperm function. Hum Reprod 1996; 11(3): 558-60.
[http://dx.doi.org/10.1093/HUMREP/11.3.558] [PMID: 8671265]

[13] Johnson L, Abdo JG, Petty CS, Neaves WB. Effect of age on the composition of seminiferous tubular boundary tissue and on the volume of each component in humans. Fertil Steril 1988; 49(6): 1045-51.
[http://dx.doi.org/10.1016/S0015-0282(16)59959-2] [PMID: 3371482]

[14] Plas E, Berger P, Hermann M, Pflüger H. Effects of aging on male fertility? Exp Gerontol 2000; 35(5): 543-51.
[http://dx.doi.org/10.1016/S0531-5565(00)00120-0] [PMID: 10978677]

[15] Sasano N, Ichijo S. Vascular patterns of the human testis with special reference to its senile changes. Tohoku J Exp Med 1969; 99(3): 269-80.
[http://dx.doi.org/10.1620/tjem.99.269] [PMID: 5363446]

[16] Dakouane Giudicelli M, Serazin V, Le Sciellour CR, Albert M, Selva J, Giudicelli Y. Increased achondroplasia mutation frequency with advanced age and evidence for G1138A mosaicism in human testis biopsies. Fertil Steril 2008; 89(6): 1651-6.
[http://dx.doi.org/10.1016/j.fertnstert.2007.04.037] [PMID: 17706214]

[17] Handelsman DJ, Staraj S. Testicular size: the effects of aging, malnutrition, and illness. J Androl 1985; 6(3): 144-51.
[http://dx.doi.org/10.1002/j.1939-4640.1985.tb00830.x] [PMID: 3997660]

[18] Yang H, Chryssikos T, Houseni M, *et al.* The effects of aging on testicular volume and glucose metabolism: an investigation with ultrasonography and FDG-PET. Mol Imaging Biol 2011; 13(2): 391-8.
[http://dx.doi.org/10.1007/s11307-010-0341-x] [PMID: 20521135]

[19] Basaria S. Reproductive aging in men. Endocrinol Metab Clin North Am 2013; 42(2): 255-70.
[http://dx.doi.org/10.1016/j.ecl.2013.02.012] [PMID: 23702400]

[20] Well D, Yang H, Houseni M, *et al.* Age-related structural and metabolic changes in the pelvic reproductive end organs. Semin Nucl Med 2007; 37(3): 173-84.
[http://dx.doi.org/10.1053/j.semnuclmed.2007.01.004] [PMID: 17418150]

[21] Zenzmaier C, Untergasser G, Berger P. Aging of the prostate epithelial stem/progenitor cell. Exp Gerontol 2008; 43(11): 981-5.
[http://dx.doi.org/10.1016/j.exger.2008.06.008] [PMID: 18639623]

[22] Jones CM, Boelaert K. The Endocrinology of Ageing: A Mini-Review. Gerontology 2015; 61(4): 291-300.
[http://dx.doi.org/10.1159/000367692] [PMID: 25471682]

[23] Gunes S, Hekim GN, Arslan MA, Asci R. Effects of aging on the male reproductive system. J Assist Reprod Genet 2016; 33(4): 441-54.
[http://dx.doi.org/10.1007/s10815-016-0663-y] [PMID: 26867640]

[24] Veldhuis JD, Keenan DM, Liu PY, Iranmanesh A, Takahashi PY, Nehra AX. The aging male hypothalamic-pituitary-gonadal axis: pulsatility and feedback. Mol Cell Endocrinol 2009; 299(1): 14-22.
[http://dx.doi.org/10.1016/j.mce.2008.09.005] [PMID: 18838102]

[25] Stone BA, Alex A, Werlin LB, Marrs RP. Age thresholds for changes in semen parameters in men. Fertil Steril 2013; 100(4): 952-8.
[http://dx.doi.org/10.1016/j.fertnstert.2013.05.046] [PMID: 23809502]

[26] Neaves WB, Johnson L, Porter JC, Parker CR Jr, Petty CS. Leydig cell numbers, daily sperm production, and serum gonadotropin levels in aging men. J Clin Endocrinol Metab 1984; 59(4): 756-63.
[http://dx.doi.org/10.1210/jcem-59-4-756] [PMID: 6434579]

[27] Pasqualotto FF, Sobreiro BP, Hallak J, Pasqualotto EB, Lucon AM. Sperm concentration and normal sperm morphology decrease and follicle-stimulating hormone level increases with age. BJU Int 2005; 96(7): 1087-91.
[http://dx.doi.org/10.1111/j.1464-410X.2005.05806.x] [PMID: 16225533]

[28] Baccarelli A, Morpurgo PS, Corsi A, *et al.* Activin A serum levels and aging of the pituitary-gonadal axis: a cross-sectional study in middle-aged and elderly healthy subjects. Exp Gerontol 2001; 36(8): 1403-12.
[http://dx.doi.org/10.1016/S0531-5565(01)00117-6] [PMID: 11602213]

[29] Comhaire FH. Andropause: hormone replacement therapy in the ageing male. Eur Urol 2000; 38(6): 655-62.
[http://dx.doi.org/10.1159/000020358] [PMID: 11111180]

[30] Brinkmann AO. Molecular basis of androgen insensitivity. Mol Cell Endocrinol 2001; 179(1-2): 105-9.
[http://dx.doi.org/10.1016/S0303-7207(01)00466-X] [PMID: 11420135]

[31] Hyde Z, Flicker L, Almeida OP, *et al.* Low free testosterone predicts frailty in older men: the health in men study. J Clin Endocrinol Metab 2010; 95(7): 3165-72.
[http://dx.doi.org/10.1210/jc.2009-2754] [PMID: 20410223]

[32] Yeap BB. Hormones and health outcomes in aging men. Exp Gerontol 2013; 48(7): 677-81.
[http://dx.doi.org/10.1016/j.exger.2012.07.012] [PMID: 22884846]

[33] Parr BA, McMahon AP. Sexually dimorphic development of the mammalian reproductive tract requires Wnt-7a. Nature 1998; 395(6703): 707-10.
[http://dx.doi.org/10.1038/27221] [PMID: 9790192]

[34] Hannema SE, Print CG, Charnock-Jones DS, Coleman N, Hughes IA. Changes in gene expression during Wolffian duct development. Horm Res 2006; 65(4): 200-9.
[PMID: 16567946]

[35] Belchetz PE, Barth JH, Kaufman JM. Biochemical endocrinology of the hypogonadal male. Ann Clin Biochem 2010; 47(Pt 6): 503-15.
[http://dx.doi.org/10.1258/acb.2010.010150] [PMID: 20956400]

[36] Jakiel G, Makara-Studzińska M, Ciebiera M, Słabuszewska-Jóźwiak A. Andropause - state of the art 2015 and review of selected aspects. Prz Menopauzalny 2015; 14(1): 1-6.
[http://dx.doi.org/10.5114/pm.2015.49998] [PMID: 26327881]

[37] Kaufman JM, Vermeulen A. The decline of androgen levels in elderly men and its clinical and therapeutic implications. Endocr Rev 2005; 26(6): 833-76.
[http://dx.doi.org/10.1210/er.2004-0013] [PMID: 15901667]

[38] Feldman HA, Longcope C, Derby CA, *et al.* Age trends in the level of serum testosterone and other hormones in middle-aged men: longitudinal results from the Massachusetts male aging study. J Clin Endocrinol Metab 2002; 87(2): 589-98.
[http://dx.doi.org/10.1210/jcem.87.2.8201] [PMID: 11836290]

[39] Pirke KM, Sintermann R, Vogt HJ. Testosterone and testosterone precursors in the spermatic vein and in the testicular tissue of old men. Reduced oxygen supply may explain the relative increase of testicular progesterone and 17 alpha-hydroxyprogesterone content and production in old age. Gerontology 1980; 26(4): 221-30.
[http://dx.doi.org/10.1159/000212418] [PMID: 7372101]

[40] Hammar M. Impaired in vitro testicular endocrine function in elderly men. Andrologia 1985; 17(5): 444-9.
[http://dx.doi.org/10.1111/j.1439-0272.1985.tb01039.x] [PMID: 3933382]

[41] Ferrini RL, Barrett-Connor E. Sex hormones and age: a cross-sectional study of testosterone and estradiol and their bioavailable fractions in community-dwelling men. Am J Epidemiol 1998; 147(8): 750-4.
[http://dx.doi.org/10.1093/oxfordjournals.aje.a009519] [PMID: 9554416]

[42] Morley JE, Kaiser FE, Perry HM III, *et al.* Longitudinal changes in testosterone, luteinizing hormone, and follicle-stimulating hormone in healthy older men. Metabolism 1997; 46(4): 410-3.
[http://dx.doi.org/10.1016/S0026-0495(97)90057-3] [PMID: 9109845]

[43] Wu FC, Tajar A, Pye SR, *et al.* Hypothalamic-pituitary-testicular axis disruptions in older men are differentially linked to age and modifiable risk factors: the European Male Aging Study. J Clin Endocrinol Metab 2008; 93(7): 2737-45.
[http://dx.doi.org/10.1210/jc.2007-1972] [PMID: 18270261]

[44] Harman SM, Metter EJ, Tobin JD, Pearson J, Blackman MR. Longitudinal effects of aging on serum total and free testosterone levels in healthy men. J Clin Endocrinol Metab 2001; 86(2): 724-31.
[http://dx.doi.org/10.1210/jcem.86.2.7219] [PMID: 11158037]

[45] Araujo AB, Esche GR, Kupelian V, *et al.* Prevalence of symptomatic androgen deficiency in men. J Clin Endocrinol Metab 2007; 92(11): 4241-7.
[http://dx.doi.org/10.1210/jc.2007-1245] [PMID: 17698901]

[46] Travison TG, Araujo AB, Kupelian V, ODonnell AB, McKinlay JB. The relative contributions of aging, health, and lifestyle factors to serum testosterone decline in men. J Clin Endocrinol Metab 2007; 92(2): 549-55.
[http://dx.doi.org/10.1210/jc.2006-1859] [PMID: 17148559]

[47] Huhtaniemi IT. Andropauselessons from the European Male Ageing Study. Ann Endocrinol (Paris) 2014; 75(2): 128-31.
[http://dx.doi.org/10.1016/j.ando.2014.03.005] [PMID: 24793989]

[48] Heller CG, Myers GB. The male climacteric, its symptomatology, diagnosis and treatment: use of urinary gonadotropins, therapeutic test with testosterone propionate and testicular biopsies in delineating the male climacteric from psychoneurosis and psychogenic impotence. JAMA 1944; 126: 472-7.
[http://dx.doi.org/10.1001/jama.1944.02850430006003]

[49] Schubert M, Jockenhövel F. Late-onset hypogonadism in the aging male (LOH): definition, diagnostic and clinical aspects. J Endocrinol Invest 2005; 28(3) (Suppl.): 23-7.
[PMID: 16042356]

[50] Huhtaniemi I, Forti G. Male late-onset hypogonadism: pathogenesis, diagnosis and treatment. Nat Rev Urol 2011; 8(6): 335-44.
[http://dx.doi.org/10.1038/nrurol.2011.47] [PMID: 21502974]

[51] Wang C, Nieschlag E, Swerdloff R, *et al.* Investigation, treatment and monitoring of late-onset hypogonadism in males. Int J Androl 2009; 32(1): 1-10.
[http://dx.doi.org/10.1111/j.1365-2605.2008.00924.x] [PMID: 18798761]

[52] Araujo AB, Dixon JM, Suarez EA, Murad MH, Guey LT, Wittert GA. Clinical review: Endogenous testosterone and mortality in men: a systematic review and meta-analysis. J Clin Endocrinol Metab 2011; 96(10): 3007-19.
[http://dx.doi.org/10.1210/jc.2011-1137] [PMID: 21816776]

[53] Bhasin S, Bagatell CJ, Bremner WJ, *et al.* Issues in testosterone replacement in older men. J Clin Endocrinol Metab 1998; 83(10): 3435-48.
[http://dx.doi.org/10.1210/jcem.83.10.5060-1] [PMID: 9768643]

[54] Sofimajidpour H, Teimoori T, Gharibi F. The Effect of Testosterone on Men With Andropause. Iran Red Crescent Med J 2015; 17(12): e19406.
[http://dx.doi.org/10.5812/ircmj.19406] [PMID: 26756004]

[55] Parsons JK, Carter HB, Platz EA, Wright EJ, Landis P, Metter EJ. Serum testosterone and the risk of prostate cancer: potential implications for testosterone therapy. Cancer Epidemiol Biomarkers Prev 2005; 14(9): 2257-60.
[http://dx.doi.org/10.1158/1055-9965.EPI-04-0715] [PMID: 16172240]

[56] Calof OM, Singh AB, Lee ML, *et al.* Adverse events associated with testosterone replacement in middle-aged and older men: a meta-analysis of randomized, placebo-controlled trials. J Gerontol A Biol Sci Med Sci 2005; 60(11): 1451-7.
[http://dx.doi.org/10.1093/gerona/60.11.1451] [PMID: 16339333]

[57] Zitzmann M, Nieschlag E. Androgen receptor gene CAG repeat length and body mass index modulate the safety of long-term intramuscular testosterone undecanoate therapy in hypogonadal men. J Clin Endocrinol Metab 2007; 92(10): 3844-53.
[http://dx.doi.org/10.1210/jc.2007-0620] [PMID: 17635942]

[58] Wang C, Swerdloff R, Kipnes M, *et al.* New testosterone buccal system (Striant) delivers physiological testosterone levels: pharmacokinetics study in hypogonadal men. J Clin Endocrinol Metab 2004; 89(8): 3821-9.
[http://dx.doi.org/10.1210/jc.2003-031866] [PMID: 15292312]

[59] Bassil N, Alkaade S, Morley JE. The benefits and risks of testosterone replacement therapy: a review. Ther Clin Risk Manag 2009; 5(3): 427-48.
[PMID: 19707253]

[60] Wang C, Harnett M, Dobs AS, Swerdloff RS. Pharmacokinetics and safety of long-acting testosterone undecanoate injections in hypogonadal men: an 84-week phase III clinical trial. J Androl 2010; 31(5): 457-65.
[http://dx.doi.org/10.2164/jandrol.109.009597] [PMID: 20133964]

[61] Bhasin S, Bremner WJ. Clinical review 85: Emerging issues in androgen replacement therapy. J Clin Endocrinol Metab 1997; 82(1): 3-8.
[PMID: 8989221]

[62] Lakshman KM, Basaria S. Safety and efficacy of testosterone gel in the treatment of male hypogonadism. Clin Interv Aging 2009; 4: 397-412.
[PMID: 19966909]

[63] Swerdloff RS, Wang C. Transdermal androgens: pharmacology and applicability to hypogonadal elderly men. J Endocrinol Invest 2005; 28(3) (Suppl.): 112-6.
[PMID: 16042369]

[64] Salehian B, Wang C, Alexander G, *et al.* Pharmacokinetics, bioefficacy, and safety of sublingual testosterone cyclodextrin in hypogonadal men: comparison to testosterone enanthatea clinical research center study. J Clin Endocrinol Metab 1995; 80(12): 3567-75.
[PMID: 8530600]

[65] Jockenhövel F, Vogel E, Kreutzer M, Reinhardt W, Lederbogen S, Reinwein D. Pharmacokinetics and pharmacodynamics of subcutaneous testosterone implants in hypogonadal men. Clin Endocrinol (Oxf) 1996; 45(1): 61-71.
[http://dx.doi.org/10.1111/j.1365-2265.1996.tb02061.x] [PMID: 8796140]

[66] Kelleher S, Conway AJ, Handelsman DJ. Influence of implantation site and track geometry on the extrusion rate and pharmacology of testosterone implants. Clin Endocrinol (Oxf) 2001; 55(4): 531-6.
[http://dx.doi.org/10.1046/j.1365-2265.2001.01357.x] [PMID: 11678837]

[67] Bhasin S, Cunningham GR, Hayes FJ, *et al.* Testosterone therapy in men with androgen deficiency syndromes: an Endocrine Society clinical practice guideline. J Clin Endocrinol Metab 2010; 95(6): 2536-59.
[http://dx.doi.org/10.1210/jc.2009-2354] [PMID: 20525905]

[68] Lawson G, Fletcher R. Delayed fatherhood. J Fam Plann Reprod Health Care 2014; 40(4): 283-8.
[http://dx.doi.org/10.1136/jfprhc-2013-100866] [PMID: 24958072]

[69] Selvaratnam JS, Robaire B. Effects of Aging and Oxidative Stress on Spermatozoa of Superoxide-Dismutase 1- and Catalase-Null Mice. Biol Reprod 2016; 95(3): 60.
[http://dx.doi.org/10.1095/biolreprod.116.141671] [PMID: 27465136]

[70] Nieschlag E, Lammers U, Freischem CW, Langer K, Wickings EJ. Reproductive functions in young fathers and grandfathers. J Clin Endocrinol Metab 1982; 55(4): 676-81. [http://dx.doi.org/10.1210/jcem-55-4-676] [PMID: 6809780]

[71] Schwartz D, Mayaux M-J, Spira A, *et al.* Semen characteristics as a function of age in 833 fertile men. Fertil Steril 1983; 39(4): 530-5. [http://dx.doi.org/10.1016/S0015-0282(16)46946-3] [PMID: 6832409]

[72] Wang C, Chan SY, Leung A, *et al.* Cross-sectional study of semen parameters in a large group of normal Chinese men. Int J Androl 1985; 8(4): 257-74. [http://dx.doi.org/10.1111/j.1365-2605.1985.tb00840.x] [PMID: 4077284]

[73] Irvine S, Cawood E, Richardson D, MacDonald E, Aitken J. Evidence of deteriorating semen quality in the United Kingdom: birth cohort study in 577 men in Scotland over 11 years. BMJ 1996; 312(7029): 467-71. [http://dx.doi.org/10.1136/bmj.312.7029.467] [PMID: 8597676]

[74] Agarwal A, Sekhon LH. Oxidative stress and antioxidants for idiopathic oligoasthenoteratospermia: Is it justified? Indian J Urol 2011; 27(1): 74-85. [http://dx.doi.org/10.4103/0970-1591.78437] [PMID: 21716893]

[75] Brahem S, Mehdi M, Elghezal H, Saad A. The effects of male aging on semen quality, sperm DNA fragmentation and chromosomal abnormalities in an infertile population. J Assist Reprod Genet 2011; 28(5): 425-32. [http://dx.doi.org/10.1007/s10815-011-9537-5] [PMID: 21287403]

[76] Sharma R, Agarwal A, Rohra VK, Assidi M, Abu-Elmagd M, Turki RF. Effects of increased paternal age on sperm quality, reproductive outcome and associated epigenetic risks to offspring. Reprod Biol Endocrinol 2015; 13: 35. [http://dx.doi.org/10.1186/s12958-015-0028-x] [PMID: 25928123]

[77] Homonnai ZT, Fainman N, David MP, Paz GF. Semen quality and sex hormone pattern of 29 middle aged men. Andrologia 1982; 14(2): 164-70. [http://dx.doi.org/10.1111/j.1439-0272.1982.tb03119.x] [PMID: 6808865]

[78] Check JH, Shanis B, Bollendorf A, Adelson H, Breen E. Semen characteristics and infertility in aging. Arch Androl 1989; 23(3): 275-7. [http://dx.doi.org/10.3109/01485018908986851] [PMID: 2694997]

[79] Gallardo E, Simón C, Levy M, Guanes PP, Remohí J, Pellicer A. Effect of age on sperm fertility potential: oocyte donation as a model. Fertil Steril 1996; 66(2): 260-4. [http://dx.doi.org/10.1016/S0015-0282(16)58450-7] [PMID: 8690113]

[80] Bujan L, Mansat A, Pontonnier F, Mieusset R. Time series analysis of sperm concentration in fertile men in Toulouse, France between 1977 and 1992. BMJ 1996; 312(7029): 471-2. [http://dx.doi.org/10.1136/bmj.312.7029.471] [PMID: 8597677]

[81] Mladenović I, Mićić S, Papić N, Genbaćev O, Marinković B. Sperm morphology and motility in different age populations. Arch Androl 1994; 32(3): 197-205. [http://dx.doi.org/10.3109/01485019408987786] [PMID: 8074574]

[82] Rolf C, Behre HM, Nieschlag E. Reproductive parameters of older compared to younger men of infertile couples. Int J Androl 1996; 19(3): 135-42. [http://dx.doi.org/10.1111/j.1365-2605.1996.tb00451.x] [PMID: 8876262]

[83] Kidd SA, Eskenazi B, Wyrobek AJ. Effects of male age on semen quality and fertility: a review of the literature. Fertil Steril 2001; 75(2): 237-48. [http://dx.doi.org/10.1016/S0015-0282(00)01679-4] [PMID: 11172821]

[84] Cooper TG, Noonan E, von Eckardstein S, *et al.* World Health Organization reference values for human semen characteristics. Hum Reprod Update 2010; 16(3): 231-45. [http://dx.doi.org/10.1093/humupd/dmp048] [PMID: 19934213]

[85] Organisation WH. WHO laboratory manual for the examination of human semen and sperm-cervical mucus interaction: Cambridge university press 1999.

[86] Cocuzza M, Athayde KS, Agarwal A, *et al.* Age-related increase of reactive oxygen species in neat semen in healthy fertile men. Urology 2008; 71(3): 490-4.
[http://dx.doi.org/10.1016/j.urology.2007.11.041] [PMID: 18342194]

[87] Mueller A, Hermo L, Robaire B. The effects of aging on the expression of glutathione S-transferases in the testis and epididymis of the Brown Norway rat. J Androl 1998; 19(4): 450-65.
[PMID: 9733148]

[88] Jervis KM, Robaire B. The effects of long-term vitamin E treatment on gene expression and oxidative stress damage in the aging Brown Norway rat epididymis. Biol Reprod 2004; 71(4): 1088-95.
[http://dx.doi.org/10.1095/biolreprod.104.028886] [PMID: 15175234]

[89] Dufaure J-P, Lareyre J-J, Schwaab V, Mattei M-G, Drevet JR. Structural organization, chromosomal localization, expression and phylogenetic evaluation of mouse glutathione peroxidase encoding genes. C R Acad Sci III 1996; 319(7): 559-68.
[PMID: 9011320]

[90] Halliwell B, Gutteridge JM. Oxygen toxicity, oxygen radicals, transition metals and disease. Biochem J 1984; 219(1): 1-14.
[http://dx.doi.org/10.1042/bj2190001] [PMID: 6326753]

[91] Baker MA, Weinberg A, Hetherington L, *et al.* Defining the mechanisms by which the reactive oxygen species by-product, 4-hydroxynonenal, affects human sperm cell function. Biol Reprod 2015. biolreprod. 114.126680.

[92] Moazamian R, Polhemus A, Connaughton H, *et al.* Oxidative stress and human spermatozoa: diagnostic and functional significance of aldehydes generated as a result of lipid peroxidation. Mol Hum Reprod 2015; 21(6): 502-15.
[http://dx.doi.org/10.1093/molehr/gav014] [PMID: 25837702]

[93] Belloc S, Benkhalifa M, Junca AM, Dumont M, Bacrie PC, Ménézo Y. Paternal age and sperm DNA decay: discrepancy between chromomycin and aniline blue staining. Reprod Biomed Online 2009; 19(2): 264-9.
[http://dx.doi.org/10.1016/S1472-6483(10)60083-1] [PMID: 19712565]

[94] Plastira K, Msaouel P, Angelopoulou R, *et al.* The effects of age on DNA fragmentation, chromatin packaging and conventional semen parameters in spermatozoa of oligoasthenoteratozoospermic patients. J Assist Reprod Genet 2007; 24(10): 437-43.
[http://dx.doi.org/10.1007/s10815-007-9162-5] [PMID: 17768675]

[95] Schmid TE, Grant PG, Marchetti F, Weldon RH, Eskenazi B, Wyrobek AJ. Elemental composition of human semen is associated with motility and genomic sperm defects among older men. Hum Reprod 2013; 28(1): 274-82.
[http://dx.doi.org/10.1093/humrep/des321] [PMID: 23042799]

[96] Barroso G, Morshedi M, Oehninger S. Analysis of DNA fragmentation, plasma membrane translocation of phosphatidylserine and oxidative stress in human spermatozoa. Hum Reprod 2000; 15(6): 1338-44.
[http://dx.doi.org/10.1093/humrep/15.6.1338] [PMID: 10831565]

[97] Ozkosem B, Feinstein SI, Fisher AB, OFlaherty C. Advancing age increases sperm chromatin damage and impairs fertility in peroxiredoxin 6 null mice. Redox Biol 2015; 5: 15-23.
[http://dx.doi.org/10.1016/j.redox.2015.02.004] [PMID: 25796034]

[98] Schulte RT, Ohl DA, Sigman M, Smith GD. Sperm DNA damage in male infertility: etiologies, assays, and outcomes. J Assist Reprod Genet 2010; 27(1): 3-12.
[http://dx.doi.org/10.1007/s10815-009-9359-x] [PMID: 20012685]

[99] Aoki VW, Emery BR, Liu L, Carrell DT. Protamine levels vary between individual sperm cells of

infertile human males and correlate with viability and DNA integrity. J Androl 2006; 27(6): 890-8. [http://dx.doi.org/10.2164/jandrol.106.000703] [PMID: 16870950]

[100] Aoki VW, Moskovtsev SI, Willis J, Liu L, Mullen JB, Carrell DT. DNA integrity is compromised in protamine-deficient human sperm. J Androl 2005; 26(6): 741-8. [http://dx.doi.org/10.2164/jandrol.05063] [PMID: 16291969]

[101] Carrell DT, Liu L. Altered protamine 2 expression is uncommon in donors of known fertility, but common among men with poor fertilizing capacity, and may reflect other abnormalities of spermiogenesis. J Androl 2001; 22(4): 604-10. [PMID: 11451357]

[102] Koppers AJ, De Iuliis GN, Finnie JM, McLaughlin EA, Aitken RJ. Significance of mitochondrial reactive oxygen species in the generation of oxidative stress in spermatozoa. J Clin Endocrinol Metab 2008; 93(8): 3199-207. [http://dx.doi.org/10.1210/jc.2007-2616] [PMID: 18492763]

[103] Bánfi B, Molnár G, Maturana A, *et al.* A Ca(2+)-activated NADPH oxidase in testis, spleen, and lymph nodes. J Biol Chem 2001; 276(40): 37594-601. [http://dx.doi.org/10.1074/jbc.M103034200] [PMID: 11483596]

[104] Eskenazi B, Wyrobek AJ, Sloter E, *et al.* The association of age and semen quality in healthy men. Hum Reprod 2003; 18(2): 447-54. [http://dx.doi.org/10.1093/humrep/deg107] [PMID: 12571189]

[105] Balasch J. Ageing and infertility: an overview. Gynecol Endocrinol 2010; 26(12): 855-60. [http://dx.doi.org/10.3109/09513590.2010.501889] [PMID: 20642380]

[106] Chianese C, Brilli S, Krausz C. Genomic changes in spermatozoa of the aging male Genetic Damage in Human Spermatozoa. Springer 2014; pp. 13-26. [http://dx.doi.org/10.1007/978-1-4614-7783-9_2]

[107] Martin AK, Robinson G, Reutens D, Mowry B. Clinical and parental age characteristics of rare copy number variant burden in patients with schizophrenia. Am J Med Genet B Neuropsychiatr Genet 2015; 168B(5): 374-82. [http://dx.doi.org/10.1002/ajmg.b.32321] [PMID: 25943776]

[108] McIntosh GC, Olshan AF, Baird PA. Paternal age and the risk of birth defects in offspring. Epidemiology 1995; 6(3): 282-8. [http://dx.doi.org/10.1097/00001648-199505000-00016] [PMID: 7619937]

[109] Zhu JL, Madsen KM, Vestergaard M, Olesen AV, Basso O, Olsen J. Paternal age and congenital malformations. Hum Reprod 2005; 20(11): 3173-7. [http://dx.doi.org/10.1093/humrep/dei186] [PMID: 16006461]

[110] Lampi KM, Hinkka-Yli-Salomäki S, Lehti V, *et al.* Parental age and risk of autism spectrum disorders in a Finnish national birth cohort. J Autism Dev Disord 2013; 43(11): 2526-35. [http://dx.doi.org/10.1007/s10803-013-1801-3] [PMID: 23479075]

[111] Sandin S, Lichtenstein P, Kuja-Halkola R, Larsson H, Hultman CM, Reichenberg A. The familial risk of autism. JAMA 2014; 311(17): 1770-7. [http://dx.doi.org/10.1001/jama.2014.4144] [PMID: 24794370]

[112] Frans EM, Sandin S, Reichenberg A, Lichtenstein P, Långström N, Hultman CM. Advancing paternal age and bipolar disorder. Arch Gen Psychiatry 2008; 65(9): 1034-40. [http://dx.doi.org/10.1001/archpsyc.65.9.1034] [PMID: 18762589]

[113] Weiser M, Reichenberg A, Werbeloff N, *et al.* Advanced parental age at birth is associated with poorer social functioning in adolescent males: shedding light on a core symptom of schizophrenia and autism. Schizophr Bull 2008; 34(6): 1042-6. [http://dx.doi.org/10.1093/schbul/sbn109] [PMID: 18796466]

[114] Hemminki K, Kyyrönen P. Parental age and risk of sporadic and familial cancer in offspring:

implications for germ cell mutagenesis. Epidemiology 1999; 10(6): 747-51. [http://dx.doi.org/10.1097/00001648-199911000-00016] [PMID: 10535790]

[115] Yip BH, Pawitan Y, Czene K. Parental age and risk of childhood cancers: a population-based cohort study from Sweden. Int J Epidemiol 2006; 35(6): 1495-503. [http://dx.doi.org/10.1093/ije/dyl177] [PMID: 17008361]

[116] Jenkins TG, Aston KI, Pflueger C, Cairns BR, Carrell DT. Age-associated sperm DNA methylation alterations: possible implications in offspring disease susceptibility. PLoS Genet 2014; 10(7): e1004458. [http://dx.doi.org/10.1371/journal.pgen.1004458] [PMID: 25010591]

[117] Milekic MH, Xin Y, ODonnell A, *et al.* Age-related sperm DNA methylation changes are transmitted to offspring and associated with abnormal behavior and dysregulated gene expression. Mol Psychiatry 2015; 20(8): 995-1001. [http://dx.doi.org/10.1038/mp.2014.84] [PMID: 25092244]

[118] Atsem S, Reichenbach J, Potabattula R, *et al.* Paternal age effects on sperm FOXK1 and KCNA7 methylation and transmission into the next generation. Hum Mol Genet 2016; 25(22): 4996-5005. [http://dx.doi.org/10.1093/hmg/ddw328] [PMID: 28171595]

[119] Vavouri T, Lehner B. Chromatin organization in sperm may be the major functional consequence of base composition variation in the human genome. PLoS Genet 2011; 7(4): e1002036. [http://dx.doi.org/10.1371/journal.pgen.1002036] [PMID: 21490963]

[120] Erkek S, Hisano M, Liang CY, *et al.* Molecular determinants of nucleosome retention at CpG-rich sequences in mouse spermatozoa. Nat Struct Mol Biol 2013; 20(7): 868-75. [http://dx.doi.org/10.1038/nsmb.2599] [PMID: 23770822]

SUBJECT INDEX

G

H

I

K

L

M

N

O

P

Q

R

S

Made in the USA
Las Vegas, NV
04 November 2026

57440791R00257